ADVANCES IN NEUROLOGY

Volume 96

ADVANCES IN NEUROLOGY

Volume 96

Behavioral Neurology of Movement Disorders

Second Edition

Editors

Karen E. Anderson, MD
*Assistant Professor
Psychiatry & Neurology
Maryland Parkinson's Disease and Movement Disorders Center
University of Maryland School of Medicine
Baltimore, Maryland*

William J. Weiner, MD
*Professor and Chairman
Department of Neurology
Director
Maryland Parkinson's Disease and Movement Disorders Center
University of Maryland School of Medicine
Baltimore, Maryland*

Anthony E. Lang, MD, FRCPC
*Professor and Director
Division of Neurology
University of Toronto
Director
Movement Disorders Centre
Toronto Western Hospital
Toronto, Canada*

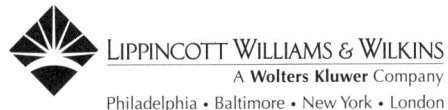

LIPPINCOTT WILLIAMS & WILKINS
A **Wolters Kluwer** Company
Philadelphia • Baltimore • New York • London
Buenos Aires • Hong Kong • Sydney • Tokyo

Acquisitions Editor: Anne M. Sydor
Developmental Editor: Sarah M. Granlund
Project Manager: Fran Gunning
Senior Manufacturing Manager: Ben Rivera
Marketing Manager: Adam Glazer
Production Services: Laserwords Private Limited
Printer: Edwards Brothers

2nd Edition
© 2005 by Lippincott Williams & Wilkins
1e, 1995, Raven Press, Ltd.
530 Walnut Street
Philadelphia, PA 19106
www.LWW.com

All rights reserved. This book is protected by copyright. No part of this book may be reproduced in any form or by any means, including photocopying, or utilizing by any information storage and retrieval system without written permission from the copyright owner, except for brief quotations embodied in critical articles and reviews.

Printed in the United States

Library of Congress Cataloging-in-Publication Data

ISBN : 0781751691
ISSN : 0091-3952

Care has been taken to confirm the accuracy of the information presented and to describe generally accepted practices. However, the authors, editors, and publisher are not responsible for errors or omissions or for any consequences from application of the information in this book and make no warranty, expressed or implied, with respect to the currency, completeness, or accuracy of the contents of the publication. Application of this information in a particular situation remains the professional responsibility of the practitioner.

The authors, editors, and publisher have exerted every effort to ensure that drug selection and dosage set forth in this text are in accordance with current recommendations and practice at the time of publication. However, in view of ongoing research, changes in government regulations, and the constant flow of information relating to drug therapy and drug reactions, the reader is urged to check the package insert for each drug for any change in indications and dosage and for added warnings and precautions. This is particularly important when the recommended agent is a new or infrequently employed drug.

Some drugs and medical devices presented in this publication have Food and Drug Administration (FDA) clearance for limited use in restricted research settings. It is the responsibility of health care providers to ascertain the FDA status of each drug or device planned for use in their clinical practice.

The publishers have made every effort to trace copyright holders for borrowed material. If they have inadvertently overlooked any, they will be pleased to make the necessary arrangements at the first opportunity.

To purchase additional copies of this book, call our customer service department at (800) 638-3030 or fax orders to (301) 824-7390. Lippincott Williams & Wilkins customer service representatives are available from 8:30 am to 6:30 pm, EST, Monday through Friday, for telephone access. Visit Lippincott Williams & Wilkins on the Internet: http://www.lww.com.

10 9 8 7 6 5 4 3 2 1

Advances in Neurology Series

Vol. 95: Myoclonic Epilepsies. *A. V. Delgado-Escueta, R. Guerrini, M. T. Medina, P. Genton, M. Bureau, and C. Dravet, eds.* 347 pp., 2005.
Vol. 94: Dystonia 4. *S. Fahn, M. DeLong, and M. Hallett, eds.* 426 pp., 2004.
Vol. 93: The Parietal Lobes. *A. Siegel, H-J. Freund, S. Anderson, and D. Spencer eds.* 396 pp., 2003.
Vol. 92: Ischemic Stroke. *H. J. M. Barnett, J. Bogoussiavsky, and H. Meldrum, eds.* 496 pp., 2003.
Vol. 91: Parkinson's Disease. *A. Gordin, S. Kaakkola, H. Teräväinen, eds.* 426 pp., 2002.
Vol. 90: Neurological Complications of Pregnancy. Second Edition. *B. Hainline and O. Devinsky, eds.* 368 pp., 2002.
Vol. 89: Myoclonus and Paroxysmal Dyskinesias. *S. Fahn, S. J. Frucht, M. Hallet, D. D. Truong, eds.* 528 pp., 2002.
Vol. 88: Neuromuscular Disorders. *R. Pourmand and Y. Harati, eds.* 368 pp., 2001.
Vol. 87: Gait Disorders. *E. Ruzicka, M. Hallett, and J. Jankovic, eds.* 432 pp., 2001.
Vol. 86: Parkinson's Disease. *D. Caine and S. Caine, eds.* 512 pp., 2001.
Vol. 85: Tourette Syndrome. *D. J. Cohen, C. Goetz, and J. Jankovic, eds.* 432 pp., 2001.
Vol. 84: Neocortical Epilepsies. *P D. Williamson, A. M. Siegel, D. W. Roberts, V M. Thadani, and M. S. Gazzaniga, eds.* 688 pp., 2000.
Vol. 83: Functional Imaging in the Epilepsies. *T R. Henry, J. S. Duncan, and S. F Berkovic, eds.* 348 pp., 2000.
Vol. 82: Corticobasal Degeneration and Related Disorders. *I. Litvan, C. G. Goetz, and A. E. Lang, eds.* 280 pp., 2000.
Vol. 81: Plasticity and Epilepsy. *H. Stefan, P Chauvel, F Anderman, and S. D. Shorvon, eds.* 396 pp., 1999.
Vol. 80: Parkinson's Disease. *G. M. Stern, ed.* 704 pp., 1999.
Vol. 79: Jasper's Basic Mechanisms of the Epilepsies. Third Edition. *A. Deigado-Escueta, W. Wilson, R. Olsen, and R. Porter eds.* 1,132 pp., 1999.
Vol. 78: Dystonia 3. *S. Fahn, C. D. Marsden, and M. R. DeLong, eds.* 1374 pp., 1998.
Vol. 77: Consciousness: At the Frontiers of Neuroscience. *eds. H. H. Jasper, L. Descarries, V. F Castellucci, and S. Rossignol, eds.* 300 pp., 1998.
Vol. 76: Antiepileptic Drug Development. *J. A. French, I. E. Leppik, and M. A. Dichter; eds.* 276 pp., 1998.
Vol. 75: Reflex Epilepsies and Reflex Seizures. *B. G. Zijkin, F Andermann, A. Beaumanoir, and A. J. Rowan, eds.* 1310 pp., 1998.
Vol. 74: Basal Ganglia and New Surgical Approaches for Parkinson's Disease. *J. A. Obeso, M. R. DeLong, C. Ohye, and C. D. Marsden, eds.* 286 pp., 1997.
Vol. 73: Brain Plasticity. *H. J. Freund, B. A. Sabei, and O. W. Witte, eds.* 448 pp., 1997.
Vol. 72: Neuronal Regeneration, Reorganization, and Repair. *F J. Seil, ed.* 416 pp., 1996.
Vol. 71: Cellular and Molecular Mechanisms of Ischemic Brain Damage. *B. K. Siesjö and T Wieloch, eds.* 560 pp., 1996.
Vol. 70: Supplementary Sensorimotor Area. *H. O. Lüders, ed.* 544 pp., 1996.
Vol. 69: Parkinson's Disease. *L. Battistin, G. Scarlato, T Caraceni, and S. Ruggieri, eds.* 752 pp., 1996.
Vol. 68: Pathogenesis and Therapy of Amyotrophic Lateral Sclerosis. *G. Serratrice and T L. Munsat, eds.* 352 pp., 1995.
Vol. 67: Negative Motor Phenomena. *S. Fahn, M. Hallett, H. O. Lüders, and C. D. Marsden, eds.* 416 pp., 1995.
Vol. 66: Epilepsy and the Functional Anatomy of the Frontal Lobe. *H. H. Jasper S. Riggio, and P S. Goldman-Rakic, eds.* 400 pp., 1995.
Vol. 65: Behavioral Neurology of Movement Disorders. *W .J. Weiner and A. E. Lang, eds.* 368 pp., 1995.
Vol. 64: Neurological Complications of Pregnancy. *O. Devinsky, E. Feldmann, and B. Hainline, eds.* 288 pp., 1994.
Vol. 63: Electrical and Magnetic Stimulation of the Brain and Spinal Cord. *O. Devinsky, A. Beric, and M. Dogali, eds.* 352 pp., 1993.

Vol. 62: Cerebral Small Artery Disease. *P. M. Pullicino, L R. Caplan, and M. Hommel, eds.* 256 pp., 1993.
Vol. 61: Inherited Ataxias. *A. E. Harding and T Deufl, eds.* 240 pp., 1993.
Vol. 60: Parkinson's Disease: From Basic Research to Treatment. *H. Narabayashi, T Nagatsu, N. Yanagisawa, and Y Muzuno, eds.* 800 pp., 1993.
Vol. 59: Neural Injury and Regeneration. *F J. Seil, ed.* 384 pp., 1993.
Vol. 58: Tourette Syndrome: Genetics, Neurobiology, and Treatment. *T N. Chase, A. J. Friedhoff, and D. J. Cohen, eds.* 400 pp., 1992.
Vol. 57: Frontal Lobe Seizures and Epilepsies. *P Chauvel, A. V Delgado-Escueta, E. Haigren, and J. Bancaud, eds.* 752 pp., 1992.
Vol. 56: Amyotrophic Lateral Sclerosis and Other Motor Neuron Diseases. *L. P Rowland, ed.* 592 pp., 1991.
Vol. 55: Neurobehavioral Problems in Epilepsy. *D. B. Smith, D. Treiman, and M. Trimbie, eds.* 512 pp., 1990.
Vol. 54: Magnetoencephalography. *S. Sato, ed.* 284 pp., 1990.
Vol. 53: Parkinson's Disease: Anatomy, Pathology, and Therapy: *M. B. Strefle, A. D. Korczyn, E. Meiamed, and M. B. H. Youdim, eds.* 640 pp., 1990.
Vol. 52: Brain Edema. Pathogenesis, Imaging, and Therapy: *D. Long, ed.* 640 pp., 1990.
Vol. 51: Alzheimer's Disease. *R. J. Wurtman, S. Corkin, J. H. Growdon, and E. Ritter-Walker eds.* 308 pp., 1990.
Vol. 50: Dystonia 2. *S. Fahn, C. D. Marsden, and D. B. Caine, eds.* 688 pp., 1988.
Vol. 49: Facial Dyskinesias. *J. Jankovic and E. Tolosa, eds.* 560 pp., 1988.
Vol. 48: Molecular Genetics of Neurological and Neuromuscular Disease. *S. DiDonato, S. DiMauro, A. Mamoli, and L P Rowland, eds.* 288 pp., 1987.
Vol. 47: Functional Recovery in Neurological Disease. *S. G. Waxman, ed.* 640 pp., 1987.
Vol. 46: Intensive Neurodiagnostic Monitoring. *R. J. Gumnit, ed.* 336 pp., 1987.
Vol. 45: Parkinson's Disease. *M. D. Yahr and K J. Bergmann, eds.* 640 pp., 1987.
Vol. 44: Basic Mechanisms of the Epilepsies: Molecular and Cellular Approaches. *A. V Deigado-Escueta, A. A. Ward Jr., D. M. Woodbury, and R. J. Porter, eds.* 1,120 pp., 1986.
Vol. 43: Myoclonus. *S. Fahn, C. D. Marsden, and M. H. Van Woert, eds.* 752 pp., 1986.
Vol. 42: Progress in Aphasiology. *F C. Rose, ed.* 384 pp., 1984.
Vol. 41: The Olivopontocerebellar Atrophies. *R. C. Duvoisin and A. Plaitakis, eds.* 304 pp., 1984.
Vol. 40: Parkinson-Specific Motor and Mental Disorders, Role of Pallidum: Pathophysiological, Biochemical, and Therapeutic Aspects. *R. G. Hassier and J. F Christ, eds.* 601 pp., 1984.
Vol. 39: Motor Control Mechanisms in Health and Disease. *J. E. Desmedt, ed.* 1,224 pp., 1983.
Vol. 38: The Dementias. *R. Mayeux and W. G. Rosen, eds.* 288 pp., 1983.
Vol. 37: Experimental Therapeutics of Movement Disorders. *S. Fahn, D. B. Caine, and I. Shouison; eds.* 339 pp., 1983.
Vol. 36: Human Motor Neuron Diseases. *L. P Rowland, ed.* 592 pp., 1982.
Vol. 35: Gilles de la Tourette Syndrome. *A. J. Friedhoff and T N. Chase, eds.* 476 pp., 1982.
Vol. 34: Status Epilepticus: Mechanism of Brain Damage and Treatment. *A. V. Delgado-Escueta, C. G. Wasterlain, D. M. Treiman, and R. J. Porter, eds.* 579 pp., 1983.
Vol. 31: Demyelinating Disease: Basic and Clinical Electrophysiology. *S. Waxman and J. Murdoch Ritchie, eds.* 544 pp., 1981.
Vol. 30: Diagnosis and Treatment of Brain Isehemia. *A. L Carney and E. M. Anderson, eds.* 424 pp., 1981.
Vol. 29: Neurofibromatosis. *V M. Riccardi and J. J. Mulvilhiil, eds.* 288 pp., 1981.
Vol. 28: Brain Edema. *J. Cervós-Navarro and R. Ferszt, eds.* 539 pp., 1980.
Vol. 27: Antiepileptic Drugs: Mechanisms of Action. *G. H. Glaser, J. K Penry, and D. M. Woodbury, eds.* 728 pp., 1980.
Vol. 26: Cerebral Hypoxia and Its Consequences. *S. Fahn, J. N. Davis, and L P Rowland, eds.* 454 pp., 1979.
Vol. 25: Cerebrovascular Disorders and Stroke. *M. Goldstein, L. Bolis, C. Fieschi, S. Gorini, and C. H. Millikan, eds.* 412 pp., 1979.
Vol. 24: The Extrapyramidal System and Its Disorders. *L. J. Poirier T L. Sourkes, and P Bédard, eds.* 552 pp., 1979.
Vol. 23: Huntington's Chorea. *T N. Chase, N. S. Wexier, and A. Barbeau, eds.* 864 pp., 1979.

Dedication

To Ted for his love, devotion, and unflagging enthusiasm for my work. KEA

For Lisa—"Up to the sky." WJW

Ten years on, missing Jane for six. To Judy—now an inspiration and always an ally, advisor, critic, and best friend. AEL

Contents

Contributing Authors xi
Preface xvii
Foreword xix
Acknowledgments xxi

Section 1: The Role of the Basal Ganglia

1. Basal Ganglia: Functional Perspectives and Behavioral Domains 1
   Jean A. Saint-Cyr

2. Behavioral Changes in Patients with Focal Lesions of the Basal Ganglia 17
   Bruno Dubois, Aurélie Funkiewiez, Bernard Pillon

Section 2: Parkinson's Disease

3. Depression in Parkinson's Disease 26
   Marc J. Mentis, Dominique Delalot

4. Anxiety Disorders in Parkinson's Disease 42
   Irene H. Richard

5. Disorders of Motivation, Sexual Conduct, and Sleep in Parkinson's Disease 56
   Dag Aarsland, Guido Alves, Jan P. Larsen

6. Parkinson's Disease as a Model for Psychosocial Issues in Chronic
   Neurodegenerative Disease 65
   Mark S. Groves, David V. Forrest

7. Early Cognitive Changes and Nondementing Behavioral Abnormalities
   in Parkinson's Disease 84
   Bonnie E. Levin, Heather Katzen

8. Dementia in Parkinson's Disease 95
   Gregory A. Rippon, Karen S. Marder

9. Behavioral Changes as Side Effects of Medication Treatment
   for Parkinson's Disease 114
   Jennifer S. Hui, Gail A. Murdock, Joseph S. Chung, Mark F. Lew

10. Psychiatric Symptoms Following Surgery for Parkinson's Disease
    with an Emphasis on Subthalamic Stimulation 130
    *Valerie Voon, Elena Moro, Jean A. Saint-Cyr, Andres M. Lozano,
    Anthony E. Lang*

Section 3: Other Akinetic Rigid Syndromes

11. Neurodegenerative Disorders with Diffuse Cortical Lewy Bodies 148
    Adam S. Fleisher, John M. Olichney

12. Cognitive and Behavioral Changes in the Parkinson-Plus Syndromes 166
    Sharon Cohen, Morris Freedman
13. Behavioral Changes in Frontotemporal Dementia with Parkinsonism 187
    Catherine E. Pace-Savitsky, Julene K. Johnson, Bruce L. Miller

Section 4: Huntington's Disease

14. Behavioral Symptoms Associated with Huntington's Disease 197
    Karen E. Anderson, Frederick J. Marshall
15. Cognitive Changes in Huntington's Disease 209
    Jane S. Paulsen, Rachel A. Conybeare
16. Psychosocial Effects of Predictive Testing for Huntington Disease 226
    Michael R. Hayden, Yvonne Bombard

Section 5: Gilles de la Tourette's Syndrome

17. Public Health Significance of Tic Disorders in Children and Adolescents 240
    Lawrence Scahill, Denis G. Sukhodolsky, Susan K. Williams, James F. Leckman
18. Obsessive–Compulsive Disorder in Tourette's Syndrome 249
    Peter G. Como, Jennifer LaMarsh, Katherine A. O'Brien

Section 6: Wilson's Disease

19. Behavioral Abnormalities in Wilson's Disease 262
    George J. Brewer

Section 7: Ataxia, Essential Tremor, and Dystonia

20. Hereditary Ataxia and Behavior 275
    Nadejda Alekseeva, Anita S. Kablinger, James B. Pinkston, Eduardo C. Gonzalez-Toledo, Alireza Minagar
21. Behavioral Symptoms Associated with Essential Tremor 284
    Elan D. Louis
22. Behavioral and Psychiatric Manifestations in Dystonia 291
    Marjan Jahanshahi

Section 8: Other Movement Disorders Associated with Behavioral Changes

23. Autoaggressive Immune-Mediated Movement Disorders 320
    Davide Martino, Gavin Giovannoni
24. Psychopathological and Cognitive Correlates of Tardive Dyskinesia
    in Patients Treated with Neuroleptics 336
    Ikwunga Wonodi, L. Elliot Hong, Gunvant K. Thaker

Section 9: Psychogenic Movement Disorders

25. Treatment Issues in Psychogenic-Neuropsychiatric Movement Disorders 350
    Daniel T. Williams, Blair Ford, Stanley Fahn

Index 365

Contributing Authors

Dag Aarsland, MD, PhD
*Professor
Geriatric Psychiatry
Psychiatric Clinic
School of Medicine
University of Bergen
Bergen, Norway*

*Consultant
Geriatric Psychiatry
Stavanger University Hospital
Stavanger, Norway*

Nadejda Alekseeva, MD
*Resident Physician
Department of Psychiatry
Louisiana State University Health Sciences Center
Shreveport, Louisiana*

Guido Alves, MD
*Research Associate
The Norwegian Centre for Movement Disorders
Stavanger University Hospital
Stavanger, Norway*

*Resident
Department of Neurology
Stavanger University Hospital
Stavanger, Norway*

Karen E. Anderson, MD
*Assistant Professor
Departments of Psychiatry and Neurology
Maryland Parkinson's Disease and Movement
  Disorders Center
University of Maryland School of Medicine
Baltimore, Maryland*

Yvonne Bombard, BSc
*Doctoral Candidate
University of British Columbia
Department of Medical Genetics
Centre for Molecular Medicine and Therapeutics
Children's and Women's Health Centre
  of British Columbia
University of British Columbia
Vancouver, Canada*

George J. Brewer MD
*Active Professor Emeritus
Department of Human Genetics
  and Department of Internal Medicine
University of Michigan Medical School
Ann Arbor, Michigan*

Joseph S. Chung, DO
*Movement Disorder Neurologist
Department of Neurology
Kaiser Permanente Southern California
Los Angeles, California*

Sharon Cohen, DSP, MD, FRCP(C)
*Assistant Professor
Department of Medicine (Neurology)
  and Graduate Department of Speech Pathology
University of Toronto
Toronto, Canada*

*Director
Toronto Memory Program
Toronto, Canada*

Peter G. Como, PhD
*Associate Professor
Departments of Neurology, Psychiatry,
  and Brain and Cognitive Science
University of Rochester Medical Center
Rochester, New York*

Rachel A. Conybeare, BS
*Research Assistant
Department of Neuropsychology
University of Iowa
Iowa City, Iowa*

Dominique Delalot, MA
*Study Coordinator
North Shore–Long Island Jewish Research Institute
Manhasset, New York*

Bruno Dubois, MD
*Professor
Department of Neurology
Hôpital de la Salpêtrière
Paris, France*

CONTRIBUTING AUTHORS

Stanley Fahn, MD
H. Houston Merritt Professor
Department of Neurology
Columbia University
New York, New York

Attending Neurologist
Department of Neurology
Neurological Institute
New York–Presbyterian Hospital
New York, New York

Adam S. Fleisher, MD
Department of Neuroscience
University of California, San Diego
La Jolla, California

Blair Ford, MD, FRCP
Associate Professor
Department of Neurology
Columbia University
New York, New York

David V. Forrest, MD
Clinical Professor of Psychiatry
Center for Psychoanalytic Training and Research
Department of Psychiatry
Columbia University
New York, New York

Attending Psychiatrist and Consultation–Liason
  Psychiatrist (Movement Disorders)
New York–Presbyterian Hospital
Neurological Institute of New York
New York, New York

Morris Freedman, MD, FRCP(C)
Professor
Department of Medicine (Neurology)
University of Toronto
Toronto, Canada

Head
Division of Neurology
Baycrest Centre For Geriatric Care
Toronto, Canada

Aurélie Funkiewiez, PhD
Postdoctoral Fellow
Hôpital de la Salpêtrière
Paris, France

Gavin Giovannoni, MBBCh, PhD
Reader in Clinical Neuroimmunology
Department of Neuroinflammation
Institute of Neurology
University College London
London, United Kingdom

Honorary Consultant Neurologist
Clinical Neurology
National Hospital for Neurology & Neurosurgery
London, United Kingdom

Eduardo C. Gonzalez-Toledo, MD, PhD
Professor and Director
Department of Radiology, Neurology,
  and Anesthesiology
Louisiana State University School of Medicine
Shreveport, Louisiana

Mark S. Groves, MD
Attending Psychiatrist in Movement Disorders
Department of Neurology and Psychiatry
Beth Israel Medical Center
New York, New York

**Michael R. Hayden, MB, ChB, PhD,
  FRCP(C), FRSC**
Professor
Department of Medical Genetics
Centre for Molecular Medicine and Therapeutics
Children's and Women's Health Centre
  of British Columbia
University of British Columbia
Vancouver, Canada

L. Elliott Hong, MD
Assistant Professor
Department of Psychiatry
University of Maryland School of Medicine
Baltimore, Maryland

Jennifer S. Hui, MD
Instructor of Clinical Neurology
Department of Neurology
Keck University of Southern California
  School of Medicine
Los Angeles, California

Marjan Jahanshahi, PhD
Principal Investigator
Sobell Department of Motor Neuroscience
  and Movement Disorders
Institute of Neurology
London, United Kingdom

Consultant Neuropsychologist
National Hospital for Neurology & Neurosurgery
London, United Kingdom

Julene K. Johnson, PhD
Assistant Professor
Department of Neurology
University of California, San Fransisco
San Francisco, California

CONTRIBUTING AUTHORS

Anita S. Kablinger, MD
Associate Professor
Departments of Psychiatry and Pharmacology
Louisiana State University Health Sciences Center
Shreveport, Louisiana

Heather Katzen, PhD
Instructor
Department of Neurology
Weill Medical College of Cornell University
Ithaca, New York

Scientific Liaison
Medical Affairs
Ortho-McNeil Neurology
Miami, Florida

Jennifer LaMarsh, BA
Psychology and Social Sciences
University of Rochester
Rochester, New York

Anthony E. Lang, MD, FRCP(C)
Professor
Department of Medicine (Neurology)
University of Toronto
Toronto, Canada

Director
Movement Disorders Clinic
Toronto Western Hospital
Toronto, Canada

Jan P. Larsen, MD, PhD
Professor
Department of Neurology
University of Bergen
Bergen, Norway

Chief
Department of Neurology
Stavanger University Hospital
Stavanger, Norway

James F. Leckman, MD
Professor
Child Study Center
Yale University School of Medicine
New Haven, Connecticut

Bonnie E. Levin PhD
Associate Professor
Department of Neurology and Psychology
University of Miami School of Medicine
Miami, Florida

Mark F. Lew, MD
Professor of Neurology
Division of Movement Disorders
Keck/University of Southern California School of Medicine
Los Angeles, California

Elan D. Louis, MD, MS
Associate Professor
Department of Neurology
Columbia University
New York, New York

Associate Attending Neurologist
Department of Neurology
New York–Presbyterian Hospital
New York, New York

Andres M. Lozano, MD, PhD, FRCS(C)
Professor
Department of Surgery (Neurosurgery)
University of Toronto
Toronto, Canada

Neurosurgeon
Toronto Western Hospital
Toronto, Canada

Karen S. Marder, MD, MPH
Professor
Department of Neurology
Taub Institute
Columbia University
New York, New York

Attending Neurologist
New York–Presbyterian Hospital
New York, New York

Frederick J. Marshall, MD
Assistant Professor
Department of Neurology
University of Rochester School of Medicine and Dentistry
Rochester, New York

Attending Neurologist, Strong Memorial Hospital
Chief of Neurology, Monroe Community Hospital
Rochester, New York

Davide Martino, MD
Research Fellow
Department of Neuroimmunology
Institute of Neurology
University College London
London, United Kingdom

Specialist Registrar in Neurology
Department of Neurologic and Psychiatric Sciences
University of Bari
Bari, Italy

Marc J. Mentis, MD
Assistant Professor
Departments of Neurology and Psychiatry
New York University
New York, New York

Attending Physician
Departments of Neurology and Psychiatry
North Shore–Long Island Jewish Research Institute
Manhasset, New York

Bruce L. Miller, MD
Professor
Department of Neurology
School of Medicine
University of California, San Francisco
San Francisco, California

Alireza Minagar, MD
Assistant Professor
Department of Neurology
Louisiana State University Health Sciences Center
Shreveport, Louisiana

Elena Moro, MD, PhD
Assistant Professor
Department of Medicine
University of Toronto
Toronto, Canada

Active Staff Physician
Department of Medicine, Division of Neurology
Toronto Western Hospital, UHN
Toronto, Canada

Gail A. Murdock, PhD
Assistant Professor of Clinical Neurology
Department of Neurology
Keck University of Southern California
  School of Medicine
Los Angeles, California

Clinical Psychologist
Leslie P. Weiner Neurologic Care
  and Research Center
University of Southern California
Los Angeles, California

Katherine A. O'Brien, BA
Brain and Cognitive Science
University of Rochester
Rochester, New York

John M. Olichney, MD
Department of Neurosciences
University of California, San Diego
La Jolla, California

Staff Physician
Neurology
VA San Diego Healthcare System
San Diego, California

Catherine E. Pace-Savitsky, MA
Researcher
Department of Neurology
Memory and Aging Center
University of California, San Francisco
San Francisco, California

Jane S. Paulsen, PhD
Director
Department of Psychiatry and Neurology
Division of Neuropsychology
University of Iowa
Iowa City, Iowa

Bernard Pillon, PhD
Director of Research
INSERM U 160

Psychologist
Fédération de Neurologie
Hôpital de la Salpêtrière
Paris, France

James B. Pinkston, PhD
Assistant Professor
Department of Neurology
Louisiana State University Health Sciences Center
Shreveport, Louisiana

Irene H. Richard, MD
Associate Professor of Neurology and Psychiatry
Department of Neurology
University of Rochester School of Medicine
  and Dentistry
Rochester, New York

Attending Physician
Strong Memorial Hospital
Rochester, New York

Gregory A. Rippon, MD, MSc
Postdoctoral Clinical Fellow
Department of Neurology
Columbia University
New York, New York

Assistant Attending Neurologist
Columbia University Medical Center
New York–Presbyterian Hospital
New York, New York

Jean A. Saint-Cyr, PhD, C.Psych
Professor
Departments of Surgery (Neurosurgery) and Psychology
University of Toronto
Toronto, Canada

Senior Scientist
Toronto Western Research Institute
University Health Network
Toronto, Canada

Lawrence Scahill, MSN, PhD
Associate Professor
Child Study Center
Yale University School of Medicine
New Haven, Connecticut

Denis G. Sukhodolsky, PhD
Associate Research Scientist
Child Study Center
Yale University School of Medicine
New Haven, Connecticut

Gunvant K. Thaker, MD
Professor
Department of Psychiatry
Maryland Psychiatric Research Center
University of Maryland School of Medicine
Baltimore, Maryland

Valerie Voon, MD
Lecturer
Department of Psychiatry
University of Toronto
Toronto, Canada

Staff psychiatrist
Psychiatry
Toronto Western Hospital, UHN
Toronto, Canada

Daniel T. Williams, MD
Clinical Professor
Department of Psychiatry
Columbia University
New York, New York

Attending Physician
Psychiatry
New York–Presbyterian Hospital
Neurological Institute of New York
New York, New York

Susan K. Williams, PhD
Postdoctoral Fellow
Child Study Center
Yale University School of Medicine
New Haven, Connecticut

Ikwunga Wonodi, MD
Assistant Professor
Maryland Psychiatric Research Center
Motor Disorders Clinic
University of Maryland School of Medicine
Baltimore, Maryland

Preface

Progress in clinical and basic neuroscience continues to add to our knowledge about movement disorders. Stunning advances in phenomenology, imaging, biochemistry, physiology, pharmacology, neuropathology, neurosurgery, molecular biology, epidemiology, and genetics have all occurred during the past several years. In this second edition of *Behavioral Neurology of Movement Disorders*, we review the contributions these developing fields have made to our understanding of behavioral changes associated with movement disorders. The array of new knowledge since publication of the first edition is reflected not only in the extensive updating that has occurred in each chapter but also in the addition of several new chapters that examine movement disorders that are newly recognized as having a prominent behavioral component to their clinical picture.

Chapters 1 and 2 address the basal ganglia's function in behavior and outline what we have learned from studying patients with focal lesions in this system. Chapters 3 to 10 provide a thorough review of psychiatric and cognitive disorders in patients with Parkinson's disease (PD). This section has been greatly expanded in this edition, with the addition of an excellent chapter that integrates brain imaging findings and neurobiologic theory with what is known about the etiology of depression in PD. This edition also features a greater focus on anxiety disorders in PD and a new chapter on the emerging area of behavioral changes caused by deep brain stimulation. Other behavioral symptoms associated with PD, including disorders of motivation, sleep disturbances, and sexual dysfunction, are addressed in a separate chapter. Material has been added in a chapter on psychotherapeutic strategies and issues in PD, which is amenable for use as a guide for therapeutic work with patients who have other movement disorders. Chapters 7 and 8 update and expand our understanding of the treatment of cognitive change in PD, with content that includes an excellent review and integration of epidemiologic, functional imaging, genetic, and neuropathologic studies in the section on PD dementia. Since the last edition, many new agents have been developed to treat motor symptoms in PD, which has necessitated that the section on behavioral changes that occur as side effects of these medications be greatly expanded. Chapters 11 to 13 examine behavioral problems in other akinetic rigid syndromes, including Lewy body dementia, Parkinson's-plus syndromes, and frontotemporal dementia with parkinsonism. Chapters 14 and 15 describe the often-devastating psychiatric and cognitive changes in Huntington's disease (HD). This section includes an excellent overview of structural and functional imaging findings in HD that relate to cognitive and functional decline, including findings in individuals who are asymptomatic gene carriers for the disorder. Chapter 16 provides an in-depth discussion of the emotional and ethical complexities of genetic testing in HD, especially for those who are asymptomatic but potentially at risk for the disorder. It additionally provides practical guidance for clinical decision making in the advent of widely available commercial testing for HD and other genetic disorders. Chapters 17 and 18 discuss behavioral abnormalities in Tourette's syndrome and describe controversies over the relationship between TS with tic disorders, TS with attention deficit hyperactivity disorder, and TS with obsessive–compulsive disorder as part of a spectrum disorder. Wilson's disease is discussed in Chapter 19, emphasizing the range of behavioral symptoms seen in the disorder and the need to diagnose it as early as feasible in patients with a purely psychiatric presentation. Chapters 20 and 21 are both new additions to this volume; Chapter 20 reviews behavioral symptoms associated with ataxias, and Chapter 21 provides an excellent, critical look at the psychiatric and cognitive changes possibly associated with essential tremor. Chapter 22 discusses the emotional symptoms seen in many patients with dystonia and addresses the issue of "nonorganic" symptomatology in these patients. A comprehensive review of the debate surrounding autoimmune-mediated movement disorders is provided in the newly added Chapter 23. Chapter 24 outlines psychopathological and cognitive changes seen in patients with tardive dyskinesia, relating these findings to underlying pathophysiology. Finally, Chapter 25 is an excellent update that addresses the challenging issues of treatment and diagnosis of psychogenic movement disorders.

Each chapter provides a comprehensive review of its topic, authored by an expert or experts in the field concerned. Some chapters address controversial topics and offer opposing points of view. Recommendations for treating these behavioral symptoms are given, often based on the authors' clinical experience, because relatively few clinical trials have been performed in this area. Individual chapters are meant to be read independently, and each section provides a thorough overview of behavioral symptoms in each disorder. The entire text is a reflection of contemporary thinking on the complex array of psychiatric and cognitive changes that often accompany movement disorders. This edition is of particular interest to neurologists, psychiatrists, psychologists, and their trainees at all levels.

We thank our contributors for their tireless efforts to produce uniformly topical, interesting, and accessible material for this text. We thank our colleagues who pursue study of behavioral changes in movement disorders, using the tools of clinical and basic neuroscience. Finally, we wish to express our gratitude to our patients and their family members. It is they who have made the greatest contributions to this text and they who on a daily basis cope with the illnesses discussed in this book. Without their understanding of the importance of clinical and basic teaching and research and their willingness to be examined and studied, this book would not have been possible. It is our hope that the sections on evaluation and diagnosis bring clarity to those clinicians who care for patients with these disorders, and that the suggestions for treatment offered in our text bring some measure of relief for their symptoms. It is also hoped that this work will stimulate further research that will reduce and eventually eliminate the suffering that these neurologic disorders cause.

KEA, WJW, AEL

Foreword

Can one imagine a doctor treating a diabetic coma correctly without knowing about the Krebs cycle or the glycogenic function of the liver? Likewise, it is now hard to imagine a movement disorder specialist treating a patient who has basal ganglia disorder without a thorough knowledge of the anatomy, physiology, and biochemistry of the brain. Some notable differences exist, however.

First, the functioning of the human brain is infinitely more complicated than that of the endocrine glands. Even so, we are beginning to understand how the brain functions. The last few years have seen remarkable progress in the field of neuroscience, and it is currently accelerating exponentially. This progress underpins the first two chapters of this book, which cover the main advances in our understanding of basal ganglia circuits and the behavioral anomalies that occur when they are impaired.

Second, when we hear the term "basal ganglia," we immediately think of motricity. In the same way, "basal ganglia lesion" conjures up the notion of involuntary abnormal movements. Yet, physiologists and clinicians have long been aware that the basal ganglia have a function in selection, adaptation, and automaticity that is not purely motor. For one thing, the movement itself, the ultimate aim of any behavior, implies the involvement of complex cognitive functions (motivation, preparation, decision, initiation) that precede performance of the movement. Moreover, the basal ganglia are complex structures that contain highly interconnected and topographically organized neuronal networks, equally involving cognitive and psychological functions. Consequently, a lesion in the basal ganglia may just as readily cause a cognitive or psychological dysfunction as a movement abnormality.

Finally, from these anatomic physiologic data, one might logically expect one or more lesions of the basal ganglia to result in motor, cognitive, or psychic disturbances, either singly or in association. This is indeed the case, a fact long observed by clinicians, even if psychic anomalies sometimes tend to go unrecognized, given the often-spectacular nature of involuntary abnormal movements such as chorea, dystonia, and hemiballismus. Nonetheless, the observation of emotional disturbances in a patient also points toward a dysfunction of deep brain structures, such as the basal ganglia. Be that as it may, emotional disturbances, especially if they do not appear in the foreground, can be extremely hard to detect, given the complexity of the symptoms, to the point where the most eminent specialists do not necessarily always agree on how to describe them.

This book provides comprehensive coverage of behavioral disorders of this type, with particular emphasis on those resulting from a wide range of brain lesions, including those in Parkinson's disease (Chapters 3 to 10) and related disorders (Chapters 11 to 13), Huntington's disease (Chapters 14–16), Tourette's syndrome (Chapters 17 and 18), Wilson's disease (Chapter 19), cerebellar ataxias (Chapter 20), essential tremor (Chapter 21), dystonias (Chapter 22), autoimmune disorders (Chapter 23), tardive dyskinesias (Chapter 24), and abnormal movements of psychogenic origin (Chapter 25). Why, then, is there a need for a book on behavioral neurology in movement disorders? Quite simply because of the remarkable scientific progress made during the past few years. On the one hand, some psychiatric disorders—even highly complex ones—have been attributed to lesions that affect limited territories of the basal ganglia, especially their limbic part. On the other hand, the perception of emotions, which may be quite elaborate, is now known to induce metabolic changes within the limbic territories of the basal ganglia. How has all this progress come about? Although the semiology of behavioral disorders, whether intellectual or emotional, is improving (through consensus meetings, precise criteria of definition, and radiologic observation of cases), the main reason lies in the great strides made in three scientific disciplines: neurophysiology, both experimental (in primates) and clinical (in both healthy subjects and patients); neuroimaging, especially functional imaging, which allows us to link precise sites within the basal ganglia to specific emotional behaviors; lastly, molecular biology, which is enabling us to develop a new nosography of neurodegenerative diseases that specifically involve the basal ganglia. In the final analysis, what is the practical importance of a thorough knowledge of the behavioral disturbances that exist in basal ganglia disorders? Its importance is twofold: for clinicians, who refine their diagnosis by adding neuropsychological and psychological analysis to their diagnostic arsenal, and will thereby be enabled to localize the responsible lesions and underlying diseases more easily; for neuroscientists, who by careful observation of abnormal behaviors—cognitive and emotional as well as motor—will be able to determine the neuropsychiatric role of the basal ganglia more precisely.

Yves Agid, MD
Centre d'Investigation Clinique
Hôpital de la Salpêtrière
Paris, France

Acknowledgments

We would like to thank the members of our respective research and clinical groups, the Maryland Parkinson's Disease and Movement Disorders Center at the University of Maryland School of Medicine, and the Movement Disorders Center at the Toronto Western Hospital. The support of the American Parkinson's Disease Association for the Parkinson's disease center at the University of Maryland and the support of the National Parkinson Foundation for the Parkinson's disease center at the Toronto Western Hospital is very much appreciated. Cheryl Grant-Johnson and Nandy Yearwood were particularly helpful in the preparation of this text. We also thank Rosalyn Newman, Morton Shulman, and Jack and Mary Clark, the special benefactors who have generously supported our research on this project as well as on many other projects related to Parkinson's disease.

1

Basal Ganglia: Functional Perspectives and Behavioral Domains

Jean A. Saint-Cyr

Departments of Surgery (Division of Neurosurgery) and Psychology, University of Toronto, Toronto, Canada

INTRODUCTION

Basal ganglia pathology engenders a wide spectrum of neurologic and neuropsychiatric symptoms (1,2). The functional domains of the basal ganglia can be grouped anatomically and clinically into three major divisions: motor (including oculomotor), associative (or cognitive), and emotional (or limbic) (3,4). The motor circuits are organized around the rostral putamen and the adjacent dorsomedial division of the caudate. The associative circuit is focused on the rest of the caudate and the caudoventral putamen, while the emotional circuits are centered in the so-called ventral striatum that includes the ventral caudate, the nucleus accumbens, and the amygdala (5).

As proposed by Alexander et al. (6), distinct anatomical and functional subcircuits exist within the basal ganglia and link up with the thalamocortical pathways. Originating from various cortical sources of input, these subcircuits can be traced through striatal relays to thalamic (and some brain stem) nuclei, finally closing the loop partially with the frontal lobes [see Reference (7) for a description of a temporal lobe component]. These subcircuits have been traced anatomically with transneuronal transport of viruses (8) and with traditional tracing techniques (3,9–12); they have also been traced physiologically (13–16). Single-unit mapping studies during human surgery for Parkinson's Disease (PD) (17–19) have also revealed these subcircuits; interestingly, in some studies, evidence has been found that somatotopy is preserved within the subthalamic nucleus (STN) (18,20) despite the dopamine (DA) loss that occurs in PD, but other studies have failed to confirm these observations (21). This discrepancy may arise from variability in on-line active and passive motor testing (especially testing of proximal joints), and in the methods used to merge data from several cases. More recently, functional imaging studies have also revealed somatotopic organization, even within the motor subcircuit (22–24). Functional imaging in PD patients has also provided a more global view of basal ganglia participation in motor and cognitive operations (25,26). At the behavioral level, dissociations between motor and associative functions have been demonstrated in patients with therapeutic focal lesions in the pallidum (27), in patients who have sustained focal vascular damage (1,28,29), and in subhuman primates in lesion and neurophysiologic experiments (30–37). The advent of functional neurosurgical interventions such as deep brain stimulation (DBS) also offers new insights into basal ganglia functions (38). Animal studies are also essential to define the basic anatomy and physiology of these circuits. Finally, disease models that mimic conditions such as PD permit studies of pathophysiology and of the efficacy of new treatment methods (16,39–43).

This chapter reviews the primary domains of basal ganglia function, using data from human and animal studies to delineate the major advances in our conceptualization of basal ganglia function. Current trends in the study of the behavioral domains of basal ganglia function are examined, with the tripartite anatomic organization as a framework.

NEUROANATOMIC ORGANIZATION

The classical nomenclature of the basal ganglia recognizes three components: the neostriatum, the paleostriatum, and the archistriatum. The neostriatum includes the caudate, the putamen, and the nucleus accumbens; the paleostriatum comprises the globus pallidus, the substantia nigra, and the pars reticulata; and the archistriatum is the amygdala. Given parallel evolution of many of these structures (44) this phylogenetic schema offers insights into function (45). However, the notion that the mammalian basal ganglia represent an avian brain with reptilian Jurassic roots (46) is not particularly enlightening although some insights can be gleaned from experiments based on those ideas (47).

Cortico-striatal projections (all of which are glutamatergic, and hence excitatory) are organized according to proximity (i.e., cortical areas project to the anatomically closest sector of the striatum), and the broad triad of functional domains has been defined on this basis (3). Conversely, trans-striatal distributions from so-called higher-order or associative cortical regions of the frontal (dorsolateral prefrontal), parietal (intraparietal sulcus), temporal (superior temporal sulcus), and anterior cingulate gyrus terminate in complex, sometimes interdigitating or patchy distributions in the striatum (10–12,48–53). The striatal terminations of these inputs, which have been described as both patchy and sparse, represent reduced information flow into the striatum, both anatomically and physiologically, down to the level of the GPi/SNr (54). Flaherty and Graybiel (55) demonstrated ipsilateral somatotopically organized inputs to the matrisomes from S1 and M1 as well as interdigitating contributions from contralateral M1 inputs, the latter strongest from axial body representation. By tracking transneuronal movement of labelled viruses (7), Middleton and Strick have demonstrated that newly identified circuit components in pallidonigral pathways can be traced through thalamic relays to finally terminate in the temporal lobes. Thus, the previous notion that the entire reascending outflow of the basal ganglia projected exclusively to the frontal lobes (6) must now be revised. However, in PD, the heterogeneity of the DA loss at the striatal level, as shown by Kish and his colleagues (56), does suggest that these temporal circuits may not be affected early in the disease.

Within the striatum, histochemical heterogeneity is evident: the DA, dynorphin, substance P, neurotensin, and acetylcholinesterase-poor striosomes are embedded in an acetylcholinesterase-rich matrix (which also stains for enkephalin and somatostatin), within which matrisomes are also present (57–61). Differential metabolic patterns have been associated with this organization, revealing that natural somato–motor behaviors activate the matrix, whereas motivational factors appear to favor the striosomes (62). In addition, cholinergic interneurons (which may also colocalize with vasoactive intestinal peptide), some of which have been identified as Tonically Active Neurons (TANs), have been anatomically and histochemically characterized (63,64). Finally, the distribution of cortical inputs also varies: In the dorsal striatum, the cortical inputs (especially from motor, somatosensory, and cingulate areas) terminate specifically in the matrix surrounding the histochemically defined striosomes (12,49, 65–67). In the ventral striatum, however, cortical inputs (especially from the prefrontal area and the insula) and some subcortical inputs (such as those from the amygdala) terminate within the striosomes themselves (58,68). TANs may establish functional bridges between striosomes and matrix regions and may participate in reinforcement-based learning in parallel with DA neurons (54,64). Piggott et al. (69) studied postmortem human striatum and found gradients of DA receptors: D1 receptors were less concentrated in the caudal putamen, D2 receptors were more concentrated in the caudal caudate and the putamen, while D3 receptors were highly concentrated in the ventral striatum; finally, D1 and D3 receptors were most concentrated in striosomes, and D2 were most concentrated in the matrix. Holt et al. (66) have demonstrated heterogeneity in normal human striatum, with a more complex and less differentiated striosome–matrix organization ventrally, extending into the nucleus accumbens. In the subhuman primate, limbic-associated membrane protein marking has the greatest density ventrally, including the accumbens (70). Other histochemical markers that localize within the striatum include calbindin, calretinin, neuropeptide Y, nitric oxide synthase, and parvalbumin, *inter alia* (70); and some of these, such as calbindin, delineate functional regions.

Examination of putamenal and pallidal projections (all of which are gabaergic, and hence inhibitory) reveals multiple branching axons. Multiple branching axons are also present in ascending STN projections (which are glutamatergic), and in other sources of input from thalamus (glutamatergic) as well as from DA cell groups (71–79). However, whether these branching patterns conform to functional domains within subcircuits remains to be determined (80). The STN, which plays a critical role in innervating the entire striatum with excitatory glutamatergic inputs, is overactive in PD, making it a key target for neurosurgical interventions with DBS (81).

Golgi and tracer studies have shown that pallidal neurons have radial dendritic arbors (73,74,77,78,82–85) that potentially enable integration of input from anatomically adjacent functional domains. Hyperdirect pathways (86) (i.e., from supplementary motor and adjacent regions to the STN), as well as the traditional direct and indirect pathways (85,87,88) (i.e., striatum to GPi/SNr and striatum to GPe, hence to STN, and lastly to GPi /SNr), provide routes for regulating the initiation and termination of action. Basal ganglia output is much more complex than the simplified traditional models suggest (89), and it can also short-circuit the classical pallido-nigral relay to the thalamus, because the GPe links directly to the reticular shell of the thalamus (90,91). The thalamic output channels are largely focused on the frontal lobes and maintain a high degree of functional segregation (8,92–95). Brain stem output channels are few but most importantly include the superior colliculus (15,96), a major node for controlling gaze shifts and voluntary saccadic eye movements. The nucleus tegmento pedunculo pontinus, pars compacta (abbreviated as TPC or PPN) and adjacent cell groups may be involved in descending motor control (97–104), but more complex roles in controlling learning and attention have also been proposed (104,105). Cerebellar influences are either channeled through thalamic relays, such as the centre médian-parafascicular complex (CM/Pf) (3), or via cortical reentrant routes (106). Cortical inputs can also act directly through CM/Pf (76,106,107). Although the CM/Pf (109) is traditionally considered to be involved in controlling arousal (108), recent studies have shown evidence that detailed sensory processing occurs in these thalamic nuclei.

The neuroanatomic organization outlined here presents several novel functional implications for the circuits described:

- They are dynamically focused and tuned for specific domains of information processing.
- They are anatomically organized to provide several information subsets from which to choose, thus permitting response selection.
- They have trans-striatal cortical inputs and ascending trans-pallidal inputs that act at multiple levels, as is the case for STN inputs, and are necessary for preparatory set and multiple loop recruitment.
- They contain TANs, which may bridge striosomes and matrisomes and which may encode new learning.
- They may also influence nonfrontal cortical targets (temporal demonstrated, suspected parietal and cingulate areas, and possibly areas that in turn project back to PFC) (53).
- They are chemically coded, with focus on compartments, such as striosomes and matrisome, and are also coded according to functional domains.

Indeed, the complexity of the basal ganglia circuitry has led to serious critiques of the box-and-arrow model used both to justify neurosurgical treatments and as a basis for our understanding of the cardinal neurologic signs and symptoms of basal ganglia lesions and diseases (54,110–112).

With regard to motor control, the basal ganglia have been proposed to be involved in orchestrating the initiation of action, either through the hyperdirect (i.e., SMA and pre-SMA projections to the STN) or the direct (i.e., cortico-putamen pathways to GPi/SNr) routes. In contrast, the indirect route, acting through the STN, has been proposed to be involved in modulatory aspects of motor control, such as linking or switching between sequences of movement, and perhaps also in aspects of termination (86,113). These proposed actions should not be divorced from motor and premotor cortical commands (37). The difficulty in attempting to "map" the motor models conceptually onto other functional domains is that some of the "cognitive" or "associative" behavioral terms are quite different or are used in contextually different frames of reference. These terms include internal navigation and response selection, establishment of preparatory set, focusing and switching attention, sequential processing, and error correction (114). In addition, the time frame extends from the millisecond range needed for the precise timing of muscular coordination to longer periods required for skill and habit acquisition (114–116). Skill and habit acquisition is related to the phasic action of DA, which can also exert a more homeostatic action (117). Working models with more specific domains, such as for oculomotor control, have also been proposed (15).

NEUROPHYSIOLOGY

Neurophysiologic studies in nonhuman primates have demonstrated the presence of multiple representations of domain-specific processing modules within the basal ganglia, each with a certain degree of anatomic segregation (11,13,44,45, 118–125).

The models proposing context-dependent functional segregation of circuits such as focalisation dynamique of Filion et al. (126), and the focused selection of Mink and Thach (127) require lateral inhibition and local disinhibition. There is no evidence, such as the presence of inhibitory interneurons, to provide a mechanism for either lateral inhibition or local disinhibition (54). In addition, as demonstrated by reports of unit data consistent with parallel distributed processing, information processing is not uniquely hierarchic and sequential (120,125,128,129). The anatomic organization is such that exuberant axonal arborizations, intersecting with radial dendritic trees, provide a basis for functionally fluid processing nodes, ideally suited for adaptive learning, sensorimotor development, habit formation, and reinforcement-based learning. The selection of actions and goals is initiated from the cortex, whereas focus and error correction is provided from ascending DA projections to the basal ganglia (37,54,117). In this context, both Hebbian and non-Hebbian mechanisms of learning have been proposed (54). Chunking of action sequences, as in visual-motor learning, may also require basal ganglia processing (130, 131). During the course of learning, the locus of control shifts dynamically, from cortex and cerebellum to striatum (producing adaptation first and then automatization) (132,133).

MODELS OF BASAL GANGLIA FUNCTION

Motor Models

The major models in current use at the clinical level are from Albin, Young, and Penny (134), Joel (87), and Wichmann and deLong (16). Although these familiar box-and-arrow models have permitted some integration of anatomic, neurochemical, and clinical information, sufficient to guide neurosurgical intervention (135,136), they have also recently come under criticism (40,54,111,112). Criticism has arisen not only because these models do not incorporate all of the now known anatomic and physiologic subtleties but also because the models fail to account for common clinical phenomena, such as tremor and dyskinesias. In addition, the specific role of the cortex is no longer seen as sending a copy of its information to the basal ganglia, but rather as sending abstracted sets of commands and goals, from both supra- and infragranular layers, to chemically coded subsets of the striatum (37,128,137,138).

Models are easiest to postulate for the sensorimotor domain. Even so, constructs—such as preparatory set, followed by initiation (which implies response selection), transitions between temporal components (which implies sequencing), and finally termination of the response (which implies activation of the antagonist and then inhibition of the agonist in order not to overshoot)—remain crude. All of these actions require an adequate motor tone (which requires normal DA levels) and are normally revealed in experimental designs with reinforcement-shaped response control (i.e., a constrained behavioral context).

For more complex behaviors, families of sequences would have to be orchestrated, requiring coordination and monitoring. The models deal with parkinsonian tremor as an internal oscillation, without specifying how this oscillation is generated. Gait abnormalities in PD are usually attributed to the TPC and the adjacent mesencephalic locomotor region, whereas rigidity is usually associated with agonist–antagonist cocontraction and hence poor timing (101,138). One problem is that the models are in large part conceptualized as modular, serial information processors with both feed-forward and feed-back elements, whereas unit recordings have found evidence for multiplexing and parallel processing. In addition, functional imaging studies in PD patients at rest all indicate substantial changes in motor cortical, parietal cortical, and cerebellar blood flow, suggesting that extrastriatal circuits contribute to both adaptive and maladaptive compensatory mechanisms (139,140).

Bergman and his colleagues (54) have been applying organizational constructs, based on recent anatomic findings and on the unit studies of Schultz and his colleagues (141,142), to modeling the pathophysiology of PD. Two predictions are that DA loss should result in inappropriate synchronization of basal ganglia unit activity and there should be overresponsiveness to sensorimotor inputs. Both predictions have now been confirmed in an experimental parkinsonian monkey preparation (40). The model proposed by Bergman and his colleagues provides a better explanation for the behavioral symptoms of tremor, bradykinesia, and dyskinesia than that previously furnished by the Albin-DeLong model.

Cognitive Domain Models

When describing the cognitive domain, one must deal with psychological constructs (attention, memory, strategic planning, learning, habits, procedures, and plasticity) and cortically based models such as the Supervisory Attentional System (143), Working Memory (144), and Cognitive Event Knowledge (145), *inter alia*. The best unit studies in this domain are those using oculomotor, memory-driven paradigms (15,146,147) or learning paradigms (63) that include the role of DA in reinforcement-based learning, a type of learning that is impaired in PD (148,149). Many of the unit delayed-response profiles previously found in the frontal lobes and in thalamic nucleus medialis dorsalis (150–152) are also found in the basal ganglia (33, 117). However, most of these studies do not attempt to integrate their findings into the "classical" models of basal ganglia circuits. Both Wise et al. (37) as well as Bar-Gad and Bergman (54) envision the cortex (read cortico-striatal) as "actor" or "teacher," with the basal ganglia DA system playing the role of "critic" or selective "reinforcement" mechanism. Thus, a reduced subset of cortically originating information (environmental state, goals) is focused through the basal ganglia, enabling appropriate actions while inhibiting competing responses. Any disparity between expected positive outcome and experience leads to a diminished DA signal, whereas fulfillment of anticipated reward engenders an increased DA signal. Schultz and his colleagues have furnished unit recording data concordant with this model (117). Brasted and Wise (153) have recently shown that learning-related unit changes occur concurrently in the dorsal premotor cortex and in the putamen during conditional visuomotor learning.

Among more recent findings in the learning literature are studies of the processing of temporal and sequential information in the basal ganglia and the chunking of information (130,131,154).

Studies have shown that PD patients are impaired in their ability to estimate time and that this impairment can be improved with STN DBS (155). However, functional imaging studies have shown that the actual temporal discrimination function is supported by the pre-SMA and cingulate cortical areas. Indeed, Ivry and Spencer (156) have argued that the basal ganglia are more involved in the decisional process than in the computational process, which may be more dependent on the cerebellum. Nevertheless, unit studies in nonhuman primates have shown that the timing of sequential operations is processed in cortico-striatal circuits (118).

Psychiatric Models

No defined models exist for the psychiatric basal ganglia domain except Mayberg's distributed depression model (157) and equally widespread concepts for schizophrenia (158) and obsessive compulsive disorder (OCD) (47,159).

At best, these models are also modular [e.g., the dorsolateral prefrontal cortex controls cognitive emotional processing and is influenced by Cognitive-Behavioral Therapy, whereas the subgenual cingulate area 25 is where direct emotional control is coordinated (157)]. These dorsolateral, prefrontal, and cingulate cortical areas project into the ventral striatum.

However, the control of emotion by the basal ganglia cannot be understood in purely neurologic terms, because it is influenced genetically [i.e., Cloninger's temperamental dimensions (160)], by developmental experience, and by lifelong social learning (161). That being said, evidence suggests that an interaction between orbitofrontal and ventral striatal circuits underlies emotional reactivity in the social–environmental context. Abulia is commonly seen after bilateral lesions of the ventral striatum (4,28,162), and the same condition can be encountered in PD patients if they are undermedicated. In addition, depression is also a common feature of PD, taking the form of either emotional lability, a reactive state, or a more chronic condition in different individuals (157,163–165). Indeed, a whole host of psychiatric conditions are known to be associated with PD, some caused by medication, others by psychosocial factors, and yet others by neurosurgical interventions (161,166).

FUNCTIONAL IMAGING

Motor System

The putamen shows changes in blood flow, glucose metabolism, and oxygen consumption [by positron emission tomography (PET) and functional magnetic resonance imaging (fMRI)], all of which reflect increased synaptic activity during motor skill learning and motor sequence learning. In general, basal ganglia activity is more engaged during activation paradigms requiring self-initiated, rather than externally triggered, behaviors (167). At rest in pathologic states, such as PD, activation of allied cortical areas (e.g., supplementary motor area) is usually decreased, a state that is reversed toward the normal pattern with effective treatment, whether it is L-dopa, targeted pallidotomy, or DBS of either the GPi or STN (25,168,169). Using activation paradigms (e.g., random joystick movements or sequential finger movements), functional imaging studies have uniformly revealed an overactivation of rostral and lateral premotor cortical areas, interpreted as an overcompensation (i.e., these cortical areas must work harder) for the PD deficits. Upon successful medical or neurosurgical treatment, these overactivations typically revert toward a more normal state.

Cognitive System

Although frontal-executive dysfunction has been correlated to decreased DA levels in the striatum (170–172), evidence of selective caudate activation in relation to a task is rarer. However, such activation has been reported in studies using spatial working memory, spatial problem-solving tasks, and virtual route navigation (26,173–175), in corroboration with neuropsychological studies. A sector is also activated during oculomotor paradigms (176). In paradigms of visuomotor sequence learning (implicit and explicit), as well as in sequential finger movement learning, the complexity of the task determines the probability of caudate recruitment to putamenal operations (132,177), whereas, in general, PD patients with executive impairment show evidence of reduced fronto-striatal activation on functional imaging (178). The ventral striatum is also activated as a function of magnitude of error and reward, in keeping with Schultz' model (179–181). The accumbens has been seen to activate during depression paradigms (157). In all of these studies, the corresponding portions of the pallidum may also show activation changes. Synaptic activity is tightly coupled to enhanced local metabolism, oxygen consumption, and blood flow; this enhancement may be associated with excitatory (e.g., glutamate-mediated), inhibitory [e.g., (gamma-amino-butyric acid) GABA-mediated], or even modulatory (e.g., DA-mediated) physiologic effects (182).

Obsessive Compulsive Disorder and Tourette's Syndrome

A connection has been recognized for some time between ventral striatal lesions and OCD symptoms (29). OCD can be viewed as the cognitive equivalent of choreoathetosis (183), because both disorders appear to be the consequences of overdriven activity. Thus, thoughts and emotions become driven, and motor automatisms are commonly driven as well. The same analogy also holds for Tourette's Syndrome, although in this case, the supposedly lesser pathology permits some degree of conscious control of tics and vocalizations (184).

Inspired by McLean's work (46), Baxter (47) has recently revived the evolutionary, or comparative, approach to decoding basal ganglia function by studying the behavior of the green anolis lizard. These behavioral and functional imaging studies have highlighted OCD-type behaviors brought about by either lesions or behavioral manipulation. Neuroanatomic homology suggests that the ventral striatum is a likely region for the locus of control of such behaviors (185). This result echoes human functional imaging studies (47,159,186). DBS of the subgenual capsule and adjacent ventral striatum is now in clinical trial for the treatment of OCD (187).

INSIGHTS FROM PARKINSON'S DISEASE

Parkinson's Disease: Analysis of Clinicopathologic Models

Motor functions have been attributed to the basal ganglia, or so-called extrapyramidal system, since the days of Kinnear Wilson and Derek Ernst Denny-Brown (2). The first explanatory models merely inferred that the basal ganglia duplicated motor cortical functions and were parallel downstream circuits. The modern era of a revised concept of basal ganglia function began with Brodal's realization that major output pathways reascended to frontal motor regions (188), but these facts were not fully incorporated into clinicopathologic models until the late 1980s (134). The opinion of James Parkinson had been that PD was not accompanied by cognitive impairment, and this view also was prevalent until the mid-1980s (189). The loss of DA at the striatal level had been recognized by Hornykiewicz in the mid-1960s (190), but again, even the dual D1 excitatory–D2 inhibitory model was not developed until recently. Because of DA's dual action, the model predicted excessive activity in both GPi/SNr and in the STN (16). Ultimately, the conclusion was that the thalamo-cortical projection was underactive in PD and overactive in the case of STN lesions. Although this model could provide some explanation for akinesia and ballism, and striatal neuronal loss could be reasonably linked with chorea in the case of Huntington's Disease, we were left in the dark when attempting to explain tremor, drug-induced dyskinesias, and cognitive impairment (54,87,112, 191). The idea that dysfunctional basal ganglia output fed error signals or inadequate information into the frontal lobes gained prominence and remains the backbone of current understanding of the pathophysiology of cognitive impairment in PD (114,189,192). In assigning functions to circuits on the basis of deficits associated with degenerative disease states or focal lesions, we must avoid logical pitfalls that are based on localizationist 19th century neurologic thinking.

If a portion of the basal ganglia is withdrawn from participation in neural processing by either a lesion or DBS, then the resulting behavioral impairment (and hence the normal control of this behavior) cannot be simply attributed to the missing elements or circuit (193). What we actually witness is the function of other circuits, deprived of the collaboration of the damaged area. However, if a circuit is malfunctioning and generating error messages, then it might be inferred that the behavior driven by that circuit could be partly controlled by that circuit; for example, the understanding that rigidity is caused by agonist–antagonist cocontraction leads us to infer that normal function arises from proper timing of the sequence of activation of the muscle groups, permitting unopposed initiation and clean termination of a precision movement. However, even that type of inference could be challenged, because the malfunction is pathologic and could be seen as being injected into the stream of normal operations that are dependent on other centers (e.g., tremor caused by oscillating circuits, with the pulsatile signal being fed into motor cortical areas). In addition, it could even be the case that tremor is driven by the cerebellum, in its attempt to regulate motor control gone awry, and arises from dysregulation of the feedback loop (194). In short, the actual pathophysiology sets up a cascade of events, some leading to primary symptoms, others partly adaptive, and the remainder inadequately compensatory. Under certain circumstances, behavior may actually look normal and be functionally so, especially after some form of treatment. However, when the patient is pushed to act more quickly or under conditions of stress or divided attention, symptoms or limitations may reappear. Assigning functions to circuits on the basis of *prima facie* inferences that correlate lesion location with behavior is therefore difficult.

The same argument holds for DBS, thought by many to simulate lesions. Thus, logic dictates that if a region of the basal ganglia is identified as being overactive, this state is corrected by reducing overactivity through lesions or high-frequency stimulation (195). Although high-frequency stimulation is now known to influence neighboring myelinated fibers at relatively low thresholds (196), lesions may interrupt fibers of passage. In either case, attributing all changes uniquely to the target structure is not possible. Therefore, all of these studies must remain correlational, because they cannot unequivocally attribute causal linkage.

Neurosurgical Treatment of PD

STN DBS possibly disconnects the dysfunctional basal ganglia from other circuits, perhaps through local liberation of GABA into the STN, which inhibits the excessive neuronal activity caused by the disease. Secondly, fiber systems that pass around the STN (e.g., fasciculus lenticularis) may very well be affected more easily by the current, and any error signal that passes through the STN, en route to targets such as the thalamus, would be jammed. Intact cortical and subcortical motor circuits would then resume normal motor control. The activation of the cerebellum and normalization of frontal cortical blood flow and oxygen consumption bear witness to that plasticity (169). The nonspecific cognitive amelioration achieved by stimulation may be partly attributable to eliminating the need to assign attentional resources to controlling symptoms, because motor control can now proceed more smoothly (197). STN DBS may have a DA-mimetic action, as is the case for motor control, and this action could directly facilitate spatial working memory (198). However, some specific functions, such as verbal fluency, are impaired by stimulation. The inference can be made that cortical compensation for that particular function is inadequate. The fact that this impairment is not reversed by the acute cessation of stimulation (219) short-term suggests that a semipermanent (because stimulation is rarely off for more than a few minutes, or at best a few hours, during so-called off-stimulation testing conditions) change in processing locus and strategy has been established during the course of the weeks and months of chronic stimulation.

Neurophysiologic studies in intact animals (14) revealed a somatotopic organization that is partly imposed by afferents from both cortex (86,113) and thalamus (65). We also have learned that DA plays a critical role in maintaining functional somatotopy within the motor zones (126). Therefore, in the absence of DA, the specificity of muscle selection is lost.

If we superimpose this model onto the cognitive sphere, then we might expect response choices to become ambivalent when DA is depleted. Normally, because phasic DA signals would selectively lead to the elimination of erroneous choices, the inefficient, error-prone, and ambiguous behavior would persist, impairing encoding of information for later retrieval. Also, any hypotheses launched from the cortex would be unfocused and would not be modified and shaped through feedback and reinforcement contingencies. Behavioral control might then be reduced to default states (199) or to the activation of preestablished strategies not appropriate or tuned to the task at hand. The use of preestablished strategies leads to perseveration. In fact, the inability to switch strategies or mental sets is one of the hallmarks of basal ganglia dysfunction.

The loss of DA also leads to a state of abulia and apathy (psychic akinesia) (162). This state is not the same as depression but is rather a paucity of emotional reactivity, initiative, drive, and motivation, with anhedonia. In the early stages of PD, perhaps complicated by medications, there may be emotional lability (165). This state is not as intense or dissociated as the emotional incontinence seen after brain stem lesions (pseudo-bulbar palsy) or in gelastic seizures. However, DBS inadvertently applied to the SNc and other areas around the STN can lead to outbursts of depression, hilarity, and aggression (200–204), perhaps stemming from remote actions along the entire basal forebrain axis, extending from the orbitofrontal cortex through the medial forebrain and lateral forebrain bundles and into the limbic midbrain [i.e., periaqueductal gray and mesencephalic tegmentum, *inter alia* (38,205–207)]. In a sense, the emotional dyscontrol seen in PD as a treatment complication can be viewed as the counterpart of bradykinesia, freezing (apathy and abulia), and dyskinesias (impulsivity, lability of mood, or emotional dysregulation). Houeto et al. (208) have noted psychiatric and behavioral decompensation in as many as 8 out of 15 patients, following STN DBS. They stressed the need for both thorough preoperative screening and systematic postoperative follow-up. Funkiewiez and colleagues in Grenoble (209) have documented mild improvement in depression, transient apathy, and thought disorders, as well as varying degrees of behavioral change, after STN DBS.

Another intriguing observation has been that some patients with PD become compulsive gamblers (161). One wonders if this phenomenon is caused by an acquired dependence on DA during the early stages of disease treatment. The mesocortical DA system associated with the ventral tegmental area of Tsai [classically considered the backbone of the reward system (210–212)] may be deteriorating in these patients. Gamblers might be seeking to enable the reward system by anticipation of gain (winning), the partial reinforcement schedule inherent in gambling, which shapes and maintains the gambling habit. Each relatively rare win would be like the crack cocaine addict's rush, leading the user to desperately seek more wins (213–215). These patients appear to become almost obsessional about seeking the gambling experience and, in this regard, resemble not only drug addicts but also patients with OCD (216).

Neuropsychological studies of STN DBS have shown little adverse effect, apart from a reduction in Verbal Fluency and Conditional Associative Learning (217–222). In a recent study, STN DBS was shown to impair working memory and response inhibition (222). Schroeder et al. (223) were able to demonstrate that STN DBS inhibited activation of the ventral striatal–frontal cortical system in the presence of increased errors in a Stroop task. These results presuppose that patients have been carefully selected, screened to rule out preoperative cognitive or psychiatric risk conditions, and are relatively young [usually 60 or less (224)]. There have also been reports that STN DBS mildly facilitated selected cognitive tasks [e.g., Trails, intradimensional shifting, and declarative memory (155,217–220, 225)]. In addition, STN DBS has also been shown to improve memory-guided saccades (226). Because outcome studies compare pre- and postoperative performance, treatments can only be said to partly restore function, as predisease performance is not known. Interestingly enough, turning off DBS may produce little effect (219), suggesting that compensatory circuits may be well established and functioning totally independent of the basal ganglia. In cases of diminished cognitive processing efficiency, one could argue that the compensation is incomplete. Conversely, in cases of improved performance, Halbig et al. (225) found that STN DBS impaired declarative memory but improved nondeclarative memory (practice effects must be strictly controlled). If the comparison is with preoperative performance, then imagine that allocation of attentional resources is increased, because patients are no longer taxed by the need to exercise voluntary control over their symptoms and to resist the distraction of their movement disorder. In the same vein, the cortical circuits, previously hampered in their collaborative function with the basal ganglia by internal error signals and reduced thalamo-cortical drive, now may function unimpeded. However, it is difficult to imagine that DBS could actually enhance performance beyond the patient's best premorbid ability.

SUMMARY

Evidence exists that the basal ganglia participate in three global functional domains: motor, associative, and emotional. The variety and complexity of the operations within these domains is inextricably linked, however, to functions of the cortical areas, especially frontal, but also integrating cerebellar, brain stem, and thalamic inputs. For example, within the frontal lobes, Petrides et al. (227,228) and others (229,230) have fractionated functions on an anatomic basis (52,106,231,232). The multiple loop model, first proposed by Alexander et al. in 1986 (233), argues that there are anatomically segregated channels funneling through the basal ganglia, which drive these types of modular circuits in a relatively independent manner. Although the point-to-point hodology does suggest some independence, the extent of dendritic and axonal arborizations as well as axonal branching patterns make total anatomic segregation impossible. Just as is the case with the organization of the motor cortical somatotopic matrix, in which functional heterogeneity arises from multiple cortical inputs as well as intrinsic local circuits (234), both a hodologic and a physiologic mechanism for dynamic focus in the basal ganglia must be invoked (54,126,127) in order to achieve modular or channeled function. Furthermore, many complex behaviors require the coactivation and coordination of more than one module, with the preparatory set defining the collection needed, which is perhaps dictated by the transstriatal cortical inputs (114). Because DA plays such a fundamental role in basal ganglia operations, and because it provides both a tonic (homeostatic) as well as a phasic action (117), should we not apply that concept across our three major behavioral domains?

Lastly, the functional boundaries between modules should not be considered as fixed or absolute, but rather as being fluid and adaptive. Thus, when motor learning begins, control appears to be cerebello–cortical, because it is conscious and constantly being monitored. Cerebello–cortical commands are relayed to the basal ganglia so that the necessary modules can be enabled and tuned through practice. Ultimately, the correct sequence is automatized and played out under more autonomous basal ganglia control (132). However, in cases where the organism has no clear strategy to apply as a set of cortical rules, but merely a general goal, what is enabled is only generalized crude behavior, which, shaped by DA-linked reinforcement and error pruning, sets limits on the subset of useful motor sequences that are then taken over under conscious cortical control. This initial strategic shaping may represent a protocognitive stage of operations, under nonconscious basal ganglia control (235). This stage of operations is not seen in functional imaging studies, because it is already established before scanning begins. However, in neuropsychological studies, inability to establish functional strategies is commonly observed in patients with basal ganglia disease, especially if the paradigms do not allow for verbal mediation (i.e., visual–spatial paradigms) (116). When verbal strategies or conscious memory processes are possible, functional imaging reveals the recruitment of hippocampal circuits to compensate for striatal insufficiency (173). Such cortical–subcortical shifts of locus of control and redistribution of processing are thought to occur naturally, depending on the task (235). In this way, the basal ganglia can be seen as functioning in concert with cortical and subcortical circuits.

ACKNOWLEDGMENTS

The preparation of this chapter was supported by a grant from the National Science and Engineering Research Council of Canada.

Anatomic organization of basal ganglia function

	Functional domains		
Role of Dopamine	Motor	Associative	Emotional
Tonic actions	Tone/selection	Attention/switching	Euthymia/regulation
Phasic actions	Initiation/sequence	Error elimination	Reward/reinforcement

REFERENCES

1. Saint-Cyr JA, Bronstein YL, Cummings JL Neurobehavioral consequences of neurosurgical treatments and focal lesions of frontal-subcortical circuits. In: Stuss D et al., eds. *Principles of frontal lobe function.* Oxford: Oxford University Press, 2002:408–427.
2. Saint-Cyr JA, Taylor AE, Nicholson K. Behavior and the basal ganglia. *Adv Neurol* 1995;65:1–28.
3. Parent A, Hazrati L-N. Functional anatomy of the basal ganglia. I. The cortico-basal ganglia-thalamo-cortical loop. *Brain Res Rev* 1995;20:91–127.
4. Mega MS, Cummings JL. Frontal-subcortical circuits and neuropsychiatric disorders. *J Neuropsychiatry Clin Neurosci* 1994;6:358–370.
5. De Olmos JS, Heimer L. The concepts of the ventral striatopallidal system and extended amygdala. *Ann N Y Acad Sci* 1999;877:1–32.
6. Alexander GE, Crutcher MD, DeLong MR. Basal ganglia-thalamocortical circuits: parallel substrates for motor, oculomotor, "prefrontal" and "limbic" functions. *Prog Brain Res* 1990;85:119–146.
7. Middleton FA, Strick PL. The temporal lobe is a target of output from the basal ganglia. *Proc Natl Acad Sci USA* 1996;93:8683–8687.
8. Middleton FA, Strick PL. New concepts about the organization of basal ganglia output. *Adv Neurol* 1997;74:57–68.
9. Ilinsky IA, Yi H, Kultas-Ilinsky K. Mode of termination of pallidal afferents to the thalamus: a light and electron microscopic study with anterograde tracers and immunocytochemistry in Macaca mulatta. *J Comp Neurol* 1997;386:601–612.
10. Saint-Cyr JA, Ungerleider LG, Desimone R. Organization of visual cortical inputs to the striatum and subsequent outputs to the pallido-nigral complex in the monkey. *J Comp Neurol* 1990;298:129–156.
11. Selemon LD, Goldman-Rakic PS. Longitudinal topography and interdigitation of cortico-striatal projections in the rhesus monkey. *J Neurol* 1985;5(3):776–794.
12. Takada M, Tokuno H, Nambu A, et al. Corticostriatal projections from the somatic motor areas of the frontal cortex in the macaque monkey: segregation versus overlap of input zones from the primary motor cortex, the supplementary meter area, and the premotor cortex. *Exp Brain Res* 1998;120:114–128.
13. Alexander GE, Crutcher MD. Preparation for movement: neural representations of intended direction in three motor areas of the monkey. *J Neurophysiol* 1990; 64:133–150.
14. Alexander GE, DeLong MR. Microstimulation of the primate neostriatum. II. Somatotopic organization of striatal microexcitable zones and their relation to neuronal response properties. *J Neurophysiol* 1985;53:1417–1430.
15. Hikosaka O, Takikawa Y, Kawagoe R. Role of the basal ganglia in the control of purposive saccadic eye movements. *Physiol Rev* 2000;80:953–978.
16. Wichmann T, DeLong MR. Functional and pathophysiological models of the basal ganglia. *Curr Opin Neurobiol* 1996;6:751–758.
17. Rodriguez-Oroz MC, Rodriguez M, Guridi J, et al. The subthalamic nucleus in Parkinson's disease: somatotopic organization and physiological characteristics. *Brain* 2001;124:1777–1790.
18. Romanelli P, Heit G, Hill BC, et al. Microelectrode recording revealing a somatotopic body map in the subthalamic nucleus in humans with Parkinson disease. *J Neurosurg* 2004;100:611–618.
19. Theodosopoulos PV, Marks WJ Jr, Christine C, et al. Locations of movement-related cells in the human subthalamic nucleus in Parkinson's disease. *Mov Disord* 2003;18:791–798.
20. Rodriguez-Oroz MC, Rodriguez M, Guridi J, et al. The subthalamic nucleus in Parkinson's disease: somatotopic organization and physiological characteristics. *Brain* 2001;124:1777–1790.
21. Abosch A, Hutchison WD, Saint-Cyr JA, et al. Movement-related neurons of the subthalamic nucleus in patients with Parkinson disease. *J Neurosurg* 2002;97:1167–1172.
22. Gerardin E, Lehéricy S, Pochon JB, et al. Foot, hand, face and eye representation in the human striatum. *Cereb Cortex* 2003;13:162–169.
23. Lehéricy S, Van de Moortele PF, Lobel E, et al. Somatotopical organization of striatal activation during finger and toe movement: a 3-T functional magnetic resonance imaging study. *Ann Neurol* 1998;44:398–404.
24. Maillard L, Ishii K, Bushara K, et al. Mapping the basal ganglia—fMRI evidence for somatotopic representation of face, hand, and foot. *Neurology* 2000;55:377–383.
25. Brooks DJ. Imaging basal ganglia function. *J Anat* 2000;196:543–554.
26. Owen AM, Doyon J. The cognitive neuropsychology of Parkinson's disease: a functional neuroimaging perspective. In: Stern GM, ed. *Parkinson's disease: advances in neurology.* Philadelphia: Lippincott Williams & Wilkins, 1999:49–56.
27. Lombardi WJ, Gross RE, Trépanier LL, et al. Relationship of lesion location to cognitive outcome following microelectrode-guided pallidotomy for Parkinson's disease—support for the existence of cognitive circuits in the human pallidum. *Brain* 2000;123:746–758.
28. Dubois B, Defontaines B, Deweer B, et al. Cognitive and behavioral changes in patients with focal lesions of the basal ganglia. *Adv Neurol* 1995;65:29–42.
29. Laplane D, Levasseur M, Pillon B, et al. Obsessive–compulsive and other behavioural changes with bilateral basal ganglia lesions. *Brain* 1989;112:699–725.
30. Boussaoud D, Kermadi I. The primate striatum: neuronal activity in relation to spatial attention versus motor preparation. *Eur J Neurosci* 1997;9:2152–2168.
31. Fernandez-Ruiz J, Wang J, Aigner TG, et al. Visual habit formation in monkeys with neurotoxic lesions of the ventrocaudal neostriatum. *Proc Natl Acad Sci USA* 2001;98:4196–4201.
32. Kermadi I, Joseph JP. Activity in the caudate nucleus of monkey during spatial sequencing. *J Neurophysiol* 1995;74:911–933.
33. Rolls ET. Neurophysiology and cognitive functions of the striatum. *Rev Neurol (Paris)* 1994;150:648–660.
34. Rolls ET, Thorpe SJ, Maddison SP. Responses of striatal neurons in the behaving monkey. 1 Head of the caudate nucleus. *Behav Brain Res* 1983;7:179–210.
35. Rosvold E. (1972) The frontal lobe system: cortical-subcortical relationships. *Acta Neurobiol Exp (Warsaw)* 1972; 32:439–460.
36. Williams GV, Rolls ET, Leonard CM, et al. Neuronal responses in the ventral striatum of the behaving macaque. *Behav Brain Res* 1993;55:243–252.
37. Wise SP, Murray EA, Gerfen CR. The frontal cortex-basal ganglia system in primates. *Crit Rev Neurobiol* 1996;10:317–356.

38. Saint-Cyr JA, Hoque T, Pereira LCM, et al. Localization of clinically effective stimulating electrodes in the human subthalamic nucleus on magnetic resonance imaging. *J Neurosurg* 2002;97:1152–1166.
39. Benazzouz A, Boraud T, Féger J, et al. Alleviation of experimental hemiparkinsonism by high-frequency stimulation of the subthalamic nucleus in primates: a comparison with L-Dopa treatment. *Mov Disord* 1996; 11:627–632.
40. Bergman H, Deuschl G. Pathophysiology of Parkinson's disease: from clinical neurology to basic neuroscience and back. *Mov Disord* 2002;17:S28–S40.
41. Boraud T, Bezard E, Bioulac B, et al. From single extracellular unit recording in experimental and human parkinsonism to the development of a functional concept of the role played by the basal ganglia in motor control. *Prog Neurobiol* 2002;66:265–283.
42. Deuschl G, Bergman H. Pathophysiology of nonparkinsonian tremors. *Mov Disord* 2002;17(Suppl. 3):S41–S48.
43. Vitek JL. Pathophysiology of dystonia: a neuronal model. *Mov Disord* 2002;17:S49–S62.
44. Sarnat HB, Netsky MG. *Evolution of the nervous system.* London: Oxford University Press, 1993.
45. Parent A. The brain in evolution and involution. *Biochem Cell Biol* 1997;75:651–667.
46. MacLean PD. *The triune brain in evolution: role in paleocerebral functions.* New York and London: Plenum Press, 1990.
47. Baxter LR Jr. Basal ganglia systems in ritualistic social displays: reptiles and humans; function and illness. *Physiol Behav* 2003;79:451–460.
48. Kemp JM, Powell TPS. The cortico-striate projection in the monkey. *Brain* 1970;93:525–546.
49. Parthasarathy HB, Schall JD, Graybiel AM. Distributed but convergent ordering of corticostriatal projections: analysis of the frontal eye field and the supplementary eye field in the macaque monkey. *J Neurosci* 1992;12:4468–4488.
50. Selemon LD, Goldman-Rakic PS. Common cortical and subcortical targets of the dorsolateral prefrontal and posterior parietal cortices in the rhesus monkey: evidence for a distributed neural network subserving spatially guided behavior. *J Neurosci* 1988;8:4049–4068.
51. Van Hoesen GW, Yeterian EH, Lavizzo-Mourey R. Widespread corticostriate projections from temporal cortex of the rhesus monkey. *J Comp Neurol* 1981; 199:205–219.
52. Yeterian EH, Pandya DN. Prefrontostriatal connections in relation to cortical architectonic organization in rhesus monkeys. *J Comp Neurol* 1991;312:43–67.
53. Yeterian EH, Van Hoesen GW. Cortico-striate projections in the rhesus monkey: the organization of certain cortico-caudate connections. *Brain Res* 1978; 139:43–63.
54. Bar-Gad I, Bergman H. Stepping out of the box: information processing in the neural networks of the basal ganglia. *Curr Opin Neurobiol* 2001;11:689–695.
55. Flaherty AW, Graybiel AM. Two input systems for body representations in the primate striatal matrix: experimental evidence in the squirrel monkey. *J Neurosci* 1993;13:1120–1137.
56. Kish SJ, Shannak K, Hornykiewicz O. Uneven pattern of dopamine loss in the striatum of patients with idiopathic Parkinson's disease. *N Engl J Med* 1988; 318:876–880.
57. Besson MJ, Graybiel AM, Nastuk MA. [3H]SCH 23390 binding to D1 dopamine receptors in the basal ganglia of the cat and primate: delineation of striosomal compartments and pallidal and nigral subdivisions. *Neuroscience* 1988;26:101–119.
58. Fudge JL, Haber SN. Defining the caudal ventral striatum in primates: cellular and histochemical features. *J Neurosci* 2002;22:10078–10082.
59. Gerfen CR. The neostriatal mosaic: multiple levels of compartmental organization in the basal ganglia. *Annu Rev Neurosci* 1992;15:285–320.
60. Nastuk MA, Graybiel AM. Patterns of muscarinic cholinergic binding in the striatum and their relation to dopamine islands and striosomes. *J Comp Neurol* 1985;237:176–194.
61. Prensa L, Giménez-Amaya JM, Parent A. Chemical heterogeneity of the striosomal compartment in the human striatum. *J Comp Neurol* 1999;413:603–618.
62. Brown LL, Feldman SM, Smith DM, et al. Differential metabolic activity in the striosome and matrix compartments of the rat striatum during natural behaviors. *J Neurosci* 2002;22:305–314.
63. Aosaki T, Kimura M, Graybiel AM. Temporal and spatial characteristics of tonically active neurons of the primate's striatum. *J Neurophysiol* 1995;73:1234–1252.
64. Saka E, Iadarola M, Fitzgerald DJ, et al. Local circuit neurons in the striatum regulate neural and behavioral responses to dopaminergic stimulation. *Proc Natl Acad Sci USA* 2002;99:9004–9009.
65. Flaherty AW, Graybiel AM. Input-output organization of the sensorimotor striatum in the squirrel monkey. *J Neurosci* 1994;14:599–610.
66. Holt DJ, Graybiel AM, Saper CB. Neurochemical architecture of the human striatum. *J Comp Neurol* 1997;384:1–25.
67. Ragsdale CW Jr, Graybiel AM. The fronto-striatal projection in the cat and monkey and its relationship to inhomogeneities established by acetylcholinesterase histochemistry. *Brain Res* 1981;208:259–266.
68. Takada M, Tokuno H, Hamada I, et al. Organization of inputs from cingulate motor areas to basal ganglia in macaque monkey. *Eur J Neurosci* 2001;14:1633–1650.
69. Piggott MA, Marshall EF, Thomas N, et al. Striatal dopaminergic markers in dementia with Lewy bodies, Alzheimer's and Parkinson's diseases: rostrocaudal distribution. *Brain* 1999;122:1449–1468.
70. Parent A, Côté PY, Lavoie B. Chemical anatomy of primate basal ganglia. *Prog Neurobiol* 1995;46:131–197.
71. Haber SN, Fudge JL, McFarland NR. Striatonigrostriatal pathways in primates form an ascending spiral from the shell to the dorsolateral striatum. *J Neurosci* 2000;20:2369–2382.
72. Parent A, Sato F, Wu Y, et al. Organization of the basal ganglia: the importance of axonal collateralization. *Trends Neurosci.* 2000;23:S20–S27.
73. Parent M, Lévesque M, Parent A. The pallidofugal projection system in primates: evidence for neurons branching ipsilaterally and contralaterally to the thalamus and brainstem. *J Chem Neuroanat* 1999;16:153–165.
74. Parent M, Lévesque M, Parent A. Two types of projection neurons in the internal pallidum of primates: single-axon tracing and three-dimensional reconstruction. *J Comp Neurol* 2001;439:162–175.
75. Prensa L, Cossette M, Parent A. Dopaminergic innervation of human basal ganglia. *J Chem Neuroanat* 2000;20:207–213.

76. Sadikot AF, Parent A, François C. Efferent connections of the centromedian and parafascicular thalamic nuclei in the squirrel monkey: a PHA-L study of subcortical projections. *J Comp Neurol* 1992;315: 137–159.
77. Sato F, Lavallée P, Lévesque M, et al. Single-axon tracing study of neurons of the external segment of the globus pallidus in primate. *J Comp Neurol* 2000;417:17–31.
78. Sato F, Parent M, Lévesque M, et al. Axonal branching pattern of neurons of the subthalamic nucleus in primates. *J Comp Neurol* 2000;424:142–152.
79. Smith Y, Bevan MD, Shink E, et al. Microcircuitry of the direct and indirect pathways of the basal ganglia. *Neuroscience* 1998;86:353–387.
80. Percheron G, Filion M. Parallel processing in the basal ganglia: up to a point. *Trends Neurosci* 1991;14:55–59.
81. Hamani C, Saint-Cyr JA, Fraser J, et al. The subthalamic nucleus in the context of movement disorders. *Brain* 2003;127:4–20.
82. Fox CA, Andrade AN, Lu QI, et al. The primate globus pallidus: a Golgi and electron microscopic study. *J Hirnforsch* 1974;15:75–93.
83. Fox CA, Rafols JA. The radial fibers in the globus pallidus. *J Comp Neurol* 1975;159:177–199.
84. Yelnik J, François C, Percheron G. Spatial relationships between striatal axonal endings and pallidal neurons in macaque monkeys. *Adv Neurol* 1997;74:45–56.
85. Parent A, Hazrati LN, Charara A. The striatopallidal fiber system in primates. *Adv Neurol* 1997;74:19–29.
86. Nambu A, Tokuno H, Takada M. Functional significance of the cortico-subthalamo-pallidal 'hyperdirect' pathway. *Neurosci Res* 2002;43:111–117.
87. Joel D, Weiner I. The connections of the primate subthalamic nucleus: indirect pathways and the open-interconnected scheme of basal ganglia-thalamocortical circuitry. *Brain Res Rev* 1997;23:62–78.
88. Onla-or S, Winstein CJ. Function of the 'direct' and 'indirect' pathways of the basal ganglia motor loop: evidence from reciprocal aiming movements in Parkinson's disease. *Cognit Brain Res* 2001;10:329–332.
89. Nakano K. Neural circuits and topographic organization of the basal ganglia and related regions. *Brain Dev* 2000;22:S5–S16.
90. Chesselet MF, Delfs JM. Basal ganglia and movement disorders: an update. *Trends Neurosci* 1996;19:417–422.
91. Parent A, Hazrati L-N. Functional anatomy of the basal ganglia. II. The place of subthalamic nucleus and external pallidum in basal ganglia circuitry. *Brain Res Rev* 1995;20:128–154.
92. Hoover JE, Strick PL. Multiple output channels in the basal ganglia. *Science* 1993;259:819–821.
93. Ilinsky IA, Jouandet ML, Goldman-Rakic PS. Organization of the nigrothalamocortical system in the rhesus monkey. *J Comp Neurol* 1985;236:315–330.
94. McFarland NR, Haber SN. Convergent inputs from thalamic motor nuclei and frontal cortical areas to the dorsal striatum in the primate. *J Neurosci* 2000;20: 3798–3813.
95. McFarland NR, Haber SN. Thalamic relay nuclei of the basal ganglia form both reciprocal and nonreciprocal cortical connections, linking multiple frontal cortical areas. *J Neurosci* 2002;22:8117–8132.
96. Hikosaka O, Wurtz RH. Visual and oculomotor functions of monkey substantia nigra pars reticulata. IV. Relation of substantia nigra to superior colliculus. *J Neurophysiol* 1983;49:1285–1301.
97. Garcia-Rill E, Homma Y, Skinner RD. Arousal mechanisms related to posture and locomotion: 1. Descending modulation. *Prog Brain Res* 2004;143:283–290.
98. Garcia-Rill E, Houser CR, Skinner RD, et al. Locomotion-inducing sites in the vicinity of the pedunculopontine nucleus. *Brain Res Bull* 1987;18:731–738.
99. Munro-Davies LE, Winter J, Aziz TZ, et al. The role of the pedunculopontine region in basal-ganglia mechanisms of akinesia. *Exp Brain Res* 1999;129:511–517.
100. Nandi D, Aziz TZ, Liu XG, et al. Brainstem motor loops in the control of movement. *Mov Disord* 2002; 17:S22–S27.
101. Pahapill PA, Lozano AM. The pedunculopontine nucleus and Parkinson's disease. *Brain* 2000;123: 1767–1783.
102. Rodríguez M, Abdala P, Barroso-Chinea P, et al. The deep mesencephalic nucleus as an output center of basal ganglia: morphological and electrophysiological similarities with the substantia nigra. *J Comp Neurol* 2001;438:12–31.
103. Skinner RD, Homma Y, Garcia-Rill E. Arousal mechanisms related to posture and locomotion: 2. Ascending modulation. *Prog Brain Res* 2004;143:291–298.
104. Winn P. Frontal syndrome as a consequence of lesions in the pedunculopontine tegmental nucleus: a short theoretical review. *Brain Res Bull* 1998;47:551–563.
105. Inglis WL, Olmstead MC, Robbins TW. Pedunculopontine tegmental nucleus lesions impair stimulus–reward learning in autoshaping and conditioned reinforcement paradigms. *Behav Neurosci* 2000;114:285–294.
106. Middleton FA, Strick PL. Basal ganglia and cerebellar loops: motor and cognitive circuits. *Brain Res Rev* 2000;31:236–250.
107. Künzle H. An autoradiographic analysis of the efferent connections from premotor and adjacent prefrontal regions (areas 6 and 9) in macaca fascicularis. *Brain Behav Evol* 1978;15:185–234.
108. Watson RT, Valenstein E, Heilman KM. Thalamic neglect. Possible role of the medial thalamus and nucleus reticularis in behavior. *Arch Neurol* 1981;38:501–506.
109. Matsumoto N, Minamimoto T, Graybiel AM, et al. Neurons in the thalamic CM-Pf complex supply striatal neurons with information about behaviorally significant sensory events. *J Neurophysiol* 2001;85:960–976.
110. Levy R, Hazrati LN, Herrero MT, et al. Re-evaluation of the functional anatomy of the basal ganglia in normal and parkinsonian states. *Neuroscience* 1997; 76:335–343.
111. Parent A, Cicchetti F. The current model of basal ganglia organization under scrutiny. *Mov Disord* 1998;13:199–202.
112. Parent A, Lévesque M, Parent M. A re-evaluation of the current model of the basal ganglia. *Parkinsonism Relat Disord* 2001;7:193–198.
113. Nambu A, Kaneda K, Tokuno H, et al. Organization of corticostriatal motor inputs in monkey putamen. *J Neurophys* 2002;88:1830–1842.
114. Saint-Cyr JA. Frontal-striatal circuit functions: context, sequence, and consequence. *J Int Neuropsychol Soc* 2003;9:103–127.
115. Graybiel AM. Building action repertoires: memory and learning functions of the basal ganglia. *Curr Opin Neurobiol* 1995;5:733–741.
116. Saint-Cyr JA, Taylor AE, Lang AE. Procedural learning and neostriatal dysfunction in man. *Brain* 1988; 111:941–959.

117. Schultz W. Getting formal with dopamine and reward. *Neuron* 2002;36:241–263.
118. Brotchie P, Iansek R, Horne MK. Motor function of the monkey globus pallidus. 2. Cognitive aspects of movement and phasic neuronal activity. *Brain* 1991;114:1685–1702.
119. Brotchie P, Iansek R, Horne MK. Motor function of the monkey globus pallidus. I. Neuronal discharge and parameters of movement. *Brain* 1991;114:1667–1683.
120. Crutcher MD, Alexander GE. Movement-related neuronal activity selectively coding either direction or muscle pattern in three motor areas of the monkey. *J Neurophysiol* 1990;64:151–163.
121. DeLong MR, Georgopoulos AP, Crutcher MD. Cortico-basal ganglia relations and coding of motor performance. In: Massion J et al., eds. *Neural coding of motor performance*. Berlin: Springer-Verlag, 1983:29–44.
122. Filion M, Tremblay L, Bédard PJ. Abnormal influences of passive limb movement on the activity of globus pallidus neurons in parkinsonian monkeys. *Brain Res* 1988;444:165–176.
123. Mink JW, Thach WT. Basal ganglia motor control II. Late pallidal timing relative to movement onset and inconsistent pallidal coding of movement parameters. *J Neurophysiol* 1991;65:301–329.
124. Mink JW, Thach WT. Basal ganglia motor control III. Pallidal ablation: normal reaction time, muscle cocontraction and slow movement. *J Neurophysiol* 1991;65:330–351.
125. Mitchell IJ, Brotchie JM, Brown GDA, et al. Modeling the functional organization of the basal ganglia. A parallel distributed processing approach. *Mov Disord* 1991;6:189–204.
126. Filion M, Tremblay L, Matsumura M. Focalisation dynamique de la convergence informationnelle dans les noyaux gris centraux. *Rev Neurol (Paris)* 1994;150:627–633.
127. Mink JW. The basal ganglia: focused selection and inhibition of competing motor programs. *Prog Neurobiol* 1996;50:381–425.
128. Alexander GE, Crutcher MD. Functional architecture of basal ganglia circuits: neural substrates of parallel processing. *Trends Neurosci* 1990;13:266–271.
129. Alexander GE, Crutcher MD. Neural representations of the target (goal) of visually guided arm movements in three motor areas of the monkey. *J Neurophysiol* 1990;64:164–178.
130. Graybiel AM. The basal ganglia and chunking of action repertoires. *Neurobiol Learn Mem* 1998;70:119–136.
131. Sakai K, Kitaguchi K, Hikosaka O. Chunking during human visuomotor sequence learning. *Exp Brain Res* 2003;152:229–242.
132. Doyon J, Penhune V, Ungerleider LG. Distinct contribution of the cortico-striatal and cortico-cerebellar systems to motor skill learning. *Neuropsychologia* 2003;41:252–262.
133. Ungerleider LG, Doyon J, Karni A. Imaging brain plasticity during motor skill learning. *Neurobiol Learn Mem* 2002;78:553–564.
134. Albin RL, Young AB, Penney JB. The functional anatomy of basal ganglia disorders. *Trends Neurosci* 1989;12:366–375.
135. Lang AE, Lozano AM. Parkinson's disease—first of two parts. *N Engl J Med* 1998;339:1044–1053.
136. Lang AE, Lozano AM. Parkinson's disease—second of two parts. *N Engl J Med* 1998;339:1130–1143.
137. Graybiel AM. The basal ganglia and cognitive pattern generators. *Schizophr Bull* 1997;23:459–469.
138. Shik ML, Orlovsky GN. Neurophysiology of locomotor automatism. *Physiol Rev* 1976;56:465–501.
139. Ceballos-Baumann AO. Functional imaging in Parkinson's disease: activation studies with PET, fMRI and SPECT. *J Neurol* 2003;250:I15–I23.
140. Turner RS, Grafton ST, McIntosh AR, et al. The functional anatomy of parkinsonian bradykinesia. *NeuroImage* 2003;19:163–179.
141. Fiorillo CD, Tobler PN, Schultz W. Discrete coding of reward probability and uncertainty by dopamine neurons. *Science* 2003;299:1898–1902.
142. Schultz W, Tremblay L, Hollerman JR. Changes in behavior-related neuronal activity in the striatum during learning. *Trends Neurosci* 2003;26:321–328.
143. Shallice T. 'Theory of mind' and the prefrontal cortex. *Brain* 2001;124:247–248.
144. Baddeley A. Working memory: looking back and looking forward. *Nat Rev Neurosci* 2003;4:829–839.
145. Zalla T, Sirigu A, Pillon B, et al. How patients with Parkinson's disease retrieve and manage cognitive event knowledge. *Cereb Cortex* 2000;36:163–179.
146. Compte A, Constantinidis C, Tegner J, et al. Temporally irregular mnemonic persistent activity in prefrontal neurons of monkeys during a delayed response task. *J Neurophysiol* 2003;90(5):3441–3454.
147. Funahashi S, Bruce CJ, Goldman-Rakic PS. Mnemonic coding of visual space in the monkey's dorsolateral prefrontal cortex. *J Neurophysiol* 1989;61:331–349.
148. Hollerman JR, Schultz W. Dopamine neurons report an error in the temporal prediction of reward during learning. *Nat Neurosci* 1998;1:304–309.
149. Kunig G, Leenders KL, Martin-Solch C, et al. Reduced reward processing in the brains of Parkinsonian patients. *NeuroReport* 2000;11:3681–3687.
150. Rolls ET. Memory systems in the brain. *Annu Rev Psychol* 2000;51:599–630.
151. Watanabe Y, Funahashi S. Neuronal activity throughout the primate mediodorsal nucleus of the thalamus during oculomotor delayed-responses II. Activity encoding visual versus motor signal. *J Neurophysiol* 2004;92(3):1756–1769.
152. Watanabe Y, Funahashi S. Neuronal activity throughout the primate mediodorsal nucleus of the thalamus during oculomotor delayed-responses. I. Cue-, delay-, and response-period activity. *J Neurophysiol* 2004;92(3):1738–1755.
153. Brasted PJ, Wise SP. Comparison of learning-related neuronal activity in the dorsal premotor cortex and striatum. *Eur J Neurosci* 2004;19:721–740.
154. Brown RG. The role of cortico-striatal circuits in learning sequential information. In: Stern GM, ed. *Parkinson's disease: advances in neurology*. Philadelphia: Lippincott Williams & Wilkins, 1999:31–39.
155. Koch G, Brusa L, Caltagirone C, et al. Subthalamic deep brain stimulation improves time perception in Parkinson's disease. *NeuroReport* 2004;15:1071–1073.
156. Ivry RB, Spencer RM. The neural representation of time. *Curr Opin Neurobiol* 2004;14:225–232.
157. Mayberg HS, Solomon DH. Depression in Parkinson's disease: a biochemical and organic viewpoint. *Adv Neurol* 1995;65:49–60.
158. Goldman-Rakic PS, Selemon LD. Functional and anatomical aspects of prefrontal pathology in schizophrenia. *Schizophr Bull* 1997;23:437–458.
159. Saxena S, Rauch SL. Functional neuroimaging and the neuroanatomy of obsessive–compulsive disorder. *Psychiatr Clin North Am* 2000;23:563–586.

160. Cloninger CR. The discovery of susceptibility genes for mental disorders. *Proc Natl Acad Sci USA* 2002; 99:13365–13367.
161. Voon V, Moro E, Saint-Cyr JA, et al. Psychiatric symptoms following surgery for Parkinson's disease with an emphasis on subthalamic stimulation. In: Weiner WJ et al., eds. *Behavioral neurology of movement disorders.* New York: Raven Press, 2004.
162. Laplane D, Dubois B. Auto-activation deficit: a basal ganglia related syndrome. *Mov Disord* 2001;16:810–814.
163. Brown R, Jahanshahi M. Depression in Parkinson's disease: a psychosocial viewpoint. *Adv Neurol* 1995; 65:61–84.
164. Starkstein SE, Petracca G, Chemerinski E, et al. Prevalence and correlates of parkinsonism in patients with primary depression. *Neurology* 2001;57:553–555.
165. Taylor AE, Saint-Cyr JA. Depression in Parkinson's disease: reconciling physiological and psychological perspectives. *J Neuropsychiatry Clin Neurosci* 1990; 2:92–98.
166. Voon V, Saint-Cyr JA, Lozano AM, et al. Suicide risk in patients with Parkinson's disease undergoing subthalamic stimulation. *Mov Disord* 2004;19:S323.
167. Taniwaki T, Okayama A, Yoshiura T, et al. Reappraisal of the motor role of basal ganglia: a functional magnetic resonance image study. *J Neurosci* 2003;23:3432–3438.
168. Ceballos-Baumann AO, Brooks DJ. Basal ganglia function and dysfunction revealed by PET activation studies. *Adv Neurol* 1997;74:127–139.
169. Limousin P, Greene J, Pollak P, et al. Changes in cerebral activity pattern due to subthalamic nucleus or internal pallidum stimulation in Parkinson's disease. *Ann Neurol* 1997;42:283–291.
170. Broussolle E, Dentresangle C, Landais P, et al. The relation of putamen and caudate nucleus 18F-Dopa uptake to motor and cognitive performances in Parkinson's disease. *J Neurol Sci* 1999;166:141–151.
171. Brucke T, Djamshidian S, Bencsits G, et al. SPECT and PET imaging of the dopaminergic system in Parkinson's disease. *J Neurol* 2000;247(Suppl. 4): IV–2–IV–7.
172. Carbon M, Marié RM. Functional imaging of cognition in Parkinson's disease. *Curr Opin Neurol* 2003; 16:475–480.
173. Dagher A, Owen AM, Boecker H, et al. The role of the striatum and hippocampus in planning—a PET activation study in Parkinson's disease. *Brain* 2001; 124:1020–1032.
174. Hartley T, Maguire EA, Spiers HJ, et al. The well-worn route and the path less traveled: distinct neural bases of route following and wayfinding in humans. *Neuron* 2003;37:877–888.
175. Lewis SJ, Dove A, Robbins TW, et al. Striatal contributions to working memory: a functional magnetic resonance imaging study in humans. *Eur J Neurosci* 2004;19:755–760.
176. Levy R, Friedman HR, Davachi L, et al. Differential activation of the caudate nucleus in primates performing spatial and nonspatial working memory tasks. *J Neurosci* 1997;17:3870–3882.
177. Catalan MJ, Ishii K, Honda M, et al. A PET study of sequential finger movements of varying length in patients with Parkinson's disease. *Brain* 1999;122:483–495.
178. Lewis SJ, Dove A, Robbins TW, et al. Cognitive impairments in early Parkinson's disease are accompanied by reductions in activity in frontostriatal neural circuitry. *J Neurosci* 2003;23:6351–6356.
179. Pagnoni G, Zink CF, Montague PR, et al. Activity in human ventral striatum locked to errors of reward prediction. *Nat Neurosci* 2002;5:97–98.
180. Pochon JB, Levy R, Fossati P, et al. The neural system that bridges reward and cognition in humans: an fMRI study. *Proc Natl Acad Sci USA* 2002;99:5669–5674.
181. Takada M, Matsumura M, Kojima J, et al. Protection against dopaminergic nigrostriatal cell death by excitatory input ablation. *Eur J Neurosci* 2000;12:1771–1780.
182. Crossman AR. Functional anatomy of movement disorders. *J Anat* 2000;196:519–525.
183. Joel D. Open interconnected model of basal ganglia-thalamocortical circuitry and its relevance to the clinical syndrome of Huntington's disease. *Mov Disord* 2001;16:407–423.
184. Comings DE. Tourette's syndrome: A behavioral spectrum disorder. *Adv Neurol* 1995;65:293–304.
185. Graybiel AM, Rauch SL. Toward a neurobiology of obsessive–compulsive disorder. *Neuron* 2000;28: 343–347.
186. Hansen ES, Hasselbalch S, Law I, et al. The caudate nucleus in obsessive–compulsive disorder. Reduced metabolism following treatment with paroxetine: a PET study. *Int J Neuropsychopharmacol* 2002;5:1–10.
187. Nuttin BJ, Gabriels L, van Kuyck K, et al. Electrical stimulation of the anterior limbs of the internal capsules in patients with severe obsessive–compulsive disorder: anecdotal reports. *Neurosurg Clin N Am* 2003; 14:267–274.
188. Brodal A. (1963) Some data and perspectives on the anatomy of the so-called "extrapyramidal system." *Acta Neurol Scand.* 39(Suppl. 4):17–38.
189. Taylor AE, Saint-Cyr JA, Lang AE. Frontal lobe dysfunction in Parkinson's disease: the cortical focus of neostriatal outflow. *Brain* 1986;109:845–883.
190. Hornykiewicz E. Dopamine miracle: from brain homogenate to dopamine replacement. *Mov Disord* 2002;17:501–508.
191. Deuschl G, Raethjen J, Lindemann M, et al. The pathophysiology of tremor. *Muscle Nerve* 2001;24:716–735.
192. Dubois B, Boller F, Pillon B, et al. Cognitive deficits in Parkinson's disease. In: Corkin S et al., eds. *Handbook of neuropsychology.* Amsterdam: Elsevier, 1991: 195–240.
193. Marsden CD, Obeso JA. The functions of the basal ganglia and the paradox of stereotaxic surgery in Parkinson's disease. *Brain* 1994;117:877–897.
194. Deuschl G, Wilms H, Krack P, et al. Function of the cerebellum in parkinsonian rest tremor and Holmes' tremor. *Ann Neurol* 1999;46:126–128.
195. Starr PA, Vitek JL, Bakay RA. Ablative surgery and deep brain stimulation for Parkinson's disease. *Neurosurgery* 1998;43:989–1013.
196. Ashby P. What does stimulation in the brain actually do? In: Lozano AM, ed. *Progress in neurological surgery.* Basel: Karger, 2000:236–245.
197. Brown RG, Dowsey PL, Brown P, et al. Impact of deep brain stimulation on upper limb akinesia in Parkinson's disease. *Ann Neurol* 1999;45:473–488.
198. Cools R, Barker RA, Sahakian BJ, et al. Enhanced or impaired cognitive function in Parkinson's disease as a function of dopaminergic medication and task demands. *Cereb Cortex* 2001;11:1136–1143.
199. Partiot A, Vérin M, Pillon B, et al. Delayed response tasks in basal ganglia lesions in man: further evidence for a striato-frontal cooperation in behavioural adaptation. *Neuropsychologia* 1996;34:709–721.

200. Bejjani BP, Damier P, Arnulf I, et al. Transient acute depression induced by high-frequency deep-brain stimulation. *N Engl J Med* 1999;340:1476–1480.
201. Bejjani BP, Houeto JL, Hariz M, et al. Aggressive behavior induced by intraoperative stimulation in the triangle of Sano. *Neurology* 2002;59:1425–1427.
202. Krack P, Kumar R, Ardouin C, et al. Mirthful laughter induced by subthalamic nucleus stimulation. *Mov Disord* 2001;16:867–875.
203. Kumar R, Krack P, Pollak P. Transient acute depression induced by high-frequency deep-brain stimulation [letter]. *N Engl J Med* 1999;341:1003–1004.
204. Okun MS, Raju DV, Walter BL, et al. Pseudobulbar crying induced by stimulation in the region of the subthalamic nucleus. *J Neurol Neurosurg Psychiatry* 2004;75:921–923.
205. Bandler R, Shipley MT. Columnar organization in the midbrain periaqueductal gray: modules for emotional expression? *Trends Neurosci* 1994;17:379–389.
206. Krack P, Ardouin C, Funkiewiez A. What is the influence of subthalamic nucleus stimulation on the limbic loop? In: Kultas-Ilinsky K, et al., eds. *Basal ganglia and thalamus in health and movement disorders*. New York: Kluwer Academic/Plenium Publishers, 2001:333–340.
207. Livingston KE, Escobar A. Anatomical bias of the limbic system concept. A proposed reorientation. *Arch Neurol* 1971;24:17–21.
208. Houeto JL, Mesnage V, Mallet L, et al. Behavioural disorders, Parkinson's disease and subthalamic stimulation. *J Neurol Neurosurg Psychiatry* 2002;72:701–707.
209. Funkiewiez A, Ardouin C, Krack P, et al. Acute psychotropic effects of bilateral subthalamic nucleus stimulation and levodopa in Parkinson's disease. *Mov Disord* 2003;18:524–530.
210. Fiorino DF, Coury A, Fibiger HC, et al. Electrical stimulation of reward sites in the ventral tegmental area increases dopamine transmission in the nucleus accumbens of the rat. *Behav Brain Res* 1993;55:131–141.
211. Williams SM, Goldman-Rakic PS. Widespread origin of the primate mesofrontal dopamine system. *Cereb Cortex* 1998;8:321–345.
212. Wise RA. Brain reward circuitry: insights from unsensed incentives. *Neuron* 2002;36:229–240.
213. Druhan JP, Fibiger HC, Phillips AG. Amphetamine-like stimulus properties produced by electrical stimulation of reward sites in the ventral tegmental area. *Behav Brain Res* 1990;38:175–184.
214. Wise RA, Leone P, Rivest R, et al. Elevations of nucleus accumbens dopamine and DOPAC levels during intravenous heroin self-administration. *Synapse* 1995;21:140–148.
215. Wise RA, Newton P, Leeb K, et al. Fluctuations in nucleus accumbens dopamine concentration during intravenous cocaine self-administration in rats. *Psychopharmacology (Berl)* 1995;120:10–20.
216. Mallet L, Mesnage V, Houeto JL, et al. Compulsions, Parkinson's disease, and stimulation. *Lancet* 2002;360:1302–1304.
217. Ardouin C, Pillon B, Peiffer E, et al. Bilateral subthalamic or pallidal stimulation for Parkinson's disease affects neither memory nor executive functions: a consecutive series of 62 patients. *Ann Neurol* 1999;46:217–223.
218. Jahanshahi M, Ardouin CMA, Brown RG, et al. The impact of deep brain stimulation on executive function in Parkinson's disease. *Brain* 2000;123:1142–1154.
219. Pillon B, Ardouin C, Damier P, et al. Neuropsychological changes between "off" and "on" STN or GPi stimulation in Parkinson's disease. *Neurology* 2000;55:411–418.
220. Woods SP, Fields JA, Troster AI. Neuropsychological sequelae of subthalamic nucleus deep brain stimulation in Parkinson's disease: a critical review. *Neuropsychol Rev* 2002;12:111–126.
221. Saint-Cyr JA, Trépanier LL, Kumar R, et al. Neuropsychological consequences of chronic bilateral stimulation of the subthalamic nucleus in Parkinson's disease. *Brain* 2000;123:2091–2108.
222. Hershey T, Revilla FJ, Wernle A, et al. Stimulation of STN impairs aspects of cognitive control in PD. *Neurology* 2004;62:1110–1114.
223. Schroeder U, Kuehler A, Haslinger B, et al. Subthalamic nucleus stimulation affects striato-anterior cingulate cortex circuit in a response conflict task: a PET study. *Brain* 2002;125:1995–2004.
224. Saint-Cyr JA, Trépanier LL. Neuropsychologic assessment of patients for movement disorder surgery. *Mov Disord* 2000;15:771–783.
225. Halbig TD, Gruber D, Kopp UA, et al. Subthalamic stimulation differentially modulates declarative and nondeclarative memory. *NeuroReport* 2004;15:539–543.
226. Rivaud-Pechoux S, Vermersch AI, Gaymard B, et al. Improvement of memory guided saccades in parkinsonian patients by high frequency subthalamic nucleus stimulation. *J Neurol Neurosurg Psychiatry* 2000;68:381–384.
227. Owen AM, Herrod NJ, Menon DK, et al. Redefining the functional organization of working memory processes within human lateral prefrontal cortex. *Eur J Neurosci* 1999;11:567–574.
228. Petrides M, Pandya DN. Dorsolateral prefrontal cortex: comparative cytoarchitectonic analysis in the human and the macaque brain and corticocortical connection patterns. *Eur J Neurosci* 1999;11:1011–1036.
229. Goldman-Rakic PS. The prefrontal landscape: implications of functional architecture for understanding human mentation and the central executive. *Philos Trans R Soc Lond B Biol Sci* 1996;351:1445–1453.
230. Levy R, Goldman-Rakic PS. Segregation of working memory functions within the dorsolateral prefrontal cortex. *Exp Brain Res* 2000;133:23–32.
231. Robbins TW. Dissociating executive functions of the prefrontal cortex. *Philos Trans R Soc Lond B Biol Sci* 1996;351:1463–1470.
232. Robbins TW. From arousal to cognition: the integrative position of the prefrontal cortex. *Prog Brain Res* 2000;126:469–483.
233. Alexander GE, DeLong MR, Strick PL. Parallel organization of functionally segregated circuits linking basal ganglia and cortex. *Annu Rev Neurosci* 1986;9:357–381.
234. Stepniewska I, Sakai ST, Qi HX, et al. Somatosensory input to the ventrolateral thalamic region in the macaque monkey: a potential substrate for parkinsonian tremor. *J Comp Neurol* 2002;455:378–395.
235. Saint-Cyr JA, Taylor AE. The mobilization of procedural learning. The "key signature" of the basal ganglia. In: Butters N et al., eds. *Neuropsychology of memory*. New York: The Guilford Press, 1992:188–202.

2

Behavioral Changes in Patients with Focal Lesions of the Basal Ganglia

Bruno Dubois, Aurélie Funkiewiez, Bernard Pillon

INSERM U 610 and Fédération de Neurologie, Hôpital de la Salpêtrière, Paris, France

The basal ganglia have been implicated in cognitive processes and in behavioral regulation on the basis of two main arguments. First, experimental studies in primates have shown that focal lesions of the striatum induce deficits in working memory, rule acquisition, and behavioral control. Second, cognitive changes have long been observed in patients with degenerative diseases that primarily involve the basal ganglia, such as Parkinson's or Huntington's diseases or progressive supranuclear palsy. From the clinical picture of these neurodegenerative disorders, the main changes postulated to result from basal ganglia dysfunction are slowing of information processing (1), dysexecutive syndrome (2), impaired memory retrieval (3), and personality changes such as inertia (4) and depressed mood (5). These symptoms have been brought together under the term *subcortical dementia* (6) to highlight the influence of deep gray-matter structures on cognition and behavior. The term is debatable, however, for at least two reasons. The clinical criteria commonly accepted by the American Psychiatric Association to define dementia do not fit well with patients whose global cognitive deficiency is mild or moderate and whose loss of autonomy can be largely attributed to associated movement disorders. Moreover, it cannot be firmly demonstrated that these deficits result from dysfunction of subcortical structures alone, because associated lesions have been described in the cerebral cortex, as in Parkinson's disease dementia (7,8) or in progressive supranuclear palsy (9). For that reason, the cognitive and behavioral functions of the basal ganglia can be better characterized by observing patients suffering from focal and isolated lesions within these structures (10,11). Such lesions induce changes that resemble the sequelae of frontal lobe damage and, to a lesser extent, some features of neuropsychiatric disorders (12), thereby raising questions about whether common underlying neuronal circuits mediate these functions and about the specific contribution of the basal ganglia to behavioral control and to cognitive processes.

BEHAVIORAL DISTURBANCES AND FOCAL LESIONS OF THE BASAL GANGLIA

Inertia

Patients suffering from bilateral lesions of the basal ganglia, and especially the globus pallidus, can show markedly reduced spontaneous activity in the absence of any motor disorder or akinesia, which can be easily but temporarily reversed by external stimulation (13). These patients tend to remain in the same place for long periods, sitting in a chair or lying in bed, taking no initiative and asking no questions, although they may respond appropriately to questions with short but adequate sentences. The first description of a patient with the inertia syndrome concerns a previously active businessman who became dramatically inactive following an encephalopathy caused by a wasp bite (14). After some time, he could initiate some routine activities like watching television or buying and reading a newspaper, but he remained inactive most of the time. When stimulated, however, he was able to perform more complex activities, like playing high-level bridge. Another patient remained in his bed for half an hour with an unlit cigarette in his mouth. When asked what he was doing, he responded: "I am waiting for a light" (15). A third patient spent 45 minutes with his hands on a lawn mower, totally unable to initiate the act of mowing (16). This "kinetic blockade" disappeared instantaneously when his son told him to mow. The most striking feature of this behavioral inertia is that it can be easily reversed by a mere incitement, which enables such patients to perform normally not only routine or overlearned activities but also complex activities. In contrast, reversing inertia in patients with frontal lobe lesions requires a more prolonged interaction that helps the patient to focus his or her attention and that provides a framework for the task to be executed (17,18).

Blunted Affect

Affect is usually flattened, with anhedonia, and emotional responses are blunted (19). Although the patients can correctly and critically assess their situation, they are not subject to self-deprecation. They admit that they have become a burden to their family, but they do so without an appropriate emotional response. They express neither drive nor anxiety but only a vague hope of recovery, which seems more of an intellectual expression than an emotionally felt one. They can react appropriately to good or bad news, but the reaction is short-lived, and they rapidly return to their usual "neutral" state. When asked about a recent accidental death in his family, one patient cried, but when asked later about recent events in his life, he did not mention the accident (19). According to the relatives of another patient, "he seemed happy, for instance, in the presence of his grand-children, [but] he did not show any affective manifestation either upon their arrival or their leaving, never asking to see them again" (20). This blunted affect may resemble a depressive state. The patients do not complain of subjective symptoms of sadness, helplessness, or desperation, however, and do not express suicidal thoughts. This state may also show some similarities to negative forms of schizophrenia, in which affective indifference is a primary symptom. However, no delirium or thought disorders have been reported except in the case of caudate lesions (21).

Mental Emptiness

The fact that patients with basal ganglia lesions can remain inactive for hours without complaining of boredom may be explained by a lack of spontaneous mental life. "My mind is empty, it's like a blank," said a patient, who was otherwise able to read or to participate in sports when encouraged to do so (19). Although purely subjective, this feeling seems to be a reliable symptom, reported in the same manner by numerous patients (22), and suggests that mental life really fades during the periods of "loneliness" and is revived by stimulation.

Autoactivation Deficit

Inertia, blunted affect, and mental emptiness are frequently encountered in patients with basal ganglia lesions. They are part of a syndrome recently described under the name *autoactivation deficit* (23), a term that draws attention to the specific contribution of the basal ganglia in activating behavior, affect, and mental life. These behavioral changes may appear only several months after the lesion occurs, but they tend to remain stable over time. The first patient described by Laplane et al. (14) developed behavioral disorders a few months after an initial coma, and these behaviors did not vary during 12 years of follow-up. This syndrome has been reported with focal lesions involving either the globus pallidus after anoxia (12) or bilateral hemorrhages (24) or the caudate nucleus after vascular accidents (ischemia, hematoma, or lacunae) (16,20). The relation between autoactivation deficits and the striatopallidal complex has been confirmed by a meta-analysis of behavioral changes following lesions of the basal ganglia: 6 of the 7 patients with pallidal lesions and 17 of the 33 patients with caudate lesions presented behavioral inertia, but none of the patients with lesions of the putamen did so (10). Thalamic lesions may also induce an autoactivation deficit: such a deficit has been reported following thalamopeduncular paramedian infarction (25). These findings suggest that both the striatopallidal complex and the thalamus may be part of a neuronal network implicated in behavioral activation. In contrast, hyperactivity, impulsiveness, or violent outbursts have been described in some cases, but only at the early stages of basal ganglia lesions that mainly involved the ventromedial region of the caudate nucleus (21,26,27), a region known to project to the orbitofrontal part of the prefrontal cortex (28).

In some cases, no behavioral change is reported after a focal lesion of the pallidum (29,30) or of the caudate nucleus (31). Two explanations can be proposed: (a) subtle behavioral changes can be ignored if they are not specifically searched for and (b) the functional consequences of basal ganglia damage may differ depending on the etiology, the precise location of the lesion, and the time of examination. In addition, it is sometimes difficult to determine the actual intensity of damage to the basal ganglia on the basis of magnetic resonance imaging (MRI) images.

Apathy and reduced spontaneous activity have also been observed in patients with degenerative diseases of the basal ganglia—Huntington's disease (32), Parkinson's disease (33,34) and, particularly, progressive supranuclear palsy (35)—using tools such as the Neuropsychiatric Inventory (36) or the Apathy Inventory (37).

Stereotyped Activities

Despite their overall decreased activity and their initiation disorder, some patients may engage in repetitive and stereotyped activities. These compulsive behaviors can be mental (generally arithmomania, such as mentally counting all the objects in the environment or repeating sentences) (14,38) or motor (snapping or sucking the fingers, making repetitive finger movements, shouting, or hand clapping). A patient with bilateral hypodensities of the internal pallidum following a brain anoxia demonstrated compulsive behavior by tapping repetitive sequences of six with a pen or a cigarette lighter, alternately opening and shutting every door that he saw for periods of 10 to 15 minutes, and swallowing each time he crossed a line on the pavement or each time the bus passed a tree (Laplane's communication). These stereotyped activities may be even more elaborate, as in the case of an amateur artist who, over a period of weeks, repeatedly painted the same type of subjects: castles, ruins, and historical portraits (13). Such stereotyped activities can resemble the compulsive acts encountered in obsessive–compulsive syndromes. The patients with basal ganglia lesions, however, manifest no distress or acute anxiety when they are asked to control their behavior, and their score is normal on the Trimble Scale of obsessive–compulsive behavior (39). Stereotyped activities or compulsions have also been reported in neurodegenerative diseases involving the basal ganglia, such as Huntington's disease (40), Parkinson's disease (41), progressive supranuclear palsy (42), and Gilles de la Tourette syndrome, in which basal ganglia dysfunction has been regularly suspected on the basis of metabolic and neuroradiological evidence (43).

Taken together, these observations implicate the basal ganglia in behavioral control, both in initiating behaviors and in suppressing automatic, uncontrolled, or stereotyped activities. This implication could at least partly explain the role of the basal ganglia in cognitive functions.

COGNITIVE DISTURBANCES AND FOCAL LESIONS OF THE BASAL GANGLIA

Global intellectual efficiency is usually preserved in patients with focal lesions of the basal ganglia. Long-term intellectual deterioration might, however, be observed after caudate infarction and be mediated through disruption of cortical projections to the caudate (44). Although the autoactivation deficit may reduce performance in some tests, the context of neuropsychological assessment and the presence of the examiner stimulate the patients. Instrumental functions are also preserved. Aphasic disorders have been described in patients with focal damage of the thalamus (45,46) but not in patients with focal lesions of the basal ganglia, except in word finding (47) or when lesions extend outside the caudate nucleus of the dominant hemisphere to the adjacent white matter (31,48). Thus, white matter pathways might be the critical structure involved in the subcortical-related language disorders (47). The neostriatum is involved, however, in modulating speech parameters and contributes to spoken output; thus, dysphonia, dysprosodia, hypophonia, and palilalia may result from damage to this region (47). Hemispatial neglect is also encountered only when the thalamus (46) or the internal capsule (49) is involved. In contrast, executive function as well as explicit and procedural memory may be impaired in focal lesions of the basal ganglia.

Executive Functions

Deficits may be observed in (a) resolving arithmetic problems that require the elaboration of complex algorithms, partly because of inertia (12); (b) the Wisconsin Card Sorting Test, which evaluates set elaboration, maintenance, and shifting (21,50), but performance on this test is not always disturbed (51); (c) the California Card Sorting Test, in which the patients experience moderate difficulties in spontaneously elaborating the sorting rules in the first part of the test but more severe difficulties in deducing the sorting rule used by the examiner in the second part of the test; (d) the Stroop test, in which patients with bipallidal (24) or striatal (52) lesions exhibit underlying difficulties with inhibiting interference; (e) lexical fluency (15,16), which suggests that the search strategies employed for long-term memory are defective. These examples from the extant literature suggest that reactive flexibility, which is required for set shifting in card sorting tests, may be disturbed following a focal lesion of the basal ganglia. These studies, in contrast with previous data, also suggest that spontaneous flexibility, which is involved in lexical fluency, may also be impaired (50). Pathological behaviors, such as prehension, utilization, and imitation, are not observed. This dysexecutive syndrome is milder than that found in Parkinson's disease (53) or progressive supranuclear palsy (54), probably because of the additional subcortical lesions that are described in these diseases.

Explicit Memory

Focal lesions of the basal ganglia induce explicit memory deficits (12), particularly when the caudate nucleus is implicated (10). However, a true amnesic syndrome is observed only as a consequence of a thalamic infarction involving the mamillothalamic tract (55). The poor free recall performance associated with basal ganglia lesions results from difficulty in activating efficient retrieval strategies rather than from a true amnesic syndrome caused by impaired memory processes. Indeed, recognition has been shown to be unimpaired despite poor free recall performance in a series of patients with vascular lesions of the caudate nucleus. These patients had been behaving as if they had "got the information but could not easily retrieve it" (21). Furthermore, implementing the same semantic cues for encoding and retrieval, as in the Grober and Buschke procedure (56), dramatically improved their recall performance, as observed in degenerative diseases of the basal ganglia (54). These results suggest that the striatopallidal complex is also implicated in activating memory processes.

Procedural Learning

Procedural learning is the ability to acquire a perceptual or motor skill or a cognitive routine through repeated exposure to a specific activity constrained by invariant rules. This ability likely involves the neostriatum (57). Although few experimental studies are available of procedural learning in patients with basal ganglia lesions, clinical observations emphasize the role of the basal ganglia in activating overlearned programs or routine procedures: these patients often have difficulty in writing, signing their name, and typing. One patient, who was previously a professional dancer, was no longer able to dance or drive a car in an automatic fashion. A deficit in mirror reading and in a serial reaction time paradigm was observed in patients with focal lesions of the caudate nucleus, whereas motor learning in the pursuit rotor task was disturbed only in a patient with a lesion restricted to the putamen. These results suggest that the basal ganglia may be involved in acquiring and automatizing new procedures and in accessing or activating motor skills and overlearned behaviors, a possibility that is supported by recent studies that show increased activity in the basal ganglia during the automatization of a new sequence of movements and during the completion of a routine procedure (58,59). According to a recent study, however, the basal ganglia could be "responsible for adjusting behavior to the general requirements of a task rather than for learning specific associations between stimuli that might be accomplished by premotor frontal areas and the cerebellum instead" (60).

DISCUSSION

The behavioral and cognitive consequences of focal lesions of the basal ganglia raise questions about the functional similarities or dissimilarities between the basal ganglia and the prefrontal cortex because both structures belong to the same neural network, which is involved in the elaboration of forthcoming actions and goal-directed behaviors. These questions already concern the processes responsible for behavioral and cognitive activation. Reward-related neuronal activity has been reported in both subcortical (striatum) and prefrontal (orbitofrontal) regions of nonhuman primates (61–63). In humans, lesions of both structures may be responsible for apathy or abulia, which can be strikingly normalized, in the case of striatopallidal lesions, by external stimulation (13). Moreover, the behavioral disturbances associated with basal ganglia lesions, such as inertia, apathy, blunted affect, and stereotyped activities, resemble those encountered in neuropsychiatric diseases, such as dysthymic and obsessive–compulsive disorders, that have been related to a dysfunction of the orbitofrontal or cingulate anterior circuits (64). In the same way, the cognitive impairments that follow focal basal ganglia lesions, that is, executive dysfunction with deficits in initiating cognitive programs, retrieving long-term memory, activating mental sets, supporting verbal fluency, and maintaining internal strategies for problem solving, are also observed after lesions of the prefrontal cortex. This observation is compatible with the mild hypometabolism observed by positron emission tomography (PET) in the frontal lobes of patients with bipallidal lesions (12) and in patients with subcortical dementia (65).

Interestingly, the description of five independent, parallel, and recurrent loops, each interconnecting specific areas of the prefrontal cortex to restricted, well-defined subregions of the basal ganglia, may support the functional continuum suggested by clinical observations of patients with focal lesions (28,66). Among these circuits, three are involved in nonmotor functions and are designated by their frontal areas of projection, namely, dorsolateral, orbitofrontal, and anterior cingulate. Specific syndromes have been associated with injury to these circuits (4). Studies of nonhuman primates and of functional magnetic resonance imaging (fMRI) in humans suggest that executive functions, such as planning and working memory, may depend on the dorsolateral circuit (67). Damage to the orbitofrontal circuit has been shown to result in impairment in decision-making tests (68) and in reversal/extinction tests (69). Lesions of the limbic loop lead to mood and motivation disorders, such as depression, apathy, and autoactivation deficit (4,23). The dysfunction of these circuits may explain the dysexecutive syndrome and the frontal lobe–type behavioral changes in patients with focal or neurodegenerative (Parkinson's disease, Huntington's disease, progressive supranuclear palsy, etc.) lesions of the basal ganglia.

Although patients with frontal lesions and those with subcortical lesions both show impairment on executive tasks, the nature of these deficits seems qualitatively different. This observation is not surprising, given that the differential and specific connections of these anatomical structures imply that they are involved in different processes. The massive convergence of striatal neurons on the pallidum also argues that information is filtered at this level. Is it thus possible to define the specificity of each structure in terms of cognitive and behavioral organization? Results of experimental studies may help to answer this question. For example, one experiment showed that patients with ischemic lesions of the dorsolateral prefrontal cortex expressed a tendency to alternate spontaneously in a delayed response task with binary choice (70). Interestingly, in contrast to normal controls, the patients were unable to subsequently change rules, because they could not suppress their spontaneous tendency to alternate. In this case, elaboration of a new goal-directed behavior was precluded by the expression of preexisting programs. In the same experiment, patients with striatal lesions or dysfunction were also impaired in rule acquisition, but for another reason—they could not maintain a new rule. Their performance was characterized by a tendency to rapidly abandon the rule they were currently implementing for the binary choice (71). These findings suggest that one of the major roles of the basal ganglia is to maintain strategies and mental sets. In line with this interpretation are clinical observations of patients with basal ganglia neurodegenerative lesions, which are characterized by a high number of nonperseverative errors in the Wisconsin Card Sorting (2), abnormal and precocious disengagement of attention in the Posner paradigm (72), increased number of alternations in the Necker cube (73), quicker readaptation after prismatic deviation (74), and impaired procedural learning (57).

The observation that lesions of the basal ganglia impair the ability to maintain a mental set suggests that the basal ganglia may be part of an anatomic network that supports the automatization of new schemas and the expression of overlearned or automatic routine behaviors that have already been proceduralized. In contrast, the frontal lobes enable the elaboration of new plans, as suggested by the tendency of patients with frontal lobe lesions to persevere in previous behaviors and by their difficulty in shifting their mental sets. On the basis of experimental and clinical evidence, we propose to segregate the functions of the basal ganglia and prefrontal cortex into two distinct and complementary systems (Fig. 2-1). On one hand, the prefrontal cortex is involved in elaborating new behavioral schemas through constant interaction with the environment, a task that requires attentional resources. The execution of this planning function, mainly organized within the dorsolateral prefrontal cortex, depends on successfully inhibiting current programs. On the other hand, one of the main functions of the basal ganglia is to proceduralize and automatize ongoing programs. Proceduralization has the advantage of freeing attentional resources that can then be made available to the prefrontal cortex to further elaborate new behavioral responses. Routine behaviors and skills are selected and activated if necessary but are repressed by the prefrontal cortex when new challenging situations require elaboration of new schemas. According to this hypothesis, the basal ganglia might be involved in stabilizing and maintaining mental sets, and they would constitute a buffer for procedural or overlearned skills. Thus, a lesion of the striatopallidal complex would disrupt the selection,

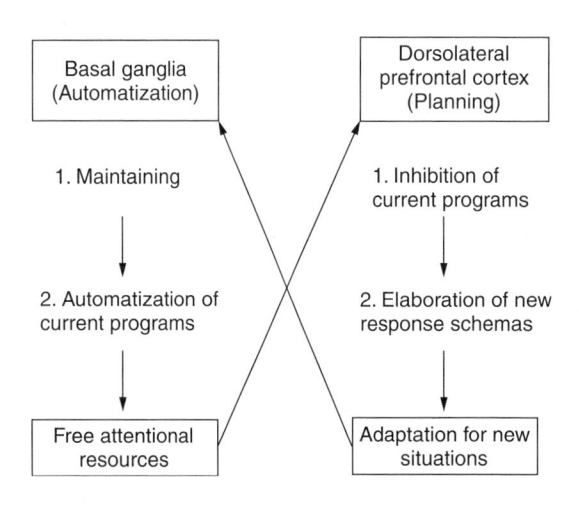

FIG. 2-1. Schematic representation of basal ganglia and dorsolateral prefrontal cortical interactions.

activation, and maintenance of procedural skills in sensorimotor, cognitive, and behavioral domains. We can therefore hypothesize that attentional resources would consequently be required for carrying out elementary cognitive processes, as has been proposed for executing automatic, overlearned movements (75). These resources would no longer be available for more strategic or complex processes, provoking the functional frontal lobe impairment that characterizes basal ganglia disorders. In addition, it is important to remember that at basal ganglia and orbitofrontal cortex levels, rewards processing is also involved in each of the functions described above, as underlined by the recent model elegantly developed by Saint-Cyr (76), who proposed to decompose the elements of basal ganglia processing along a temporal continuum, including the context (attention and working memory), the sequences (control of action), and the consequences (reinforcement and implicit learning). We now need to specify the functional contribution of the different parts of the basal ganglia and prefrontal cortex in this organization. Functional imaging studies in normal subjects and in patients with focal, subcortical, or cortical lesions will enable anatomofunctional correlation and will help us to understand how these different areas interact.

REFERENCES

1. Dubois B, Pillon B, Legault F, et al. Slowing of cognitive processing in progressive supranuclear palsy. A comparison with Parkinson's disease. *Arch Neurol* 1988;45:1194–1199.
2. Taylor AE, Saint-Cyr JA, Lang AE. Frontal lobe dysfunction in Parkinson's disease—the cortical focus of neostriatal outflow. *Brain* 1986;109:845–883.
3. Pillon B, Deweer B, Agid Y, et al. Explicit memory in Alzheimer's, Huntington's and Parkinson's diseases. *Arch Neurol* 1993;50:374–379.
4. Cummings JL. Frontal-subcortical circuits and human behavior. *Arch Neurol* 1993;50:873–880.
5. Mayeux R, Stern Y, Rosen J, et al. Depression, intellectual impairment and Parkinson's disease. *Neurology* 1981;31:645–650.
6. Albert ML, Feldman RG, Willis AL. The subcortical dementia of progressive supranuclear palsy. *J Neurol Neurosurg Psychiatry* 1974;37:121–130.
7. Vermersch P, Delacourte A, Javoy-Agid F, et al. Dementia in Parkinson's disease. *Ann Neurol* 1993;33:445–450.
8. Apaydin H, Ahlskog JE, Parisi JE, et al. Parkinson's disease neuropathology: later-developing dementia and loss of the levodopa response. *Arch Neurol* 2002;59:102–112.
9. Hauw JJ, Verny M, Delaere P, et al. Constant neurofibrillary changes in the neocortex in progressive nuclear palsy. Basic differences with Alzheimer's disease and aging. *Neurosci Lett* 1990;119:182–186.
10. Bhatia KP, Marsden CD. The behavioural and motor consequences of focal lesions of the basal ganglia in man. *Brain* 1994;117:859–876.
11. Dubois B, Défontaines B, Deweer B, et al. Cognitive and behavioral changes in patients with focal lesions of the basal ganglia. In: Weiner WJ, Lang AE, eds. *Behavioral neurology of movement disorders*, Vol. 65, *Advances in neurology*. New York: Raven Press, 1995;29–41.
12. Laplane D, Levasseur M, Pillon B, et al. Obsessive–compulsive and other behavioral changes with bilateral basal ganglia lesions. A neuropsychological, magnetic resonance imaging and positron tomography study. *Brain* 1989;112:699–725.
13. Laplane D, Baulac M, Widlocher D, et al. Pure psychic akinesia with bilateral lesion of the basal ganglia. *J Neurol Neurosurg Psychiatry* 1984;47:377–385.
14. Laplane D, Widlocher D, Pillon B, et al. Comportement compulsif d'allure obsessionnelle par nécrose circonscrite bilatérale pallido-striatale: encéphalopathie par piqûre de guêpe. *Rev Neurol* 1981;137:269–276.
15. Ali-Chérif A, Royère ML, Gosset A, et al. Troubles du comportement et de l'activité mentale après intoxication oxycarbonée. Lésions pallidales bilatérales. *Rev Neurol* 1984;140:401–405.
16. Trillet M, Croisile B, Tourniaire D, et al. Perturbation de l'activité motrice volontaire et lésions des noyaux caudés. *Rev Neurol* 1990;146:338–344.
17. Luria AR, Tsvetkova LS. The program of constructive activity in local brain injuries. *Neuropsychologia* 1964;2:95–107.
18. Stuss DT, Benson DF. *The frontal lobes*. New York: Raven Press, 1986.
19. Laplane D, Baulac M, Pillon B, et al. Perte de l'auto-activation psychique. Activité compulsive d'allure obsessionnelle. Lésion lenticulaire bilatérale. *Rev Neurol* 1982;138:137–141.
20. Habib M, Poncet M. Perte de l'élan vital, de l'intérêt et de l'activité (syndrome athymormique) au cours de lésions lacunaires des corps striés. *Rev Neurol* 1988;144:571–577.
21. Mendez MF, Adams NL, Lewandowski KS. Neurobehavioral changes associated with caudate lesions. *Neurology* 1989;39:349–354.
22. Habib M. Disorders of motivation. In: Bogousslavsky J, Cummings JL, eds. *Behavior and mood disorders in focal brain lesions*. Cambridge: Cambridge University Press, 2000:261–284.
23. Laplane D, Dubois D. Auto-activation deficit: a basal ganglia related syndrome. *Mov Disord* 2001;16:810–814.
24. Strub RL. Frontal lobe syndrome in a patient with bilateral globus pallidus lesions. *Arch Neurol* 1989;46:1024–1027.
25. Bogousslavsky J, Regli F, Delaloye B, et al. Loss of psychic self-activation with bithalamic infarction. Neurobehavioral, CT, MRI, and SPECT correlates. *Acta Neurol Scand* 1991;83:309–316.
26. Richfield EK, Twyman R, Berent S. Neurological syndrome following bilateral damage to the head of the caudate nuclei. *Ann Neurol* 1987;22:768–771.

27. Penisson-Besnier I, Le Gall D, Dubas F. Comportement compulsif d'allure obsessionnelle (arithmomanie). Atrophie des noyaux caudés. *Rev Neurol* 1992;148: 262–267.
28. Alexander GE, De Long MR, Strick PL. Parallel organization of functionally segregated circuits linking basal ganglia and cortex. *Annu Rev Neurosci* 1986;9: 357–381.
29. Klawans H, Stein RW, Tanner CM, et al. A pure parkinsonism syndrome following acute carbon monoxide intoxication. *Arch Neurol* 1982;39:302–304.
30. Fève AP, Fenelon G, Wallays C, et al. Axial motor disturbances after hypoxic lesions of the globus pallidus. *Mov Disord* 1993;8:321–326.
31. Stein R, Kase C, Hier D, et al. Caudate hemorrhage. *Neurology* 1984;34:1549–1554.
32. Caine ED, Fisher JM. Dementia in Huntington's disease. In: Vinken PJ, Bruyn GW, Frederiks JA, eds. *Handbook of clinical neurology*, Vol. 46, *Neurobehavioral disorders*. Amsterdam: Elsevier Science Publishers, 1985:305–310.
33. Pluck GC, Brown RG. Apathy in Parkinson's disease. *J Neurol Neurosurg Psychiatry* 2002;73:636–642.
34. Czernecki V, Pillon B, Houeto JL, et al. Motivation, reward and Parkinson's disease: influence of dopatherapy. *Neuropsychologia* 2002;40:2257–2267.
35. Litvan I, Paulsen JS, Mega MS, et al. Neuropsychiatric assessment of patients with hyperkinetic and hypokinetic movement disorders. *Arch Neurol* 1998; 55:1313–1319.
36. Cummings JL, Mega M, Gray K, et al. The Neuropsychiatric Inventory: comprehensive assessment of psychopathology in dementia. *Neurology* 1994;44: 2308–2314.
37. Robert PH, Clairet S, Benoit M, et al. The apathy inventory: assessment of apathy and awareness in Alzheimer's disease, Parkinson's disease and mild cognitive impairment. *Int J Geriatr Psychiatry* 2002;17:1099–1105.
38. Laplane D, Boulliat J, Baron JC, et al. Comportement compulsif d'allure obsessionnelle par lésion bilatérale des noyaux lenticulaires. Un nouveau cas. *Encéphale* 1988;14:27–32.
39. Frankel M, Jeffrey L, Cummings MD, et al. Obsessions and compulsions in Gilles de la Tourette's syndrome. *Neurology* 1986;36:378–382.
40. Litvan I, Paulsen JS, Mega MS, et al. Neuropsychiatric assessment of patients with hyperkinetic and hypokinetic movement disorders. *Arch Neurol* 1998; 55:1313–1319.
41. Mallet L, Mesnage V, Houeto JL, et al. Compulsions, Parkinson's disease and stimulation. *Lancet* 2002;360: 1302–1304.
42. Destée A, Gray F, Parent M, et al. Comportement compulsif d'allure obsessionnelle et paralysie supranucléaire progressive. *Rev Neurol* 1990;146:12–18.
43. Jankovic JJ. Tics and Tourette's syndrome. In: Jankovic JJ, Tolosa E, eds. *Parkinson's disease and movement disorders*, 4th ed. Philadelphia: Lippincott Williams & Wilkins, 2002:311–330.
44. Bokura H, Robinson RG. Long-term cognitive impairment associated with caudate lesions. *Stroke* 1997;28:970–975.
45. Puel M, Cardebat D, Demonet JF, et al. Le role du thalamus dans les aphasies sous-corticales. *Rev Neurol* 1986;142:431–440.
46. Karussis D, Leker RR, Abramsky O. Cognitive dysfunction following thalamic stroke: a study of 16 cases and review of the literature. *J Neurol Sci* 2000; 172:25–29.
47. Alexander MP, Naeser MA, Palumbo CL. Correlations of subcortical CT lesion sites and aphasia profiles. *Brain* 1987;110:961–991.
48. Caplan LR, Schmahmann JD, Kase CS, et al. Caudate infarcts. *Arch Neurol* 1990;47:133–143.
49. Ferro JM, Kertez A, Black SE. Subcortical neglect: quantification, anatomy, and recovery. *Neurology* 1987; 37:1487–1492.
50. Eslinger PJ, Grattan LM. Frontal lobe and frontal-striatal substrates for different forms of human cognitive flexibility. *Neuropsychologia* 1993;31:17–28.
51. Godefroy O, Rousseaux M, Leys D, et al. Frontal lobe dysfunction in unilateral lenticulo-striate infarcts. *Arch Neurol* 1992; 49:1285–1289.
52. Weilburg JB, Mesulam MM, Xeitraub S, et al. Focal striatal abnormalities in a patient with obsessive–compulsive disorder. *Arch Neurol* 1989;46:233–235.
53. Pillon B, Boller F, Levy R, et al. Cognitive deficits and dementia in Parkinson's disease. In: Boller F, Grafman J, eds. *Handbook of neuropsychology*, Vol. 6, *Aging and dementia*. Amsterdam: Elsevier, 2001:311–371.
54. Dubois B, Pillon B. Cognitive and behavioral aspects of basal ganglia diseases. In: Jankovic JJ, Tolosa E, eds. *Parkinson's disease and movement disorders*, 4th ed. Philadelphia: Lippincott William & Wilkins, 2002:530–545.
55. Van der Werf TD, Witter MP, Uylings HB, et al. Neuropsychology of infarctions of the thalamus: a review. *Neuropsychologia* 2000;38:613–627.
56. Grober E, Buschke H. Genuine memory deficits in dementia. *Dev Neuropsychol* 1987;3:13–36.
57. Sarazin M, Deweer B, Merkl A, et al. Procedural learning and striato-frontal dysfunction in Parkinson's disease. *Mov Disord* 2002;17:265–273.
58. Doyon J, Laforce R, Bouchard G, et al. Role of the striatum, cerebellum and frontal lobes in the automatization of a repeated visuomotor sequence of movements. *Neuropsychologia* 1998;36:625–641.
59. Doyon J, Penhune V, Ungerleider LG. Distinct contribution of the cortico-striatal and cortico-cerebellar system to motor skill learning. *Neuropsychologia* 2003; 41:252–262.
60. Exner C, Koschack J, Irle E. The differential role of premotor frontal cortex and basal ganglia in motor sequence learning: evidence from focal basal ganglia lesions. *Learn Mem* 2002;9:376–386.
61. Tremblay L, Hollerman JR, Schultz W. Modifications of reward expectation-related neuronal activity during learning in primate striatum. *J Neurophysiol* 1998; 80:964–977.
62. Tremblay L, Schultz W. Relative reward preference in primate orbitofrontal cortex. *Nature* 1999;398:704–708.
63. Schultz W, Dayan P, Montague PR. A neural substrate of prediction and reward. *Science* 1997;275:1593–1599.
64. Adler CM, McDonough-Ryan P, Sax KW, et al. fMRI of neuronal activation with symptom provocation in unmedicated patients with obsessive compulsive disorder. *J Psychiatr Res* 2000;34:317–324.
65. D'Antona R, Baron JC, Samson Y, et al. Subcortical dementia. Frontal cortex hypometabolism detected by positron tomography in patients with progressive supranuclear palsy. *Brain* 1985;108:785–799.

66. Alexander GE, Crutcher MD, DeLong MR. Basal ganglia-thalamocortical circuits: parallel substrates for motor, oculomotor, "prefrontal" and "limbic" functions. *Prog Brain Res* 1990;85:119–146.
67. Pochon JB, Levy R, Poline JB, et al. The role of dorsolateral prefrontal cortex in the preparation of the forthcoming actions: an fMRI study. *Cereb Cortex* 2001;11:260–266.
68. Bechara A, Damasio H, Damasio AR, et al. Different contributions of the human amygdala and ventromedial prefrontal cortex to decision-making. *J Neurosci* 1999;19:5473–5481.
69. Rolls ET, Hornak J, Wade D, et al. Emotion-related learning in patients with social and emotional changes associated with frontal lobe damage. *J Neurol Neurosurg Psychiatry* 1994; 57:1518–1524.
70. Vérin M, Partiot A, Pillon B, et al. Delayed response tasks and prefrontal lesions in man. *Neuropsychologia* 1993;31:1379–1396.
71. Partiot A, Vérin M, Pillon B, et al. Delayed response tasks in basal ganglia lesions in man. Further evidence for a striato-frontal cooperation in behavioural adaptation. *Neuropsychologia* 1996;34:709–721.
72. Wright MJ, Burns RJ, Geffen GM, et al. Covert orientation of visual attention in Parkinson's disease: an impairment in the maintenance of attention. *Neuropsychologia* 1990;28:151–159.
73. Talland GA. Cognitive function in Parkinson's disease. *J Nerv Ment Dis* 1962;135:196–205.
74. Stern Y, Mayeux R, Hermann A, et al. Prism adaptation in Parkinson's disease. *J Neurol Neurosurg Psychiatry* 1988;51:1584–1587.
75. Marsden CD. The mysterious motor function of the basal ganglia: The Robert Wartenberg Lecture. *Neurology* 1982; 32:514–539.
76. Saint-Cyr JA. Frontal-striatal circuit functions: context, sequence, and consequence. *J Int Neuropsychol Soc* 2003;9:103–127.

3
Depression in Parkinson's Disease

Marc J. Mentis[1] and Dominique Delalot[2]

[1]*Department of Neurology and Psychiatry,*
New York University Hospital, New York, New York
North Shore–Long Island Jewish Research Institute, Manhasset, New York;
[2]*Research Assistant, North Shore–Long Island*
Jewish Research Institute, Manhasset,
New York

INTRODUCTION

In 1817, James Parkinson described not only the motor symptoms exhibited by his patients with the "shaking palsy," but also a comorbid "melancholy" that substantially affected their lives (1). Cummings, in an excellent review of Parkinson's disease, written in 1992, stated, "Depression is the most common neuropsychiatric disturbance of Parkinson's disease (PD), but its frequency, characteristics, course, treatment, responsiveness, and neurobiological substrates are at best only partially established" (2). Although progress has been made in all of these domains during the past decade, nonetheless, Cummings' observation remains frustratingly true. PD affects about one million Americans, and depression has been identified by PD patients, caregivers, and physicians in six countries as a more important factor than disease severity or medication in quality of life ratings (3–5). For these reasons, the National Institute of Neurological Disorders and Stroke at the National Institutes of Health, at the request of Congress, has developed a five-year research agenda to further the understanding of depression in PD (6).

The lack of a single accepted and valid nosology is central to much of the variability and debate surrounding depression research in PD. Therefore, this chapter, unless otherwise stated, uses the definitions given by the *The Diagnostic and Statistical Manual of Mental Disorders,* 4th edition (DSM-IV) for depression. Major depression requires five or more of nine symptoms during a two-week period. These symptoms must include depressed mood or anhedonia. The other seven symptoms are weight loss or gain, sleep increase or decrease, psychomotor agitation or retardation, fatigue or loss of energy, feelings of worthlessness and guilt, poor concentration and indecisiveness, and suicidal ideation. Compared to the symptoms of major depression, the symptoms in dysthymia are less severe but more chronic, whereas the symptoms in minor depression have the same chronicity as in major depression but are less severe or less numerous.

DEMOGRAPHICS

In every decade since 1922, estimates of the prevalence of depression in PD have varied consistently (7), ranging from 4% to 75% (8,9). This variability has been attributed to several potential causes: a reactive (lower prevalence estimates) versus a biological (higher estimates) theoretical construct, clinical diagnosis (lower) versus use of standardized scales (higher), scripted interviews (lower) versus self-rated scales (higher), community-based studies (lower) versus studies from research centers (higher), and studies performed abroad (lower) versus studies performed in the United States (higher). Results have also differed because of inconsistent definitions of depression, the use of different instruments to measure depression, the use of different cutoffs within the same instrument, different populations (idiopathic PD and secondary PD), and sampling bias. Although there is truth to all of these observations, they are unfortunate products of a more fundamental problem: because the motor and cognitive symptoms of PD overlap with the symptoms of depression, diagnosing depression in PD is difficult. Further, there is no consensus on how to assign an overlap symptom for PD motor, PD cognitive, or PD depression categories. Finally, there is no validated, sensitive, and specific instrument designed specifically to identify and quantify depression in PD.

Euthymic PD patients can appear depressed because they may have masked facies and bradykinesia, psychomotor retardation, fatigue, sleep disturbances, and weight loss (when medication fails and symptoms increase) that mimic the somatic symptoms of depression. Patients may also appear withdrawn from society because loss of motor function can reduce social participation. Finally, cognitive symptoms including apathy, impaired concentration, poor attention, and memory loss often masquerade as depression.

Slaughter (7) analyzed 11 papers published from 1984 through 2000 that used DSM-II or DSM-III-R criteria. Dysthymia was present in 22.5% of PD patients (48 of 213 patients) (10–13); minor depression was present in 36.6% (155 of 423) (14–16); and major depression was present in 24.8% (278 of 1,119) (10–18). When dysthymia, minor depression, and major depression were combined, the overall prevalence of all depressive symptoms was 42.4% (500 of 1,179 PD patients). In an ongoing Global Parkinson's Disease Survey including 1,000 patients, 200 clinicians, and 187 caregivers in five countries (including the USA), about 50% of patients were found to have substantial depressive symptoms (3). In contrast to prevalence rates of around 40% from research centers in the United States, prevalence rates in community-based studies are lower elsewhere, 5.1% in Norway (14), 19.6% in the United Kingdom (19), 24% in Finland (5), and 16.5% in China (20). In contrast, Meara et al. (21) found depression in 64% of their patients in North Wales.

PRESENTATION AND BIOLOGICAL ASSOCIATIONS

Symptoms

Many of the overlap symptoms between depressed and euthymic PD patients are somatic (see above). Leentjens et al. (22) reported that nonsomatic (psychic) items on the Montgomery–Asberg Depression Rating Scale (MADRS) (23) and the Hamilton Depression Rating Scale (HDRS) (24) correlated better with the diagnosis of depression than did somatic items. There is general agreement with Brown et al. (25) that the nonsomatic symptoms of depression in PD are subtly different from those of primary depression. In PD, nonsomatic depression is expressed primarily as sadness, dysphoria, irritability, pessimism about the future, and suicidal ideation, with less guilt, self-reproach, or feelings of failure than in primary depression (26–28). Whether PD patients with depression are more apathetic than euthymic patients, or whether their poor mood is more dependent upon an external locus of control, remains to be confirmed (29,30). Depression precedes motor symptoms in 12% to 37% of PD patients (26), a statistic often cited as supporting a biological rather than a "reactive" etiology.

Anxiety symptoms are common in the depression of PD and can be severe (31,32). Sixty-seven percent of depressed PD patients experience considerable anxiety. In a case-controlled study, Shiba et al. (33) found that both depressive and anxiety symptoms could precede motor symptoms. Both depression and anxiety were observed in 15% of PD patients, versus 7% of controls, and anxiety preceded depression in 72% of the PD patients. However, both irritability and anxiety occur with increased frequency in depression in older patients (32,34).

Although suicidal ideation is common in PD depression, completed suicide is not (2). In a review of 458 PD patients, Stenager at al. (35) found no increase in suicide compared to the general population. The reason for this phenomenon is unknown. Although not extensively researched, the incidence of delusions and hallucinations in PD depression appears to be low (36,37).

Severity

For the reasons stated above, estimates of symptom severity in PD depression vary considerably. In their analysis of reports published from 1967 through 1990 that used DSM and other instruments, Cummings et al. (2) found that among PD patients with depression, 54% had moderate-to-severe symptoms (major depression; range 9%–81%), and 45% had mild symptoms (dysthymia or minor depression; range 11%–91%). In contrast, extrapolating from Slaughter's review of 11 studies that used DSM criteria [see above (7)], major depression was about half as common as dysthymia and minor depression.

Course

Although the literature is scant, Cummings (2) suggests that depression divides PD patients into two groups that are relatively stable over time: those patients with depressive symptoms and those without. Brown et al. (25), in a 14-month follow-up study, observed that 16% of PD patients were depressed and 61% were euthymic, both at baseline and approximately one year later. Further, 11% of the depressed patients resolved over the 14-month period, whereas 11% of the euthymic patients became depressed. Mayeux et al. (38), in a study of 49 PD patients for a mean of 30 months, found that major depression and dysthymia resolved in 7% (one of 14 patients) and 45% (one of three patients) respectively. None of the 28 euthymic patients developed depression.

Risk Factors and Clinical Associations

PD patients with a history of depression (39,40) and impaired functional activity are at risk for both major and minor depression (20). In contrast, a family history of depression and duration of PD (2) confers no increased risk of depression. Age of PD symptom onset is a controversial risk factor, with some studies showing greater risk for depression when onset is in younger patients (15,18), others showing greater risk in older patients (41), and still others failing to identify age of onset as a factor (31,42–44). Likewise, recent reports have not resolved the issue of whether female sex conveys an increased risk (2), with some studies finding women at increased risk (41), and others not (14,21).

Starkstein et al. (40) and Direnfeld et al. (45) felt that patients with more left brain damage (right hemiparkinsonism) were at greater risk for depression. However, Barber et al. (46) and Huber (47) failed to show any effect of laterality. Left brain damage after stroke may be associated with depression (48); however, in trauma, right frontal damage may be more important. Neither structural nor functional imaging studies in PD have shown lesion lateralization associated with major (49) or minor (50) depression.

Most studies that have compared the level of depression in PD with the level of depression in non-CNS diseases that cause comparable disabilities have found levels of depression to be greater in PD (42,51–53), although a few have not (31). This disparity is often cited as evidence that depression in PD has a biological basis and is not simply a "response" to disability. Further, a reliable association between depression and Hoehn and Yahr stage of PD (54) has not been established. Most investigators show no relation (43,51,55); others claim a complex nonlinear relationship (40,56).

Most studies fail to show a strong correlation between depression and motor symptoms (rigidity, bradykinesia, and tremor) (10,15,40,51,57, 58). Two studies suggest that, compared to patients with "classic" PD (tremor present), patients with akinetic rigid PD (11) or severe postural instability and gait difficulty (59) may experience depression more often. Because these non-tremor signs are more responsive than tremor to dopamine replacement, these findings imply that dopamine loss plays a role in causing depression.

Another motor phenomenon that suggests a role for the dopamine system in depression is the "on-off" phenomenon. "Off" refers to a patient who is frozen and unable to move. "On" refers to a patient who is able to move, and who usually also has increased involuntary movements or dyskinesias. As PD progresses, after being "on," patients can go "off" when the efficacy of levodopa therapy wears off. With time, going "off" occurs more quickly after taking levodopa, and levodopa must be administered more frequently. The "on-off" phenomenon can also be unrelated to medication ingestion. In this case, the "on-off" condition is thought to reflect changing sensitivity to dopamine, and to release of dopamine from synaptic clefts that occur as the disease progresses. Racette et al. (60) have shown a positive correlation between depression and the "on-off" phenomenon. Short-lived episodes of dysphoria may also occur during the "off" phase (29,61–66). The most common interpretation is that mood fluctuations result from severe motor fluctuations (61,62,64,65). However, two methodologically detailed studies have shown dissociation in the timing between mood changes and motor changes (67,68), suggesting that the mood changes are neither a psychological reaction to the motor changes nor a physiological reaction to dopamine administration.

Cognitive impairment is common in PD; about 30% of PD patients become demented (69), and, although estimates vary, if appropriate frontal lobe tasks are tested, up to 90% of PD patients show signs of cognitive impairment (70). The relation between dementia and depression remains controversial. Because of overlap between cognitive (poor attention, shortened concentration, memory loss, confusion, indecisiveness) and depressive symptoms, the results of studies correlating depression with cognitive dysfunction have nosological difficulties (i.e., "pseudodementia" vs. dementia) and such results invite multiple interpretations. Likely, depression is equally common in PD with and without dementia (55,71–73). Whatever the mechanism ("pseudo" vs. "real" dementia), subjects with depression exhibit more cognitive impairment than euthymic patients do, particularly in "frontal lobe/executive" tasks (39,74–76). Starkstein et al. (75) suggest that major depression predicts greater decline in cognitive function, activities of daily living, and even motor signs. Further, depression that occurs early in PD is associated with a more rapid cognitive decline (74) and an increased incidence of dementia (77,78). The reverse may also be true, in that cognitive impairment correlates positively with depression (41). Dementia and depression combined is associated with lower levels of 5-hydroxyindole acetic acid (5-HIAA), a metabolite of serotonin, in cerebrospinal fluid (CSF) than either dementia or depression alone (17). Although these findings are beyond the scope of this chapter, they provoke debate on whether the underlying pathophysiology of depression and cognitive dysfunction in PD involves dysfunction within different parallel frontal corticostriatal–putaminal–thalamic–cortical (CSPTC) loops (79), or dysfunction within a common loop that results in multiple behavioral expressions.

Because symptoms of hypothyroidism (poor concentration, fatigue, flat affect, bradykinesia, and depression) and testosterone deficiency (anhedonia, fatigue, and sexual dysfunction) overlap with PD symptoms, these diagnoses can be missed in PD. The incidence of hypothyroidism is increased in PD (80–82), and PD drugs may inhibit thyrotropin-secreting hormone, masking hypothyroidism and making laboratory diagnosis in PD difficult (82,83). Replacement therapy for hypothyroidism and testosterone deficiency (84) can improve refractory cognitive and depressive symptoms in PD.

Diagnosis

The diagnostic difficulty and high prevalence of depression in PD requires that clinicians be aware of the overlap of depression and motor-cognitive symptoms and have a high index of suspicion to make the diagnosis accurately. Rating scales are a useful tool for both clinical practice and research. There are more than 100 depression instruments (85), none of them specific for depression in PD, and only a few have been validated in PD. The Beck Depression Inventory (BDI) (86), the Montgomery–Asberg Depression Rating Scale (MADRS) (23), and the Hamilton Depression Rating Scale (HDRS) (24) have been most commonly used. However, they have somatic crossover items that can result in diagnosis of depression in euthymic PD patients. Levin et al. (27) have shown, using a cluster analysis, that the BDI provides a valid score for depression in PD. Leentjens et al. (87), using receiver-operating characteristic curves to evaluate sensitivity and specificity, found that a BDI cutoff score of 8/9 identified most depressed patients, while a cutoff of 13/14 maximized separation of depression and euthymia. Evaluated in similar fashion (88), the MADRS showed acceptable sensitivity and specificity at 14/15, whereas the HAMD-17 had acceptable sensitivity at 11/12 and specificity at 13/14.

DSM-IV appears to be evolving as the gold standard for evaluating depression in PD. Although a single scale will go a long way toward resolving many of the nosological issues that have plagued PD-depression research, this approach is problematic. The DSM forces a subjective decision as to whether a symptom is part of a primary depressive disorder or secondary to another disease. This decision requires an understanding of the underlying pathophysiology, and the clinical capability to separate identical symptoms into diagnostic categories of primary depression, depression in PD, and euthymic PD diagnostic categories. This distinction is precisely the information that is not known, and this tautology is at the heart of many controversies surrounding PD and depression. To ensure that selection and diagnostic criteria do not contaminate results, researchers attempting to understand these relations need to finesse this DSM-IV tautology appropriately.

Biological Markers

Neuropathology and Biochemistry

Compared to euthymic PD patients, those with depression have shortened rapid eye movement sleep latency (Bu-26). This condition likely results from pedunculopontine degeneration, but it may be considered a marker for more widespread brainstem pathology. Further, depressed PD patients exhibit reduced echogenicity on transcranial ultrasonography and altered magnetic resonance imaging signal intensity in midline brainstem structures (Bu-27). Nuclei in this region include the ventral tegmental area (VTA, dopaminergic neurons), the midline raphe nuclei (serotonergic neurons), and locus caeruleus (LC, norepinephric neurons). Because of relevant animal findings that have shed light on depression in non-PD patients, these nuclei and brain regions modulated by these neurotransmitters have been most researched as causative factors in PD depression. The possible contributions from other transmitters or peptides (including glutamate, metenkephalin, leu-enkephalin, substance P, and bombesin) that are also reduced in PD (89) are not yet established.

Dopamine System

Morphological studies in PD, although results vary, generally show cell loss in the VTA (89–94). Some investigators have found disproportionate degeneration in the VTA of PD patients with depression and dementia (95)—more extensive than in euthymic and non-demented PD patients— although this degeneration may correlate better with cognitive than mood disorder (96). Dopamine depletion is also evident in VTA mesocortical and mesolimbic projection areas (97). Imaging studies show that these regions have impaired function (see *Neuroimaging*). The fact that methylphenidate fails to induce a euphoriant effect in depressed PD patients but succeeds in euthymic PD patients, and in those with primary depression (98), may indicate that dopamine mesocorticolimbic neurons are dysfunctional in PD depression. However, homovanillic acid levels in CSF correlate poorly with depression (99), and dopamine therapy has little effect on mood (100).

Serotonin System

Although cell loss has been reported in the dorsal raphe nuclei in PD depression (101), studies evaluating brain stem, cortical, and CSF concentrations of serotonin and its metabolite 5-HIAA in depression have been inconsistent. However, in PD, serotonin levels in nuclei and projection areas have been shown to be reduced (102–104). Positron emission tomography (PET) studies have demonstrated that 5-HT$_{1A}$ receptor binding is reduced in the raphe nuclei of PD patients, with a trend for binding to be lowest in those PD patients who were depressed (105). CSF 5-HIAA levels have been observed to be lower in depressed PD patients than in euthymic PD patients in some (10,38), but not all, studies

(106). Overall, neither CSF 5-HIAA nor platelet receptor levels are sensitive or specific enough to be sole markers for depression in PD. Some improvement in depression has been seen after 5-hydroxytryptophan and l-tryptophan administration that correlated with increased CSF 5-HIAA levels (99,107). Genetic studies are also beginning to implicate the serotonin system in depression in PD. The short allele of a functional polymorphism in the serotonin transporter results in reduced levels of serotonin in the synaptic cleft and is associated with depression (108,109). Elevating synaptic serotonin levels with selective serotonin reuptake inhibitors (SSRIs) appears to alleviate PD and primary depressions equivalently [see *Specific Serotonin Reuptake Inhibitors (SSRIs)*].

Norepinephrine System

Cell loss occurs in the locus caeruleus in PD (92). Some evidence suggests that depressed PD patients have greater LC cell loss than euthymic patients, particularly caudally in the nucleus (110). However, caudal LC projects to the spinal chord, whereas other LC projections to the limbic cortex and subcortical nuclei would be more likely to play a role in depression. The dorsal ascending NE (norepinephrine) pathway (111) is abnormal in PD, and reduced levels of alpha-2 adrenoceptors (112) have been found in platelets of untreated patients. Because NE dysfunction is important in anxiety disorders in non-PD patients (113), these findings suggest a role for underlying NE dysfunction in the anxiety symptoms commonly associated with depression in PD (see above). Elevating synaptic norepinephrine levels with tricyclic antidepressants (TCAs) improves PD and primary depressions equally.

Surgery

Deep brain stimulation surgery (DBS) offers unique insights into brain networks that might be involved in depression in PD. DBS of the thalamus or the globus pallidus interna (GPi) affects motoric systems but has not been associated with changes in mood. By contrast, DBS in and around the subthalamic nucleus (STN), in addition to affecting motor symptoms, has been associated with acute and delayed depressive and euphoric mood changes (114,115). The STN is heterogeneous, with motor, limbic, and associative regions that project topographically, and to some extent separately, to different regions of the pallidum and striatum (116). Thus, anatomical circuits passing through the STN may underlie acute mood changes (115) or may be associated with chronic local and distal adaptive changes that result in depression (114,117). The fact that mood changes are not observed during DBS of the thalamus and GPi, and further, that DBS can cause mood changes without causing any motor changes, suggests that regional brain circuits (CSPTC and other loops) that subtend motor and mood functions are different and have weak functional interconnections.

Neuroimaging

Dopamine depletion in the substantia nigra results in a net disinhibition of the striatum. This disinhibition is reflected as increased fluorodeoxyglucose use and blood flow in posterolateral basal ganglia (118), and these changes in the basal ganglia are proportional to motor symptoms. Further, when a multivariate analysis of PET data is performed (Scaled Subprofile Model) that can extract groups of regions that covary together and that differentiate PD from healthy controls, in addition to the basal ganglia, prefrontal and parieto-occipital regions are identified as markers for PD (119). The authors hypothesized that CSPTC loops passing through these nonmotor regions (prefrontal, parieto–occipital) and basal ganglia might be associated with nonmotor symptoms in PD. Mayberg et al. (120) showed that compared to euthymic PD patients and euthymic controls, PD patients with major depression had reduced metabolism in the caudate, the orbital and inferior frontal cortex, and the anterior temporal pole (Fig. 3-1A). Further, reduced metabolism in the orbitofrontal cortex correlated with the severity of depression, but not with cognitive changes. Other blood flow studies of major depression in PD have emphasized dorsolateral frontal (121), medial frontal, and anterior cingulate (122) brain regions. These regional differences may reflect

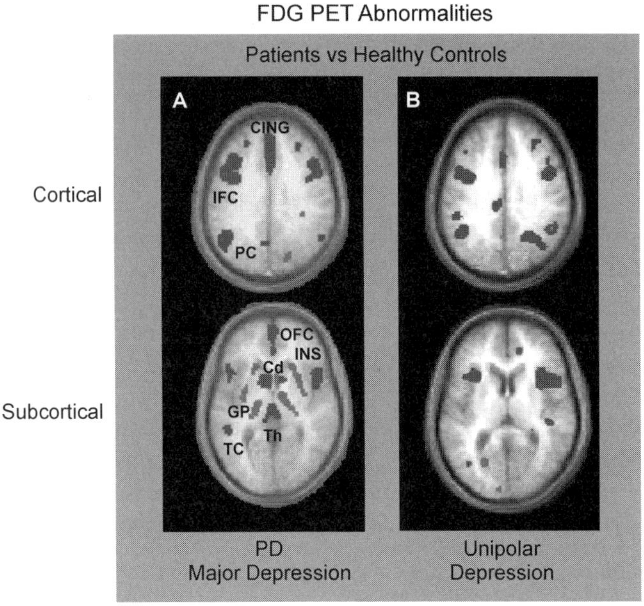

FIG. 3-1. FDG PET Abnormalities. Brain regions associated with depression are similar in Parkinson's disease and unipolar depression. FDG, fluoro-deoxyglucose scan; PET, positron emission tomography; CING, cingulated; IFC, inferior frontal cortex; PC, parietal cortex; OFC, orbital frontal cortex; INS, insula; Cd, caudate nucleus; GP, globus pallidus; Th, thalamic nucleus; TC, temporal cortex. This figure was provided by Helen Mayberg, M.D., Department of Psychiatry, Emory University.

biases inherent in specific imaging and analytic techniques rather than conflicting results (122). The anatomical location of functional abnormality associated with major depression in PD is similar to, although not identical with, that seen in primary depression (Fig. 3-1B) (123–125), post-stroke depression (48,126), and other basal ganglia diseases (120,127).

Minor depression has not been extensively studied in PD. Starkstein et al. (75) found that compared to euthymic patients or patients with minor depression, PD patients with major depression had greater cognitive decline, deterioration in activities of daily living, and motor symptoms, suggesting a qualitative rather than quantitative difference between minor and major depression. However, Mentis et al. (50) showed that the regions correlating with minor depression and dysphoria were similar to those associated with major depression in PD (Fig. 3-2A) (120). Further, Mentis et al. demonstrated that brain regions associated with cognitive dysfunction less severe than dementia were different from, and did not overlap with, those regions associated with minor depression, dysthymia, or major depression (Fig. 3-2B). Together these data suggest that the functional anatomy underlying major depression is similar, whether the pathology is PD, unipolar depression, other basal ganglia disease, or stroke. Further, the functional anatomy underlying PD depression symptoms is different from that underlying PD cognitive symptoms.

ETIOLOGY

Ultimately, we do not understand the mechanism by which objective structural, chemical, or network changes in the brain are subjectively experienced as moods or thoughts. Therefore, it is useful to examine the etiology of depression from a "necessary/sufficient" perspective. If depression had a single unique cause, that cause would be both necessary and sufficient; that is, that cause would have to be present in every case of depression, and that cause, acting on its

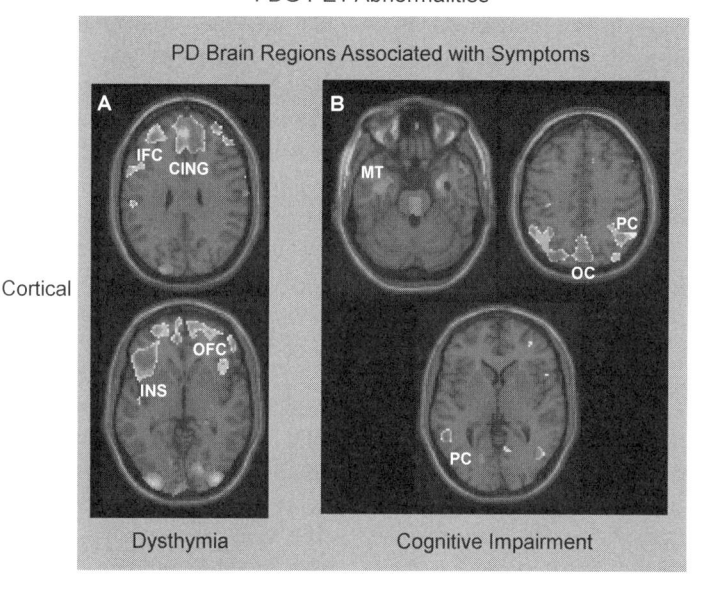

FIG. 3-2. FDG PET Abnormalities. In Parkinson's disease, brain regions associated with dysthymia (Fig. 3-2 panel A) are similar to brain regions associated with major depression (Fig. 3-1 panel A), but they differ from brain regions associated with cognitive symptoms (Fig. 3-2 panel B). FDG, fluoro-deoxyglucose scan; PET, positron emission tomography; IFC, inferior frontal cortex; CING cingulated; OFC, orbital frontal cortex; INS, insula; MT, medial temporal cortex; PC, parietal cortex; OC, occipital cortex. This figure was adapted from Mentis MJ, et al. Relationships among the metabolic patterns that correlate with mnemonic, visuospatial, and mood symptoms in Parkinson's disease. *Am J Psychiatry* 2002;159(5):746–754, with permission.

own, would cause depression in every instance. Should depression have multiple causes, each cause would be sufficient, but any one cause need not be present (necessary) for depression to manifest. Should the cause of depression require mandatory modification (i.e., a genetic predisposition requiring an environmental event), such modification would be necessary, but on its own, not sufficient to cause depression.

Although correlations need not be causative, the associations between brain changes and depression in PD presented above make a compelling argument that changes in the brain caused by PD pathology can be experienced as depression. On the other hand, the fact that depression in PD likely has a biological cause does not exclude the possibility that other causes exist as well. Theoretically, a depressed mood may be a reaction to the motor, cognitive, and social losses that result from PD ("reactive depression"), or it may result from PD medication.

This theory would imply that a biological, reactive, or drug cause may be sufficient but not necessary for depression to develop.

Biological

Because PD pathology is primarily subcortical and affects the aminergic nuclei, biological theories of PD depression have focused on these nuclei, their corticopetal and corticofugal tracts, and the brain regions they modify. Although serotonin, dopamine, and norepinephrine have been most studied, abnormalities occur in many other neural chemicals that may potentially be important. Recent insights have enriched newer biological hypotheses. First, the identification by Alexander et al. (79) of separate "motor," "oculomotor," "prefrontal," and "limbic" CSPTC loops provided the concept of anatomical networks whereby subcortical lesions might affect complex "higher" cortical functions such as mood and cognition. Subsequent to the description of CSPTC loops, a great deal of research has evaluated the mechanisms by which they function (128). Second, contrary to previous ideas, it is now generally agreed that the basal ganglia do not simply perform some rudimentary sensory or motor transformation but rather orchestrate complex operations on multiple aspects of cognition and mood (129). Because the aminergic neurotransmitters affected by PD pathology act within and upon these CSPTC loops and basal ganglia, the major subcortical and cortical dysfunction resulting from aminergic dysfunction may be experienced as abnormalities in domains as diverse as mood, cognition, and motor function. Another observation theorists have focused upon is the large individual variability of pathology among the subcortical nuclei. This variability may be the substrate for the observed heterogeneity of symptoms among PD patients—the low level of correlation observed within and among motor, mood, and cognitive symptoms.

Cummings (2) focused on the dopamine system in his theory of depression in PD. Neuronal loss, particularly in the VTA, resulted in dopamine depletion within mesolimbic and mesocortical pathways. Because animal studies have shown impaired mesolimbic function to be associated with decreased reward mediation, environmental dependency, and inadequate stress response, Cummings argued that failure within this system in humans might be responsible for the apathy, worthlessness, hopelessness, helplessness, and dysphoria seen in depression. Further, dysfunction within the mesocortical pathway may underlie the cognitive symptoms of PD. Supporting this hypothesis are the numerous biological abnormalities within the dopamine system. However, although dopamine abnormalities may be present in varying degrees in patients with PD and depression, replacing dopamine does not cure depression. Thus, although dopamine depletion may be necessary to cause depression in PD, in isolation it is not sufficient.

Mayberg et al. (130) argued for a unifying hypothesis of depression in PD that was based on the interaction between two subcortico–cortical networks and decreased aminergic function. Monoamine degeneration (primarily in the VTA) resulted in remote changes in basotemporal limbic structures (the orbital and inferior frontal cortex and the temporal pole; see Fig. 3-2A) that disrupted anterograde or retrograde CSPTC loops. The function of serotonergic neurons was impaired secondarily because of dysfunction within the orbital-to-dorsal raphe outflow. Although this hypothesis is heuristically elegant because it explains many biological and imaging findings, at present, there is no way to confirm whether this process is both necessary and sufficient for PD depression to manifest.

Several recent hypotheses (131,132) have been less anatomically and biochemically specific. They suggest that some relationship, the details of which are unknown, exists between depletion of dopamine, serotonin, norepinephrine, and acetylcholine and motor, cognitive, and mood symptoms. Likely, some genetic modulation also occurs. Further, the heterogeneity of symptoms, severity, and course among PD patients is a consequence of the heterogeneity of pathology among these nuclei.

The drugs taken by PD patients are an unlikely cause for depression. Dopamine depletion by reserpine causes depression (65), dopamine agonists (levodopa and amantadine) and MAO-B inhibitors (selegiline) are weak antidepressants (2,66,67), whereas D2 dopamine receptor agonists (pramipexole) are somewhat effective antidepressants (133), and anticholinergics cause euphoria rather than depression. The relationship between levodopa administration and mood changes in the "on-off" phenomenon has been discussed above.

Reactive

PD patients have many problems: physical loss (motor symptoms), cognitive loss (poor memory, attention loss, and impaired concentration and visuospatial function), social loss (job problems, marital discord, and isolation) and the knowledge that the disease has no cure. Acute sadness in response to these losses is expected, and sustained depression is a possibility. Early onset PD patients (<65 years old) have higher depression rates than patients with later onset (13,134). Perhaps, compared to older patients, these patients suffer greater consequences from the social problems, lose more function in the physical and cognitive domains, and thus are more susceptible to a reactive depression. However, the observations that depression can occur before motor or cognitive symptoms, that depression severity does not correlate with motor or cognitive function, and that other illnesses with equivalent disabilities have lower incidences of depression suggest that although a reaction to symptoms may be sufficient to cause depression in some patients, it is not necessary for depression to occur.

Toward an Etiological Synthesis

Given the information provided above, we think it likely that reduced levels of dopamine, serotonin, norepinephrine, and acetylcholine within CSPTC loops and basal ganglia and the resultant corticofugal and corticopetal regional dysfunction are important in causing the depressive, cognitive, and motor symptoms of PD. We think it likely that each neurotransmitter can affect all symptoms (depressive, cognitive, and motor). We think it likely that the heterogeneity of brain pathology is expressed as a heterogeneity within and between depressive, motor, and cognitive symptoms. Perhaps each neurotransmitter is associated more with some symptoms than others; for example, dopamine (motor, psychosis), serotonin (depression), norepinephrine (anxiety), and acetylcholine (cognition). However, the exact relationship and mechanisms by which this complex functional anatomy relates to symptoms remains to be empirically determined. We propose that the biological abnormality underlying minor depression and dysthymia is a less severe version of the biological abnormality that underlies major depression—a quantitative rather than a qualitative effect. Further, this biological abnormality is similar whether depressive symptoms occur in PD depression, unipolar depression, other basal ganglia diseases, stroke, or other medical diseases. Although further exploration is beyond the scope of this chapter, we speculate that the neural networks that underlie the acute sad response to the limitations of PD might feed back onto the subcortical amine nuclei and result in depression by causing a *functional* impairment of the nuclei even in the absence of any PD pathology within the nuclei.

TREATMENT

Drugs

A large multicenter double-blind, placebo-controlled study using sensitive and specific diagnostic instruments for depression in PD does not exist. This article has addressed the difficulties of diagnosing depression in PD and the problems with commonly used instruments not designed for depression in this disease. There are, however, controlled studies of various drugs used to treat depression in PD. Unfortunately they all have limitations, including small sample size, heterogeneous populations (idiopathic PD mixed with secondary parkinsonism), subjective rating scales, arbitrary cutoff points for diagnosing depression that differ among studies, and poorly delineated subtypes of depression (major, minor, and dysthymia). Notwithstanding this lack of definitive data, it appears that drug therapy for depression in PD, with respect to drug class, dose, course, side effects, and efficacy, is comparable to drug therapy for unipolar depression. (This finding is not surprising, if indeed a similar pathophysiology of depression exists, regardless of etiology.) Further research is required to determine if therapeutic differences exist between depression in PD and other depressions, or between different depression subtypes within PD.

Tricyclic Antidepressants (TCAs)

As in unipolar depression, these drugs are effective in treating depression in PD. However, their side effects are more troublesome to PD patients than to patients with unipolar depression because PD pathology itself causes autonomic and cholinergic dysfunction. Thus, orthostatic hypotension (alpha adrenergic action) can be severe, and impaired cognition, constipation, dry mouth, urinary retention, and other cholinergic side effects are augmented in PD patients. Conversely, using a TCA to induce sedation (through histamine H1 action) in a patient with PD sleep impairment may be beneficial.

Double-blind, placebo-controlled trials of imipramine (135) and desipramine have been conducted (136). Motor symptoms and scores on the BDI were improved; however, standardized rating scales were not used, and the study populations were heterogeneous. In a double-blind, placebo-controlled crossover study of nortriptyline (137), depression improved, and there was no adverse effect on motor symptoms; however, standardized rating scales were not used.

Specific Serotonin Reuptake Inhibitors (SSRIs)

SSRIs are effective in treating depression in PD and are better tolerated by PD patients than the TCAs. Given the number of recent studies of SSRIs for this purpose, these agents now appear to be the drugs of first choice for depression in PD. Side effects of SSRIs are similar in PD and unipolar patients and include insomnia, agitation, nausea, and sexual dysfunction. A theoretical concern is that SSRIs could increase serotonin inhibition of dopaminergic neurons in the substantia nigra (138,139) and thus increase motor symptoms in PD. Studies are mixed with some showing an increase in motor symptoms (138–144) and others showing no change (145–151). Another concern is inducing a possibly fatal serotonin syndrome by combining an SSRI and a monoamine oxidase A (MOA-A) inhibitor. At the low doses used in PD, selegiline is only supposed to inhibit MOA-B, and thus theoretically the combination of an SSRI and selegiline should be safe. However, at higher doses, selegiline can inhibit both MOA-A and MOA-B enzymes. In a survey of physicians belonging to the Parkinson's Disease Study Group, Richard et al. (152) found that 75% of the physicians had used an SSRI in combination with selegiline. Serotonin syndrome–like symptoms developed in 0.24% of patients, and the symptoms were considered serious in 0.04%. Fortunately no fatalities occurred.

Several non–placebo-controlled studies have shown that the SSRIs improve depression in PD and do not adversely affect motor symptoms. In an open-label study using the BDI and HDRS, Ceravolo et al. (146) showed that paroxetine improved major depression and dysthymia and that motor function was not impaired. In other studies, sertraline improved BDI scores (148), and fluvoxamine improved major depression (149).

Serotonin Norepinephrine Reuptake Inhibitors (SNRIs)

This group of drugs share norepinephrine and serotonin reuptake inhibition with the TCAs, but have no alpha 1 (orthostatic hypotension), cholinergic (cognitive loss, constipation, dry eyes, urinary retention) or histamine H_1 blocking (sedation) side effects. Theoretically, venlafaxine and other members of this group should be excellent antidepressants in PD. They should have the efficacy of the TCAs without their side effects. Further, their effect on norepinephrine may be particularly effective in controlling the anxiety symptoms associated with depression in PD. These theoretical advantages await research confirmation.

Serotonin 2 Antagonist/Reuptake Inhibitors (SARIs)

Nefazodone and other drugs of this class have strong 5-HT_2 antagonism, with weaker serotonin reuptake inhibition, and thus have some theoretical advantage over drugs with stronger and nonspecific serotonin reuptake inhibition, including the SSRIs. SSRIs increase serotonin's effect at all receptors. At 5-HT_{1A} receptors, this effect will likely be antidepressant, but it will also increase serotonin's action at 5-HT_2 receptors in the forebrain, which may increase anxiety and agitation, or 5-HT_2 receptors in the spinal chord, which may result in sexual dysfunction. SARIs likely have a net antagonism at 5-HT_2 receptors and agonism at other 5-HT receptors that may result in fewer side effects than are produced by the SSRIs. No studies have determined the efficacy of the SARIs for depression in PD nor whether their side-effects profile is better than that of the SSRIs.

Norepinephrine Dopamine Reuptake Blockers (NDRIs)

In a study designed to evaluate motor function rather than depression, bupropion improved depressive symptoms in 5 of 12 PD patients (153).

Depression category was not specified, and the drug was not administered for antidepressive effects.

Others

Electroconvulsive therapy (ECT) increases 5-HT and DA neurotransmission in animals (154), and has been shown to be effective across many PD symptoms, including depression, psychosis, and motor symptoms (155–158). The effect on motor symptoms lasts only days to weeks. Studies of transcranial magnetic stimulation (TMS) have showed some improvement in both mood and motor symptoms in PD (159,160). Behavioral therapies likely are also effective in treating depression in PD (161). These studies are small, and further research is needed to identify any specific PD indications or subpopulations that would benefit from these approaches.

SUMMARY

In contrast to depression, motor symptoms in PD have been extensively researched. The result is a detailed understanding of the pathophysiology of abnormal movements (162). Commitment to, and funding for, a well thought-out depression research plan, such as that presented by the working group at the National Institutes of Health (6), will bring similar theoretical understanding and patient relief for the most disabling of all PD symptoms (3–5)—depression.

REFERENCES

1. Parkinson J. *An essay on the shaking palsy*. London: Neely and Jones, 1817.
2. Cummings JL. Depression and Parkinson's disease: a review. *Am J Psychiatry* 1992;149(4):443–454.
3. Global Parkinson's Disease Survey Steering Committee. Factors impacting on quality of life in Parkinson's disease: results from an international survey. *Mov Disord* 2002;17:60–67.
4. Karlsen KH, Larsen JP, Tandberg E, et al. Influence of clinical and demographic variables on quality of life in patients with Parkinson's disease. *J Neurol Neurosurg Psychiatry* 1999;66(4):431–435.
5. Kuopio AM, Marttila RJ, Helenius H, et al. The quality of life in Parkinson's disease. *Mov Disord* 2000;15:216–223.
6. Edwards E, Kitt C, Oliver E, et al. Depression and Parkinson's disease: a new look at an old problem. *Depress Anxiety* 2002;16(1):39–48.
7. Slaughter JR, Slaughter KA, Nichols D, et al. Prevalence, clinical manifestations, etiology, and treatment of depression in Parkinson's disease. *J Neuropsychiatry Clin Neurosci* 2001;13(2):187–196.
8. Allain H, Schuck S, Mauduit N. Depression in Parkinson's disease. *Br Med J* 2000;320(7245):1287–1288.
9. Ranoux D. Depression and Parkinson disease. *Encephale* 2000;26 Spec No 3:22–26.
10. Mayeux R, Stern Y, Cote L, et al. Altered serotonin metabolism in depressed patients with Parkinson's disease. *Neurology* 1984;34(5):642–646.
11. Starkstein SE, Petracca G, Chemerinski E, et al. Depression in classic versus akinetic-rigid Parkinson's disease. *Mov Disord* 1998;13(1):29–33.
12. Mayeux R, Williams JB, Stern Y, et al. Depression and Parkinson's disease. *Adv Neurol* 1984;40:241–250.
13. Cole SA, Woodard JL, Juncos JL, et al. Depression and disability in Parkinson's disease. *J Neuropsychiatry Clin Neurosci* 1996;8(1):20–25.
14. Tandberg E, Larsen JP, Aarsland D, et al. The occurrence of depression in Parkinson's disease. A community-based study. *Arch Neurol* 1996;53(2):175–179.
15. Starkstein SE, Berthier ML, Bolduc PL, et al. Depression in patients with early versus late onset of Parkinson's disease. *Neurology* 1989;39(11):1441–1445.
16. Hantz P, Caradoc-Davies G, Caradoc-Davies T, et al. Depression in Parkinson's disease. *Am J Psychiatry* 1994;151(7):1010–1014.
17. Sano M, Stern Y, Williams J, et al. Coexisting dementia and depression in Parkinson's disease. *Arch Neurol* 1989;46(12):1284–1286.
18. Santamaria J, Tolosa E, Valles A. Parkinson's disease with depression: a possible subgroup of idiopathic parkinsonism. *Neurology* 1986;36(8):1130–1133.
19. Schrag A, Jahanshahi M, Quinn N. What contributes to quality of life in patients with Parkinson's disease? *J Neurol Neurosurg Psychiatry* 2000;69(3):308–312.
20. Liu CY, Wang SJ, Fuh JL, et al. The correlation of depression with functional activity in Parkinson's disease. *J Neurol* 1997;244(8):493–498.
21. Meara J, Mitchelmore E, Hobson P. Use of the GDS-15 geriatric depression scale as a screening instrument for depressive symptomatology in patients with Parkinson's disease and their carers in the community. *Age Ageing* 1999;28(1):35–38.
22. Leentjens AF, Marinus J, Van Hilten JJ, et al. The contribution of somatic symptoms to the diagnosis of depressive disorder in Parkinson's disease: a discriminant analytic approach. *J Neuropsychiatry Clin Neurosci* 2003;15(1):74–77.
23. Montgomery SA, Asberg M. A new depression scale designed to be sensitive to change. *Br J Psychiatry* 1979;134:382–389.
24. Hamilton M. A rating scale for depression. *J Neurol Neurosurg Psychiatry* 1960;23:56–62.
25. Brown RG, MacCarthy B, Gotham AM, et al. Depression and disability in Parkinson's disease: a follow-up of 132 cases. *Psychol Med* 1988;18(1):49–55.
26. Taylor AE, Saint-Cyr JA, Lang AE, et al. Parkinson's disease and depression. A critical re-evaluation. *Brain* 1986;109(Pt 2):279–292.
27. Levin BE, Llabre MM, Weiner WJ. Parkinson's disease and depression: psychometric properties of the Beck Depression Inventory. *J Neurol Neurosurg Psychiatry* 1988;51(11):1401–1404.

28. Huber SJ, Freidenberg DL, Paulson GW, et al. The pattern of depressive symptoms varies with progression of Parkinson's disease. *J Neurol Neurosurg Psychiatry* 1990;53(4):275–278.
29. Brown RG, Marsden CD, Quinn N, et al. Alterations in cognitive performance and affect-arousal state during fluctuations in motor function in Parkinson's disease. *J Neurol Neurosurg Psychiatry* 1984;47(5):454–465.
30. Henderson R, Kurlan R, Kersun JM, et al. Preliminary examination of the comorbidity of anxiety and depression in Parkinson's disease. *J Neuropsychiatry Clin Neurosci* 1992;4(3):257–264.
31. Gotham AM, Brown RG, Marsden CD. Depression in Parkinson's disease: a quantitative and qualitative analysis. *J Neurol Neurosurg Psychiatry* 1986;49(4):381–389.
32. Schiffer RB, Kurlan R, Rubin A, et al. Evidence for atypical depression in Parkinson's disease. *Am J Psychiatry* 1988;145(8):1020–1022.
33. Shiba M, Bower JH, Maraganore DM, et al. Anxiety disorders and depressive disorders preceding Parkinson's disease: a case-control study. *Mov Disord* 2000;15(4): 669–677.
34. Stein MB, Heuser IJ, Juncos JL, et al. Anxiety disorders in patients with Parkinson's disease. *Am J Psychiatry* 1990;147(2):217–220.
35. Stenager EN, Wermuth L, Stenager E, et al. Suicide in patients with Parkinson's disease. An epidemiological study. *Acta Psychiatr Scand* 1994;90(1):70–72.
36. Brown RG, MacCarthy B. Psychiatric morbidity in patients with Parkinson's disease. *Psychol Med* 1990; 20(1):77–87.
37. Rafal R. Mental disorders in Parkinson's disease. *R I Med J* 1986;69(7):323–326.
38. Mayeux R, Stern Y, Sano M, et al. The relationship of serotonin to depression in Parkinson's disease. *Mov Disord* 1988;3(3):237–244.
39. Mayeux R, Stern Y, Rosen J, et al. Depression, intellectual impairment, and Parkinson disease. *Neurology* 1981;31(6):645–650.
40. Starkstein SE, Preziosi TJ, Bolduc PL, et al. Depression in Parkinson's disease. *J Nerv Ment Dis* 1990; 178(1):27–31.
41. Tandberg E, Larsen JP, Aarsland D, et al. Risk factors for depression in Parkinson disease. *Arch Neurol* 1997; 54(5):625–630.
42. Warburton JW. Depressive symptoms in Parkinson patients referred for thalamotomy. *J Neurol Neurosurg Psychiatry* 1967;30(4):368–370.
43. Celesia GG, Wanamaker WM. Psychiatric disturbances in Parkinson's disease. *Dis Nerv Syst* 1972; 33(9):577–583.
44. Dooneief G, Mirabello E, Bell K, et al. An estimate of the incidence of depression in idiopathic Parkinson's disease. *Arch Neurol* 1992;49(3):305–307.
45. Direnfeld LK, Albert ML, Volicer L, et al. Parkinson's disease. The possible relationship of laterality to dementia and neurochemical findings. *Arch Neurol* 1984; 41(9):935–941.
46. Barber J, Tomer R, Sroka H, et al. Does unilateral dopamine deficit contribute to depression? *Psychiatry Res* 1985;15(1):17–24.
47. Huber SJ, Freidenberg DL, Shuttleworth EC, et al. Neuropsychological similarities in lateralized parkinsonism. *Cortex* 1989;25(3):461–470.
48. Robinson RG, Starkstein SE, Price TR. Post-stroke depression and lesion location. *Stroke* 1988;19(1):125–126.
49. Mayberg HS, Starkstein SE, Sadzot B, et al. Selective hypometabolism in the inferior frontal lobe in depressed patients with Parkinson's disease. *Ann Neurol* 1990;28(1):57–64.
50. Mentis MJ, McIntosh AR, Perrine K, et al. Relationships among the metabolic patterns that correlate with mnemonic, visuospatial, and mood symptoms in Parkinson's disease. *Am J Psychiatry* 2002;159(5):746–754.
51. Ehmann TS, Beninger RJ, Gawel MJ, et al. Depressive symptoms in Parkinson's disease: a comparison with disabled control subjects. *J Geriatr Psychiatry Neurol* 1990;3(1):3–9.
52. Singer E. The effect of treatment with levodopa on Parkinson patients' social functioning and outlook on life. *J Chronic Dis* 1974;27(11-12):581–594.
53. Horn S. Some psychological factors in Parkinsonism. *J Neurol Neurosurg Psychiatry* 1974;37(1):27–31.
54. Hoehn M, Yahr M. Parkinsonism: onset, progression, and mortality. *Neurology* 1967;17:427–442.
55. Bieliauskas LA, Glantz RH. Depression type in Parkinson disease. *J Clin Exp Neuropsychol* 1989;11(5): 597–604.
56. Brown R, Jahanshahi M. Depression in Parkinson's disease: a psychosocial viewpoint. *Adv Neurol* 1995; 65:61–84.
57. Vogel HP. Symptoms of depression in Parkinson's disease. *Pharmacopsychiatria* 1982;15(6):192–196.
58. Kostic VS, Djuricic BM, Covickovic-Sternic N, et al. Depression and Parkinson's disease: possible role of serotonergic mechanisms. *J Neurol* 1987;234(2):94–96.
59. Jankovic J, McDermott M, Carter J, et al., The Parkinson Study Group. Variable expression of Parkinson's disease: a base-line analysis of the DATATOP cohort. *Neurology* 1990;40(10):1529–1534.
60. Racette BA, Hartlein JM, Hershey T, et al. Clinical features and comorbidity of mood fluctuations in Parkinson's disease. *J Neuropsychiatry Clin Neurosci* 2002;14(4):438–442.
61. Cantello R, Gilli M, Riccio A, et al. Mood changes associated with "end-of-dose deterioration" in Parkinson's disease: a controlled study. *J Neurol Neurosurg Psychiatry* 1986;49(10):1182–1190.
62. Friedenberg DL, Cummings JL. Parkinson's disease, depression, and the on-off phenomenon. *Psychosomatics* 1989;30(1):94–99.
63. Girotti F, Carella F, Grassi MP, et al. Motor and cognitive performances of parkinsonian patients in the on and off phases of the disease. *J Neurol Neurosurg Psychiatry* 1986;49(6):657–660.
64. Hardie RJ, Lees AJ, Stern GM. On-off fluctuations in Parkinson's disease. A clinical and neuropharmacological study. *Brain* 1984;107(Pt 2):487–506.
65. Nissenbaum H, Quinn NP, Brown RG, et al. Mood swings associated with the 'on-off' phenomenon in Parkinson's disease. *Psychol Med* 1987;17(4): 899–904.
66. Menza MA, Sage J, Marshall E, et al. Mood changes and "on-off" phenomena in Parkinson's disease. *Mov Disord* 1990;5(2):148–151.
67. Maricle RA, Nutt JG, Carter JH. Mood and anxiety fluctuation in Parkinson's disease associated with levodopa infusion: preliminary findings. *Mov Disord* 1995; 10(3):329–332.
68. Richard IH, Justus AW, Kurlan R. Relationship between mood and motor fluctuations in Parkinson's disease. *J Neuropsychiatry Clin Neurosci* 2001;13(1):35–41.

69. Aarsland D, Tandberg E, Larsen JP, et al. Frequency of dementia in Parkinson disease. *Arch Neurol* 1996;53(6):538–542.
70. Pirozzolo FJ, Hansch EC, Mortimer JA, et al. Dementia in Parkinson disease: a neuropsychological analysis. *Brain Cogn* 1982;1(1):71–83.
71. Lieberman A, Dziatolowski M, Kupersmith M, et al. Dementia in Parkinson disease. *Ann Neurol* 1979;6(4):355–359.
72. Freedman M, Oscar-Berman M. Selective delayed response deficits in Parkinson's and Alzheimer's disease. *Arch Neurol* 1986;43(9):886–890.
73. Huber SJ, Shuttleworth EC, Paulson GW. Dementia in Parkinson's disease. *Arch Neurol* 1986;43(10):987–990.
74. Starkstein SE, Bolduc PL, Mayberg HS, et al. Cognitive impairments and depression in Parkinson's disease: a follow-up study. *J Neurol Neurosurg Psychiatry* 1990;53(7):597–602.
75. Starkstein SE, Mayberg HS, Leiguarda R, et al. A prospective longitudinal study of depression, cognitive decline, and physical impairments in patients with Parkinson's disease. *J Neurol Neurosurg Psychiatry* 1992;55(5):377–382.
76. Starkstein SE, Robinson RG. Dementia of depression in Parkinson's disease and stroke. *J Nerv Ment Dis* 1991;179(10):593–601.
77. Hughes TA, Ross HF, Musa S, et al. A 10-year study of the incidence of and factors predicting dementia in Parkinson's disease. *Neurology* 2000;54(8):1596–1602.
78. Stern Y, Marder K, Tang MX, et al. Antecedent clinical features associated with dementia in Parkinson's disease. *Neurology* 1993;43(9):1690–1692.
79. Alexander GE, Crutcher MD, DeLong MR. Basal ganglia-thalamocortical circuits: parallel substrates for motor, oculomotor, "prefrontal" and "limbic" functions. *Prog Brain Res* 1990;85:119–146.
80. Berger JR, Kelley RE. Thyroid function in Parkinson disease. *Neurology* 1981;31(1):93–95.
81. Otake K, Oiso Y, Mitsuma T, et al. Hypothalamic dysfunction in Parkinson's disease patients. *Acta Med Hung* 1994;50(1-2):3–13.
82. Tandeter HB, Shvartzman P. Parkinson's disease camouflaging early signs of hypothyroidism. *Postgrad Med* 1993;94(5):187–190.
83. Lefebvre J, Loeuille GA, Steinling M, et al. Comparative action of L-dopa and bromocriptine on thyreostimulating hormone (T.S.H.) in primary hypothyroidism (author's transl). *Nouv Presse Med* 1979;8(38):3033–3036.
84. Okun MS, McDonald WM, DeLong MR. Refractory nonmotor symptoms in male patients with Parkinson disease due to testosterone deficiency: a common unrecognized comorbidity. *Arch Neurol* 2002;59(5):807–811.
85. Beekman ATF. Diagnostic procedures in depression in Parkinson's disease. In: Wolster EC, Scheltens P, Berendse HW, eds. *Mental dysfunction in Parkinson's disease*, Vol. II. 1999:263–271.
86. Beck A, Ward C, Mendelson M, et al. An inventory for measuring depression. *Arch Gen Psychiatry* 1961;4:561–571.
87. Leentjens AF, Verhey FR, Luijckx GJ, et al. The validity of the Beck Depression Inventory as a screening and diagnostic instrument for depression in patients with Parkinson's disease. *Mov Disord* 2000;15(6):1221–1224.
88. Leentjens AF, Verhey FR, Lousberg R, et al. The validity of the Hamilton and Montgomery-Asberg depression rating scales as screening and diagnostic tools for depression in Parkinson's disease. *Int J Geriatr Psychiatry* 2000;15(7):644–649.
89. Javoy-Agid F, Agid Y. Is the mesocortical dopaminergic system involved in Parkinson disease? *Neurology* 1980;30(12):1326–1330.
90. Damier P, Hirsch EC, Agid Y, et al. The substantia nigra of the human brain. II. Patterns of loss of dopamine-containing neurons in Parkinson's disease. *Brain* 1999;122(Pt 8):1437–1448.
91. Agid Y, Cervera P, Hirsch E, et al. Biochemistry of Parkinson's disease 28 years later: a critical review. *Mov Disord* 1989;4(Suppl. 1):S126–S144.
92. Jellinger K. Overview of morphological changes in Parkinson's disease. *Adv Neurol* 1987;45:1–18.
93. Hornykiewicz O. Biochemical abnormalities in some extrastriatal neuronal systems in Parkinson's disease. In: Rinne UK, Klinger M, Stamm G, eds. *Parkinson's disease: current progress, problems, and management.* 1980.
94. Uhl GR, Hedreen JC, Price DL. Parkinson's disease: loss of neurons from the ventral tegmental area contralateral to therapeutic surgical lesions. *Neurology* 1985;35(8):1215–1218.
95. Torack RM, Morris JC. The association of ventral tegmental area histopathology with adult dementia. *Arch Neurol* 1988;45(5):497–501.
96. Rinne JO, Rummukainen J, Paljarvi L, et al. Dementia in Parkinson's disease is related to neuronal loss in the medial substantia nigra. *Ann Neurol* 1989;26(1):47–50.
97. Charlton CG. Depletion of nigrostriatal and forebrain tyrosine hydroxylase by S-adenosylmethionine: a model that may explain the occurrence of depression in Parkinson's disease. *Life Sci* 1997;61(5):495–502.
98. Cantello R, Aguggia M, Gilli M, et al. Major depression in Parkinson's disease and the mood response to intravenous methylphenidate: possible role of the "hedonic" dopamine synapse. *J Neurol Neurosurg Psychiatry* 1989;52(6):724–731.
99. Mayeux R, Stern Y, Williams JB, et al. Clinical and biochemical features of depression in Parkinson's disease. *Am J Psychiatry* 1986;143(6):756–759.
100. Marsh GG, Markham CH. Does levodopa alter depression and psychopathology in Parkinsonism patients? *J Neurol Neurosurg Psychiatry* 1973;36(6):925–935.
101. Paulus W, Jellinger K. The neuropathologic basis of different clinical subgroups of Parkinson's disease. *J Neuropathol Exp Neurol* 1991;50(6):743–755.
102. Barbeau, A. Parkinson's disease: clinical features and etiopathology. In: Vinken PJ, Bruyn GW, Klawans HL, eds. *Handbook of clinical neurology*, Vol. 5(49), *Extrapyramidal disorders*. New York: Elsevier, 1986.
103. D'Amato RJ, Zweig RM, Whitehouse PJ. Aminergic systems in Alzheimer's disease and Parkinson's disease. *Ann Neurol* 1987;22:229–236.
104. Raisman R, Cash R, Agid Y. Parkinson's disease: decreased density of 3H-imipramine and 3H-paroxetine binding sites in putamen. *Neurology* 1986;36(4):556–560.
105. Doder M, Rabiner EA, Turjanski N, et al. Brain serotonin 1a receptors in Parkinson's disease with and without depression measured by positron emission tomography with 11-WAY 100635. *Mov Disord* 2000;15:213.
106. Kuhn W, Muller T, Gerlach M, et al. Depression in Parkinson's disease: biogenic amines in CSF of "de novo" patients. *J Neural Transm* 1996;103(12):1441–1445.

107. Coppen A, Metcalfe M, Carroll JD, et al. Levodopa and L-tryptophan therapy in Parkinsonism. *Lancet* 1972;1(7752):654–658.
108. Menza MA, Palermo B, DiPaola R, et al. Depression and anxiety in Parkinson's disease: possible effect of genetic variation in the serotonin transporter. *J Geriatr Psychiatry Neurol* 1999;12(2):49–52.
109. Mossner R, Henneberg A, Schmitt A, et al. Allelic variation of serotonin transporter expression is associated with depression in Parkinson's disease. *Mol Psychiatry* 2001;6(3):350–352.
110. Chan-Palay V, Asan E. Alterations in catecholamine neurons of the locus coeruleus in senile dementia of the Alzheimer type and in Parkinson's disease with and without dementia and depression. *J Comp Neurol* 1989;287(3):373–392.
111. Weiner W, Lang A. *Movement disorders: a comprehensive survey.* Mount Kisco, NY: Futura, 1989.
112. Villeneuve A, Berlan M, Lafontan M, et al. Platelet alpha 2 adrenoceptors in Parkinson's disease: decreased number in untreated patients and recovery after treatment. *Eur J Clin Invest* 1985;15(6):403–407.
113. Nutt D, Lawson C. Panic attacks. A neurochemical overview of models and mechanisms. *Br J Psychiatry* 1992;160:165–178.
114. Houeto JL, Mesnage V, Mallet L, et al. Behavioural disorders, Parkinson's disease and subthalamic stimulation. *J Neurol Neurosurg Psychiatry* 2002;72(6):701–707.
115. Bejjani BP, Damier P, Arnulf I, et al. Transient acute depression induced by high-frequency deep-brain stimulation. *N Engl J Med* 1999;340(19):1476–1480.
116. Rodriguez-Oroz MC, Rodriguez M, Guridi J, et al. The subthalamic nucleus in Parkinson's disease: somatotopic organization and physiological characteristics. *Brain* 2001;124(Pt 9):1777–1790.
117. Mayberg HS, Lozano AM. Penfield revisited? Understanding and modifying behavior by deep brain stimulation for PD. *Neurology* 2002;59(9):1298–1299.
118. Eidelberg D, Moeller JR, Dhawan V, et al. The metabolic anatomy of Parkinson's disease: complementary [18F]fluorodeoxyglucose and [18F]fluorodopa positron emission tomographic studies. *Mov Disord* 1990;5(3):203–213.
119. Moeller JR, Nakamura T, Mentis MJ, et al. Reproducibility of regional metabolic covariance patterns: comparison of four populations. *J Nucl Med* 1999;40(8):1264–1269.
120. Mayberg HS, Starkstein SE, Peyser CE, et al. Paralimbic frontal lobe hypometabolism in depression associated with Huntington's disease. *Neurology* 1992;42(9):1791–1797.
121. Jagust WJ, Reed BR, Martin EM, et al. Cognitive function and regional cerebral blood flow in Parkinson's disease. *Brain* 1992;115(Pt 2):521–537.
122. Ring HA, Bench CJ, Trimble MR, et al. Depression in Parkinson's disease. A positron emission study. *Br J Psychiatry* 1994;165(3):333–339.
123. Baxter LR, Schwartz JM, Phelps ME, et al. Reduction of prefrontal cortex glucose metabolism common to three types of depression. *Arch Gen Psychiatry* 1989;46:243–250.
124. Buchsbaum MS, Wu J, DeLisi LE, et al. Frontal cortex and basal ganglia metabolic rates assessed by positron emission tomography with [18F]2-deoxyglucose in affective illness. *J Affect Disord* 1986;10(2):137–152.
125. Post RM, DeLisi LE, Holcomb HH, et al. Glucose utilization in the temporal cortex of affectively ill patients: positron emission tomography. *Biol Psychiatry* 1987;22(5):545–553.
126. Starkstein SE, Robinson RG, Price TR. Comparison of cortical and subcortical lesions in the production of poststroke mood disorders. *Brain* 1987;110(Pt 4):1045–1059.
127. Mayberg, HS, Neuro-imaging studies of depression in neurological disease. In: Starkstein SE, Robinson RG, eds. *Depression in neurologic diseases.* 1993:186–216.
128. Wichmann T, DeLong MR. Functional and pathophysiological models of the basal ganglia. *Curr Opin Neurobiol* 1996;6(6):751–758.
129. Brown, RG. The role of cortico-striatal circuits in learning sequential information. In: GM Stern, ed. *Parkinson's disease: advances in neurology.* Philadelphia: Lippincott Williams & Wilkins, 1999:31–39.
130. Mayberg HS, Solomon DH. Depression in Parkinson's disease: a biochemical and organic viewpoint. *Adv Neurol* 1995;65:49–60.
131. McDonald WM, Richard IH, DeLong MR. Prevalence, etiology, and treatment of depression in Parkinson's disease. *Biol Psychiatry* 2003;54(3):363–375.
132. Burn DJ. Beyond the iron mask: towards better recognition and treatment of depression associated with Parkinson's disease. *Mov Disord* 2002;17(3):445–454.
133. Corrigan MH, Denahan AQ, Wright CE, et al. Comparison of pramipexole, fluoxetine, and placebo in patients with major depression. *Depress Anxiety* 2000;11(2):58–65.
134. Kostic VS, Filipovic SR, Lecic D, et al. Effect of age at onset on frequency of depression in Parkinson's disease. *J Neurol Neurosurg Psychiatry* 1994;57(10):1265–1267.
135. Strong, R. Imipramine in the treatment of parkinsonism: a double blind placebo study. *Br Med J* 1965;2:33–34.
136. Laitinen L. Desipramine in treatment of Parkinson's disease. A placebo-controlled study. *Acta Neurol Scand* 1969;45(1):109–113.
137. Andersen J, Aabro E, Gulmann N, et al. Anti-depressive treatment in Parkinson's disease. A controlled trial of the effect of nortriptyline in patients with Parkinson's disease treated with L-DOPA. *Acta Neurol Scand* 1980;62(4):210–219.
138. Jimenez-Jimenez FJ, Tejeiro J, Martinez-Junquera G, et al. Parkinsonism exacerbated by paroxetine. *Neurology* 1994;44(12):2406.
139. Meltzer HY, Young M, Metz J, et al. Extrapyramidal side effects and increased serum prolactin following fluoxetine, a new antidepressant. *J Neural Transm* 1979;45(2):165–175.
140. Bouchard R, Pourcher E, Vincent P. Fluoxetine and extrapyramidal side effects. *Am J Psychiatry* 1989;146:1352–1353.
141. Hesselink JM. Serotonin and Parkinson's disease. *Am J Psychiatry* 1993;150(5):843–844.
142. Simons JA. Fluoxetine in Parkinson's disease. *Mov Disord* 1996;11(5):581–582.
143. Steur EN. Increase of Parkinson disability after fluoxetine medication. *Neurology* 1993;43(1):211–213.
144. Tate JL. Extrapyramidal symptoms in a patient taking haloperidol and fluoxetine. *Am J Psychiatry* 1989;146(3):399–400.
145. Caley CF, Friedman JH. Does fluoxetine exacerbate Parkinson's disease? *J Clin Psychiatry* 1992;53(8):278–282.

146. Ceravolo R, Nuti A, Piccinni A, et al. Paroxetine in Parkinson's disease: effects on motor and depressive symptoms. *Neurology* 2000;55(8):1216–1218.
147. Dell'Agnello G, Ceravolo R, Nuti A, et al. SSRIs do not worsen Parkinson's disease: evidence from an open-label, prospective study. *Clin Neuropharmacol* 2001;24(4):221–227.
148. Hauser RA, Zesiewicz TA. Sertraline for the treatment of depression in Parkinson's disease. *Mov Disord* 1997;12(5):756–759.
149. Montastruc JL, Fabre N, Blin O, et al. Does fluoxetine aggravate Parkinson's disease? A pilot prospective study. *Mov Disord* 1995;10(3):355–357.
150. Rampello L, Chiechio S, Raffaele R, et al. The SSRI, citalopram, improves bradykinesia in patients with Parkinson's disease treated with L-dopa. *Clin Neuropharmacol* 2002;25(1):21–24.
151. Richard IH, Maughn A, Kurlan R. Do serotonin reuptake inhibitor antidepressants worsen Parkinson's disease? A retrospective case series. *Mov Disord* 1999;14(1):155–157.
152. Richard IH, Kurlan R. Parkinson Study Group. A survey of antidepressant drug use in Parkinson's disease. *Neurology* 1997;49(4):1168–1170.
153. Goetz CG, Tanner CM, Klawans HL. Bupropion in Parkinson's disease. *Neurology* 1984;34(8):1092–1094.
154. Yoshida K, Higuchi H, Kamata M, et al. Single and repeated electroconvulsive shocks activate dopaminergic and 5-hydroxytryptaminergic neurotransmission in the frontal cortex of rats. *Prog Neuropsychopharmacol Biol Psychiatry* 1998;22(2):435–444.
155. Aarsland D, Larsen JP, Waage O, et al. Maintenance electroconvulsive therapy for Parkinson's disease. *Convuls Ther* 1997;13(4):274–277.
156. Fall PA, Granerus AK. Maintenance ECT in Parkinson's disease. *J Neural Transm* 1999;106(7-8):737–741.
157. Moellentine C, Rummans T, Ahlskog JE, et al. Effectiveness of ECT in patients with parkinsonism. *J Neuropsychiatry Clin Neurosci* 1998;10(2):187–193.
158. Wengel SP, Burke WJ, Pfeiffer RF, et al. Maintenance electroconvulsive therapy for intractable Parkinson's disease. *Am J Geriatr Psychiatry* 1998;6(3):263–269.
159. Dragasevic N, Potrebic A, Damjanovic A, et al. Therapeutic efficacy of bilateral prefrontal slow repetitive transcranial magnetic stimulation in depressed patients with Parkinson's disease: an open study. *Mov Disord* 2002;17(3):528–532.
160. Mally J, Stone TW. Therapeutic and "dose-dependent" effect of repetitive microelectroshock induced by transcranial magnetic stimulation in Parkinson's disease. *J Neurosci Res* 1999;57(6):935–940.
161. Poewe W, Luginger E. Depression in Parkinson's disease: impediments to recognition and treatment options. *Neurology* 1999;52(7 Suppl 3):S2–S6.
162. Wichmann T, DeLong MR. Models of basal ganglia function and pathophysiology of movement disorders. *Neurosurg Clin North Am* 1998;9(2):223–236.

4

Anxiety Disorders in Parkinson's Disease

Irene H. Richard

University of Rochester School of Medicine and Dentistry
Rochester, New York

INTRODUCTION

The fact that anxiety symptoms are highly prevalent among patients with Parkinson's Disease (PD) will come as no surprise to most clinicians caring for these patients on a regular basis, yet the topic has received little attention from researchers. This chapter focuses on available information that supports a relationship between PD and anxiety. Treatment for anxiety is addressed, but the lack of available clinical research data will be readily apparent.

To meet criteria for an anxiety disorder, symptoms must generally be of great enough magnitude to cause substantial distress or disability. The anxiety disorders are distinguished from one another by their constellation of symptoms, responses to medications, and, in some cases, presumed etiologic mechanisms. DSM-IV (*The Diagnostic and Statistical Manual of Mental Disorders*, 4th edition) (1) includes the categories of anxiety disorders, but criteria such as those outlined in DSM-IV may or may not be applicable to patients with PD, and the symptoms of PD itself may overlap with those of certain anxiety disorders (e.g., shaking). This combination of factors can make diagnosing anxiety disorders in patients with PD difficult and certainly poses a challenge for investigators conducting research in this area.

Prevalence of Anxiety in PD

Studies suggest that 25% to 50% of all people with PD experience anxiety disorders (2,3). In addition to exceeding prevalence rates in the general population, rates of anxiety disorders in patients with PD have been found by most (but not all) investigators to be higher than in patients with other neurologic or medical illnesses.

Stein and co-workers (2) systematically evaluated 24 patients with PD for the presence of DSM-III-R Axis I syndromes. Clinically important anxiety disorders were diagnosed in nine subjects (38%), a rate that is much greater than the incidence in the general population (5%–15%), in primary care clinics (10%), or in patients with chronic medical conditions (11%). Vazquez et al. (3) found that 31 of 131 patients with PD (24%) had experienced recurrent panic attacks that fulfilled most DSM-III-R criteria (4) for panic disorder.

Schiffer et al. (5) carried out structured clinical psychiatric interviews for 16 depressed patients with PD and 20 depressed patients with multiple sclerosis and found that anxiety disorders were more common in the patients with PD. Seventy-five percent of the patients with PD met criteria for past or present generalized anxiety disorder (GAD) or panic disorder, whereas only 10% of patients with multiple sclerosis met these criteria.

Menza et al. (6) compared 42 patients with PD and 21 matched medical control subjects (patients with chronic debilitating osteoarthritis, matched for age and length of illness) using DSM-III-R criteria and a variety of psychiatric rating scales. Twelve patients with PD (29%), but only one medical control subject (5%), had a formal anxiety disorder. In a subsequent study of 104 patients with PD and 61 medical control subjects with equal disability, Menza and Mark (7) noted that patients with PD scored higher than control subjects on measures of depression and anxiety.

Not all studies confirm the notion that anxiety is more common in patients with PD than in other medically ill patients. Gotham et al. (8) found that anxiety was more common in patients with PD than among healthy control subjects but was not more common than it was among patients with chronic arthritis. Berrios et al. (9) suggested that autonomic symptoms in patients with PD might be misconstrued as anxiety and could result in overdiagnosis of anxiety disorders in this population (10). However, because "significance persisted after the autonomic items were removed from the Hamilton scales," it seems more likely that patients with PD have a common neurobiological abnormality that can result in both emotional and autonomic dysfunction.

Clinical Features of Anxiety Disorders

A Range of Disorders

A wide range of anxiety disorders has been reported in patients with PD. Generalized anxiety disorder, panic disorder, and social phobia appear to be the most frequently reported. obsessive–compulsive disorder (OCD) has been reported to a lesser degree. Of course, as with depressive symptoms, many patients experience symptoms of anxiety that are not frequent or severe enough to meet criteria for an anxiety disorder but are distressing nonetheless. Also, many patients experience anxiety in the setting of a depressive disorder.

Menza et al. (6) noted that primary diagnoses in patients with PD are clustered among panic disorder, phobic disorder, and GAD. Schiffer et al. (5) reported the presence of panic disorder and GAD, whereas Vazquez et al. (3) described only panic disorder. Stein et al. (2) observed that patients with PD can experience more than one anxiety disorder (as well as comorbid depressive disorders).

The distribution of anxiety disorders may be somewhat different in familial parkinsonism. Lauterbach and Duvoisin (11) described anxiety disorders in patients with familial parkinsonism and noted that the rate of GAD they observed was similar to that reported by Stein et al. (2) in their study of patients with PD, whereas rates of panic disorder were lower, and rates of social phobia and OCD were higher.

GAD

According to DSM-IV, GAD is characterized by excessive anxiety and worry about a number of activities and is associated with restlessness, fatigue, difficulty in concentrating, irritability, muscle tension, or sleep disturbance. In GAD, the focus of the anxiety and worry should not be confined to features of an Axis I disorder (e.g., panic) and should not occur exclusively in the setting of a depressive disorder (1).

Panic Disorder

Patients with panic disorder experience recurrent, unexpected panic attacks. A panic attack is characterized by a discrete period of intense fear or discomfort, in which a variety of symptoms develop abruptly and reach a peak within 10 minutes. The symptoms include palpitations, sweating, shaking, shortness of breath, dizziness, depersonalization, and fear of dying. Patients with panic disorder experience persistent concern about having additional attacks or about exhibiting a major change in behavior related to the attacks (1).

In reviewing the epidemiology and comorbidity of anxiety disorders among the elderly, Flint (10) concluded that GAD and phobias account for most of the anxiety disorders in late life and that panic disorders are rare. Thus, the onset of panic in late age, in association with PD, is contrary to the expected natural course of this condition and favors an etiologic link between the two disorders. Notably, however, some authors believe that underdiagnosis of anxiety in late life may contribute to low prevalence estimates in the elderly population (12,13) and that other medical conditions (e.g., chronic obstructive pulmonary disease, COPD) might also have a role in the onset of late-life panic disorder.

Social Phobia

According to DSM-IV, social phobia is characterized by a marked and persistent fear of one or more social situations. The individual fears that he or she will act in a way (or show anxiety symptoms) that will be embarrassing but recognizes that the fear is excessive. The DSM-IV criteria specify that the fear need not be related to a medical disorder; an example given is tremor in patients with PD (1).

Some patients' fear of social situations appears to be directly related to their PD symptoms. Others have more diffuse social phobia unrelated to, and at times even predating, the diagnosis of PD. In their study of patients with familial parkinsonism, Lauterbach and Duvoisin (11) noted 5 of 28 patients who experienced embarrassment about PD symptoms but found that 12 of their patients with familial parkinsonism who were diagnosed with social phobia experienced anxiety symptoms before motor features were diagnosed. Stein et al. (4) commented that four of the patients in whom they diagnosed social phobia had self-consciousness that was not related to their PD symptoms. Three additional patients had symptoms of social phobia that appeared to be secondary to self-consciousness about PD symptoms. These patients would meet DSM-IV criteria for "Anxiety Disorder, Not Otherwise Specified" (1).

OCD

OCD is characterized by complaints of persistent or repetitive thoughts (obsessions) or behaviors (compulsions). The person feels compelled to continue, despite an awareness that the thoughts or behaviors may be inappropriate, and feels distress if he stops them. OCD must be distinguished from obsessive–compulsive personality disorder (OCP, an Axis II disorder), in which the thoughts and behaviors are generally not perceived as unreasonable or distressing (1).

One recent study suggests that neither OCD nor obsessive–compulsive symptoms (OCS) are more common in patients with PD than in matched controls (14). In another study, Muller et al. (15) evaluated the characteristics of OCS in Tourette's syndrome (TS), OCD, and PD. The OCD and TS patients had higher scores on obsessive–compulsive inventories than normal controls, whereas patients with PD merely scored higher on one subscale (ordering) of one inventory. Alegret et al. (16) administered two inventories to a sample of nondemented and nondepressed patients with PD. Patients with severe PD showed more obsessive traits than normal controls (particularly in checking, doubting, and cleaning subscales), whereas patients with mild disease did not differ from normal controls. The authors suggested that OC symptoms may be related to a subset of neurochemical changes in the basal ganglia circuitry as the disease progresses.

Relationship of Anxiety to Antiparkinsonian Medications

The issue of whether antiparkinsonian medications might be responsible for some of the anxiety symptoms seen in patients with PD remains unsettled. Not much research has been conducted in this area since we reviewed the subject in 1996 (17). Henderson et al. (18) noted that 44% of PD subjects taking levodopa and reporting anxiety experienced the onset of anxiety before beginning levodopa, and 56% experienced it after treatment was initiated. Stein et al. (2) found no significant difference between anxious and nonanxious patients with PD with regard to the cumulative dose of levodopa. The authors did note, however, that many subjects were taking other antiparkinsonian medications such as anticholinergics, amantadine, and bromocriptine and that potential influences of these drugs could not be excluded.

Siemers et al. (19) studied the anxiety state and motor performance of 19 patients with idiopathic PD. All 19 patients were taking levodopa or carbidopa, and most were also receiving adjunctive antiparkinsonian medications, including dopamine receptor agonists, selegiline (deprenyl), and anticholinergics. Two patients were taking benzodiazepines. The authors found no statistical differences in motor, depression, or anxiety scores based on the presence or absence of the additional medications. In the study by Menza et al. (6), levodopa dose did not significantly correlate with anxiety measures. The authors also found that measures of anxiety did not differ between patients receiving or not receiving selegiline or pergolide. Rondot et al. (20) found that anxious patients with PD received doses of levodopa comparable to those given in the general PD population. In contrast to the above reports, Vazquez et al. (3) concluded that panic attacks were related to levodopa therapy but not to other agonist drugs. The authors found that 24% of patients with PD who were receiving long-term levodopa therapy had experienced recurrent panic attacks. They also noted that the patients with PD who had panic disorder were started on levodopa earlier than the patients with PD who did not have panic disorder and that the patients with panic disorder needed higher dosages.

Relationship between Anxiety and Motor Fluctuations

Some authors have reported higher degrees of anxiety in patients who experience "on-off" motor fluctuations than in other patients with PD (6,18,21), whereas others have failed to confirm this relationship (2,11,22). One could conjecture that the unpredictable nature of the on-off states might result in anxiety behavior similar to that which occurs in laboratory animals after they are exposed to unpredictable aversive stimuli (23). Riley and Lang (24) include anxiety as one of the psychiatric disturbances that vary with parkinsonian motor fluctuations. Most authors have noted that in patients who do experience the on-off phenomenon, anxiety tends to occur most often during the "off" phase (2,3, 18,19). In 1976, Marsden and Parkes (25) commented that "the off period may be accompanied by panic, flushing and sweating, and leg pain." One study revealed that in most patients, mood or anxiety improved significantly from "off" to "on" but then worsened again in the "on" state when dyskinesias appeared (26), leading the authors to conclude that the behavioral responses of most patients probably reflect an emotional reaction to their motor symptoms. An alternative explanation might be that an optimal level of dopamine is necessary to prevent depressed mood and anxiety. In their levodopa infusion studies, Maricle et al. (27) found that mood, anxiety, and motor fluctuations tended to correlate, in that patients experienced greater anxiety and depression during periods of poor mobility, and vice versa. They did not find that patients' anxiety and depression recurred with the onset of dyskinesias. Vazquez et al. (3) found that in 90.3% of the patients, panic attacks were associated with the "off" period. However, in one patient, panic attacks coincided with the "on" period (with or without dyskinesias), and in two other patients, panic attacks were unrelated to motor fluctuations (28). Our ongoing research of mood and anxiety fluctuations in PD supports heterogeneity among patients in patterns of anxiety, mood, and motor fluctuations (29). It is possible that variations in brain levels of levodopa are responsible for anxiety fluctuations (at least in some patients), although some authors have suggested that changes in serotonin (19) or norepinephrine (3) may play a role. Further studies are needed to clarify the relationship between motor state and anxiety in patients with PD and to uncover pathogenetic mechanisms.

Relationship between Anxiety and Depression

In psychiatric populations, anxiety and depressive disorders commonly coexist (30); this coexistence may be particularly prevalent in the elderly (28). The relationship between anxiety and depression appears to be particularly strong, however, in elderly patients with PD. In a review of depression in PD, Cummings (31) notes that the depression in patients with PD is distinguished from other depressive disorders by greater anxiety and less self-punitive ideation. After discovering that the diagnoses of anxiety and panic disorder were significantly more common among depressed patients with PD than among depressed patients with multiple sclerosis, Schiffer et al. (5) suggested that patients with PD may experience an "atypical" depression. One study showed that 92% of patients with PD who had an anxiety disorder also had a depressive disorder and that 67% of those with a depressive disorder also had an anxiety disorder (6). Another study compared patients with PD with age-matched, healthy spouse controls and noted that the report of depression plus panic or anxiety (as compared with either condition alone) best distinguished the two populations (18). In the study by Vazquez et al., the subgroup of patients with PD who also experienced panic attacks had a higher rate of concomitant depression (28).

We conducted a yohimbine challenge study involving patients with PD (32). Those with anxiety disorders developed panic attacks at frequencies comparable to those of primary psychiatric patients with panic disorders. Of particular interest was the finding that a PD patient with a history of major depression alone (without an anxiety disorder) experienced a yohimbine-induced panic attack. Although major depression and panic disorder overlap considerably, studies in psychiatric populations have shown that patients with major depression alone do not develop panic attacks with provocative measures (30). Our observation of yohimbine-induced panic in a patient with PD and major depression alone supports the notion that depression in patients with PD may truly be "atypical" (5,30) and more closely linked to anxiety and panic than is depression in primary psychiatric patients.

Although other studies have also shown a close correlation between depression and anxiety in patients with PD (3,33), anxiety can clearly occur in the absence of depression. A study by Lui et al. (34) revealed that, although the degrees of anxiety and depression assessed by standardized rating scales were generally correlated, 14 of 58 patients with PD who lacked depressive symptoms fulfilled DSM-III-R criteria for GAD.

Relationship between Anxiety and Dementia

Although some evidence exists that the rate of anxiety is increased in primary dementia disorders (35), the relationship between anxiety and dementia in patients with PD is not clear [as noted in our previous review article (17)]. Depression appears to be equally common in PD patients with and without dementia (30). Iruela et al. (36) hypothesized that anxiety may actually lessen in patients with PD if they become demented; brain levels of norepinephrine are substantially decreased in demented patients with PD (37), and abnormal activity of noradrenergic cells in the locus caeruleus has been hypothesized to cause anxiety. Addressing this issue, however, Lauterbach (38) studied 38 patients with familial parkinsonism and found no relationship between dementia and anxiety symptoms. Most of the studies that examined anxiety in patients with PD either failed to comment on the cognitive status of the patients (5,18) or deliberately excluded patients with dementia (2,6,19), so definite conclusions cannot be reached regarding a relationship between anxiety and cognitive decline in this illness. Fleminger (33) noted that two groups of patients with PD who differed with regard to the presence of anxiety did not differ in their performance on two tests of cognitive function (National Adult Reading Test and Information, Memory, and Concentration Test). Vazquez et al. (3) found that anxious and nonanxious patients with PD did not differ with respect to their severity of dementia as assessed by the Unified Parkinson's Disease Rating Scale (UPDRS) but noted that more formal measures of cognitive function were not performed and also that the degree of mental impairment was low in both groups.

Etiology of Anxiety in PD

Anxiety Is a Manifestation of the Disease Itself

Evidence supporting the notion that anxiety is not simply a reaction to the motor deficits in patients with PD include the following observations: (a) most studies have shown that depression in patients with PD is not closely correlated with the severity of motor symptoms or the degree of disability (30); (b) in the levodopa-infusion study conducted by Maricle et al. (27), the emotional changes generally preceded the motor changes by several minutes, thereby making it unlikely that the anxiety and depression represented an emotional reaction to motor impairment; (c) patients who experienced anxiety and panic attacks during an experimental yohimbine challenge had no measurable worsening of their parkinsonian motor function (39); and (d) although some investigators who have assessed patients with idiopathic PD have observed that anxiety symptoms tend to appear after the diagnosis of PD has been established (2,3,18), others have found that anxiety occurs before motor symptoms (11), including a recent case–control study by Shiba et al. (40), which suggests that anxiety disorders in patients with PD precede onset of motor symptoms by years.

The main neurotransmitters implicated in the pathogenesis of anxiety in primary psychiatric populations include norepinephrine, serotonin, and gamma-aminobutyric acid (GABA) (41–43). More recently, evidence suggests that cholecystokinin (CCK) may be involved in the pathogenesis of panic disorder (44) and that dopamine may have a role in the development of social phobia. Many biologic abnormalities demonstrated in patients with PD may not only explain the frequent occurrence of anxiety in this disorder but also contribute to our understanding of the mechanisms of anxiety in psychiatric patients.

Norepinephrine

Strong evidence implicates noradrenergic dysfunction, particularly of the alpha-2 adrenergic receptors, and perhaps of the locus caeruleus itself, in the development of primary anxiety disorders, especially panic disorder (41,42,45–49). Interestingly, many abnormalities of the noradrenergic system have also been discovered in patients with PD (50). The dorsal ascending noradrenergic pathway is particularly affected (47–49, 51) and changes appear to occur in both central (52) and peripheral adrenergic receptors (52,53). Lauterbach (38), Lauterbach and Duvoisin (11), and Vazquez et al. (3) independently provided data in PD suggesting that locus caeruleus disinhibition may lead to secondary panic attacks, whereas locus caeruleus degeneration and subsequent incompetence might explain attenuation of primary panic attacks.

Further support for a noradrenergic role in anxiety associated with PD comes from our pilot study of experimental yohimbine-induced panic. Oral yohimbine (an alpha-2 antagonist) was administered to six patients with PD who had a history of anxiety or depression, two parkinsonian patients without psychiatric illness, and two normal controls. Patients with PD who had a history of anxiety developed panic attacks at frequencies comparable to those of primary psychiatric patients with panic disorder. Regardless of their history of anxiety or depression, parkinsonian patients demonstrated a vulnerability to yohimbine-induced somatic and autonomic symptoms (31,39).

Serotonin

Alterations in the serotonin neurotransmitter system have also been postulated to play a role in anxiety disorders, particularly in OCD but also in social phobia (51,52), posttraumatic stress disorder, GAD, and perhaps panic disorder (53). Abnormalities of the serotonergic system have been noted in patients with PD (54–56). A genotype–phenotype correlation study involving 32 patients by Menza et al. (57) suggests that the short allele of the serotonin transporter gene may represent an important risk factor for the development of anxiety and depression in patients with PD. It is possible that interactions between noradrenergic and serotonergic systems may be relevant to the expression of certain anxiety disorders, because serotonin can decrease locus caeruleus firing by 5-hydroxytryptamine (5-HT2) serotonin receptors (53).

GABA

The potential role of GABA in the genesis of anxiety is suggested by the efficacy of benzodiazepines in treating panic disorder and GAD; these drugs produce their effects by activating GABA receptors in the brain (53). In most of the PD brains examined, an increased concentration of GABA in the putamen and pallidum and a decreased concentration in cortical areas have been observed (50).

Dopamine

Both dopamine and serotonin systems may be involved in OCD (58,59) and some authors have postulated a dopaminergic dysregulation in panic disorder (60,61). Mounting evidence, including two single photon emission computed tomography (SPECT) neuroimaging studies (62–64), supports a role for abnormalities in striatal dopaminergic function in patients with social phobia (54). Genetic studies of dopamine receptor and dopamine transporter polymorphisms have yet to establish a genetic linkage or association to panic disorder (55,64).

The levodopa infusion studies in patients with PD that were performed by Maricle et al. (27) clearly implicate a dopaminergic deficiency state in anxiety, at least anxiety that is associated with motor fluctuations. Tomer et al. (56) hypothesized that reduced dopaminergic activity in the striatum may be responsible for OCD in patients with PD. Dopamine decreases the firing rate of the locus caeruleus (65). Several investigators have hypothesized that the dopamine deficiency in PD might result in an alteration of noradrenergic systems and could be responsible for certain anxiety disorders in patients with this illness (3,36,38).

Brain Localization

Some evidence suggests that lateralized cerebral factors may be important in the genesis of anxiety. Imaging studies have revealed right hemispheric abnormalities in panic disorders (66), and new-onset panic disorder after a right thalamic infarct has been reported (67). No imaging studies such as these have been reported that specifically examined anxiety in patients with PD. Evidence does exist, however, that involvement of the right side of the brain is greater in patients with PD who have anxiety symptoms. Fleminger (33) examined 17 patients with PD whose symptoms were worse on the right side of the body (right-sided hemiparkinsonism, RHP) and 13 patients whose symptoms were worse on the left side of the body (left-sided hemiparkinsonism, LHP). Present State Examination symptoms that were more common in the LHP group were panic with autonomic features, depressed mood, and social withdrawal. Similarly, Rubin et al. (68) noted that panic–anxiety disorder in patients with PD was associated with early left–right asymmetry of PD motor features. Investigators have noted correlations between the frequency (14) and severity (56) of OCS and left-sided motor symptoms in PD, particularly for symmetry and ordering/arranging (14).

Brain imaging studies in psychiatric patients with anxiety have shown abnormalities in the basal ganglia (69–71). Potts et al. (72) noted an age-related reduction in putamen volumes in patients with social phobia. The authors conjectured that social phobia might be a manifestation of a dopamine-deficiency state and that some social phobic patients as they age may be at greater risk of developing the manifestations of parkinsonism. Neuropsychological testing has also demonstrated that patients with OCD and PD have deficits attributable to basal ganglia dysfunction (72,73). These findings suggest that basal ganglia disturbances in PD might explain the development of anxiety in patients suffering from this illness.

Treatment of Anxiety in Parkinson's Disease

Pharmacotherapy

The drugs most commonly used to treat anxiety disorders include benzodiazepines, buspirone, selective serotonin reuptake inhibitors (SSRIs) and, more recently, the combined serotonin and norepinephrine reuptake inhibitors (SNRIs). The traditional tricyclic antidepressants (TCAs) and nonselective monoamine oxidase inhibitors (MAOIs) are generally not first-line treatments, because of concerns regarding tolerability. Very few clinical trials have examined medication treatment for anxiety in the elderly (74), and no studies have specifically addressed the optimal treatment of anxiety in patients with PD. Elderly patients may be more sensitive than younger ones to anxiolytic medications by virtue of their altered metabolism, tendency toward falls and oversedation, and concomitant medical conditions (13,75,76).

Antiparkinsonian Agents

If anxiety occurs exclusively during the "off" period, it would be reasonable to first try to minimize "off" time by adjusting the antiparkinsonian medication regimen. Some preliminary studies have also suggested that the dopamine agonist pramipexole might be effective in alleviating depressive symptoms (77–79). Effects of this medication on anxiety have not yet been studied.

Selegiline (deprenyl and Eldepryl) is a selective monoamine oxidase (MAO) type B inhibitor when used at low doses and it does not induce hypertensive crisis in patients with PD who are treated with dopaminergic agents. The drug is commonly used in PD to prolong the duration of levodopa action in patients with motor fluctuations and also because of controversial reports that this drug may slow the progression of PD. The drug has been found to be an effective antidepressant agent in psychiatric populations, but only at higher doses, with which its MAO-B selectivity is lost. Although selegiline has not been specifically tested for its antianxiety effects, depressed patients with anxiety or panic actually responded less well in one study to selegiline than those without anxiety symptoms (80). In an open-label pilot study conducted to determine whether amantadine helps treatment-resistant depression, eight patients (without PD) who were given amantadine over a period of 4 weeks demonstrated an improvement in both depression and anxiety scores (81).

Benzodiazepines

Stein et al. (2) comments that anxiety disorders in PD may respond to pharmacotherapy with antidepressants and benzodiazepines. Benzodiazepines can provide relief of symptoms associated with panic, GAD, and social phobia but are not indicated for OCD. Alprazolam was shown to be effective for anxiety symptoms in mixed anxiety-depressive disorder in patients who are more than 60 years old and who had just undergone bypass surgery (13).

However, Lauterbach and Duvoisin (11) cautioned that benzodiazepines can at times worsen parkinsonian symptoms, and benzodiazepines can also be problematic, because they can impair arousal, cognition, and balance. In their prospective assessment of falls among patients with PD, Bloem et al. (82) found that recurrent falls were more common among persons taking benzodiazepines.

In fact, animal studies have demonstrated that benzodiazepines can lower the levels of dopamine in the striatum, and one pilot study suggests that GABA antagonism may actually result in improved motor function (83). On the other hand, a comparison by Van de Vijver et al. (84) of rates of increase of antiparkinsonian drug treatment found no statistically significant difference between those patients who started a benzodiazepine and those who did not.

Buspirone

Buspirone can be effective for GAD but is unlikely to help panic, OCD, or social phobia (13). A study of buspirone in patients with PD, which was designed to investigate possible antiparkinsonian effects of the drug, showed that the agent was well tolerated in doses up to 60 mg but actually caused increased anxiety and worsening of motor function at doses of 100 mg per day. Antianxiety effects were not observed at the well-tolerated doses, but patients were not selected for the presence of anxiety (85). Another study investigating the efficacy of buspirone for dyskinesias in patients with PD revealed no change in depression or anxiety scores at a dosage of 20 mg per day. However, patients were not selected on the basis of psychological symptoms (86).

SSRIs

SSRIs are generally well tolerated and can be effective for almost all types of anxiety, including panic, OCD, and social phobia. Their role in treating GAD is less clear (13), although Wylie et al. (87) conducted an open-label trial of fluvoxamine (median daily dosage: 200 mg) that suggested efficacy in the treatment of GAD, panic disorder, and OCD in 19 older outpatients (mean age, 66.8).

Open-label studies of sertraline (88) and paroxetine (89,90) for *depressive* symptoms suggest that these agents may be well tolerated in patients with PD. In an article reviewing depression in PD, Slaughter et al. (91) describe their own unpublished experience with 10 consecutive patients on open-label sertraline. Nine of ten patients had moderate to complete resolution of depression. However, one patient reported an increase in anxiety and motor restlessness, requiring discontinuation of sertraline and introduction of lorazepam. After being treated for anxiety, this patient resumed sertraline, and the depressive symptoms resolved.

There are case reports of SSRIs increasing the level of motor disability in patients with PD (92–94), although other authors have reported that the drug does not appear to be associated with exacerbations of parkinsonian signs and symptoms (95–97). It is advisable to use an SSRI if deemed appropriate but to monitor motor function and discontinue the SSRI (gradually tapering the dosage to avoid a possible withdrawal syndrome) if it appears to have been associated with a worsening motor status. The issue of whether SSRIs result in motor dysfunction awaits a formal clinical trial, which would also address the issue of antidepressant and perhaps anxiolytic efficacy of these generally well-tolerated agents in patients with PD.

SNRIs

Very few clinicians use TCAs as first-line (or even second-line) agents because of their propensity to induce anticholinergic side effects and worsen orthostatic hypotension and because they can cause serious cardiac toxicity. No clinical trials of the SNRIs have been conducted in patients with PD. One SNRI, venlafaxine, has been shown to be effective in treating primary anxiety disorders and appears to be particularly effective in reducing anxiety symptoms in depressed patients (98). Data from several controlled trials support the safety and efficacy of venlafaxine for *depression* in geriatric populations (99). Venlafaxine can (rarely) be associated with an increase in blood pressure (99), which may be a benefit in the PD population, in whom pharmacologic and nonpharmacologic techniques are frequently used to increase blood pressure. Emerging data also suggest that venlafaxine may be helpful in neuropathic and other pain syndromes, an effect that may also be relevant in patients with PD (who may experience pain as a "nonmotor" symptom of PD) (99). There have been no published reports of venlafaxine worsening parkinsonian motor function.

Another frequently used SNRI is mirtazapine, a presynaptic alpha-2 antagonist (100). Mirtazapine is of particular interest in PD because it has been reported (in a case series involving 5 patients) to improve tremor and levodopa-induced dyskinesias (101). However, there are some conflicting reports regarding the effects of mirtazapine on motor function. Mirtazapine has been reported to be helpful in neuroleptic-induced akathisia (102,103), but it has also been reported to induce akathisia (104). Furthermore, although it is reported to be helpful for tremor and dyskinesias, it has also been reported to induce dystonia (105). Mirtazapine has been reported to both induce (106) and treat the serotonin syndrome (107) and may increase the propensity toward restless legs syndrome (108). Mirtazapine has also been associated with REM behavior disorder (RBD) (109) and psychosis (110) in parkinsonian patients (both of which are already problematic in many patients with PD). No controlled studies of this agent have been performed in patients with PD, but Pahwa and Lyons (111) conducted a randomized, double-blind, placebo-controlled crossover study of mirtazapine in 17 patients with essential tremor (ET). Most patients with ET did not benefit from mirtazapine. Adverse effects were common and included drowsiness, confusion, dry mouth, weight gain, polyuria, gait and balance problems, and blurred vision. Subjects were not selected based on the presence of anxiety, however; the aim of the therapy was to reduce tremor.

Cholinesterase Inhibitors

In his review of depression in patients with PD, Burn (112) brings up the possibility that cholinesterase inhibitors, currently used to treat dementia, may also have anxiolytic properties. He describes a randomized, double-blind, placebo-controlled study by McKeith et al. (113) of rivastigmine in patients with dementia with Lewy bodies (DLB), wherein anxiety (as measured using the Neuropsychiatric Inventory, or NPI) (114) improved in those subjects taking an active drug.

Potential Medication Interactions

Specific aspects of PD, especially the use of antiparkinsonian medications, may importantly influence the choice of medications used to treat anxiety in patients with this illness. For instance, nonselective MAOIs are contraindicated in patients receiving levodopa because of the risk of hypertensive crisis, and physicians are cautioned against the combined use of TCAs and SSRIs (and now SNRIs) with selegiline because of the potentially serious central nervous system (CNS) toxicity that may represent the serotonin syndrome. Manifestations of the serotonin syndrome vary but may include changes in motor and autonomic function and in mental status. Several years ago, we surveyed members of the Parkinson Study Group (PSG) and reviewed published case reports and adverse experiences reported to the US Food and Drug Administration and the manufacturer of Eldepryl. Serious adverse experiences resulting from the combined use of selegiline and antidepressants in patients with PD appeared to be quite rare, and occurrence of the true "serotonin syndrome" was even rarer (115). One patient treated with selegiline developed hypertensive crisis when given buspirone (86). A conservative approach would be to avoid selegiline in any PD patient who requires a TCA, an SSRI, an SNRI or, perhaps, buspirone for treatment of anxiety or depression. We believe that careful monitoring of patients on this combination is important and that patients should be informed of potential risks. We would not, however, consider the risks unacceptable if the patient could benefit from the combination of deprenyl and an antidepressant medication (115).

Surgery

The full effect that surgical therapies for PD may have on psychiatric symptoms is not clear. In one study of the effect of unilateral pallidotomy on cognition, patients reported significantly fewer symptoms of anxiety after surgery (116). In a study by Scott et al. (117), 20 consecutive patients who underwent posteroventral pallidotomy (8 bilateral and 12 unilateral procedures) were assessed 4 weeks before and 3 to 4 months after surgery, with minimal changes in medications. Motor function improved and, as a group, pallidotomy patients reported improved quality of life, reduced functional disability, and reduced anxiety and depression. Straits-Troster et al. (118) evaluated 23 subjects who underwent pallidotomy, 9 who underwent pallidal deep brain stimulation (DBS), and 7 who underwent thalamic DBS before surgery and 3 months after surgery. All three groups experienced significant improvement in motor function as measured by the UPDRS. Pallidal DBS patients had statistically significant improvements in symptoms of depressed mood and anxiety. The post-surgical changes in the pallidotomy group's depression and anxiety scale scores approached significance, but scores for patients with tremor-predominant PD who underwent thalamic DBS did not change significantly. The authors noted that it would be important to assess these changes over time to determine whether these mood changes were sustained or perhaps reflected post-surgical relief from anticipatory anxiety. Higginson et al. (119) evaluated 39 patients with PD 1 month before and 4 months after surgery (24 unilateral pallidotomy, 10 pallidal DBS, 4 thalamic DBS, and 1 unilateral thalamotomy). They noted statistically significant reductions of Beck Anxiety Inventory (BAI) (120) total score as well as neurophysiologic, autonomic, and subjective factors from the BAI. The panic factor did not significantly change after surgery; the authors suggested that this finding was possibly an artifact of limited power afforded by the sample size. The authors concluded that surgery reduces anxiety symptoms in a way that is independent of its effect on PD symptoms. Some investigators have noted improvements in OCD symptoms after high-frequency subthalamic stimulation (121) and after unilateral posteroventral pallidotomy (122). However, new onset mental automatisms (e.g., compulsive mental counting) have been reported after bilateral contemporaneous posteroventral pallidotomy (123).

SUMMARY

Anxiety disorders frequently occur in association with PD and may be important causes of morbidity. Actual prevalence rates are uncertain, but estimates suggest that up to 40% of patients with PD experience substantial anxiety. This percentage is greater than expected, particularly for an elderly population. In addition, the age at onset of anxiety in PD (and particularly panic disorder) is later than would be expected from current information regarding the natural course of anxiety disorders.

Virtually all of the types of anxiety disorders have been described in PD, but panic disorder, GAD, and social phobia appear to be the ones most commonly encountered. Although most patients with motor fluctuations experience greater anxiety during the "off" phase, this is not a universal phenomenon.

Anxiety frequently develops before the motor features do, suggesting that anxiety may not represent psychological and social difficulties in adapting to the illness but rather may be linked to specific neurobiologic processes that occur in PD.

Most evidence points to disturbances in central noradrenergic systems, but other neurotransmitters (e.g., serotonin, dopamine) may be involved as well. Studies suggest that right hemispheric disturbances may be particularly important for the genesis of anxiety, especially panic and OCD. Whether antiparkinsonian medications themselves contribute to anxiety needs clarification.

Anxiety and depression frequently coexist in PD. It remains to be determined whether anxiety in patients with PD reflects one of the following pathologies: (a) an underlying depressive mood disorder, (b) a particular subtype of depression (atypical depression, anxious or agitated depression), or (c) an independent psychiatric disturbance. The relationship between anxiety and dementia in PD is not clear, but current evidence suggests that cognitive dysfunction is not related to the presence of anxiety symptoms in this disorder.

The optimal pharmacologic treatment for anxiety in patients with PD has not been established, nor has the effect of PD surgery on anxiety symptoms.

ACKNOWLEDGMENTS

Dr. Richard's research has been supported by the National Institute of Neurological Disorders and Stroke (#1 K23 NS 02184) and by a Young Investigator Award from the National Alliance for Research in Schizophrenia and Depression (NARSAD). I would like to thank Donna LaDonna for her help preparing the manuscript.

REFERENCES

1. American Psychiatric Association. *Diagnostic and statistical manual of mental disorders*, 4th ed. Washington, DC, 1994.
2. Stein M, Henser I, Juncos J, et al. Anxiety disorders in patients with Parkinson's disease. *Am J Psychiatry* 1990;147:217–220.
3. Vazquez A, Jimenez-Jimenez F, Garcia-Ruiz P, et al. "Panic attacks" in Parkinson's disease: a long-term complication of levodopa therapy. *Acta Neurol Scand* 1993;87:14–18.
4. American Psychiatric Association. *Diagnostic and statistical manual of mental disorders*, 3rd ed. Washington, DC, 1987.
5. Schiffer R, Kurlan R, Rubin A. Evidence for atypical depression in Parkinson's disease. *Am J Psychiatry* 1988;145:1020–1022.
6. Menza M, Robertson-Hoffman D, Bonapace A. Parkinson's disease and anxiety: comorbidity with depression. *Biol Psychiatry* 1993;34:465–470.
7. Menza M, Mark M. Parkinson's disease and depression: the relationship to disability and personality. *J Neuropsychiatry Clin Neurosci* 1994;6:165–169.
8. Gotham A-M, Brown R, Marsden C. Depression in Parkinson's disease: a quantitative and qualitative analysis. *J Neurol Neurosurg Psychiatry* 1986;49:381–389.
9. Berrios GE, Campbell C, Politynska BE. Autonomic failure, depression and anxiety in Parkinson's disease. *B J Psychiatry* 1995;166;789–792.
10. Flint A. Epidemiology and comorbidity of anxiety disorders in the elderly. *Am J Psychiatry* 1994;151:640–649.
11. Lauterbach E, Duvoisin R. Anxiety disorders and familial Parkinsonism [Letter]. *Am J Psychiatry* 1992;148:274.
12. Palmer B, Jeste D, Sheikh J. Anxiety disorders in the elderly: DSM-IV and other barriers to diagnosis and treatment. *J Affect Disord* 1997;46(3):183–190.
13. Small G. Recognizing and treating anxiety in the elderly. *J Clin Psychiatry* 1997;58:41–47.
14. Maia A, Pinto A, Barbosa E, et al. obsessive–compulsive symptoms, obsessive–compulsive disorder, and related disorders in Parkinson's disease. *J Neuropsychiatry Clin Neurosci* 2003;15:371–374.
15. Muller N, Putz A, Kathmann N, et al. Characteristics of obsessive–compulsive symptoms in Tourette's syndrome, obsessive–compulsive disorder and Parkinson's disease. *Psychiatry Res* 1997;70:105–114.
16. Alegret M, Junque C, Valldeoriola F, et al. obsessive–compulsive symptoms in Parkinson's disease. *J Neurol Neurosurg Psychiatry* 2001;70:394–396.
17. Richard I, Schiffer R, Kurlan R. Anxiety and Parkinson's disease. *J Neuropsychiatry Clin Neurosci* 1996; 8:383–392.
18. Henderson R, Kurlan R, Kersun J. Preliminary examination of the comorbidity of anxiety and depression in Parkinson's disease. *J Neuropsychiatry Clin Neurosci* 1992;4:257–264.

19. Seimers E, Shekhar A, Quaid K, et al. Anxiety and motor performance in Parkinson's disease. *Mov Disord* 1993;8:501–506.
20. Rondot P, deRecondo J, Colgnet A, et al. Mental disorders in Parkinson's disease after treatment with L-dopa. *Adv Neurol* 1984;40:259–269.
21. Factor S, Molho E, Podskalny G, et al. Parkinson's disease: drug-induced psychiatric states. In: Weiner W, Lang A, eds. *Behavioral neurology of movement disorders*. New York: Raven Press, 1995.
22. Nissenbaum H, Quinn N, Brown R, et al. Mood swings associated with the "on-off" phenomenon in Parkinson's disease. *Psychol Med* 1987;17:899–904.
23. Seligman M. Chronic fear produced by unpredictable shock. *J Comp Physiol Psychol* 1968;66:402–411.
24. Riley D, Lang A. The spectrum of levodopa-related fluctuations in Parkinson's disease. *Neurology* 1993;43:1459–1464.
25. Marsden C, Parkes J. "On-off" effects in patients with Parkinson's disease on chronic levodopa therapy. *Lancet* 1976;1:292–296.
26. Menza M, Sage J, Marshall E, et al. Mood changes and "on-off" phenomena in Parkinson's disease. *Mov Disord* 1990;5:148–151.
27. Maricle R, Nutt J, Valentine R, et al. Dose-response relationship of levodopa with mood and anxiety in fluctuating Parkinson's disease: a double-blind, placebo controlled study. *Neurology* 1995;45:1757–1760.
28. Jimenez-Jimenez F, Vazquez A, Molina J. Nonmotor fluctuations in patients with Parkinson's disease. *Neurology* 1997;49:1472.
29. Richard I, Justus A, Kurlan R. The relationship between mood and motor fluctuations in Parkinson's disease. *J Neuropsychiatry Clin Neurosci* 2001;3:35–41.
30. Targum S. Differential responses to anxiogenic challenge studies in patients with major depressive disorder and panic disorder. *Biol Psychiatry* 1990;28:21–34.
31. Cummings J. Depression and Parkinson's disease. A review. *Am J Psychiatry* 1992;149:443–454.
32. Richard I, Szegethy E, Lichter D, et al. Parkinson's disease: a preliminary study of yohimbine challenge in patients with anxiety. *Clin Neuropharmacol* 1999;22:172–175.
33. Fleminger S. Left-sided Parkinson's disease is associated with greater anxiety and depression. *Psychol Med* 1991;21:629–638.
34. Lui C, Yang S, Fuh J, et al. The correlation of depression with functional activity in Parkinson's disease. *J Neurol* 1997;244:493–498.
35. Wands K, Merskey H, Hachinski V, et al. A questionnaire investigation of anxiety and depression in early dementia. *J Am Geriatr Soc* 1990;38:535–538.
36. Iruela L, Ibanez-Rojo V, Immaculada P, et al. Anxiety disorders and Parkinson's disease [Letter]. *Am J Psychiatry* 1992;149:719–720.
37. Cash R, Dennis T, L'Heureux R, et al. Parkinson's disease and dementia: norepinephrine and dopamine in locus ceruleus. *Neurology* 1987;37:42–46.
38. Lauterbach E. The locus ceruleus and anxiety disorders in demented and nondemented familial parkinsonism [Letter]. *Am J Psychiatry* 1993;150:994.
39. Kurlan R, Lichter D, Schiffer R. Panic/anxiety in Parkinson's disease: yohimbine challenge [Abstract]. *Neurology* 1989;39(Suppl. 1):421.
40. Shiba M, Bower J, Maraganore D, et al. Anxiety disorders and depressive disorders preceding Parkinson's disease: a case-control study. *Mov Disord* 2000;15:669–677.
41. Nutt D, Lawson C. Panic attacks: a neurochemical overview of models and mechanisms. *Br J Psychiatry* 1992;160:165–178.
42. Heninger G, Charney D. Monoamine receptor systems and anxiety disorders. *Psychiatr Clin North Am* 1988;11:309–326.
43. Owens M, Nemeroff C. The role of corticotropin-releasing factory in the pathophysiology of affective and anxiety disorders: laboratory and clinical studies. *Ciba Found Symp* 1993;172:296–308.
44. Hattori E, Ebihara M, Yamada K, et al. Identification of a compound short tandem repeat stretch in the 5'-upstream region of the cholecystokinin gene, and its association with panic disorder but not with schizophrenia. *Mol Psychiatry* 2001;6:465–470.
45. Charney D, Heninger G, Brief A. Noradrenergic function in panic anxiety: effects of yohimbine in healthy subjects and patients with agoraphobia and panic disorder. *Arch Gen Psychiatry* 1984;41:751–763.
46. Charney D, Heninger G. Abnormal regulation of noradrenergic function in panic disorders: effects of clonidine in healthy subjects and patients with agoraphobia and panic disorder. *Arch Gen Psychiatry* 1986;43:1042–1054.
47. Charney D, Woods S, Goodman W, et al. Neurobiological mechanisms of panic anxiety: biochemical and behavioral correlates of yohimbine-induced panic attacks. *Am J Psychiatry* 1987;144:1030–1036.
48. Uhde T, Stein M, Vittone B, et al. Behavioral and physiologic effects of short-term and long-term administration of clonidine in panic disorder. *Arch Gen Psychiatry* 1989;46:170–177.
49. Nutt D. Altered alpha-2-adrenoceptor sensitivity in panic disorder. *Arch Gen Psychiatry* 1989;46:165–169.
50. Agid Y, Cervera P, Hirsch E, et al. Biochemistry of Parkinson's disease 28 years later: a critical review. *Mov Disord* 1989;4(Suppl. 1):S126–S144.
51. Insel T, Zohar J, Benkelfat C, et al. Serotonin in obsessions, compulsions, and the control of aggressive impulses. *Ann N Y Acad Sci* 1990;600:574–585.
52. Miner C, Davidson J. Biological characterization of social phobia [Review]. *Eur Arch Psychiatry Clin Neurosci* 1995;244:304–308.
53. Charney D, Woods S, Krystal J, et al. Serotonin function in human anxiety disorders. *Ann N Y Acad Sci* 1990;600:558–572.
54. Potts N, Davidson J. Social phobia: biological aspects and pharmacotherapy. *Prog Neuropsychopharmacol Biol Psychiatry* 1992;16:635–646.
55. Hamilton S, Haghighi F, Heiman G, et al. Investigation of dopamine receptor (DRD4) and dopamine transporter (DAT) polymorphisms for genetic linkage or association to panic disorder. *Am J Med Genet* 2000;96:324–330.
56. Tomer R, Levin B, Weiner W. obsessive–compulsive symptoms and motor asymmetries in Parkinson's disease. *Neuropsychiatry Neuropsychol Behav Neurol* 1993;6:26–30.
57. Menza M, Palermo B, DiPaola R, et al. Depression and anxiety in Parkinson's disease: possible effect of genetic variation in the serotonin transporter. *J Geriatr Psychiatry Neurol* 1999;12:49–52.

58. McDougle C, Goodman W, Price L. Dopamine antagonists in tic-related and psychotic spectrum obsessive compulsive disorder [Literature Review]. *J Clin Psychiatry* 1994;55 (Suppl. 3):24–31.
59. Marazziti D, Hollander E, Lensi P, et al. Peripheral markers of serotonin and dopamine function in obsessive–compulsive disorder. *Psychiatry Res* 1992;42:41–51.
60. Pitchot W, Ansseau M, Gonzalez Moreno A, et al. Dopaminergic function in panic disorder: comparison with major and minor depression. *Biol Psychiatry* 1992;32:1004–1011.
61. Argyl N. Panic attacks in chronic schizophrenia. *Br J Psychiatry* 1990;157:430–433.
62. Tiihonen J, Kuikka J, Bergstrom K, et al. Dopamine reuptake site densities in patients with social phobia. *Am J Psychiatry* 1997;154:239–242.
63. Schneier F, Liebowitz M, Abi-Dargham A, et al. Low dopamine D(2) receptor binding potential in social phobia. *Am J Psychiatry* 2000;157:457–459.
64. Kennedy J, Neves-Pereira M, King N, et al. Dopamine system genes not linked to social phobia. *Psychiatr Gen* 2001;11:213–217.
65. Cedarbaum J, Aghajanian G. Catecholamine receptors on locus ceruleus neurons: pharmacological characterization. *Eur J Pharmacol* 1977;44:375–385.
66. Fountaine R, Breton G, Dery R, et al. Temporal lobe abnormalities in panic disorder: an MRI study. *Biol Psychiatry* 1990;27:304–310.
67. Woodman C, Tabatabai F. New-onset panic disorder after right thalamic infarct. *Psychosomatics* 1998;39:165–167.
68. Rubin A, Kurlan R, Schiffer R. Atypical depression in Parkinson's disease [Abstract]. *Ann Neurol* 1986;20:150.
69. Faulstich M, Sullivan D. Positron emission tomography in neuropsychiatry. *Invest Radiol* 1991;26:184–194.
70. Davidson J, Krishnan K, Charles H, et al. Magnetic resonance spectroscopy in social phobia: preliminary findings. *J Clin Psychiatry* 1993;54(Suppl. 12):19–24.
71. Potts N, Davidson J, Krishnan K, et al. Magnetic resonance imaging in social phobia. *Psychiatry Res* 1994;52:35–42.
72. Hollander E, Cohen L, Richards M, et al. A pilot study of the neuropsychology of obsessive–compulsive disorder and Parkinson's disease: basal ganglia disorders. *J Neuropsychiatry Clin Neurosci* 1993;5:104–107.
73. Saint-Cyr J, Taylor A, Nicholson K. Behavior and the basal ganglia [Literature Review]. *Adv Neurol* 1995;65:1–28.
74. Pearson J. Research in late-life anxiety. Summary of a National Institute of Mental Health Workshop on late-life anxiety. *Psychopharmacol Bull* 1998;34:127–138.
75. Salzman C. Anxiety in the elderly: treatment strategies. *J Clin Psychiatry* 1990;51(Suppl. 10):18–21.
76. Stoudemire A, Moran M. Psychopharmacologic treatment of anxiety in the medically ill elderly patient: special considerations. *J Clin Psychiatry* 1993;54 (Suppl. 5):27–33.
77. Pogarell O, Kunig G, Oertel W. A non-ergot dopamine agonist, pramipexole, in the therapy of advanced Parkinson's disease: improvement of parkinsonian symptoms and treatment-associated complications. A review of three studies. *Clin Neuropharmacol* 1997;20:S28–S35.
78. Corrigan M, Evans CM, DL. Pramipexole, a dopamine agonist, in the treatment of major depression. Abstract presented at annual American Society of Neuropsychology meeting, Honolulu, 1997.
79. Szegedi A, Hillert A, Wetzel H, et al. Pramipexole, a dopamine agonist, in major depression: antidepressant effects and tolerability in an open-label study with multiple doses. *Clin Neuropharmacol* 1997;20:S36–S45.
80. Mann J, Aarons S, Wilner P, et al. A controlled study of the antidepressant efficacy and side effects of (-) deprenyl. *Arch Gen Psychiatry* 1989;46:45–50.
81. Stryjer R, Strous R, Shaked G, et al. Amantadine as augmentation therapy in the management of treatment-resistant depression. *Int Clin Psychopharmacol* 2003;18:93–96.
82. Bloem B, Grimbergen Y, Cramer M, et al. Prospective assessment of falls in Parkinson's disease. *J Neurol* 2001;248:950–958.
83. Ondo, H. Flumazenil, a GABA antagonist, may improve features of Parkinson's disease. *Mov Disord* 2003;18:683–685.
84. Van de Vijver D, Roos R, Jansen P, et al. Influence of benzodiazepines on antiparkinsonian drug treatment in levodopa users. *Acta Neurol Scand* 2002;105:8–12.
85. Ludwig C, Weinberger D, Bruno G, et al. Buspirone, Parkinson's disease, and the locus ceruleus. *Clin Neuropharmacol* 1986;9:373–378.
86. Bonifati V, Fabrizio E, Cipriani R, et al. Buspirone in levodopa-induced dyskinesias. *Clin Neuropharmacol* 1994;17:73–82.
87. Wylie M, Miller M, Shear M, et al. Fluvoxamine pharmacotherapy of anxiety disorders in later life: preliminary open-trial data. *J Geriatr Psychiatry and Neurology* 2000;13:43–48.
88. Hauser R, Zesiewicz T. Sertraline for the treatment of depression in Parkinson's disease. *Mov Disord* 1997;12:756–759.
89. Ceravolo R, Nuti A, Piccinni A, et al. Effects on motor and depressive symptoms. *Neurology* 2000;55:1216–1218.
90. Tesei S, Antonini A, Canesi M, et al. Tolerability of paroxetine in Parkinson's disease: a prospective study. *Mov Disord* 2000;15:986–989.
91. Slaughter J, Slaughter K, Nichols D, et al. Prevalence, clinical manifestations, etiology, and treatment of depression in Parkinson's disease. *J Neuropsychiatry Clin Neurosci* 2001;13:187–196.
92. Jansen Steur H. Increase of Parkinson disability after fluoxetine medication. *Neurology* 1993;43:211–213.
93. Chouinard G, Sultan S. A case of Parkinson's disease exacerbated by fluoxetine. *Hum Psychopharmacol* 1992;7:63–66.
94. Jimenez-Jimenez F, Tejeiro J, Martinez-Junquera G, et al. Parkinsonism exacerbated by paroxetine. *Neurology* 1994;44:2406.
95. Caley C, Friedman J. Does fluoxetine exacerbate Parkinson's disease? *J Clin Psychiatry* 1992;53:278–282.
96. Montastruc J-L, Fabre N, Blin O. Does fluoxetine aggravate Parkinson's disease? A pilot prospective study. *Mov Disord* 1995;10:355–357.
97. Shulman L, Singer C, Liefert R, et al. Therapeutic effects of sertraline in patients with Parkinson's disease. *Mov Disord* 1996;11:603.
98. Davidson J, Meoni P, Harudiequet V, et al. Achieving remission with venlafaxine and fluoxetine in major depression: its relationship to anxiety symptoms. *Depress Anxiety* 2002;16:4–13.
99. Staab J, Evans D. Efficacy of venlafaxine in geriatric depression. *Depress Anxiety* 2000;12:63–68.

100. Fawcett J, Barkin R. Review of the results from clinical studies on the efficacy, safety and tolerability of mirtazapine for the treatment of patients with major depression. *J Affect Disord* 1998;51:267–285.
101. Pact V, Giduz T. Mirtazapine treats resting tremor, essential tremor, and levodopa-induced dyskinesias. *Neurology* 1999;53:1154.
102. Poyurovsky M, Shardorodsky M, Fuchs C, et al. Treatment of neuroleptic-induced akathisia with the 5-HT2 antagonist mianserin. Double-blind, placebo-controlled study. *Br J Psychiatry* 1999;174:238–242.
103. Poyurovsky M, Weizman A. Mirtazapine for neuroleptic-induced akathisia. *Am J Psychiatry* 2001;158:819.
104. Girishchandra B, Johnson L, SCresp R, et al. Mirtazapine-induced akathisia. *Med J Aust* 2002; 176:242.
105. Lu R, Hurley A, Gourley M. Dystonia induced by mirtazapine. *J Clin Psychiatry* 2002;63:452–453.
106. Hernandez J, Ramos F, Infante J, et al. Severe serotonin syndrome induced by mirtazapine monotherapy. *Ann Pharmacother* 2002;36:641–643.
107. Hoes M, Zeijpveld J. Mirtazapine as treatment for serotonin syndrome. *Pharmacopsychiatry* 1996;29:81.
108. Bahk W, Pae C, Chae J, et al. Mirtazapine may have the propensity for developing a restless legs syndrome? A case report. *Psychiatry Clin Neurosci* 2002;56:209–210.
109. Onofrj M, Luciano A, Thomas A, et al. Mirtazapine induces REM sleep behavior disorder (RBD) in parkinsonism. *Neurology* 2003;60:113–115.
110. Normann C, Hesslinger B, Frauenknecht S, et al. Psychosis during chronic levodopa therapy triggered by the new antidepressive drug mirtazapine. *Pharmacopsychiatry* 1997;30:263–265.
111. Pahwa R, Lyons K. Mirtazapine in essential tremor: a double-blind, placebo-controlled pilot study. *Mov Disord* 2003;18:584–587.
112. Burn D. Beyond the iron mask: towards better recognition and treatment of depression associated with Parkinson's disease. *Mov Disord* 2002;17:445–454.
113. McKeith I, Del Ser T, Spano P, et al. Efficacy of rivastigmine in dementia with Lewy bodies: a randomised, double-blind, placebo-controlled international study. *Lancet* 2000;356:2031–2036.
114. Cummings J, Mega M, Gray K, et al. The neuropsychiatric inventory: comprehensive assessment of psychopathology in dementia. *Neurology* 1994;44: 2308–2314.
115. Richard I, Kurlan R, Tanner C, et al. Serotonin syndrome and the combined use of deprenyl and an antidepressant in Parkinson's disease. *Neurology* 1997; 48:1070–1077.
116. Troster A, Fields J, Wilkinson S, et al. Unilateral pallidal stimulation for Parkinson's disease: neurobehavioral functioning before and 3 months after electrode implantation. *Neurology* 1997;49:1078–1083.
117. Scott R, Gregory R, Hines N, et al. Neuropsychological, neurological and functional outcome following pallidotomy for Parkinson's disease: a consecutive series of eight simultaneous bilateral and twelve unilateral procedures. *Brain* 1998;121:659–675.
118. Straits-Troster K, Fields J, Wilkinson S, et al. Health-related quality of life in Parkinson's disease after pallidotomy and deep brain stimulation. *Brain Cogn* 2000; 42:399–416.
119. Higginson C, Fields J, Troster A. Which symptoms of anxiety diminish after surgical interventions for Parkinson's disease? *Neuropsychiatry Neuropsychol Behav Neurol* 2001;14:117–121.
120. Beck A, Epstein N, Brown G, et al. An inventory for measuring clinical anxiety: psychometric properties. *J Consult Clin Psychol* 1988;56:893–897.
121. Mallet L, Mesnage V, Houeto J, et al. Compulsions, Parkinson's disease, and stimulation. *Lancet* 2002; 360:1302–1304.
122. Junque C, Alegret M, Nobbe F, et al. Cognitive and behavioral changes after unilateral posteroventral pallidotomy: relationship with lesional data from MRI. *Mov Disord* 1999;14:780–789.
123. Dhika J, Ghika-Schmid F, Fankhauser H, et al. Bilateral contemporaneous posteroventral pallidotomy for the treatment of Parkinson's disease: neuropsychological and neurological side effects. Report of four cases and review of the literature. *J Neurosurg* 1999;91: 313–321.

5

Disorders of Motivation, Sexual Conduct, and Sleep in Parkinson's Disease

Dag Aarsland,[1] Guido Alves,[2] Jan P. Larsen[3]

[1]Stavanger University Hospital, Psychiatric Clinic and School of Medicine, University of Bergen, Norway; [2]Stavanger University Hospital, Department of Neurology; [3]Stavanger University Hospital, Department of Neurology and School of Medicine

Mediated through its four major pathways, the mesolimbic, the mesocortical, the tuberoinfundibular, and the nigrostriatal pathways, dopamine exerts effects on a wide spectrum of human behaviors and disorders, ranging from mood, motivation, emotions, working memory, reward mechanisms, sleep, hallucinations, and sexual functioning, in addition to motor functioning. Other neurotransmitter systems involved in human behavior, such as serotonin and noradrenalin pathways, as well as limbic and frontal cortices, are also affected in Parkinson's disease (PD) (1). Thus, it is not surprising that PD and dopaminergic therapies are associated with a wide range of behavioral alterations and psychiatric symptoms.

Depression, anxiety, irritability, and visual hallucinations are among the most common psychiatric symptoms in PD (2–4) and have received much scientific focus during the last decade. This chapter will discuss some of the less commonly described behavioral manifestations encountered in patients with PD, such as apathy and fatigue, sexual disturbances, mania, sleep disturbances, personality changes, pathologic gambling, and addiction to antiparkinsonian agents. The limited evidence available to guide treatment of these symptoms will be briefly reviewed.

APATHY

Apathy consists of lack of motivation with diminished goal-directed behavior, reduced goal-directed cognition, and decreased emotional engagement. Validated apathy rating scales include the apathy evaluation scale (5) and the Starkstein Apathy Scale (6), and assessment of apathy is included in the Neuropsychiatric Inventory (NPI) (7). Although symptoms of apathy may overlap those of depression, there is evidence that apathy is separable from depression (8,9), and a considerable proportion of patients with PD exhibit apathy in the absence of depression (10). Patients with apathy without depression do not show key symptoms of depression, such as sadness and feelings of helplessness, hopelessness, and worthlessness.

Apathy occurs in neurodegenerative diseases such as frontotemporal dementia, Alzheimer's disease, dementia with Lewy bodies (DLB), and progressive supranuclear palsy (8,11). Many factors potentially contribute to apathetic behavior, including parietal, limbic, and frontal pathologies (11). Across diagnostic groups, apathy is related to functional disturbance of the anterior cingulum (12–14), an area with reciprocal connections with limbic and frontal cortices and basal ganglia structures.

Several studies have explored the prevalence of apathy in patients with PD, and findings range from 17% to 70% (3,4,6,8,10,15) (see Table 5-1). This variability probably reflects the different instruments used to assess apathy, different cut-off values for defining apathy, and different populations of patients with PD. In particular, because apathy is associated with cognitive

TABLE 5-1. *Prevalence of apathy in PD*

Study (reference)	Sample	N	Mean MMSE score	Instrument	% with apathy	Higher than control group
Aarsland 1999 (3)	Community-based	139	25.2	NPI	17	No control group
Ringman 2002 (4)	Hospital-based	40	22.5	NPI	40	Yes (nonneurological patients)
Isella 2002 (10)	Hospital-based	33	#	AES	70 (43)*	Yes (healthy)
Starkstein 1992 (6)	Hospital-based	50	25–28	SAS	42	No control group
Levy 1998 (8)	Hospital-based	40	27.9	NPI	33	No (other degenerative brain disease)
Pluck 2002 (15)	Hospital-based	45	27.8	AES	38	Yes (osteoarthritis)

MMSE, Mini-Mental State Examination; NPI, Neuropsychiatric Inventory (7); AES, Apathy evaluation scale (5); SAS, Starkstein Apathy Scale (6).
*After adjusting cutoff score.
MMSE score not given. Mean cognitive scores suggest only mild impairment.

impairment (8,10,15), the reported prevalence of apathy will vary according to whether patients with dementia are included or not. A strong correlation between apathy and executive dysfunction has been reported (10,15). Although the prevalence varies among studies, there is consistency between studies in that apathy is more common and severe in patients with PD than in healthy subjects or patients without brain disease (10,15,16), although apathy in PD is less common and less severe than in patients with Alzheimer's disease, frontotemporal dementia, and progressive supranuclear palsy (8,16–18) (Table 5-1).

To control for the possibility that apathy is a psychological reaction or adaptation to nonspecific disability (15), apathy scores in patients with PD were compared with those of patients with osteoarthritis with a similar level of functional impairment. Apathy increased significantly among patients with PD, compared to those with osteoarthritis, suggesting that apathy is a direct consequence of disease-related physiologic changes.

The dopaminergic reward system might be implicated in the pathogenesis of apathy in patients with PD; thus, dopaminergic drugs may improve this syndrome. Controlled clinical trials focusing on apathy have not been reported; however, in an uncontrolled study, dopaminergic therapy was associated with improved motivation (19). In a randomized trial, anecdotal reports indicated decreased apathy during treatment with pramipexole (20), a dopamine agonist with a preferential affinity for the D3 receptors, which induces clinically relevant changes in orbitofrontal and anterior cingulate cortices (21). A case report suggested that methylphenidate may improve apathy in patients with PD (22). Finally, open-label trials indicate that cholinergic agents may improve apathy in patients with PD (23): in a placebo-controlled trial of rivastigmine in DLB, a disorder clinically and neurobiologically similar to PD with dementia, apathy was among the neuropsychiatric symptoms that differed significantly between the treatment groups (24).

FATIGUE

Fatigue, defined as an overwhelming sense of tiredness, lack of energy, and feeling of exhaustion (25), can appear as a mental and physical symptom (26,27). It is a common symptom in several neurologic, psychiatric, and systemic diseases of unknown etiology. Pathologic cytokines in certain areas of the brain, frontal lobe dysfunction, and dopaminergic dysfunction in limbic structures may play a role in the pathogenesis of fatigue in PD (28–30).

Several clinical studies have shown prevalence rates of fatigue of more than 40% of patients with PD (31–34). Up to one third of patients with PD described fatigue as their most disabling symptom (31,32), with a negative effect on quality of life (35). Its subjective nature and the comorbidity with other common nonmotor features may confound the measurement of fatigue in patients with PD. However, it can be distinguished from depression, in which lack of self-esteem, despair, and feelings of hopelessness are prominent features (34).

In a randomized crossover study, levodopa significantly improved physical fatigue in finger tapping and force generation in patients with PD (27), supporting the hypothesis that physical fatigue in patients with PD is at least partially related to dopaminergic deficiency. Modafinil, a novel wake-promoting agent, improved fatigue in a crossover trial in patients with multiple sclerosis (36), but not in patients with PD (37).

SEXUAL DISTURBANCES

Dopamine is involved in the complex neurochemical regulation of sexual function, either directly through the putative relation between libido and orgasm and the mesolimbic dopaminergic "reward center" (38), or by influencing the pituitary secretion of prolactin and by stimulating the release of oxytocin, which is directly involved in the physical and emotional components of the sexual response (39). Thus, it is not surprising that sexual disturbances are common among both men and women with PD. They are more commonly reported by male patients and their female spouses (40). The most commonly reported disturbances are impotence and reduced libido in men, whereas women may report difficulty in achieving arousal and orgasm. Sildenafil may improve erectile dysfunction in male PD subjects (41), and in many cases, antiparkinsonian treatment may improve these disturbances. However, in a few patients, dopaminergic agents may induce hypersexuality and paraphilias, although the exact prevalence is not known. In a review of the early literature, Cummings (42) reported hypersexuality in 3% of patients with PD who were receiving dopaminergic therapy and noted that most cases involved treatment with levodopa. In an early review, Goodwin reported hypersexual behavior in 0.9% of patients with PD (43). Other authors have suggested that the dopamine agonist pergolide may impressively improve sexual disturbances but also induce hypersexuality. Seven of 32 male patients with advanced PD who received pergolide in addition to levodopa reported important changes in their sexual functions, such as hypersexuality and hyperlibidinous behavior (44). Reversible transvestic fetishism was described in a 72-year-old man with a long history of levodopa-treated PD, after selegiline was added (45). The covert nature of paraphilic behavior until accidentally reported by family members in several of the cases suggests that in many patients with PD, such complications may remain undetected. Dose reduction and psychotherapy usually alleviates the behavior disturbance, although this approach may be difficult because of the worsening of motor symptoms (44).

DISTURBANCES OF SLEEP

During the last 10 years, the scientific understanding of the sleep/wake regulation in the brain has entered a new era. The functions of several brainstem nuclei, with their communicating pathways in the ascending arousing system through the hypothalamus and thalamus to the cortex, have been clarified (46). In patients with PD, Lewy bodies and neuronal cell loss may often be found in these brainstem areas—outside the classical lesions in the substantia nigra. Therefore, patients with PD can be expected to experience a number of sleep disorders, such as insomnia, daytime somnolence, and parasomnias including rapid eye movement (REM) sleep behavior disorder (rapid eye movement behavior disorder, RBD) (47,48). In addition to the influence of the cerebral pathology of the disease, dopaminergic medication and coexisting behavioral pathologies, like depression, may contribute to the much higher than expected frequencies of sleep disorders in patients with PD.

Insomnia is a common and important complaint of patients with PD. We found that 60% of patients reported frequent nocturnal sleeping problems, and about 25% of them rated their overall nighttime problem as moderate to severe. The most common problems were frequent awakening (sleep fragmentation) and early awakening (49), and these problems were more important contributors to impaired quality of life than the motor symptoms (50). Increasing the dosage of dopaminergic treatment will often increase sleep disruption and should be avoided unless the patient's sleep is primarily disturbed by the motor manifestations of parkinsonism during the night. Depression should be looked for and, if appropriate, be treated in patients with insomnia.

Excessive daytime sleepiness (EDS) is also common in patients with PD (51). Family and social interactions often decrease, and driving may be limited or stopped completely. EDS is thought to be primarily caused by the cerebral lesions of PD itself (52), but dopaminergic agents contribute as well (53). In sleep attacks, that is, sudden-onset sleep episodes, the dopaminergic treatment may be the more likely cause, and patients with PD should be informed about the possibility of developing sleep problems during the day when new drugs are prescribed. The results from 2 crossover studies, which included 21 and 15 patients with PD (37 and 54, respectively), suggest that modafinil improves EDS in patients with PD to the same degree as that shown in patients with narcolepsy. Modafinil should be considered in patients with severe problems that do not respond when dopaminergic treatment is reduced.

RBD is one of several parasomnias that occur in PD, and is characterized by loss of skeletal muscle atonia during REM sleep, with prominent motor activity and dreaming. The typical clinical features of RBD include vocalizations ranging from mumbles and screaming to intelligible speech. Movement can vary from single limb jerks to complex behaviors such as walking and even punching. The dream content is often frightening. Because most REM sleep occurs in the latter half of the night, RBD tends to occur in the early morning hours. Recent studies have shown that patients with RBD have a predilection for neurodegenerative disorders characterized by alpha-synucleinopathy, such as DLB, multiple system atrophy (MSA), and PD.

In a clinicopathologic study of 15 patients who had showed RBD, all patients had synucleinopathy: DLB ($n = 6$), MSA ($n = 2$), or PD ($n = 2$) (55). In many cases, RBD begins years before parkinsonism evolves (56). The underlying pathophysiology of RBD in patients with PD is complex and not known in detail. Several pontine and midbrain nuclei are involved, such as the pedunculus-pontine nucleus and locus caeruleus, as are dopaminergic, noradrenergic, serotonergic, and cholinergic neurotransmission (57). The involvement of the dopamine system is supported by the connection between RBD and reduction of striatal dopamine transporters (58) and the improvement of RBD with levodopa treatment (59).

Although controlled trials of RBD have not been reported, the mainstay of treatment has been a dose of 0.5 to 1.0 mg per day of clonazepam in addition to ensuring safety in the sleep environment (60). In one open-label study, 12 of 14 patients with RBD improved with melatonin, after having experienced side effects or lack of improvement with clonazepam (61). Although cholinesterase inhibitors may occasionally aggravate RBD and induce parasomnias in some patients, these drugs may improve RBD in other patients (62).

MANIA

Although depression is the most common neuropsychiatric symptom in PD (2–4), behavioral changes in the opposite direction may occur in some patients. Such changes can vary from simple euphoria with feelings of well being to fully developed manic episodes with elation, increased psychomotor activity, risk-taking behaviors, and decreased need for sleep. On the basis of early literature, Cummings estimated the prevalence of mania in PD to be about 1% of the patients who were treated with dopaminergic agents (42). For example, Goodwin reported hypomania in 1.5% of patients with PD (43). The emergence of mania on dopaminergic drugs is consistent with the hypothesis that dopaminergic neurotransmission is increased in bipolar disorder, and with the possible improvement of depression during treatment with the D3-preferring agonist pramipexole in patients with PD (63) as well as those without PD

(64). A bipolar affective syndrome occurs in some patients with PD, usually after 3 to 5 years of dopaminergic therapy, and may develop after dose increase (65). In some cases, remission of PD may occur during manic episodes (65).

Little is known regarding the treatment of manic symptoms in patients with PD. The dosage of dopaminergic agents should be reduced, and antidepressants must be withdrawn immediately when manic symptoms occur. Atypical antipsychotics should be considered if manic symptoms are accompanied by hallucinations or delusions (65). Successful antimanic treatment has been reported with mood-stabilizing drugs, such as lithium and clozapine (66), but one should proceed with caution in patients with PD, since lithium may cause severe side-effects, and neither has been systematically tested in patients with PD.

Recently, several reports have described the development of mania after deep brain stimulation, particularly stimulation involving the lower electrodes caudal to the subthalamic nucleus area (67,68) and after pallidotomy, particularly lesions involving the anterior, nonmotor portion of the pallidum (69).

IS THERE A PARKINSONIAN PERSONALITY?

It has been suggested that PD is associated with a specific personality type, described as compulsive, industrious, introverted, serious, inflexible (70). Prospective studies that use validated personality assessments are needed to address this question. Some studies have indicated that patients with PD score lower than controls on a personality trait called *novelty seeking* (71), which is hypothesized to be dopamine driven and is similar to the characteristics described above. This personality profile has been found to be associated with dopaminergic function in the left caudate (72) in patients with PD. However, other studies have not found that novelty seeking differs in patients with PD compared to other groups (73). In the largest positron-emission tomography (PET) study to date exploring this hypothesis, novelty seeking was mildly associated with unmedicated patients with PD but was not associated with dopaminergic function in the striatum or frontal lobe (74). However, patients with PD scored higher on a trait called *harm avoidance*, characterized by being fearful, pessimistic, and shy, and this trait was associated with dopaminergic function in the right caudate. The authors suggest that this trait is not disease specific, but rather represents an effect of chronic disease, depression, or both (74).

PATHOLOGIC GAMBLING AND ABUSE

The mesocortical dopamine system is critical for the reward system. Pathology of this reward system may cause behavioral changes such as addiction to drugs and alcohol, compulsions, and pathologic gambling. Pathologic gambling in the general population, associated with a disturbance of the dopaminergic system (75,76), has been reported in patients with advanced PD, with prevalences ranging between 0.05% (77) and 5% (78). Pathologic gambling usually begins after starting levodopa therapy (78) or with an increase in dopaminergic therapy with dopamine agonists (77) and tends to occur most often during the "on" period in patients with motor fluctuations (78). Associations have been reported between pathologic gambling and alcohol abuse or dependence, compulsions, and affective disturbances (77–79). Anecdotal evidence suggests that reducing dopaminergic therapy and using subthalamic stimulation, serotonergic medication, and psychosocial and educative strategies may ameliorate this behavior (77–79).

Neuropharmacological similarities exist between antiparkinsonian agents and centrally acting stimulants that act on the mesolimbic dopaminergic system. Thus, antiparkinsonian agents have a theoretical potential for dependence and abuse, and data from animal studies suggest that these agents induce behavioral changes similar to those induced by psychostimulants (80). In fact, several case reports show that levodopa abuse and the withdrawal symptoms that may emerge can have devastating behavioral and social consequences in some cases (81–83), even in people who do not have PD (84). Levodopa addiction may co-occur with pathologic gambling and obsessive–compulsive symptoms (79,83). Patients with a history of heavy alcohol consumption or illegal drug use seem to be at a high risk of developing a problem with abuse, and social isolation and depression before or after the onset of PD may exacerbate the syndrome (80). Clinical criteria for the syndrome, called *dopamine dysregulation syndrome*, have been proposed (81); see (80) for an excellent review on this topic.

The literature contains little information concerning the management of pathologic gambling and addiction to dopaminergic agents. Nonspecific procedures such as reducing the dopaminergic therapy should be employed, and the underlying mechanisms should be carefully explained to the patient and family members. Psychotherapy, psychosocial support, and even drug addiction rehabilitation programs may be helpful for selected patients. Suggestions for preventing addiction include prescribing the lowest doses of long-acting agents and avoiding intermittent subcutaneous apomorphine in patients thought to be susceptible to addiction (80).

SUMMARY

Apathy and fatigue, sexual disturbances, mania, sleep disturbances, personality changes, pathologic gambling, and addiction to antiparkinson agents occur in patients with PD and may pose considerable stress on the patients themselves and their caregivers.

With the exception of apathy and fatigue, little is known regarding the prevalence of these symptoms in patients with PD. The pathophysiologic mechanisms are unknown, although disturbances of the mesolimbic and mesocortical dopaminergic pathways are probably involved. Antiparkinsonian drugs or surgery seem to be

TABLE 5-2. *Prevalence of and medications for selected psychiatric symptoms in PD*

	Prevalence (%)	Etiology	Drug treatment*	Efficacy*
Apathy	40	Mesocortical D deficiency	Levodopa (level III), D agonists (level I), methylphenidate (level III), cholinesterase inhibitors (level III)	Insufficient evidence
Fatigue	40	Cytokines mesolimbic D deficiency	Levodopa (level I), modafinil (in MS: level I: positive; in PD: level I: negative)	Likely efficacious; insufficient evidence
Excessive daytime sleepiness	20	D agents brain stem pathology	Modafinil (level 1)	Likely efficacious
RBD	30	Striatal D deficiency	Clonazepam (level III), melatonin (level III), cholinesterase inhibitors (level III)	Insufficient evidence
Hypersexuality	1	Dopaminergic therapy	Reduction of dosage or withdrawal, psychotherapy (level III)	Insufficient evidence
Hypomania	1	Dopaminergic therapy	Withdrawal, mood stabilizers, atypical antipsychotics (level III)	Insufficient evidence
Pathologic gambling	0.05–5	Dopaminergic therapy	Reduction of dosage, psychotherapy (level III)	Insufficient evidence
Addiction to dopaminergic therapy	Rare	Dopaminergic therapy	Reduction of dosage, psychotherapy (level III)	Insufficient evidence

D, Dopamine.

*Classification of evidence, rating of study quality, and efficacy conclusions are based on the methods described in reference (85). In brief, level I studies are randomized controlled trials; level II studies are controlled clinical trials or observational controlled studies such as cohort or case–control studies; and level III studies are noncontrolled studies like case series. The efficacy conclusion "likely efficacious" requires support from data from any level I trial without conflicting level I data.

the main etiologic factors for sexual disturbance, hypomania, addiction, and pathologic gambling, whereas hypodopaminergic states may contribute to symptoms such as apathy, fatigue, RBD, and possibly personality changes. Although some placebo-controlled trials have been published recently, no established treatments are currently available for these symptoms (85) (see Table 5-2), and thus future clinical trials are needed.

REFERENCES

1. Braak H, Braak E. Pathoanatomy of Parkinson's disease. *J Neurol* 2000;247(Suppl. 2):II3–II10.
2. Brown RG, MacCarthy B. Psychiatric morbidity in patients with Parkinson's disease. *Psychol Med* 1990; 20:77–87.
3. Aarsland D, Larsen JP, Lim NG, et al. Range of neuropsychiatric disturbances in patients with Parkinson's disease. *J Neurol Neurosurg Psychiatry* 1999;67: 492–496.
4. Ringman JM, Diaz-Olavarrieta C, Rodriguez Y, et al. The prevalence and correlates of neuropsychiatric symptoms in a population with Parkinson's disease in Mexico. *Neuropsychiatry Neuropsychol Behav Neurol* 2002;15:99–105.
5. Marin RS, Biedrzycki RC, Firinciogullari S. Reliability and validity of the apathy evaluation scale. *Psychiatry Res* 1991;38:143–162.
6. Starkstein SE, Mayberg HS, Preziosi TJ, et al. Reliability, validity, and clinical correlates of apathy in Parkinson's disease. *J Neuropsychiatry Clin Neurosci* 1992;4:134–139.
7. Cummings JL, Mega M, Gray K, et al. The neuropsychiatric inventory: comprehensive assessment of psychopathology in dementia. *Neurology* 1994;44: 2308–2314.
8. Levy ML, Cummings JL, Fairbanks LA, et al. Apathy is not depression. *J Neuropsychiatry Clin Neurosci* 1998;10:314–319.
9. Marin RS, Firinciogullari S, Biedrzycki RC. Group differences in the relationship between apathy and depression. *J Nerv Ment Dis* 1994;182:235–239.
10. Isella V, Melzi P, Grimaldi M, et al. Clinical, neuropsychological, and morphometric correlates of apathy in Parkinson's disease. *Mov Disord* 2002;17:366–371.
11. Cummings J. *The neuropsychiatry of Alzheimer's disease and related dementias*. London: Martin Dunitz Ltd, 2003.
12. Craig AH, Cummings JL, Fairbanks L, et al. Cerebral blood flow correlates of apathy in Alzheimer disease. *Arch Neurol* 1996;53:1116–1120.
13. Benoit M, Koulibaly PM, Migneco O, et al. Brain perfusion in Alzheimer's disease with and without apathy: a SPECT study with statistical parametric mapping analysis. *Psychiatry Res* 2002;114:103–111.
14. Sarazin M, Michon A, Pillon B, et al. Metabolic correlates of behavioral and affective disturbances in frontal lobe pathologies. *J Neurol* 2003;250:827–833.
15. Pluck GC, Brown RG. Apathy in Parkinson's disease. *J Neurol Neurosurg Psychiatry* 2002;73:636–642.
16. Robert PH, Clairet S, Benoit M, et al. The apathy inventory: assessment of apathy and awareness in Alzheimer's disease, Parkinson's disease and mild cognitive impairment. *Int J Geriatr Psychiatry* 2002;17:1099–1105.
17. Aarsland D, Litvan I, Larsen JP. Neuropsychiatric symptoms of patients with progressive supranuclear palsy and Parkinson's disease. *J Neuropsychiatry Clin Neurosci* 2001;13:42–49.
18. Aarsland D, Cummings JL, Larsen JP. Neuropsychiatric differences between Parkinson's disease with dementia and Alzheimer's disease. *Int J Geriatr Psychiatry* 2001; 16:184–191.
19. Czernecki V, Pillon B, Houeto JL, et al. Motivation, reward, and Parkinson's disease: influence of dopatherapy. *Neuropsychologia* 2002;40:2257–2267.
20. Lieberman A, Ranhosky A, Korts D. Clinical evaluation of pramipexole in advanced Parkinson's disease: results of a double-blind, placebo-controlled, parallel-group study. *Neurology* 1997;49:162–168.
21. Black KJ, Hershey T, Koller JM, et al. A possible substrate for dopamine-related changes in mood and behavior: prefrontal and limbic effects of a D3-preferring dopamine agonist. *Proc Natl Acad Sci USA* 2002;99: 17113–17118.
22. Chatterjee A, Fahn S. Methylphenidate treats apathy in Parkinson's disease. *J Neuropsychiatry Clin Neurosci* 2002;14:461–462.
23. Aarsland D, Hutchinson M, Larsen JP. Cognitive, psychiatric and motor response to galantamine in Parkinson's disease with dementia. *Int J Geriatr Psychiatry* 2003;18:937–941.
24. McKeith I, Del Ser T, Spano P, et al. Efficacy of rivastigmine in dementia with Lewy bodies: a randomised, double-blind, placebo-controlled international study. *Lancet* 2000;356:2031–2036.
25. Krupp LB, Pollina DA. Mechanisms and management of fatigue in progressive neurological disorders. *Curr Opin Neurol* 1996;9:456–460.
26. Garber CE, Friedman JH. Effects of fatigue on physical activity and function in patients with Parkinson's disease. *Neurology* 2003;60:1119–1124.
27. Lou JS, Kearns G, Benice T, et al. Levodopa improves physical fatigue in Parkinson's disease: a double-blind, placebo-controlled, crossover study. *Mov Disord* 2003; 18:1108–1114.
28. Nagatsu T, Mogi M, Ichinose H, et al. Cytokines in Parkinson's disease. *J Neural Transm Suppl* 2000; 143–151.
29. Abe K, Takanashi M, Yanagihara T. Fatigue in patients with Parkinson's disease. *Behav Neurol* 2000;12: 103–106.
30. Abe K, Takanashi M, Yanagihara T, et al. Pergolide mesilate may improve fatigue in patients with Parkinson's disease. *Behav Neurol* 2001;13:117–121.
31. Friedman J, Friedman H. Fatigue in Parkinson's disease. *Neurology* 1993;43:2016–2018.
32. van Hilten JJ, Weggeman M, van der Velde EA, et al. Sleep, excessive daytime sleepiness and fatigue in Parkinson's disease. *J Neural Transm Park Dis Dement Sect* 1993;5:235–244.
33. Shulman LM, Taback RL, Bean J, et al. Comorbidity of the nonmotor symptoms of Parkinson's disease. *Mov Disord* 2001;16:507–510.
34. Karlsen K, Larsen JP, Tandberg E, et al. Fatigue in patients with Parkinson's disease. *Mov Disord* 1999; 14:237–241.

35. Herlofson K, Larsen JP. The influence of fatigue on health-related quality of life in patients with Parkinson's disease. *Acta Neurol Scand* 2003;107:1–6.
36. Rammohan KW, Rosenberg JH, Lynn DJ, et al. Efficacy and safety of modafinil (Provigil) for the treatment of fatigue in multiple sclerosis: a two centre phase 2 study. *J Neurol Neurosurg Psychiatry* 2002;72:179–183.
37. Adler CH, Caviness JN, Hentz JG, et al. Randomized trial of modafinil for treating subjective daytime sleepiness in patients with Parkinson's disease. *Mov Disord* 2003;18:287–293.
38. Stahl S. *Essential psychopharmacology*. Cambridge, MA: Cambridge University Press, 2000.
39. Nappi RE, Detaddei S, Veneroni F, et al. Sexual disorders in Parkinson's disease. *Funct Neurol* 2001;16:283–288.
40. Lambert D, Waters CH. Sexual dysfunction in Parkinson's disease. *Clin Neurosci* 1998;5:73–77.
41. Raffaele R, Vecchio I, Giammusso B, et al. Efficacy and safety of fixed-dose oral sildenafil in the treatment of sexual dysfunction in depressed patients with idiopathic Parkinson's disease. *Eur Urol* 2002;41:382–386.
42. Cummings JL. Behavioral complications of drug treatment of Parkinson's disease. *J Am Geriatr Soc* 1991;39:708–716.
43. Goodwin FK. Psychiatric side effects of levodopa in man. *JAMA* 1971;218:1915–1920.
44. Kanovsky P, Bares M, Pohanka M, et al. Penile erections and hypersexuality induced by pergolide treatment in advanced, fluctuating Parkinson's disease. *J Neurol* 2002;249:112–114.
45. Riley DE. Reversible transvestic fetishism in a man with Parkinson's disease treated with selegiline. *Clin Neuropharmacol* 2002;25:234–237.
46. Saper CB, Chou TC, Scammell TE. The sleep switch: hypothalamic control of sleep and wakefulness. *Trends Neurosci* 2001;24:726–731.
47. Poewe W, Hogl B. Parkinson's disease and sleep. *Curr Opin Neurol* 2000;13:423–426.
48. Larsen JP. Sleep disorders in Parkinson's disease. *Adv Neurol* 2003;91:329–334.
49. Tandberg E, Larsen JP, Karlsen K. A community-based study of sleep disorders in patients with Parkinson's disease. *Mov Disord* 1998;13:895–899.
50. Karlsen KH, Larsen JP, Tandberg E, et al. Influence of clinical and demographic variables on quality of life in patients with Parkinson's disease. *J Neurol Neurosurg Psychiatry* 1999;66:431–435.
51. Tandberg E, Larsen JP, Karlsen K. Excessive daytime sleepiness and sleep benefit in Parkinson's disease: a community-based study. *Mov Disord* 1999;14:922–927.
52. Gjerstad MD, Aarsland D, Larsen JP. Development of daytime somnolence over time in Parkinson's disease. *Neurology* 2002;58:1544–1546.
53. Brodsky MA, Godbold J, Roth T, et al. Sleepiness in Parkinson's disease: a controlled study. *Mov Disord* 2003;18:668–672.
54. Hogl B, Saletu M, Brandauer E, et al. Modafinil for the treatment of daytime sleepiness in Parkinson's disease: a double-blind, randomized, crossover, placebo-controlled polygraphic trial. *Sleep* 2002;25:905–909.
55. Boeve BF, Silber MH, Parisi JE, et al. Synucleinopathy pathology and REM sleep behavior disorder plus dementia or parkinsonism. *Neurology* 2003;61:40–45.
56. Schenck CH, Mahowald MW. REM sleep parasomnias. *Neurol Clin* 1996;14:697–720.
57. Boeve BF, Silber MH, Ferman TJ, et al. REM sleep behavior disorder in Parkinson's disease, dementia with Lewy bodies, and multiple system atrophy. In: Bedard MA, ed. *Mental and behavioral dysfunction in movement disorders*. Totowa, NJ: Humana Press, 2003:383–399.
58. Eisensehr I, Linke R, Tatsch K, et al. Increased muscle activity during rapid eye movement sleep correlates with decrease of striatal presynaptic dopamine transporters. IPT and IBZM SPECT imaging in subclinical and clinically manifest idiopathic REM sleep behavior disorder, Parkinson's disease, and controls. *Sleep* 2003;26:507–512.
59. Tan A, Salgado M, Fahn S. Rapid eye movement sleep behavior disorder preceding Parkinson's disease with therapeutic response to levodopa. *Mov Disord* 1996;11:214–216.
60. Boeve BF, Silber MH, Ferman TJ. Current management of sleep disturbances in dementia. *Curr Neurol Neurosci Rep* 2002;2:169–177.
61. Boeve BF, Silber MH, Ferman TJ. Melatonin for treatment of REM sleep behavior disorder in neurologic disorders: results in 14 patients. *Sleep Med* 2003;4:281–284.
62. Ringman JM, Simmons JH. Treatment of REM sleep behavior disorder with donepezil: a report of three cases. *Neurology* 2000;55:870–871.
63. Rektorova I, Rektor I, Bares M, et al. Pramipexole and pergolide in the treatment of depression in Parkinson's disease: a national multicentre prospective randomized study. *Eur J Neurol* 2003;10:399–406.
64. Perugi G, Toni C, Ruffolo G, et al. Adjunctive dopamine agonists in treatment-resistant bipolar II depression: an open case series. *Pharmacopsychiatry* 2001;34:137–141.
65. Cannas A, Spissu A, Floris GL, et al. Bipolar affective disorder and Parkinson's disease: a rare, insidious and often unrecognized association. *Neurol Sci* 2002;23(Suppl . 2):S67–S68.
66. Kim E, Zwil AS, McAllister TW, et al. Treatment of organic bipolar mood disorders in Parkinson's disease. *J Neuropsychiatry Clin Neurosci* 1994;6:181–184.
67. Kulisevsky J, Berthier ML, Gironell A, et al. Mania following deep brain stimulation for Parkinson's disease. *Neurology* 2002;59:1421–1424.
68. Funkiewiez A, Ardouin C, Krack P, et al. Acute psychotropic effects of bilateral subthalamic nucleus stimulation and levodopa in Parkinson's disease. *Mov Disord* 2003;18:524–530.
69. Okun MS, Bakay RA, DeLong MR, et al. Transient manic behavior after pallidotomy. *Brain Cogn* 2003;52:281–283.
70. Hubble JP, Koller WC. The parkinsonian personality. *Adv Neurol* 1995;65:43–48.
71. Menza MA, Golbe LI, Cody RA, et al. Dopamine-related personality traits in Parkinson's disease. *Neurology* 1993;43:505–508.
72. Menza MA, Mark MH, Burn DJ, et al. Personality correlates of [18F]dopa striatal uptake: results of positron-emission tomography in Parkinson's disease. *J Neuropsychiatry Clin Neurosci* 1995;7:176–179.
73. Jacobs H, Heberlein I, Vieregge A, et al. Personality traits in young patients with Parkinson's disease. *Acta Neurol Scand* 2001;103:82–87.
74. Kaasinen V, Nurmi E, Bergman J, et al. Personality traits and brain dopaminergic function in Parkinson's disease. *Proc Natl Acad Sci USA* 2001;98:13272–13277.

75. Comings DE, Rosenthal RJ, Lesieur HR, et al. A study of the dopamine D2 receptor gene in pathological gambling. *Pharmacogenetics* 1996;6:223–234.
76. Bergh C, Eklund T, Sodersten P, et al. Altered dopamine function in pathological gambling. *Psychol Med* 1997;27:473–475.
77. Driver-Dunckley E, Samanta J, Stacy M. Pathological gambling associated with dopamine agonist therapy in Parkinson's disease. *Neurology* 2003;61:422–423.
78. Molina JA, Sainz-Artiga MJ, Fraile A, et al. Pathologic gambling in Parkinson's disease: a behavioral manifestation of pharmacologic treatment? *Mov Disord* 2000;15:869–872.
79. Gschwandtner U, Aston J, Renaud S, et al. Pathologic gambling in patients with Parkinson's disease. *Clin Neuropharmacol* 2001;24:170–172.
80. Lawrence AD, Evans AH, Lees AJ. Compulsive use of dopamine replacement therapy in Parkinson's disease: reward systems gone awry? *Lancet Neurol* 2003;2:595–604.
81. Giovannoni G, O'Sullivan JD, Turner K, et al. Hedonistic homeostatic dysregulation in patients with Parkinson's disease on dopamine replacement therapies. *J Neurol Neurosurg Psychiatry* 2000;68:423–428.
82. Spigset O, von Scheele C. Levodopa dependence and abuse in Parkinson's disease. *Pharmacotherapy* 1997;17:1027–1030.
83. Serrano-Dueñas M. Chronic dopaminergic drug addiction and pathologic gambling in patients with Parkinson's disease—presentation of four cases. *German J Psychiatry* 2002;5:62–66.
84. Steiner I, Wirguin I. Levodopa addiction in non-parkinsonian patients. *Neurology* 2003;61:1451.
85. Lang AE, Lees A. Management of Parkinson's disease: an evidence-based review. *Mov Disord* 2002;17:S1–S166.

6
Parkinson's Disease as a Model for Psychosocial Issues in Chronic Neurodegenerative Disease

Mark S. Groves[1] and David V. Forrest[2]

[1]*Beth Israel Medical Center, New York, New York;* [2]*Psychoanalytic Center, Department of Psychiatry, Columbia University, New York, New York*

Neurodegenerative diseases such as Parkinson's disease (PD) exert profound effects on patients' daily lives. Throughout the course of illness, from the diagnosis to late stages, patients are confronted by multiple challenges. Some challenges are confined to specific stages of illness, but others span the entire course of illness (1). The substantial variability between individuals in course of illness precludes the physician's ability to predict a specific patient's clinical course accurately. Pharmacologic treatments play a critical role in treating PD. As the illness unfolds and develops over time, the neurologist or other health care provider will adjust treatment to address new complications or changes in the patient's symptoms. However, the neurologist or other health care provider should also be open to suggesting opportunities for psychosocial interventions that can dramatically affect the patient's quality of life (2–5).

The neurologist or PD clinician in a busy clinical practice may prefer to assign the task of psychosocial interventions to other professionals, such as psychiatric colleagues or social workers. This division of roles may often be necessary or advisable, given the distinct skills and training of various health professionals. However, the primary PD clinician (whether neurologist, nurse practitioner, or other health care provider) is allocated particular authority by his or her patient and, therefore, may be able to affect quality of life considerably with even the briefest interventions. For the patient with PD, the primary PD clinician sustains hope, and this doctor–patient relationship itself can be as important as medication. Many neurologists and other PD clinicians undervalue the importance of their relationships with patients or the effect that their interactions and words alone can have. Skilled diagnosticians often feel uncomfortable shifting the focus of their interactions with patients from diagnosis and treatment to the patients' subjective and emotional experiences of illness.

In this chapter, we outline a number of psychosocial issues confronted by patients with PD across various stages of the illness. Although other neurodegenerative diseases and movement disorders bring unique challenges, many observations in this chapter can be generalized to these other conditions. PD is not a perfect model for these other neurodegenerative diseases, however. Many effective symptomatic treatments are available for PD, in contrast to some other neurodegenerative diseases for which few effective treatments are currently available. PD is also much more common than many other neurodegenerative diseases, so patients can readily access educational materials, support groups, and other resources that can counteract fear, misunderstanding by others, and a sense of isolation. Cognitive deficits and dementia, although severe in a subset of patients with PD, are less prominent and global in PD than in some other neurodegenerative diseases (6,7). PD, unlike Huntington's Disease (HD) or spinocerebellar ataxias (SCA), is also usually not inherited, at least not in a familial pattern we can identify. Thus, some psychosocial interventions such as psychotherapy may be more appropriate for a specific patient with PD than for a patient with a different neurodegenerative disease (e.g., Huntington's disease in its late stages).

For convenience, we divide the course of PD into three stages: early (diagnosis/mildly symptomatic), middle (moderately symptomatic, without major treatment complications), and late (highly symptomatic, with major treatment complications). Certainly, considerable overlap occurs between these stages—some of the psychosocial issues and challenges we discuss persist throughout the course of illness and are not confined to a single stage of illness. Nevertheless, we find it useful to organize the psychosocial issues, and their respective treatment interventions, by the stages of PD during which they most commonly occur. For easy reference, this chapter provides summary tables for each stage (see Tables 6-1 through 6-3).

Space limitations preclude discussing all of the psychosocial issues confronted by patients with PD or addressing every possible psychosocial intervention. The generalizations offered herein must be tailored to individual patients and their personalities or preferences. Other alternatives may be more appropriate or effect greater results. A pragmatic approach is warranted, and various interventions can be attempted sequentially. When satisfactory results cannot be accomplished after a number of attempts or interventions, outside consultation is indicated.

Although many psychosocial interventions identified in this chapter may seem obvious, intuitive, or nonspecific, keeping them in mind and applying them appropriately can have profound effects on quality of life. An overly exclusive focus on treating the motor symptoms of PD is inadequate (4,5,8–10). In fact, numerous recent studies have shown that the greatest predictors of quality of life in PD lie outside the motor realm, such as the presence of depression (11–16). Caregivers and patients alike can easily be seduced by the excitement and promise of new biologic and technologic interventions; one role of providers is to keep desperate patients from pursuing dangerous experimental "cures." A broader focus on modulating the patient's experience of living with PD, rather than an exclusive focus on targeting the disease itself, will bring the greatest benefit to the patient's quality of life (8,14,16–20).

THE EARLY STAGE OF PD: DIAGNOSIS/MILDLY SYMPTOMATIC

Accepting the Diagnosis

Accepting the diagnosis of a chronic neurodegenerative disease such as PD is an individualized process that takes time (21). Because PD is relatively common, though usually not familial, patients often will have friends or family members with this disease; their memories of these people may be very upsetting. Depending on the degree of symptoms at the time of the diagnosis and the patient's fears, the diagnosis can come as a shock, or even a relief, because it provides an explanation for symptoms and offers the possibility of symptomatic treatment. Patients vary considerably in their coping skills and readiness for education about the disease. Some will have many questions and promptly seek out more information. Others will need more time to let the diagnosis "sink in" and will prefer to avoid being overloaded with information initially. The PD caregiver must respect the patient's readiness to accept the diagnosis and allow the patient to proceed with the process at his or her own pace. "Denial" should be considered problematic only when it prevents the patient from receiving essential treatment. As a progressive neurodegenerative disease without a cure, PD does not require a patient to receive treatment before he or she is ready. Some patients will use denial to ameliorate the impact of a diagnosis and facilitate gradual acceptance. "Breaking through" denial is generally counterproductive, because it only increases the anxiety and fear that the patient is attempting to ward off. Education about PD should occur over a number of visits (3,22). At the time of diagnosis, a patient may be unable to hear or process detailed information. Handouts, brochures, and books can be helpful, because they enable the patient to absorb the material at his or her own pace when emotionally ready (3,22). However, they may contain disturbing material about advanced stages, which may increase the patient's anxiety unnecessarily.

The PD clinician should work to achieve a number of goals during the period of care surrounding diagnosis (3,23,24). First, establishing a treatment alliance between the clinician and patient is critical. The treatment alliance enables the patient to feel safe and increases the likelihood that the patient will adhere to treatment recommendations. Listening empathically to the patient's concerns and questions is critical and is perhaps the most effective way to build rapport. It is usually advisable for the provider to sit down through most of the interview, because remaining seated conveys a willingness and readiness to listen. Ask the patient about his or her internal reactions to diagnosis. Do not assume that the patient will experience any particular reaction. Give permission for the patient, when appropriate, to express an array of emotional reactions: anger, fear, sadness, and so on, and assure the patient that these emotions are normal.

Providing information and education about PD to patients as they are ready to hear it will help diminish their fear of the unknown—another important goal for the provider in this period (25). Look for inappropriate self-blame. Patients may feel that they developed PD because of previous behaviors or could have prevented the disease in some way. Correcting these erroneous beliefs will help diminish inappropriate guilt. Even if illicit drug use is thought to have caused the disorder, as in the case of some patients with drug-induced parkinsonism (a distinct entity from idiopathic PD), the patient did not know that this result could occur, and guilt is counterproductive.

Although some sadness is common during the period while the diagnosis is being accepted, it is not universal, and the PD clinician should evaluate depression, not accept it as "reactive" and normal (26–28). Ask patients about all depressive symptoms (mood, ability to obtain pleasure in activities, sleep, energy, appetite, etc.), especially suicidal ideation (29). Referral to counseling or psychiatric treatment may be indicated.

It is essential to instill and sustain hope (4). Emphasizing that PD progresses slowly and that many symptomatic treatments, supports, and resources are available will facilitate greater hopefulness. Mentioning the possibility of further advances in treatment during the patient's course of illness is also helpful. A realistically optimistic outlook is important—patients will often be very sensitive to their providers' outlooks and affects.

Changing Self-identity

Receiving a diagnosis of a chronic neurodegenerative disease requires affected individuals to change their views of themselves (18,21,30–32). Many patients are diagnosed with PD late in life when they already have other medical conditions. Early onset patients, however, may still consciously or unconsciously hold on to views of themselves as invulnerable—a diagnosis of PD forces them to accept their mortality and relinquish these fantasies of invulnerability (33,34). The PD clinician should empathize with the patient through his or her process of narcissistic injury and illness-identity change. Preventing the patient from equating the diagnosis with an imminent death sentence is important, to counteract distorted catastrophic thinking and maintain hope. Educating the patient about many of the skills and functions unaffected by PD is helpful, as is encouraging him or her to maintain regular daily routines and activities—a concrete experiential reminder to the patient that "life goes on" even after a diagnosis of PD (32).

Symptom Searching and Checking

Some patients in the early stages of PD will anxiously fear progression and attribute minor incidents, such as dropping objects or other events, to progression of disease (appropriately, at times). Self-consciousness about tremor can lead to anxiety, which exacerbates the tremor further (31,35). Certainly, treatment will be offered if symptoms are troublesome enough to warrant it. However, the PD clinician can offer gentle reassurance, when appropriate, and encourage the patient to "hand over" responsibility for monitoring progression to the provider, who can offer to follow up with the patient at regular intervals. Even when many months elapse between visits, regular follow-up can be supportive and decrease the patient's anxiety. When the patient's anxiety about progression fails to respond to these initial measures, further treatment may be warranted, including psychotherapy or medications or both (18,35). Exploring the patient's specific fears will often be revealing and therapeutic for the patient. Selective serotonin reuptake inhibitor (SSRI) antidepressants, such as escitalopram and sertraline, can be helpful in targeting prominent symptoms of anxiety, depression, or both in PD. The PD clinician should be aware that anxiety and depression are particularly common in PD (35–38).

Dependency Fears and Conflicts

A nearly universal psychosocial challenge for patients throughout the course of PD is confronting dependency fears and conflicts (31,39, 40). Some patients have obsessional personality styles—they like to be in control, can be stubborn or obstinate, and they often value order, predictability, and independence. To these individuals, a neurodegenerative illness represents a loss of control and a tremendous threat to their highly valued independence. Dependence on others is threatening, uncomfortable, and a blow to self-esteem for these individuals. Empathizing with these fears and actively encouraging autonomy and continued independence in the early stages of illness can be helpful. However, it is also important to encourage patients to reach out to friends and loved ones for emotional support (32). Discomfort with the idea of dependence on others may prevent these individuals from seeking needed support.

Patients' support networks vary in number and strength; some patients will fear that they will not have anyone to depend on as their disease progresses, or they may fear abandonment by their primary caregivers. Listening empathically to these fears is important, as is emphasizing that the treatment team will be available to support them throughout their course of illness. Encouraging patients to broaden their support networks and maintain social contacts is important (31). One way of allaying anxiety is to increase the patient's sense of control by making him or her the boss or executive who "assembles a team" of neurologist, psychiatrist, physical therapist, and a variety of personal trainers for everything from muscle strength to voice and facial expression. An increased sense of control can greatly influence the well-being of patients with PD (41). Advising patients to join support groups can be helpful, if groups are available that are well matched to a patient's age and severity of illness (42).

Alienation from "Well" Others

In the midst of coping with a new diagnosis of PD, patients often feel alienated from peers who do not have PD. Such alienation is heightened if the patient is depressed, and those around him or her appear to be going about daily life with minimal fears and concerns. The PD clinician can assist the patient in decreasing this sense of alienation and prevent social withdrawal through a number of interventions. First, empathize with the patient's sense of alienation from the "well." Feeling understood decreases a sense of alienation and is supportive. Second, foster the patient's participation in PD support groups, which can be tremendously helpful because other members of the group likely have had similar experiences, and patients can give each other useful advice on coping with this illness. Support groups are not universally helpful, however (1). Group members may relate upsetting stories that increase fear or mistrust of caregivers, give bad drug advice on the basis of their own nongeneralizable experience, or foster increased pessimism. Therefore, support groups must be selected carefully. On-line support groups and chat rooms can also be helpful, though they lack face-to-face human contact. Third, patients may hesitate to share their concerns and feelings with friends and family because of a fear that they will burden others or that they will not be understood. However, the sense of alienation and isolation is exacerbated by hiding one's emotions and inner experiences from others, and patients should be encouraged to "open up" to friends and family members, even if they suspect they will be disappointed. A common fear is that family members may exaggerate the patients' mental incapabilities and conspire to take over their affairs and resources. This fear may be a rationalization for avoiding useful psychiatric contact. Patients with such fears should be told mental incapacity is unlikely and that the psychiatrist and the psychiatric record will be able to stand by the patient and prove his or her capacity if such a situation arises.

Exposing and Concealing Symptoms

In the early stages of illness, patients often do not want co-workers or other peers to know about their diagnosis of PD. On the job, they might realistically fear discrimination. Or they may feel uncomfortable with the idea of others feeling sorry for them or conceiving of them as fragile or ill. In exploring a patient's fear of exposure or desire to conceal symptoms, the role of shame must be distinguished from the roles of other concerns, such as fear of discrimination (34). Ask patients what they fear others will think, or how they will respond when others recognize their PD. Look for opportunities to challenge shameful conceptions of illness or distortions and emphasize that PD does not define who the patient is or diminish his or her value as an individual (18,30,43). Identifying some of the patient's strengths can help bolster the patient's self-esteem and energize him or her in more effectively coping with PD. An ashamed, deflated patient may avoid treatment or social contact, which can make things worse.

Of course, a patient's desire to diminish symptoms may be warranted if the symptoms are impairing daily functioning. A particularly disabling symptom early in the course of PD is diminished facial expressivity (29,44). Especially for the patient who wishes to "pass" as normal, coaching in facial expressiveness is indicated. Forrest and Pullman are developing diagnostic and therapeutic techniques (unpublished personal communication). In such cases, treatment will target the motor symptoms that are present. Look for and treat any psychiatric symptoms, such as depression or anxiety, that may be contributing to or worsening the patient's symptoms or function (35,45). For the patient who is biased against psychiatric treatment, education about the interaction between psychiatric symptoms and motor symptoms can make treatment with an antidepressant more palatable. Most patients will readily acknowledge, when asked, that they have noticed an increase in motor symptoms during periods of high anxiety. At times, adequate treatment of anxiety or depression can improve the patients' motor symptoms and functional disability dramatically (35,36,45,46).

Effect on Relationships

A diagnosis of a chronic neurodegenerative disease such as PD can exert tremendous strain on a patient's primary relationships and may necessitate shifts in roles that can dramatically upset previous patterns (31,43,47). These role shifts can be very uncomfortable to one or both individuals in a relationship. A patient who was the "backbone" of a family, always available to support others in their times of need, may suddenly need to receive support from those others when faced with a neurodegenerative disease. This change in roles within the family may be upsetting to family members who depended heavily on the patient's support and perhaps took it for granted. Patients may fear they will be a burden on their families, or they may fear abandonment (39). Depending on the nature of a patient's relationships, such fears may or may not be warranted; early on, they are often exaggerated. In any case, empathize with the patient's fears and normalize the stress that illness exerts on relationships. When indicated and desired, referrals to individual, couple, or family counseling can help alleviate strain on the patient's relationships and facilitate open communication. Caregivers can benefit substantially from referral to caregivers' support groups and other resources such as on-line chatrooms, websites, and so on, and they should be encouraged to take vacations and seek pleasure (42). Preventing caregiver burnout is in the caregiver's and patient's best interests and is especially important in later stages of illness, when the patient's symptoms are worse and the patient is, out of necessity, more dependent on his or her caregiver (42,43,48).

Issues of sexuality must also be addressed and generally will not be revealed by the patient unless explicitly invited. Sexual dysfunction in PD may stem from psychological or biologic factors (49,50). The patient recently diagnosed with PD may feel defective and less attractive. Additionally, sexual problems may be an expression of other relationship difficulties or conflicts. Alternatively, medications may affect libido, arousal, or orgasm. A peculiarity of treatments for PD is that they may *increase* sexual drive (50). By introducing sexual concerns as

TABLE 6-1. *The early stage of PD: Diagnosis—Mildly symptomatic*

Psychosocial challenges	Goal(s)	Interventions
Acceptance of diagnosis	Foster doctor–patient alliance	Inquire about patient's reactions to diagnosis. Listen and provide him/her with sufficient time to express these reactions. Empathize with the individual's experience; normalize when appropriate.
	Diminish fear of the unknown	Educate about PD: symptoms, treatment, course of illness, etc. Provide written materials and recommend websites/books.
	Correct erroneous self-blame	Educate about etiology; actively defuse patient self-blame/guilt.
	Assess depressive symptoms and treat if indicated	Ask about all depressive symptoms, especially suicidal tendency, and assess severity. Avoid tendency to view depression as normal. Counseling/treatment may be indicated. Follow symptoms to ensure remission.
	Instill/sustain hope	Emphasize the slow progression of the disease, the availability of treatments and supports/resources, and likelihood of future treatments/advances in research.
Change in self-identity	Foster realistic acceptance of mortality and relinquishment of fantasies of invulnerability	Empathize with the individual's experience. Normalize when appropriate. Prevent patient from equating diagnosis with a death sentence.
	Prevent patient from collapsing identity to the disease itself: "person with PD" v. "Parkinsonian"	Emphasize importance of maintaining interests/activities and daily routine. Educate about the array of skills that are generally unaffected by PD.
Symptom searching/checking	Diminish somatic preoccupations and fears of progression	Reassure when appropriate; schedule regular visits to remove responsibility of symptom finding from patient and to bolster supportive effects of treatment relationship.
Dependency fears/conflicts	Encourage patients to achieve comfort and balance between the opposing needs for independence/autonomy and dependence on others for support	Promote independent functioning and autonomy, while encouraging patients to reach out to friends and loved ones for emotional support through the early stages of illness.
	Diminish fear of increased dependency in the future	Empathize with patients' fears. Normalize when appropriate. Reassure patients that treatment will aim to maintain independent functioning as long as possible, but when greater assistance is necessary, it will be arranged. The PD treatment team will ensure appropriate services are provided; the patient will not go through the illness alone. Mobilize supports; encourage patient to expand his/her support network—e.g., joining support groups, and participation in other social activities.
Exposure/concealment of symptoms; alienation from "well" others	Prevent social withdrawal, alienation, and isolation	Empathize with patient's sense of alienation from the "well." Foster participation in support groups (matching patient, whenever possible, to group similar in age and level of functioning) to combat alienation. On-line support groups/chat rooms can also be helpful. Encourage patient to discuss fears with friends and loved ones. Although responses from others vary in helpfulness and degree of empathy, sharing feelings in itself can decrease the sense of alienation from others.

(continues)

TABLE 6-1. *Continued*

Psychosocial challenges	Goal(s)	Interventions
	Challenge shameful conceptions of illness	Explore patient's desire to conceal symptoms and beliefs about what the symptoms mean and how they are interpreted by others. Correct distortions or unhelpful conceptions.
	Bolster self-esteem	Challenge shameful feelings, emphasizing that the illness does not define who the patient is. Naming some of the patient's personal strengths and admirable qualities (when valued by the patient and genuinely expressed by the caregiver) can bolster self-esteem.
	Decrease symptoms with treatment, when possible and desired	The presence of early symptoms, such as tremor, may prove problematic for patients, especially in occupational settings. Offer treatment for such symptoms when appropriate and desired. Address psychiatric symptoms, such as anxiety, that may be contributing to worsening of symptoms.
Impact on relationships	Assess patient's relationship(s), looking for strain/conflicts that could be ameliorated	Inquire about patient's relationships, his/her fear of being a burden, or fear of abandonment. Offer empathy and normalize the challenges that illness presents to a relationship. Offer referrals for group or individual counseling. Refer caregiver to caregiver support groups and other resources.
	Openly invite discussion of issues of sexuality	Emphasize how common sexual concerns are in the context of major illness to diminish shame and foster increased comfort in discussing these issues. Invite patients to discuss fears, questions, and problems and offer treatment and/or reassurance, when indicated.

common among patients with medical illness, the PD clinician can diminish shame and foster a more comfortable setting for patients to reveal their concerns or questions. A full discussion of sexual issues and their treatment is beyond the scope of this chapter, but several excellent reviews of this important (and often neglected) clinical issue are available in the literature (20,50,51).

THE MIDDLE STAGE OF PD: MODERATELY SYMPTOMATIC WITHOUT MAJOR TREATMENT COMPLICATIONS

By the middle stage of PD, most patients' symptoms will be prominent enough that they will require dopaminergic medications (52). In earlier stages, a dopamine agonist may be used alone, but by the middle stage of PD, most patients will have started carbidopa-levodopa. Increasing medication and adding new ones symbolizes the progression of this disease, and some patients will choose to avoid starting certain medications out of a desire to deny the extent of their disease progression. Most patients, however, are so uncomfortable when "parkinsonized" that medication nonadherence is probably far less common in PD than in many other chronic illnesses such as diabetes or HIV infection. Many of the psychosocial issues that are present in the early stage of illness persist through the middle stage. Even the process of accepting the diagnosis can extend throughout the course of illness. Patients vary in how effectively they work through various psychosocial challenges.

Exposing and Concealing Symptoms

Motor symptoms of PD are increasingly prominent by the middle stage of illness. Looking for and treating any psychiatric symptoms that may be exacerbating motor symptoms or impairing function remains important. If the patient continues to hold shameful conceptions of illness, discuss and challenge these beliefs (30). They are not unfounded. Parkinsonian movements are often aped by actors ridiculing aged foolish characters, and society lionizes graceful movements such as those displayed by professional athletes or ballet dancers. Patients may choose at this stage to tell more people about their PD diagnosis, as the symptoms become more prominent and impair daily life to a greater degree than in the early stage of illness.

Decreased Physical Stamina and Increased Fatigue

As PD progresses, patients will notice decreased physical stamina and increased fatigue (32,39, 53–55). To individuals who previously valued physical exercise or activities highly, the decreased stamina will be particularly frustrating. Fatigue can easily become a reason for patients to avoid social activities and stay at home instead (13,54). A vicious cycle of decreased activity and deconditioning can ensue, however, that should be prevented as much as possible by encouraging patients to stay as active as they can and to participate in social activities regularly (32,56). Physical and occupational therapy can be instrumental in maintaining range of motion, preventing deconditioning, and reducing the risk of falls and should be recommended when indicated. Some patients, for whom vigorous exercise has never been an important part of life, will have greater trouble than others finding motivation to participate in exercise programs and will need more encouragement and coaching. Depression can impair motivation and, when present, should be treated with medication, psychotherapy, or both.

Loss of Physical Abilities and Ability to Perform Certain Tasks

Impairment of fine-motor skills, also inevitable in PD, is another loss patients must bear. Challenge patient's "I can't do that anymore" statements, because they may readily give up activities or hobbies because of frustration with a decreased level of skill. Finding creative ways around new difficulties, with the help of an occupational therapist, can increase patients' sense of self-esteem and autonomy. Empathy for the losses and frustrations is indicated and can be helpful in reducing distress. Motor difficulties may be increasingly global, however, affecting sedentary hobbies as well as those requiring great physical effort.

Fear of Falls

Gait instability is a cardinal symptom of PD, so some fear of falling is probably appropriate, and likely beneficial, because it may lead patients to be more cautious when walking in inclement weather or to avoid unstable or dangerous paths. The degree of avoidance can become problematic, however, if patients overly restrict their activities and avoid leaving the house. Physical therapy and gait training are important, as is the use of assistive devices. Because balance is worse at night, as visual cues decrease and medication wears off, heavy carpeting or even playground rubber mats can be placed between bed and bath to decrease the risk of injury from falls. Undergarments with hip pads can prevent fractures. Adequate pharmacologic treatment of motor symptoms can help patients to maintain better function. Home care or assistance may be necessary. When avoidance exists to an excessive degree, behavioral approaches may be indicated to diminish an exaggerated fear of falls. Purchasing emergency contact devices for patients to wear, in case they fall and are unable to get up, can somewhat alleviate patient and caregiver fears.

Insomnia and Daytime Somnolence

A comprehensive discussion of the causes and treatments of insomnia in PD is beyond the scope of this chapter, but several studies cover this topic (57–60). This common area is listed as a psychosocial issue because it can dramatically affect the psychosocial functioning of patient and caregiver alike. Few individuals are able to cope effectively when chronically sleep deprived. Daytime somnolence, which can also be a major obstacle to maintaining social contact and activities, should also be addressed (60). Many sleep problems in the patient with PD are caused by the PD itself or a related condition such as REM (rapid eye movement) sleep behavior disorder or are exacerbated by medications used to treat PD (57). However, education about the basic tenets of good sleep hygiene remains useful. For example, the patient who is unable to sleep should get up for a period of relaxing activity. Encouraging daytime activity can help reduce excessive daytime napping, which can perpetuate nighttime insomnia, but exercise should not be performed an hour or two prior to bedtime.

Role Transition: Retirement

The timing of retirement will, of course, vary among individuals and different professions, but many patients will retire at some point in the middle stage of illness, perhaps earlier than originally intended or than the peer group (47). This major life transition is an important stressor, even when perceived as a relief, and takes considerable adjustment (61,62). To those individuals whose self-esteem and personal satisfaction was highly connected to their occupations, retirement may be experienced as an especially major loss (32). Encouraging patients to find other means of feeling productive and useful can counteract feelings of uselessness and worthlessness that may ensue.

Dependency Fears and Conflicts

An increased need to depend on the assistance of others frequently accompanies the decline in physical stamina, increased propensity to fatigue, loss of certain physical abilities, and progression of motor symptoms of PD (32,39,40). Whereas dependency fears in the early stage of PD may have focused on the unknown future of disability, patients in the middle stage of PD may begin to directly experience these difficulties. Patients should be encouraged to strive for as much independent functioning as possible and simultaneously helped to develop comfort in requesting and receiving help when it is needed. Some patients will resist depending on others, whereas others will give up their independence too readily. The goals of the PD clinician are to balance these extremes and match this balance to the degree of physical functioning. Psychotherapy may help patients work through dependency fears and conflicts that impair help-seeking, diminish social contact, or strain personal relationships. Patients facing chronic neurodegenerative diseases such as PD commonly experience frustrations related to the loss of independence, the need to depend on others, the fear of being a burden to others, and the fear of inadequate support (32,39). Patient support groups are particularly useful for facilitating discussion of these fears and conflicts and for providing support and understanding.

Alienation from "Well" Others; Social Isolation

Preventing social isolation should be a major psychosocial goal of the PD clinician. As symptoms of PD increase, so can the sense of alienation from others who are well. This sense of alienation can contribute to loneliness and depression and should be addressed. Fostering patient participation in support groups is important. Patients should be matched by age and degree of illness whenever possible, because groups are more effective when members perceive that others are facing similar stresses and can identify with each other. Listening empathically to patients' experiences is important and can diminish the sense of alienation.

Effect on Relationships

Relationships are affected substantially by PD (39,43). The strain on a relationship will often increase with the severity of symptoms and with the decline in a patient's ability to function (48,63). Continue to inquire about patients' relationships and other sources of support; refer couples, families, or caregivers to counseling or support groups when such referrals are likely to be helpful. Additionally, issues of sexuality should still be discussed and addressed as indicated (50,51).

TABLE 6-2. *The middle stage of PD: Moderately symptomatic without significant treatment complications*

Psychosocial challenges	Goal(s)	Interventions
Exposure/concealment of symptoms	Decrease symptoms with treatment	Treat motor symptoms with medications. Look for psychiatric symptoms such as anxiety that may be exacerbating the motor symptoms.
	Continue to challenge shameful conceptions of illness and bolster self-esteem	Explore patient's concerns about worsening motor symptoms and beliefs about how these symptoms are interpreted by others. Correct distortions or unhelpful conceptions. Emphasize that PD does not define the patient. Encourage continued activities that foster a sense of productivity and personal satisfaction.
Decreased physical stamina/fatigue	Build strength and prevent deconditioning in order to allow patient to remain active	Physical therapy/occupational therapy. Provide education about stretching and exercises. Encourage patient to find enjoyable ways to stay physically active. Empathize with patient's decreased stamina/energy.
	Prevent withdrawal from social activities	Empathize with patient's tendency to avoid situations that will likely be fatiguing but emphasize the importance of maintaining social contacts and staying as active as possible.
Loss of physical abilities/ ability to perform certain tasks	Assist patient in adapting to diminished physical abilities	Occupational therapy and physical therapy. Encourage patient to find new ways to perform skilled motor activities that are becoming difficult. Empathize with patient's loss of physical skills/abilities.
	Prevent patient from too readily giving up tasks or responsibilities to others	Challenge patient's "I can't do that anymore" statements when appropriate. Encourage independent functioning and autonomy.
Fear of falls	Improve balance/gait	Physical therapy/gait training. Teach patient to use assistive devices and other techniques to prevent falls. Avoid medications that worsen balance. Treat motor symptoms.
	Diminish exaggerated fear in order to prevent avoidance of activities	Training and education will build confidence and diminish fear. If necessary, behavioral approaches to prevent excessive avoidance can extinguish an exaggerated fear of falls. Home care or assistance from others can be helpful.
Insomnia/daytime somnolence	Diminish daytime somnolence and nighttime insomnia in order to facilitate physical and social functioning during the day	Adjust medication regimen as appropriate to facilitate sleep at night and wakefulness during the day. Adjunctive use of hypnotic agents or wakefulness agents may be indicated.
		Diagnose and treat, if present, conditions that may be exacerbating insomnia such as REM sleep behavior disorder or sleep apnea.
		Teach patient good sleep hygiene. Encourage increased daytime physical activity commensurate with current abilities.
Role transition: retirement	Assist patient in coping with the major role transitions of retirement	Inquire about the patient's feelings about retirement. Explore ways that he/she can continue to feel productive through activities outside work. Empathize with patient's sense of loss (if present).

(continues)

TABLE 6-2. *Continued*

Psychosocial challenges	Goal(s)	Interventions
Dependency fears/conflicts	Encourage patients to achieve comfort and balance between the opposing needs for independence/autonomy and dependence on others for support	Continue to promote as much independent functioning as possible while helping patient adjust to increased need to depend on others. Empathize with patient's experience adjusting to increasing dependency.
	Diminish fear of increased dependency in the future	Empathize with patients' fears. Normalize when appropriate. Reassure patients that all efforts will be made to help them maintain independent functioning as long as possible, but when greater assistance is necessary, it will be arranged. Remind patients that the team will ensure that required services are provided and they will not go through the illness alone. Continue to mobilize supports and encourage expansion of social networks. Support groups can be helpful in this stage. If indicated, home care can be arranged.
Alienation from "well" others/social isolation	Prevent social withdrawal, alienation, and isolation	Empathize with patient's greater sense of alienation from those who are "well." Foster participation in support groups (matching patient, whenever possible, to groups similar in age and level of functioning) to combat alienation. On-line support groups/chat rooms can be helpful. Encourage patient to openly discuss fears with friends and loved ones.
Impact on relationships	Assess patient's relationship(s), looking for strain/conflicts that could be ameliorated	Inquire about relationships, inviting discussion of fear of being a burden, or fear of abandonment. Offer empathy and normalize the increasing challenges that PD presents a relationship and the shifts in roles. Offer referrals for group or individual counseling. Refer caregiver to caregiver support groups and other resources.
	Openly invite discussion of issues of sexuality	Invite patients to discuss fears, questions, and problems. Offer treatment and/or reassurance.

Midstage, relationships will begin to be affected by a perceived lack of emotional responsiveness because of the facial motor impairment (48). Loved ones and caretakers should be reminded that the patient appreciates them, and patients should be reminded to say so.

THE LATE STAGE OF PD: HIGHLY SYMPTOMATIC WITH SUBSTANTIAL TREATMENT COMPLICATIONS

The late stage of PD is marked by numerous new stressors, and the disease tends to dominate daily life to a greater degree than ever before, taxing the coping resources of even the most highly adapted individuals. Whereas in the early stages, symptomatic treatment benefits patients with minimal complications, the late stage of PD is marked by decreasing efficacy of symptomatic treatment and problematic side effects, such as motor fluctuations and prolonged "off" periods (64,65). Psychosocial interventions are critical during this period to support both patient and caregiver.

Structuring Life Around Medication and "On" Periods; Coping with Motor Complications

In the late stage of PD, patients develop complications of treatment with dopaminergic medications—the "on/off" phenomenon, medications "wearing off," dyskinesias, and so on. The duration of "on" periods shortens, and patients must increase the dose and frequency of medications to maximize motor functioning. Cumbersome medication schedules begin to structure patients' daily lives and interfere with social functioning. Activities must be planned within increasingly narrow windows of "on" periods—many patients begin to stop planning social activities, and increased social isolation is common, contributing to depression and worsened function (64). The PD clinician aims to maximize "on" periods through careful adjustments in the medication regimen and schedule. Educating patients and caregivers about these motor complications and their treatment is critical. Patients can feel that their illness is increasingly out of control; for these individuals, taking a collaborative approach to treatment planning can be useful, giving the patient a number of treatment options, if available, from which to choose. As always, teasing out the potential contribution of psychiatric symptoms to decreased functioning is important, and when such symptoms are present, treatment should be instituted. Overall quality of life, not simply improved motor function, is the primary goal. If extensive adjustments of medications fail to adequately improve motor function, or treatment side effects (primarily severe dyskinesias) are too disabling, patients can be referred for deep brain stimulation (DBS) surgery, if they are deemed appropriate candidates. Extensive education is required to correct patients' potentially unrealistic expectations about DBS, and preoperative assessment should include not merely cognitive assessments, because additional cognitive deficits may result from the procedure, but also some psychiatric screening. Psychiatric screening is important to assess any comorbid psychiatric conditions that may be inadequately treated, to identify those patients who may be at particular risk of psychiatric complications by nature of their histories and thus warrant closer preoperative and postoperative monitoring, and to ensure that patients' understanding of the risks and benefits is adequate to confer capacity to consent to the procedure.

Loss of Further Physical Capacities and Ability to Perform Tasks

The progression of PD inevitably leads to further loss of physical skills and abilities, thus decreasing patients' capacities for independent function. Losses of function, like other losses in life, must be mourned and assimilated and can precipitate depression. The PD clinician's interventions should aim to assist patients in physically adapting to diminished physical abilities (e.g., through enlisting the expertise and assistance of occupational and physical therapists) and emotionally adapting to these losses (through empathic understanding, counseling, and other supportive interventions such as groups); interventions should also ensure that patients are not prematurely relinquishing tasks and responsibilities. Home-care services should be arranged, when appropriate, to assist the patient and decrease caregiver burden.

Loss of Independence; Dependency Fears and Conflicts

Through each stage of PD, patients must confront anew issues of dependency and shift their balance between conflicting needs for independence and autonomy and the increasing need to depend on others for support. To the patients whose self-conceptions are centered on independence and being able to care for others, this progressive surrender of responsibilities is particularly distressing. Empathy for their frustrations and sense of loss is helpful and should come from multiple sources. Yet, empathy may be inadequate for some patients who feel stuck in regret and anger about their illness and struggle to accept these losses. For these individuals, a more formal course of psychotherapy may assist them to work through these issues.

Speech Problems, Drooling, and Facial Masking

Throughout this chapter, we have emphasized repeatedly the importance of attending to the effect PD has on patients' social functioning and relationships, because we feel that social isolation and withdrawal is one of the major psychosocial issues that affect patient quality of life. In addition to the fatigue, alienation, motor symptoms, and psychiatric symptoms such as depression and anxiety, other symptoms of PD can interfere with social function. These symptoms include speech problems, drooling, and facial masking. Speech problems, in particular, such as hypophonia and articulation difficulties, can be extremely disabling and frustrating to patients, because these problems impede effective communication, and patients may have difficulty expressing their desires and needs to their caregivers (20,30,43,44,66). Drooling can be embarrassing, and patients may choose to avoid social situations because of this symptom (39). It is worsened by stooped posture. Facial masking certainly can be present in earlier stages of illness as well. Patients may be misread by others because they lack the full range of usual facial expressions that accompany emotional states (29,44). Their appearances may be misread as depressed, disinterested, or even mildly astonished, but their internal states may contrast considerably with their outward appearances. Even more than usual, it becomes essential to directly ask how a patient is feeling rather than attempting to infer the patient's emotional state from his or her appearance. The loss of a patient's liveliness and full range of emotional expression to facial masking (and, in some patients, apathy) can be a particularly difficult loss for caregivers and family members (48). Caregivers should be educated about these three symptoms, and interventions may be indicated, such as speech therapy for the speech difficulties, or medicated mouthwashes for drooling.

Decreased Physical Stamina and Increased Fatigue

Fatigue and decreased stamina worsen over the course of illness, and physical and occupational therapy remain important to prevent deconditioning, maintain full range of motion, diminish the risk of falls, and facilitate social functioning. Physical therapists will tailor the exercises to patients' abilities. Extreme slowing is particularly frustrating for partners and caregivers.

Fear of Falls

Although fear of falls is often appropriate, given gait instability, freezing, and other motor problems, excessive fear of falls can lead patients to abandon activities and retreat to a home-bound existence. At some point, such a retreat may be unavoidable, but this fear should be challenged, and patients should be taught how to use assistive devices to increase safety and maintain mobility. Motorized go-carts and wheelchairs may enable interesting excursions for patient and caregiver. Medications that can impair balance should be avoided whenever possible. Anxiety disorders, when present, should be treated, so that they do not contribute to and magnify fears about loss of balance (35).

Psychiatric Complications of Medications: Hallucinations and Paranoia

Psychiatric complications of medications can be particularly disturbing to caregivers and family members. We will not address herein their causes or treatment, as this subject is well covered elsewhere (67,68). However, we wish to emphasize the importance of educating family members about symptoms such as hallucinations and paranoia. When understood, these symptoms will be less disturbing, and caregivers must be encouraged to keep PD clinicians informed about these symptoms so that medication can be adjusted, or, when necessary, antipsychotic medications with a low propensity to worsen PD symptoms, such as quetiapine, can be added or adjusted. One peculiarity of dopamine-driven visual hallucinosis is its tolerability in many patients. Overmedication with antipsychotics should be eschewed.

Derangement of Sleep–Wake Cycle

As dopaminergic medications are increased in quantity and frequency to target worsened motor symptoms of PD, sleep is frequently impaired further. Insomnia can be tremendously frustrating to patients and their caregivers (69). Daytime somnolence often also exists, in part because of medications, and exacerbates nighttime insomnia, leading to an even further derangement of the sleep–wake cycle. Wakefulness during the day and sleep at night are two separate, though somewhat related, goals that should be targeted with a number of interventions. Hypnotic agents and wakefulness-promoting agents may be prescribed, medication dosing regimens adjusted, and diagnosis of other conditions that affect sleep, such as sleep apnea, REM sleep behavioral disorder, anxiety disorders, and depression, should be considered (59,70). The patient and caregivers should continue to be educated about the principles of sleep hygiene, and daytime activity should be increased whenever possible. Exposure to light during the day is also important, to reset circadian rhythms.

Prominent Cognitive Deficits; Dementia

Unlike other chronic neurodegenerative diseases such as Alzheimer's disease and Huntington's disease, PD fortunately does not inevitably and universally entail dementia (6). For those patients who do develop PD dementia, Dementia with Lewy bodies, or comorbid Alzheimer's disease, however, multiple additional psychosocial issues arise for the patient and caregivers (71). The overarching goal of interventions is to diminish the effect of cognitive deficits on daily functioning. A number of approaches can be useful. Teaching patients mnemonic techniques, such as keeping a notebook with reminders, can prolong functioning when deficits are not yet severe. Educating caregivers about cognitive deficits is also important, so that memory problems are not misinterpreted as willful refusals and expectations of the patient remain realistic (48). Reducing the complexity of the environment and maintaining daily routines can be very helpful in organizing the patient and preventing problems. As always, medication regimens should be examined closely to reduce any anticholinergic burden that could be exacerbating memory deficits. Excessively sedating medications can also impair cognition, as can opiates. Depression or anxiety, if present, should be treated, because they can also exacerbate or even mimic cognitive deficits. If appropriate, use of pharmacologic agents for dementia, such as cholinesterase inhibitors or N-methyl D-aspartate receptor antagonists, should be considered. Adequate support services in the home are essential to maintain safety and assist in activities of daily living. Home safety should be inspected and monitored closely. Dementia added to the motor symptoms of PD is an especially heavy burden for patients and caregivers to bear—extra support in every form is indicated for these individuals and for their caregivers (63,71).

Effect on Relationships; Caregiver Burnout

The progression of illness and further decline in functioning magnify the stressors accompanying PD, and thus, the strain on relationships is intensified. Continued inquiring about patients' relationships and prescribe interventions to assist both patient and caregiver(s) (48). Caregiver support groups are especially critical tools in helping refuel caregivers in their continued efforts to support patients with PD. When patients have dedicated caregivers, the PD clinician's interventions may be best directed to the caregiver, rather than the patient, to prevent caregiver burnout and maintain this critical source of support (43,48,72). Caregivers will often need to be given explicit permission to take care of themselves (and to relinquish some responsibilities to others, such as home health attendants) (42,43, 63,73). They can feel trapped in a 24-hours-a-day, 7-days-a-week role, and the unhealthiness of this nonstop responsibility should be emphasized.

Adding to the difficulty of caregiving for patients with PD can be a change in the patient's personality, arising from dementia and involving increased irritability, excessive demands, or paranoia (48). Some patients will accuse their caregivers of neglect or abuse or even develop delusions that their spouse caregivers are having affairs with others. Such accusations, if baseless, and lack of appreciation add substantially to the burden of caregiving and can deplete the resources of even the most highly adapted caregiver. Empathy and maximum support should be offered to refuel the caregivers in their thankless and exhausting efforts. It remains important to inquire about and address sexual problems or concerns, if they are present. At the same time, swindling, theft, and elder abuse is possible, and, in any case, the doctor should model for the caregivers an esteeming, respectful stance about the patient.

TABLE 6-3. *The late stage of PD: Highly symptomatic with significant treatment complications*

Psychosocial challenges	Goal(s)	Interventions
Structuring life around medication and "on" periods; coping with motor complications: dyskinesias, "on/off," and wearing off	Maximize "on" periods and diminish motor complications as much as possible so as to facilitate maximal physical and social functioning	Adjust medication regimen as necessary. Educate about motor complications and their treatment. Empathize with patient's frustrations. To facilitate an increased sense of control, make patient a partner in treatment decisions, if appropriate. Encourage patient to schedule activities at "best" times and plan for "off" periods or fluctuations. Look for and treat psychiatric symptoms that contribute to poor physical or social functioning. If medication adjustments fail to adequately relieve motor complications and improve functioning, consider referral for DBS surgery, if clinically appropriate.
Loss of further physical capacities/ability to perform tasks	Assist patient in adapting to diminished physical abilities Prevent patient from too readily giving up tasks or responsibilities to others	Occupational therapy and physical therapy. Empathize with patient's loss of physical skills/abilities. Challenge patient's "I can't do that anymore" statements when appropriate. Offer empathy and encourage patient to enlist help/support of others. Arrange home care services and monitor caregiver burden.
Loss of independence; dependency fears/conflicts	Assist patients to adjust to an increasing need to depend on others for support	Empathize with patient's experience adjusting to increasing dependency. Facilitate maximal independent functioning and autonomy. Ensure adequate support services, including home care, are provided. Participation in support groups can be helpful.
Speech problems, drooling, and facial masking	Diminish impact these symptoms, if present, have on social functioning	Speech therapy, if indicated. Prescribe other treatments as indicated, e.g., for drooling. Educate caregivers about these symptoms and how to deal with them. Empathize with patient's frustrations with respect to others' reactions to these symptoms.
Decreased physical stamina/fatigue	Continue to prevent deconditioning in order to allow patient to remain active	Physical therapy/occupational therapy. Teach exercises tailored to patient's level of motor functioning. Encourage patient to stay as physically active as possible. Empathize with patient's painful recognition of decreased stamina/energy.
Fear of falls	Improve balance/gait as much as possible; increase safety to prevent falls.	Physical therapy/gait training. Teach patient to use assistive devices and other techniques that can help prevent falls. Avoid medications that can worsen balance. Treat motor symptoms as indicated.
Social isolation	Prevent withdrawal from social activities, when possible	Emphasize the importance of maintaining social contacts and staying as active as possible. Empathize with patient's sense of loss at having to give up many activities. When available, and if the patient is interested, refer patient to adult day health programs with provided transportation.
Psychiatric complications of medications: hallucinations and paranoia	Reduce psychiatric complications of medications Educate family members about these symptoms	Adjust PD medications to reduce complications. Adjunctive use of atypical antipsychotics, e.g., quetiapine, may be necessary. These symptoms may disturb caregivers more than the patient. Educate the patient and caregivers about these symptoms and their treatment. Empathize with patients' and caregivers' experiences.

(continues)

TABLE 6-3. *Continued*

Psychosocial challenges	Goal(s)	Interventions
Derangement of sleep/wake cycle	Diminish daytime somnolence and improve nighttime insomnia in order to facilitate physical and social functioning during the day	Adjust medication regimen as appropriate to facilitate sleep at night and wakefulness during the day. Adjunctive use of hypnotic agents or wakefulness agents may be indicated. Diagnose and treat, if present, conditions that can exacerbate insomnia such as REM sleep behavior disorder or sleep apnea. Teach patient good sleep hygiene. Encourage increased daytime physical activity commensurate with current abilities. Refer to sleep center if treatment responses are inadequate.
Prominent cognitive deficits/dementia (if present)	Diminish impact of cognitive deficits on daily functioning	Teach patient techniques to assist with memory deficits, e.g., keeping a notebook with reminders. Educate caregivers and family members about cognitive deficits/dementia. Empathize with their frustrations. Examine anticholinergic burden of medication regimen and discontinue any agents that could be exacerbating deficits. Treat comorbid psychiatric symptoms that can affect cognitive function, such as depression or anxiety. If appropriate, consider use of pharmacologic agents for dementia/cognitive deficits. Ensure adequate support services are available and that medication adherence is being monitored. Ensure home environment is safe.
Impact on relationships	Assess patient's relationship(s), looking for strain/conflicts that could be ameliorated	Inquire about relationships, inviting discussion of the patient's fear of being a burden, or fear of abandonment. Offer empathy and normalize the challenges that worsening PD presents to a relationship and the shifts in roles. Offer referrals for group or individual counseling. Refer caregiver to caregiver support groups and other resources.
	Openly invite discussion of issues of sexuality	Invite patients to discuss fears, questions, and problems and offer treatment and/or reassurance.
Caregiver burnout	Help caregivers 'refuel' and prevent their burnout	Ask caregivers how they are coping and empathically listen to their frustrations. Encourage caregivers to make use of support services to enable them to maintain their own social contacts and activities as much as possible. Ensure caregivers are able to get sufficient sleep. Some may need to be given permission to sleep in a separate bed or room. Refer caregivers to counseling, support groups, and/or psychiatric treatment if indicated. Caregiver support groups and on-line resources are useful in diminishing guilt feelings and helping caregivers learn coping techniques from each other.

SUMMARY

Throughout the course of PD, opportunities abound for psychosocial interventions that can improve a patient's quality of life. The psychosocial challenges accompanying PD vary by stage of illness, though some challenges persist throughout the course of illness. As illustrated in the tables in this chapter, many of these interventions involve empathic listening and inquiry, education, challenging distorted or overly helpless thoughts and self-conceptions, and facilitating social contact and functioning. Others directly address the needs of caregivers who are confronted with the devastating effects of PD on their loved ones. Although many of the recommendations in this chapter are nonspecific and intuitive, their potential effect should not be underestimated. Although we have been unable to address all of the psychosocial issues confronted by patients facing PD, we hope that this chapter serves as a useful guide for providers looking for additional opportunities for psychosocial interventions designed to increase patient quality of life. These interventions can be delegated to other members of the team, and the assistance of psychiatrists or social workers may be warranted, but PD clinicians themselves can have the most dramatic effect on their patients because of their allocated authority and their salutary alliance with the patient.

FURTHER READING

Forrest DV. Psychotherapy for patients with neuropsychiatric disorders. In: Yudofsky SC, Hales RE, eds. *The American Psychiatric Press Textbook of Neuropsychiatry and Clinical Neurosciences*, Fourth edition. Washington, DC: American Psychiatric Publishing Inc, 2002.

REFERENCES

1. *Mov Disord* Psychosocial counseling in Parkinson's disease. 2002;17 (Suppl. 4):S160–S162.
2. Krakow K, Haltenhof H, Buhler KE. Coping with Parkinson's disease and refractory epilepsy: a comparative study. *J Nerv Ment Dis* 1999;187:503–508.
3. Pentland B, Barnes MP, Findley LJ, et al. Parkinson's disease: the spectrum of disabilities. *J Neurol Neurosurg Psychiatr* 1992;55(Suppl):32–35.
4. Jacopini G. The experience of disease: psychosocial aspects of movement disorders. *J Neurosci Nurs* 2000; 32:263–265.
5. Ellgring H, Seiler S, Perleth B, et al. Psychosocial aspects of Parkinson's disease. *Neurology* 1993;43(12 Suppl 6):S41–S44.
6. Levy G, Marder K. Prevalence, incidence, and risk factors for dementia in Parkinson's disease. In: Bédard MA, Agid Y, Chouinard S et al., eds. *Mental and behavioral dysfunction in movement disorders*. Totowa, NJ: Humana Press, 2003:259–270.
7. Stout JC, Paulsen JS. Assessing cognition in movement disorders. In: Bédard MA, Agid Y, Chouinard S et al., eds. *Mental and behavioral dysfunction in movement disorders*, Totowa, NJ: Humana Press, 2003:85–100.
8. Aarsland D, Larsen JP, Lim NG, et al. Range of neuropsychiatric disturbances in patients with Parkinson's disease. *J Neurol Neurosurg Psychiatr* 1999;67: 492–496.
9. Friedman JH. Behavioral dysfunction in Parkinson's disease. *Clin Neurosci* 1998;5:87–93.
10. Marinus J, Visser M, Martinez-Martin P, et al. A short psychosocial questionnaire for patients with Parkinson's disease: the SCOPA-PS. *J Clin Epidemiol* 2003; 56:61–67.
11. Weintraub D, Moberg PJ, Duda JE, et al. Effect of psychiatric and other nonmotor symptoms on disability in Parkinson's disease. *J Am Geriatr Soc* 2004;52:784–788.
12. Bhatia K, Brooks DJ, Burn DJ, et al. Updated guidelines for the management of Parkinson's disease. *Hosp Med (London)* 2001;62:456–470.
13. Wolters EC. Psychiatric complications in Parkinson's disease. *J Neural Transm Suppl* 2000;60:291–302.
14. Karlsen KH, Tandberg E, Aarsland D, et al. Health related quality of life in Parkinson's disease: a prospective longitudinal study. *J Neurol Neurosurg Psychiatr* 2000;69:584–589.
15. Burn DJ. Beyond the iron mask: toward better recognition and treatment of depression associated with Parkinson's disease. *Mov Disord* 2002;17:445–454.
16. Schrag A, Selai C. Medical and psychosocial determinants of quality of life in Parkinson's disease. In: Bédard MA, Agid Y, Chouinard S et al., eds. *Mental and behavioral dysfunction in movement disorders*. Totowa, NJ: Humana Press, 2003:501–516.
17. Martinez-Martin P. An introduction to the concept of "quality of life in Parkinson's disease." *J Neurol* 1998; 245(Suppl. 1):S2–S6.
18. Habermann B. Continuity challenges of Parkinson's disease in middle life. *J Neurosci Nurs* 1999;31:200–207.
19. Schrag A, Jahanshahi M, Quinn N. How does Parkinson's disease affect quality of life? A comparison with quality of life in the general population. *Mov Disord* 2000;15:1112–1118.
20. Fitzsimmons B, Bunting LK. Parkinson's disease: quality of life issues. *Nurs Clin North Am* 1993;28:807–818.
21. Habermann B. Day-to-day demands of Parkinson's disease. *West J Nurs Res* 1996;18:397–413.
22. Montgomery EB Jr, Lieberman A, Singh G, et al. Patient education and health promotion can be effective in Parkinson's disease: a randomized controlled trial. *Am J Med* 1994;97:429–435.
23. Lieberman A. An integrated approach to patient management in Parkinson's disease. *Neurol Clin* 1992;10: 553–565.

24. Koller WC. Treatment of early Parkinson's disease. *Neurology* 2002;58(4 Suppl 1):S79–S86.
25. Oertel WH, Ellgring H. Parkinson's disease—medical education and psychosocial aspects. *Patient Educ Couns* 1995;26:71–79.
26. Cummings JL. Depression and Parkinson's disease: a review. *Am J Psychiatry* 1992;149:443–454.
27. McDonald WM, Richard IH, DeLong MR. Prevalence, etiology, and treatment of depression in Parkinson's disease. *Biol Psychiatry* 2003;54:363–375.
28. Kostic VS, Stefanova E, Dragasevic N, et al. Diagnosis and treatment of depression in Parkinson's disease. In: Bédard MA, Agid Y, Chouinard S et al., eds. *Mental and behavioral dysfunction in movement disorders*. Totowa, NJ: Humana Press, 2003:351–368.
29. Slaughter JR, Slaughter KA, Nichols D, et al. Prevalence, clinical manifestations, etiology, and treatment of depression in Parkinson's disease. *J Neuropsychiatry Clin Neurosci* 2001;13:187–196.
30. Abudi S, Bar-Tal Y, Ziv L, et al. Parkinson's disease symptoms—patients' perceptions. *J Adv Nurs* 1997; 25:54–59.
31. Backer JH. Stressors, social support, coping, and health dysfunction in individuals with Parkinson's disease. *J Gerontol Nurs* 2000;26:6–16.
32. Marr JA. The experience of living with Parkinson's disease. *J Neurosci Nurs* 1991;23:325–329.
33. McCall B. Young-onset Parkinson's disease: a guide to care and support. *Nurs Times* 2003;99(30):28–31.
34. Strain JJ, Grossman S. Psychological reactions to medical illness and hospitalization. In: Strain JJ, Grossman S, eds. *Psychological care of the medically ill: a primer in liaison psychiatry*. New York: Appleton-Century-Crofts, 1975:25.
35. Dakof GA, Mendelsohn GA. Parkinson's disease: the psychosocial aspects of a chronic illness. *Psychol Bull* 1986;99:375–387.
36. Siemers ER, Shekhar A, Quaid K, et al. Anxiety and motor performance in Parkinson's disease. *Mov Disord* 1993;8:501–506.
37. Menza MA, Robertson-Hoffman DE, Bonapace AS. Parkinson's disease and anxiety: comorbidity with depression. *Biol Psychiat* 1993;34:465–470.
38. Henderson R, Kurlan R, Kersun JM, et al. Preliminary examination of the comorbidity of anxiety and depression in Parkinson's disease. *J Neuropsychiatry Clin Neurosci* 1992;4:257–264.
39. Frazier LD. Coping with disease-related stressors in Parkinson's disease. *Gerontologist* 2000;40:53–63.
40. Tison F, Barberger-Gateau P, Dubroca B, et al. Dependency in Parkinson's disease: a population-based survey in nondemented elderly subjects. *Mov Disord* 1997; 12:910–915.
41. Wallhagen MI, Brod M. Perceived control and well-being in Parkinson's disease. *West J Nurs Res* 1997;19: 11–25.
42. Habermann B. Spousal perspective of Parkinson's disease in middle life. *J Adv Nurs* 2000;31:1409–1415.
43. Calne SM. The psychosocial impact of late-stage Parkinson's disease. *J Neurosci Nurs* 2003;35:306–313.
44. Ring H. Psychological and social problems of Parkinson's disease. *Br J Hosp Med* 1993;49:111–116.
45. Liu CY, Wang SJ, Fuh JL, et al. The correlation of depression with functional activity in Parkinson's disease. *J Neurol* 1997;244:493–498.
46. Cole SA, Woodard JL, Juncos JL, et al. Depression and disability in Parkinson's disease. *J Neuropsychiatry Clin Neurosci* 1996;8:20–25.
47. Schrag A, Hovris A, Morley D, et al. Young- versus older-onset Parkinson's disease: impact of disease and psychosocial consequences. *Mov Disord* 2003;18: 1250–1256.
48. Carter JH, Stewart BJ, Archbold PG, et al. Living with a person who has Parkinson's disease: the spouse's perspective by stage of disease. Parkinson's Study Group. *Mov Disord* 1998;13:20–28.
49. Brown RG, Jahanshahi M, Quinn N, et al. Sexual function in patients with Parkinson's disease and their partners. *J Neurol Neurosurg Psychiatry* 1990;53:480–486.
50. Bronner G, Royter V, Korczyn AD, et al. Sexuality and Parkinson's disease. In: Bédard MA, Agid Y, Chouinard S et al., eds. *Mental and behavioral dysfunction in movement disorders*. Totowa, NJ: Humana Press, 2003:517–526.
51. Welsh M, Hung L, Waters CH. Sexuality in women with Parkinson's disease. *Mov Disord* 1997;12:923–927.
52. Fahn S. Description of Parkinson's disease as a clinical syndrome. *Ann N Y Acad Sci* 2003;991:1–14.
53. Herlofson K, Larsen JP. The influence of fatigue on health-related quality of life in patients with Parkinson's disease. *Acta Neurol Scand* 2003;107:1–6.
54. Lou JS, Kearns G, Oken B, et al. Exacerbated physical fatigue and mental fatigue in Parkinson's disease. *Mov Disord* 2001;16:190–196.
55. Shulman LM, Taback RL, Bean J, et al. Comorbidity of the nonmotor symptoms of Parkinson's disease. *Mov Disord* 2001;16:507–510.
56. Fahn S. Medical treatment of Parkinson's disease. *J Neurol* 1998;245 (11 Suppl 3):P15–P24.
57. Trenkwalder C. Sleep dysfunction in Parkinson's disease. *Clin Neurosci* 1998;5:107–114.
58. Askenasy JJ. Sleep disturbances in Parkinsonism. *J Neural Transm* 2003;110:125–150.
59. Menza MA, Rosen RC. Sleep in Parkinson's disease. The role of depression and anxiety. *Psychosomatics* 1995;36:262–266.
60. Rye DB, Daley JT, Freeman AA, et al. Daytime sleepiness and sleep attacks in idiopathic Parkinson's disease. In: Bédard MA, Agid Y, Chouinard S et al., eds. *Mental and behavioral dysfunction in movement disorders*. Totowa, NJ: Humana Press, 2003:527–538.
61. Whetter-Goldstein K, Sloan F, Kulas E, et al. The burden of Parkinson's disease on society, family, and the individual. *J Am Geriatr Soc* 1997;45:844–849.
62. Clarke CE, Zobkiw RM, Gullaksen E. Quality of life and care in Parkinson's disease. *Br J Clin Pract* 1995; 49:288–293.
63. Edwards NE, Scheetz PS. Predictors of burden for caregivers of patients with Parkinson's disease. *J Neurosci Nurs* 2002;34:184–190.
64. Adler CH. Relevance of motor complications in Parkinson's disease. *Neurology* 2002;58(4 Suppl 1):S51–S56.
65. Raudino F. Non motor off in Parkinson's disease. *Acta Neurol Scand* 2001;104:312–315.

66. Cohen H. Disorders of speech and language in Parkinson's disease. In: Bédard MA, Agid Y, Chouinard S et al., eds. *Mental and behavioral dysfunction in movement disorders*. Totowa, NJ: Humana Press, 2003:125–134.
67. Juncos JL. Management of psychotic aspects of Parkinson's disease. *J Clin Psychiat* 1999;60(Suppl. 8):42–53.
68. Aarsland D, Larsen JP. Diagnosis and treatment of hallucinations and delusions in Parkinson's disease. In: Bédard MA, Agid Y, Chouinard S et al., eds. *Mental and behavioral dysfunction in movement disorders*. Totowa, NJ: Humana Press, 2003:369–382.
69. Stocchi F, Barbato L, Nordera G, et al. Sleep disorders in Parkinson's disease. *J Neurol* 1998;245(Suppl. 1):S15–S18.
70. Boeve BF, Silber MH, Ferman TJ, et al. REM sleep behavior disorder in Parkinson's disease, dementia with Lewy bodies, and multiple system atrophy. In: Bédard MA, Agid Y, Chouinard S et al., eds. *Mental and behavioral dysfunction in movement disorders*. Totowa, NJ: Humana Press, 2003:383–398.
71. Korczyn AD. Dementia in Parkinson's disease. *J Neurol* 2001;248 (Suppl. 3):III1–III4.
72. Berry RA, Murphy JF. Well-being of caregivers of spouses with Parkinson's disease. *Clin Nurs Res* 1995; 4:373–386.
73. O'Reilly F, Finnan F, Allwright S et al., The effects of caring for a spouse with Parkinson's disease on social, psychological and physical well-being. *Br J Gen Pract* 1996;46:507–512.

7

Early Cognitive Changes and Nondementing Behavioral Abnormalities in Parkinson's Disease

Bonnie E. Levin[1] and Heather L. Katzen[2]

[1]*Department of Neurology, University of Miami School of Medicine, Miami, Florida;*
[2]*Department of Neurology, Weill Medical College of Cornell University, Ithaca, New York*

Despite a large number of studies in the literature that examine neuropsychologic deficits in Parkinson's disease (PD), relatively few studies have specifically addressed the issue of early cognitive changes. Most studies examine heterogenous PD samples, in which disease duration, age, motor symptom severity, and treatment regimens vary. Studying patients in the earlier stages of the disease provides important insights into discrete cognitive changes associated with selective basal ganglia dysfunction (1). Furthermore, the potentially confounding factors that exist in the advanced stages of the disease, such as medication side effects, global cognitive impairment, and severe motor symptoms, are less likely to be prominent.

A definition of "early PD" is controversial because short disease duration and mild disease severity each represent an early stage of the disorder. For the purpose of this chapter, early PD is defined as a recent-onset disease (five years' duration or less) or as symptom severity at Hoehn and Yahr stages I and II. Studies that combine patients with early PD and patients with more advanced PD are not reviewed in this chapter unless patients with earlier PD can be examined as a separate group.

CLINICAL CORRELATES OF COGNITIVE DECLINE

Dementia, as defined by *The Diagnostic and Statistical Manual of Mental Disorders*, 4th edition (DSM-IV) criteria, is rare in early PD; mild cognitive changes are more prevalent but remain the subject of controversy. One problem is that cognition in PD cannot be studied independently from other clinical parameters that influence the type and pattern of cognitive change. These clinical correlates include age and age of onset, motor symptom severity, side of onset, and medication effects.

Age and Age of Onset

Early-onset PD was once believed to produce more severe clinical symptoms (2,3), but other well-controlled studies comparing the effects of early (<50 years) and later (>70 years) age of onset now indicate that the opposite may be true: Compared with younger patients with PD, older patients exhibit a higher incidence of cognitive impairment and overall dementia and a more rapid course of disease progression. First described by Celesia and Wanamaker (4), these findings have subsequently been observed by other investigators (5), including those using standardized neuropsychological tests (6–10).

Some studies have been criticized for examining subjects at only one point in time, thus bypassing the question of whether the older subjects were nondemented in their younger years and deteriorated with advancing age. Longitudinal studies have now documented a similar outcome associated with advanced age. Biggins et al. (11) conducted serial assessments of cognition, mood, and motor symptomatology at 9-month intervals on 87 patients with PD and 50 control subjects. Initially, 6% of the patients with PD were demented (based on DSM-III-R), but 54 months later, the cumulative incidence of dementia among the patients with PD was 19%, whereas none of the control subjects were demented. Biggins et al. found that patients with PD who became demented were older, had PD longer, and had an older age of onset. In a prospective cohort study of 250 patients with PD, Stern et al. (12) found advanced age to be one of the antecedent risk factors for dementia. Locascio et al. (13) also reported select cognitive deficits that appeared earlier in the disease for patients with late-onset PD. More recently, Marras et al. (5) reviewed a series of studies to identify predictors of prognosis in PD and found, with only one exception, older age at onset to be an adverse prognostic factor associated with rapid decline.

Medication Effects

Consensus regarding the effect of pharmacologic treatment on cognition in PD patients is lacking. Levodopa treatment has been shown to result in improved performance on tasks of delayed verbal memory (14), choice reaction time (15), and attention (16) but may interfere with other tasks associated with frontal lobe functions (17). Still other studies find modest effects on cognitive function and psychiatric status (18) or report an initial improvement on levodopa in overall cognitive functioning that gradually reverts to baseline performance levels (19–21).

A similar lack of consensus exists regarding the effects of anticholinergic treatment on memory function in PD, with some studies showing impaired recent and recognition memory (22–24), whereas others find no evidence of memory deterioration (25).

The lack of consistency between these studies is attributable to a host of factors that prevent interstudy comparisons. These factors include differing drugs, dosages, modes of administration, and length of treatment. Other methodologic confounds include lack of consistency in the type of method used to assess each of the cognitive domains, and differences between subjects' ages, disease durations, and disease severities.

Few studies have examined the effects of pharmacologic treatment in the early stages of PD. Canavan (26) found that anticholinergic medication did not disrupt either associative learning performance or conceptual set shifting in early PD. Levin et al. (25) compared four groups of patients with early PD ($n = 54$) on two verbal memory measures and one visuospatial recognition task. Subjects were either unmedicated, taking anticholinergics or dopamine alone, or taking a combination of these drugs. No significant differences were observed between the four groups on any of the memory measures.

Cooper et al. (27) tested 82 patients with newly diagnosed PD, who had never received drug therapy, with a full battery of neuropsychological measures. Subjects were then randomly assigned to one of three monotherapy treatment groups—levodopa, bromocriptine, or anticholinergic drugs—and retested approximately 4 months later. The investigators found that although levodopa and anticholinergic medication improved motor control, their effects on cognitive function differed. Anticholinergic medication impaired short-term memory, specifically the registration of new information, whereas dopaminergic medication improved performance scores on a working memory task. Although the study by Cooper et al. underscores the importance of controlling for treatment variables, it is also clear that for some patients with PD, medication may exert a highly selective influence on cognitive performance early in the illness.

Motor Symptoms and Side of Onset

Studies of cognitive function and cardinal motor signs in patients with PD reveal several consistent trends. Prominent tremor is associated with normal or near normal mental status, whereas bradykinesia and rigidity correlate with a wide range of intellectual deficits. Furthermore, it is now recognized that the side of motor onset may influence cognitive outcome (5,28,29). Tomer et al. (30) compared 48 subjects with right-sided motor onset with 40 patients whose motor signs began on the left side of the body. The left-sided onset group performed consistently more poorly than the right-sided onset group on multiple neuropsychological measures, including immediate and delayed verbal memory, word retrieval, semantic verbal fluency, visuospatial analysis, abstract reasoning, attention span, and mental tracking. These findings imply that cognitive deterioration is linked to an asymmetric disturbance of dopamine pathways, which are established early in the early process.

Language

The degree to which language is affected in PD is difficult to evaluate, because many tasks require competency in nonlinguistic abilities, such as attention, memory, and executive function (31). Nevertheless, there is general consensus that frank aphasias are not part of the parkinsonian symptom complex. There are, however, several studies that find subtle qualitative differences in the higher-order linguistic tasks during the early stages of the illness.

Lees and Smith (32) found that patients with early PD gave a higher number of perseverative intrusions compared to age-matched controls on a word fluency task. The authors interpreted this finding as evidence that patients with PD experience difficulty in shifting between categories under time constraints. Illes (33) analyzed spontaneous language production in five patients with mild PD as defined by Websters' rating scale. Although syntax was intact, they noted the presence of silent hesitations at the beginning of sentences, a finding interpreted as evidence of difficulty in planning upcoming linguistic sequences. In addition, they found an elevated number of open class optional phrases and postulated that this may be an adaptive strategy in generating as much information as possible in a single sentence.

Levin et al. (34) found that patients with early PD did not differ from age-matched and education-matched control subjects on fund of vocabulary, word retrieval, and two measures of verbal fluency. However, these patients performed one of the categoric fluency measures and the recitation of months backwards significantly worse than controls did.

Grossman et al. (35) examined sentence comprehension and praxis in 22 patients with early PD who were receiving either minimal or no antiparkinsonian medication. They found that patients with PD, compared with control subjects, exhibited significantly more difficulty answering syntactically embedded questions. Patients with PD also exhibited compromised ability to perform learned gestures, according to measures of representational and nonrepresentational praxis. The investigators noted that substitution of a body part for the object was a common error type on representational praxis items. Other studies, such as Lees and Smith (32), did not find evidence of apraxia in the early stages of PD.

Cooper et al. (36) studied 60 nondemented patients, newly diagnosed with PD, who had never received pharmacologic therapy for their disease. These patients were compared with 40 healthy control subjects of comparable age, sex, and premorbid IQ based on the New Adult Reading Test (NART) and the Wechsler Adult Intelligence Scale-Revised (WAIS-R) vocabulary. Patients were rigorously screened for other medical and psychiatric conditions, alcoholism, and head injury. The investigators examined word retrieval (Boston Naming Test), expressive language (Reporter's Test), comprehension (Token Test), and semantic fluency (inanimate objects, animals category alternation using colors and birds). The only differences noted between the two groups were in language expression, object word fluency, and the category alternation tasks, in which patients with PD showed mild deficits compared with controls.

These studies support other research on individuals with more advanced stages of the disease, indicating that language ability is largely preserved in PD. No study to date that has employed a comprehensive test battery has found a pervasive language disturbance. When language impairments are found, they are highly circumscribed, subtle, and may involve organizational or fluency skills. Thus, the question arises whether these deficits represent a specific language impairment or are symptoms of a more generalized executive disturbance involving frontal systems.

Visuospatial Skills

Visuospatial abnormalities are among the most common and the most controversial neuropsychological deficits reported in PD. Conceptual and methodologic questions make this area of research a subject of ongoing controversy. A major problem is that researchers do not agree on the definition of visuospatial deficit. Most studies rely on a particular task to define the construct. As a result, the label "visuospatial deficit" has been applied to patients with PD who have difficulty in any one of a number of spatial tasks including facial recognition, visual analysis and synthesis, visual discrimination, visual recognition, spatial memory, personal space, spatial planning, visuomotor integration, visual attention, and visual orientation (37).

Another problem is how visuospatial abnormalities are assessed. Many visuospatial tasks, particularly those used in earlier studies, are timed and require adept manual dexterity to reach a successful solution. Only recently have investigators employed tasks that are motorfree and untimed, two factors that allow visuospatial deficits to be studied independently from the motor abnormalities associated with the disease.

Very few studies have focused on visuospatial skills in the early stage of PD. Canavan et al. (38) administered three visuospatial tasks to patients with early PD, patients with focal frontal or temporal lobe lesions, and healthy age-matched controls. Their measures included a spatial delayed alternation task, a street plan test of left–right orientation, and a prism adaptation task. They found that three groups of patients, those with PD, frontal lobe lesions, and postoperative right temporal lobectomy, required significantly more trials to reach the criterion on the prism adaptation task than either the healthy controls or patients who had undergone left temporal lobectomy. Interestingly, patients with PD who had predominantly left-sided parkinsonian signs (right basal ganglia pathology) performed worse on this measure than patients with PD who had either bilateral or predominantly right-sided motor symptomatology. No group differences were observed on the other visual–spatial measures.

Montgomery et al. (39) compared 24 mildly impaired (stages I and II) and 24 moderately impaired (stage III) patients with PD with 35 age-matched control subjects on judgment of line orientation and a spatial updating task. The spatial updating task required subjects to maintain their sense of direction after being moved in their environment while relying on either visual or vestibular sensory information. In the visual condition, subjects were moved in a wheelchair while wearing a headbox that permitted a view of the walls and ceiling but not the floor. In the vestibular condition, subjects were guided through the same route but were blindfolded, leaving only vestibular and somatosensory input. The authors found that difficulty with the visual condition of the spatial updating task correlated with poor performance in judging line orientation, a finding that they interpreted as evidence for mild visual perceptual problems in select patients with early PD.

Cooper et al. (36) found that patients with early PD showed visuomotor constructive deficits when copying a complex geometric figure (Rey Osterrieth Complex Figure) but performed normally on a visuoconstructive task using a three-dimensional model.

Levin et al. (40) administered six visuospatial measures to 184 patients with PD of varying duration and to 90 control subjects matched by age and education. The visuospatial battery consisted of facial recognition (Benton's Facial Recognition Task), line orientation (Judgment of Line Orientation), mental object assembly (a modified version of the Hooper Visual Organization Task), verbal embedded figures (Ghent Embedded Figures), nonverbal embedded figures, and a modified block design test (only 2 × 2 matrix designs were included). The group with early PD ($n = 84$; disease duration = 1.0–4.0 years) performed as well as control subjects on all of the visuospatial measures except facial recognition. However, Dujardin (41) found deficits in decoding emotional facial expressions in a group of patients with early PD who had not been treated with antiparkinsonian medication.

Although impaired visuospatial skills are commonly found in PD and appear to be independent of motor abnormalities associated with the disease, it is unclear how prominent these changes are in the early stages of the disease. Prism adaptation, recognition of embedded facial figures, copying complex geometric designs, and spatial updating require active planning and strategy as well as a host of other skills, which are not necessarily unique to spatial cognition. It is possible that the earliest visuospatial changes reflect an executive dysfunction and not a true visuospatial deficit per se. This view is compatible with the view that visuospatial deficits in the earliest stages of PD emerge when tasks involve set shifting, another aspect of executive function (42,43).

MEMORY

Memory impairment has been found in the early stages of PD and appears to be independent of dementia. Taylor et al. (44) compared 15 newly diagnosed, untreated patients with PD and 15 healthy control subjects matched by age and verbal IQ. Multiple memory skills were assessed, including short-term and delayed recall of logical discourse and semantically related word lists, recognition span for spatial position, incremental verbal list learning of unrelated words, priming effects, and source memory.

Patients with PD performed comparably with control subjects on immediate and delayed recall of logical discourse and semantically unrelated words, and on delayed recognition of spatial position. However, important differences emerged between the two groups in their spontaneous organization of the stimuli. Patients with PD were consistently worse than control subjects in their recall of semantically related words [California Verbal Learning Test (CVLT)] and used clustering, a strategy presumed to facilitate learning, less often and less efficiently on the five immediate recall conditions. Patients with PD also exhibited deficient source memory, relative to control subjects, and increased sensitivity to interference effects during learning. Taylor et al. interpreted these findings as evidence that recall difficulties among patients with PD result from a basic planning deficit, stemming from frontostriatal dysfunction, that interferes with the acquisition of novel stimuli.

Cooper et al. (45) found that patients with newly diagnosed PD were more impaired than age- and sex-matched controls on backward digit span, immediate and delayed recall of the logical memory passages, and paired associate learning. These investigators also used the Brown–Peterson Distractor Task, a paradigm that assesses patients' ability to recall consonant trigrams after varying distractor-filled intervals. Patients with PD performed as well as control subjects on the immediate recall condition (no distractor) but performed more poorly on each of the five different distractor-filled intervals. Fischer et al. (46) studied recency and primacy recognition in patients with early PD and healthy control subjects, matched by age, education, and sex, using a modified version of Milner's temporal ordering task. Of the 29 patients in their sample, 23 were in stages I and II. Subjects were presented with 22 black-and-white line drawings and were then asked to indicate the first (primacy) and last (recency) picture from four choices. Patients with PD had more difficulty recalling the recency items than healthy control subjects did. More recent research supports these initial findings. Stoffers (47) found deficits in sequential visuospatial memory, and Pillon et al. (48) reported deficient memory for spatial location in patients with early PD who had not been treated with antiparkinsonian medication.

The issue of memory impairment in PD is complicated, because memory is composed of a diverse group of skills that may be functionally distinct and do not necessarily deteriorate in a uniform fashion. Therefore, what is called "memory impairment" may involve one or more individual deficits, each of which may show a different rate of decline. Yet, despite what appears to be a heterogeneous collection of deficits, much of the research shares a common theme: Early memory dysfunction may stem from a more generalized executive deficit that is not specific to a particular stimulus modality but disrupts the memorization process. Difficulties with anticipation, planning, sequencing, and organization would lead to problems attending to and maintaining information, making it difficult to process and recall stimuli. More recent research points to a problem in working memory, a term first proposed by Fuster (49) to describe the executive process by which the subject holds information on-line for the purpose of maintaining an active representation to guide later action. Fuster proposed that working memory depends on the integrity of the prefrontal cortex. Goldman-Rakic (50), who proposed an experimental model linking working memory to the prefrontal cortex, suggested that this model might explain some of the cognitive impairments in nonfocal pathologies such as PD.

Executive Functions

There has been a recent surge of interest in executive function deficits associated with PD. Executive functions are an integral part of many cognitive tasks, because they include anticipation, planning, goal selection, monitoring, and using feedback to guide behavior (51). Executive deficits are believed to reflect frontal lobe dysfunction. Early cognitive dysfunction has been linked to executive deficits associated with frontostriatal disturbance. Canavan et al. (52) compared patients with PD and patients who had frontal lobe lesions. Patients with early PD (symptom range, 6–86 months) were compared with healthy control subjects, and with patients who had documented lesions involving either the frontal or temporal lobes, in their ability to reproduce sequences of digits, spatial positions, and hand gestures. The group with PD performed comparably to control subjects on all of the sequencing tasks. Only subjects with frontal lobe lesions and right (but not left) temporal lobectomies showed select performance deficits on motor sequencing and the span tasks.

Canavan (26) also compared the same patient groups on two conditional associative learning tasks, a visual motor task requiring subjects to learn associations between six colors and six movements of a handle, and a visual–visual task requiring subjects to learn associations between color and shapes. The authors also administered the Wisconsin Card Sorting Task (WCST), a set shifting task based on three categoric sorting rules. No differences were noted between patients with PD and age-matched controls on any of the associative learning tasks. Although patients with PD did not differ from control subjects in the number of categories achieved on the WCST, they made more perseverative errors. An important observation noted in this study was that whereas most patients with PD showed no impairments on the learning tasks, an older subset of patients with PD performed consistently poorly on most measures. This finding supports other studies, such as that by Dubois et al. (10), who found that age has a negative effect on cognition in patients with PD.

Downes et al. (53) reported that patients with both early, nonmedicated and more advanced, medicated PD performed more poorly than healthy control subjects on a discriminative learning task that involved an extradimensional shift. These researchers did not find that patients with PD were more perseverative, nor did they find evidence of a more basic defect in arousal functions. Rather, they argued that patients with early PD have a highly specific attentional dysfunction, characterized by problems ignoring irrelevant stimulus dimensions, that leads to an unpredictable response set and ultimately an increase in errors.

Owen et al. (54) studied 44 patients with idiopathic PD, 15 of whom were nonmedicated (13 in stages I and II; 2 in stage III) and 29 of whom were medicated and had PD that was either mild to moderate ($n = 15$) or severe ($n = 14$). Medicated patients were screened for dementia and depression. The three PD groups were compared with three groups of healthy control subjects, matched by age and premorbid IQ using the NART. Subjects were given a battery of computerized tests sensitive to frontal lobe functions, which included a modified Tower of London test to assess planning performance and an attentional set-shifting task. The set-shifting task required subjects to discern, based on computerized feedback, which of two stimulus dimensions was relevant. On the Tower of London task, the nonmedicated patients with PD were no different from control subjects in terms of their accuracy and initial thinking time. However, all PD groups had difficulty with the attentional set shifting. These subjects not only had impaired set shifting but difficulty formulating and maintaining the correct response set.

Cooper et al. (36) administered several measures of executive function, including the WCST, timed and untimed Picture Arrangement, and a digit-ordering task. On the WCST, the group with PD did not differ from the control group on the number of categories achieved, overall correct responses, "other" or unique errors, percentage of conceptual responses, or ability to maintain set.

However, patients with PD did require significantly more cards to achieve the first category and performed more poorly on Picture Arrangement and digit ordering. The investigators also found that patients with PD and depression made more qualitative errors on Picture Arrangement and scored fewer categories and made more errors on the WCST than nondepressed patients with PD did.

In sum, executive deficits have been repeatedly found in early PD. Because many cognitive tasks rely on one or more executive components, it would follow that patients with PD, even in the earliest stages, may show impairments in a variety of cognitive areas.

Cognitive Processing Time

Although bradykinesia has been extensively studied in PD, whether patients with PD also require longer processing time when solving cognitive tasks remains unknown. Disentangling these two components is difficult, because many cognitive measures use a motor component. Two studies have specifically examined cognitive processing speed in patients with early PD. Zimmermann et al. (55) studied simple and choice reaction time in 10 untreated patients with early PD (duration of illness, 3–24 months), 9 patients with more advanced PD (duration, 2–12 years), and 17 healthy control subjects matched by age, sex, education, and IQ. Three reaction-time tasks were employed, one involving a simple motor response, and two others (choice reaction time) that presented cues requiring different degrees of cognitive processing to complete the task. In all groups, reaction time increased as cognitive load increased. Untreated patients with PD responded similarly to control subjects on the simple and choice reaction-time tasks when cognitive loading was either absent or low.

However, the patients with early PD performed more slowly than control subjects and comparably to medicated patients with PD in the length of decision-making time required for choice reaction-time tasks that incorporated the highest cognitive loading. These findings suggest that decision-making processing is compromised early in PD when cognitive demands are high.

Jordan et al. (56) investigated the extent to which attentional focusing and temporal predictability could explain prolonged response time in patients with PD. These authors compared 32 patients with newly diagnosed PD, 34 patients with PD who were taking medication, and 24 healthy control subjects on two simple reaction-time measures. Both groups with PD showed evidence of increased reaction time on each reaction-time measure but demonstrated normal effects of variable cue stimulus intervals. They hypothesized that the prolonged response time in early PD may be nondopaminergic in origin.

SPECIAL SENSORY CHANGES: OLFACTION AND CONTRAST SENSITIVITY

Loss of olfactory function in PD patients was first noted in 1980 by Korten and Meulstee (57). Although standardized testing was not performed, they reported that 41 of 80 patients with PD under their care were "unable to smell adequately."

Doty et al. (58,59) reported that olfactory dysfunction occurs early in the course of PD and is independent of stage, disease duration, and other cognitive and neurologic manifestations of the illness. They (60) examined 81 patients, of whom 43 were in stage I or II. Although patients with early PD were not studied separately, 75% of the patients showed less sensitivity than control subjects on a threshold detection measure. When patients were given the University of Pennsylvania Smell Identification Test (UPSIT), 90% of the group with PD scored lower than control subjects. No differences were noted between sides of the nose, indicating odor dysfunction was symmetric.

Olfaction deficits in PD may be secondary to use of antiparkinsonian medication. However, Doty et al. (60) compared medicated and unmedicated patients with early PD, all of whom were in stages I and II (except for one subject who was in stage III), and found olfaction deficits in both groups.

Contrast sensitivity deficits are another special sensory change that has been reported in patients with early PD. This deficit is of particular interest to investigators employing behavioral measures that examine the ability to detect varying degrees of luminance. Bulens et al. (61) studied 39 patients with PD, all but three of whom were in stage I and II, and found that 64% showed contrast sensitivity loss in one or both eyes. Abnormal contrast sensitivity curves were not related to disease severity or visual acuity.

DEPRESSION

The association between depression and PD was recognized in 1817 by Parkinson (62) in his original essay. Although many descriptive reports of depression in PD followed, only relatively recently have changes in mood been systematically assessed using standardized rating scales and structured interviews based on DSM-III criteria. These studies indicate that depression is prevalent in PD, affecting between 30% and 50% of patients and may, even in patients with early PD, exacerbate cognitive deficits (63). Two subtypes have been noted: major depression (moderate to severe symptoms) and dysthymia (mild symptoms). Most patients with PD exhibit a mild to moderate chronic depressed mood. Severe depression in patients with PD is uncommon. A third category that is beginning to receive recognition is subsyndromal depression, a milder form that does not meet strict DSM-IV criteria but is characterized by depression symptoms. Estimates of depressed mood likely are substantially higher when subsyndromal depression is taken into account (64).

The repeated observation that symptoms of depression frequently begin before the onset of PD motor symptoms is especially striking. Mayeux et al. (65) did not specifically examine early PD, but noted that 43% of depressed patients with PD exhibited evidence of depression before their motor symptoms appeared. Santamaria et al. (66) carried out a structured interview based on DSM-III criteria for depression and administered the Beck Depression Inventory (BDI) to 34 patients with early PD (duration between 0.5 and 4 years) and 23 healthy control subjects of comparable age and sex. They reported that patients with PD showed a higher frequency of dysthymia ($n = 10$) and major depression ($n = 1$) compared with control subjects ($n = 4$). For 15 patients (44%), the first episode of depression began 1.5 to 36 years before the onset of motor symptoms. This subgroup of patients tended to be younger at PD onset and exhibited less severe parkinsonism. No relationship was observed between depression (BDI scores) and disease severity or duration.

Depression in PD may in part be related to asymmetric hemispheric involvement. Starkstein et al. (67) found a relationship between depression and lateralization of PD motor symptoms. When left hemiparkinsonism (LHP) patients were compared with right hemiparkinsonism (RHP) patients, the RHP group showed a higher incidence of depression and scored higher on three depression indices, the Hamilton Rating Scale for Depression, the BDI, and the Present State Examination (PSE).

Depression may be related to the stage of PD. Cummings (68) found that young patients with PD in the early stages of their disease might be more vulnerable to depression than older patients with PD. However, Starkstein et al. (69) found that depression was disproportionately represented in the early and later stages, but for different reasons: Whereas early PD depression may be associated with structural and biochemical changes associated with left basal ganglia pathology, later PD-related depression may arise from progressive deterioration and impairment in activities of daily living (ADLs).

HYPOTHESIS REGARDING NEUROCHEMICAL CORRELATES OF COGNITIVE DECLINE

There is general consensus that parkinsonian symptoms begin after approximately 80% of dopaminergic neurons have been depleted. The mesocortical dopamine system is believed to be less depleted than the nigrostriatal dopamine projections (70). Lewis et al. (71) used event-related functional magnetic resonance imaging (fMRI) to compare cognitively impaired and unimpaired patients with early PD and found a significant signal reduction in the striatal and frontal lobe regions among patients with working memory deficits.

Although degeneration of dopaminergic pathways is believed to be directly related to cognitive decline, some evidence indicates that the pathophysiology may be more complex. The array of neuropsychologic deficits, even in the earliest stages of the disease, likely cannot be explained by a decline in any one neurotransmitter system. Clinicopathologic correlations are usually obtained from individuals in more advanced stages of the disease. Currently, animal studies provide the best model of early PD, but these data may be limited in their generalizability to human subjects.

In addition to the predominant dopamine deficiency, there are also other alterations in the ascending noradrenergic system, selective and perhaps sporadic serotonergic involvement in the raphe nuclei, and various changes in neuropeptidergic systems. Particular attention has been focused on the locus ceruleus pathology that is seen in PD and that disrupts the cerulocortical noradrenergic systems, resulting in decreased norepinephrine concentrations in the amygdala, hippocampus, and frontal cortex. Although the functions of the cerulocortical pathway are not understood, selective lesions of the locus caeruleus have been reported to produce attentional and memory impairment (72). Furthermore, involvement of serotonergic-raphe neurons in patients with PD has been related to depression and possibly cognitive dysfunction in some patients (73). Cholinergic dysfunction, which may begin quite early in PD patients, also may contribute to cognitive impairment (74).

SUMMARY

Early cognitive changes in patients with PD are often subtle and influenced by factors that interact with the disease process, including age of disease onset, medication, and the specific constellation of motor symptoms.

These factors notwithstanding, ample evidence exists that specific cognitive changes occur early in the course of PD. This evidence does not imply that cognitive deficits are pervasive during the early stages. To the contrary, they are usually subtle and often difficult to detect without formal neuropsychological testing. Executive-function deficits are the most frequently reported cognitive problems and, given that executive skills are an integral part of many tasks, it follows that subtle difficulties may be seen on a wide range of cognitive measures, particularly in working memory and visuospatial dysfunction, two areas that rely heavily on executive skills. Whereas apraxia and language processing deficits occur infrequently, subtle changes in olfaction and contrast sensitivity have also been repeatedly observed. Finally, depressive symptoms are also common in the early stages of the disease. The significance of the early behavioral changes and their prognostic implications are largely unknown. Prospective studies are needed to understand the longitudinal course of early cognitive changes to determine whether they remain as circumscribed impairments or represent a precursor to a more widespread dementia.

REFERENCES

1. Marsden CD. The mysteries of motor functions of the basal ganglia: the Robert Wartenburg lecture. *Neurology* 1982;32:514–539.
2. Mjones H. Paralysis agitans: a clinical and genetic study. *Acta Psychiatry Neurol* 1949;54 (Suppl):1–195.
3. Lesser RD, Fahn S, Snider SR, et al. Analysis of the clinical problems in parkinsonism and the complications of longterm levodopa therapy. *Neurology* 1979;29:1253–1260.
4. Celesia GG, Wanamaker WM. Psychiatric disturbances in Parkinson's disease. *Dis Nerv Syst* 1972;33:577–583.
5. Marras C, Rochon P, Lang AE. Predicting motor decline and disability in Parkinson's disease: a systematic review. *Arch Neurol* 2002;59(11):1724–1728.
6. Marttila RJ, Rinne UK. Dementia in Parkinson's disease. *Acta Neurol Scand* 1976;54:431–441.
7. Heitanen M, Teravainen H. The effect of age of disease onset on neuropsychology performance in Parkinson's disease. *J Neurol Neurosurg Psychiatry* 1988;51:244–249.
8. Ebmeier KP, Calder SA, Crawford JR, et al. Clinical features predicting dementia in idiopathic Parkinson's disease: a follow up study. *Neurology* 1990;40:1222–1224.
9. Elizan TS, Sroka H, Maker H, et al. Dementia in idiopathic Parkinson's disease: variables associated with its occurrence in 203 patients. *J Neural Transm* 1986;65:285–302.
10. Dubois B, Pillon B, Sternic N. Age-induced cognitive disturbances in Parkinson's disease. *Neurology* 1990;40:38–41.
11. Biggins CA, Boyd JL, Harrop FM, et al. A controlled, longitudinal study of dementia in Parkinson's disease. *J Neurol Neurosurg Psychiatry* 1992;55:566–571.
12. Stern Y, Marder K, Tang MX, et al. Antecedent clinical features associated with dementia in Parkinson's disease. *Neurology* 1993;43:1690–1692.
13. Locascio JJ, Corkin S, Growden JH. Relation between clinical characteristics of Parkinson's disease and cognitive decline. *J Clin Exp Neuropsychol* 2003;25(1):94–109.

14. Mohr E, Fabbrini G, Ruggieri S, et al. Cognitive concomitants of dopamine system stimulation in parkinsonian patients. *J Neurol Neurosurg Psychiatry* 1987;50:1192–1196.
15. Pullman SL, Watts RL, Juncos JL, et al. Dopaminergic effects of single and choice reaction time performance in Parkinson's disease. *Neurology* 1988;38:249–254.
16. Bowen FP, Kamienny RS, Burns MM, et al. Parkinsonism: effects of levodopa treatment on concept formation. *Neurology* 1975;25:701–704.
17. Gotham AM, Brown RG, Marsden CD. "Frontal" cognitive function in patients with Parkinson's disease "on" and "off" levodopa. *Brain* 1988;111:299–321.
18. Growden JH, Kieburtz K, McDermott MP et al., Parkinson Study Group. Levodopa improves motor function without impairing cognition in mild non-demented Parkinson's disease patients. *Neurology* 1998;50(5):1327–1331.
19. Riklan M, Whelitian W, Cullinan T. Levodopa and psychometric test performance in parkinsonism—5 years later. *Neurology* 1976;26:173–179.
20. Portin R, Rinne UK. Neuropsychological responses of parkinsonian patients to longterm levodopa treatment. In: Rinne UK, Klinger M, Stamm G, eds. *Parkinson's disease: current progress, problems and management*. Amsterdam: Elsevier North Holland, 1980.
21. Porton R, Rinne UK. Predictive factors for cognitive deterioration and dementia in Parkinson's disease. *Adv Neurol* 1986;45:413–416.
22. Dubios B, Danze F, Pillon B, et al. Cholinergic dependent cognitive deficits in Parkinson's disease. *Ann Neurol* 1987;22:26–30.
23. Koller W. Disturbances of recent memory function in parkinsonian patients on anticholinergic therapy. *Cortex* 1984;20:307–311.
24. Sadah M, Braham J, Madan M. Effects of anticholinergic drugs on memory in Parkinson's disease. *Arch Neurol* 1982;39:666–667.
25. Levin BE, Llabre MM, Reisman S. A retrospective analysis of the effects of anticholinergic medication on memory performance in Parkinson's disease. *J Neuropsychiatry Clin Neurosci* 1991;3:412–416.
26. Canavan AGM. The performance on learning tasks of patients in the early stages of Parkinson's disease. *Neuropsychologia* 1989;27:141–156.
27. Cooper JA, Sagar HJ, Doherty SM, et al. Different effects of dopaminergic and anticholinergic therapy on cognitive and motor function in Parkinson's disease. *Brain* 1992;115:1701–1725.
28. Aarsland D, Andersen K, Larsen JP, et al. Prevalence and characteristics of dementia in Parkinson's disease: an 8-year prospective study. *Arch Neurol* 2003;60(3):387–392.
29. Levin BE, Tomer R, Rey G. Clinical correlates of cognitive impairments in Parkinson's disease. In: Huber SJ, Cummings JL, eds. *Parkinson's disease: neurobehavioral aspects*. New York: Oxford Press, 1992.
30. Tomer R, Levin BE, Weiner WJ. Side of onset of motor symptoms influence cognition in Parkinson's disease. *Ann Neurol* 1993;579–584.
31. Bayles K. Language and Parkinson's disease. *Alzheimer's Dis Assoc Disord* 1990;4:171–180.
32. Lees AJ, Smith E. Cognitive deficits in the early stages of Parkinson's disease. *Brain* 1983;106:257–270.
33. Illes J. Neurolinguistic features of spontaneous language production dissociate three forms of neurodegenerative disease. *Brain Lang* 1989;37:628–642.
34. Levin BE, Llabre M, Weiner WJ. Cognitive impairments associated with early Parkinson's disease. *Neurology* 1989;39:557–561.
35. Grossman M, Carvell S, Gollomp S, et al. Sentence comprehension and praxis deficits in Parkinson's disease. *Neurology* 1991;41:1620–1626.
36. Cooper JA, Sagar HJ, Jordan N, et al. Cognitive impairment in early untreated Parkinson's disease and its relationship to motor disability. *Brain* 1991;114:2095–2122.
37. Levin BE. Spatial cognition in Parkinson's disease. *Alzheimer's Dis Assoc Disord* 1990;4:161–170.
38. Canavan AGM, Passingham RE, Marsden CD, et al. Prism adaptation and other tasks involving spatial abilities in patients with Parkinson's disease, patients with frontal lobe lesions and patients with unilateral temporal lobectomies. *Neuropsychologia* 1990;28:969–984.
39. Montgomery P, Silverstein P, Wichmann R, et al. Spatial updating in Parkinson's disease. *Brain Cogn* 1993;23:113–126.
40. Levin BE, Llabre MM, Reisman S, et al. Visuospatial impairment in Parkinson's disease. *Neurology* 1991;41:365–369.
41. Dujardin K, Blairy S, Defebvre L, et al. Deficits in decoding emotional facial expressions in Parkinson's disease. *Neuropsychologia* 2004;42(2):239–250.
42. Brown RG, Marsden CD. Visuospatial function in Parkinson's disease. *Brain* 1986;109:987–1002.
43. Farina E, Gattellaro G, Pomati S, et al. Researching a differential impairment of frontal functions and explicit memory in early Parkinson's disease. *Eur J Neurol* 2000;7(3):259–267.
44. Taylor AE, Saint-Cyr JA, Lang AE. Memory and learning in early Parkinson's disease. *Brain Cogn* 1990;2:211–232.
45. Cooper JA, Sagar HJ, Sullivan EV. Short-term memory and temporal ordering in early Parkinson's disease: effects of disease chronicity and medication. *Neuropsychologia* 1993;31:933–949.
46. Fischer P, Kendler P, Goldenberg G. Recency primacy recognition in Parkinson's disease. *J Neural Transm* 1990;2:71–77.
47. Stoffers D, Berendse HW, Deijen JB, et al. Deficits on Corsi's block-tapping task in early stage Parkinson's disease. *Parkinsonism Relat Disord* 2003;10(2):107–111.
48. Pillon B, Ertle S, Deweer B, et al. Memory for spatial location in 'de novo' parkinsonian patients. *Neuropsychologia* 1997;35(3):221–228.
49. Fuster JM. *The prefrontal cortex: anatomy, physiology and neuropsychology of the frontal lobe*. New York: Raven Press, 1980.
50. Goldman-Rakic PS. Circuitry of primate prefrontal cortex and regulation of behavior by representational memory. In: Plum F, Mountcastle V, eds. *Handbook of physiology, the nervous system*. Bethesda, MD: American Physiological Society, 1978.
51. Stuss DT, Benson DF. *The frontal lobes*. New York: Raven Press, 1986.
52. Canavan AGM, Passingham RE, Marsden CD, et al. Sequencing ability in parkinsonians, patients with frontal lobe lesions and patients who have undergone unilateral temporal lobectomies. *Neuropsychologia* 1989;27:787–798.

53. Downes JJ, Roberts AC, Sahakian BJ, et al. Impaired extradimensional shift performance in medicated and unmedicated Parkinson's disease: evidence for a specific attentional dysfunction. *Neuropsychologia* 1989;27:1329–1343.
54. Owen AM, James M, Leigh PN, et al. Fronto-striatal cognitive deficits at different stages of Parkinson's disease. *Brain* 1992;115:1727–1751.
55. Zimmermann P, Sprengelmeyer R, Fimm B, et al. Cognitive slowing in decision tasks in early and advanced Parkinson's disease. *Brain Cogn* 1992;18:60–69.
56. Jordan N, Sagar HJ, Cooper JA. Cognitive components of reaction time in Parkinson's disease. *J Neurol Neurosurg Psychiatry* 1992;55:658–664.
57. Korten JJ, Meulstee J. Olfactory disturbances in parkinsonism. *Clin Neurosurg* 1980;82:113–118.
58. Doty RI, Deems DA, Stellar S. Olfactory dysfunction in parkinsonism. *Neurology* 1988;38:1237–1244.
59. Doty RL, Riklan M, Deems DA, et al. The olfactory and cognitive deficits of Parkinson's disease: evidence for independence. *Ann Neurol* 1989;25:166–171.
60. Doty RL, Stern MB, Pfeiffer C, et al. Bilateral olfactory dysfunction in early stage treated and untreated idiopathic Parkinson's disease. *J Neurol Neurosurg Psychiatry* 1992;55:138–142.
61. Bulens SC, Meerwaldt JD, Wildt GJvd, et al. Contrast sensitivity in Parkinson's disease. *Neurology* 1986;36:1121–1125.
62. Parkinson J. *An essay on the shaking palsy*. London: Sherwood, Neely and Jones, 1817.
63. Uekermann J, Daum I, Peters S, et al. Depressed mood and executive dysfunction in early Parkinson's disease. *Acta Neurol Scand* 2003;107(5):341–348.
64. Marsh L, Berk A. Neuropsychiatric aspects of Parkinson's disease: recent advances. *Curr Psychiatry Rep* 2003;5:680–676.
65. Mayeux R, Stern Y, Rosen J, et al. Depression, intellectual impairment and Parkinson's disease. *Neurology* 1981;31:645–650.
66. Santamaria J, Tolosa E, Valles A. Parkinson's disease with depression: a possible subgroup of idiopathic parkinsonism. *Neurology* 1986;36:1130–1133.
67. Starkstein SE, Berthier TJ, Bolduc PL, et al. Depression in Parkinson's disease. *J Nerv Ment Dis* 1990;178:27–31.
68. Cummings JL. Depression in Parkinson's disease. *Am J Psychiatry* 1992;149:443–454.
69. Starkstein SE, Berthier ML, Bolduc PL, et al. Depression in patients with early versus late onset of Parkinson's disease. *Neurology* 1989;39:1441–1445.
70. Agid Y, Javoy-Agid F, Ruberg M. Biochemistry of neurotransmitters in Parkinson's disease. In: Marsden CD, Fahn S, eds. *Movement disorders*, Vol. 2. London: Butterworth, 1987:166–230.
71. Lewis SJ, Dove A, Robbins TW, et al. Cognitive impairments in early Parkinson's disease are accompanied by reductions in activity in frontostriatal neural circuitry. *J Neurosci* 2003;23(15):6351–6356.
72. Iverson S. Cortical monoamines and behavior. In: Descarries L, Reader LA, Jasper HH, eds. *Monoamine innervation of the cerebral cortex*. New York: Alan Liss, 1984:349.
73. Mayeux R, Stern Y, Cote L, et al. Altered serotonin metabolism in depressed patients with Parkinson's disease. *Neurology* 1984;34:642–646.
74. Dubois B, Ruberg M, Javory-Agid F, et al. A subcortical-cortical cholinergic system is affected in Parkinson's disease. *Brain Res* 1983;288:213–218.

8

Dementia in Parkinson's Disease

Gregory A. Rippon and Karen S. Marder

Department of Neurology, Columbia University, New York, New York

INTRODUCTION

In 1817, in his initial description of paralysis agitans, James Parkinson stated, "the senses and intellect remain uninjured" (1). Since that description of the disease that subsequently came to bear his name, many have questioned his assumption (2,3). Increasingly recognized, dementia as a manifestation of idiopathic Parkinson's disease (PD) has been associated with abbreviated survival (3,4), reduced quality of life (QOL) (5), nursing home placement (6), and increased caregiver burden (7). This chapter reviews the epidemiology, clinical aspects, diagnosis and management, neurochemistry, and neuropathology associated with cognitive impairment in PD.

EPIDEMIOLOGY

Prevalence of PDD

Early prevalence estimates of Parkinson Disease Dementia (PDD) ranged from 7% to 81% (3, 8–24), resulting in an average estimate of 35.1% (25). In 1984, Brown and Marsden (25) identified several difficulties in ascertaining the prevalence of PDD, such as lack of consistent diagnostic criteria for dementia, varied methods of assessing cognitive function, sampling variability (subjects came from clinics, hospitals, institutions, and psychiatric referrals), and lack of rigor in the diagnosis of idiopathic PD.

Absence of a clear definition of dementia or relaxed criteria for its diagnosis can lead researchers to overestimate prevalence. For example, Martin et al. (17) estimated the prevalence of PDD to be 81%. Criteria for a diagnosis of dementia in that study did not exclude acute confusional states, and only a small number of errors on a screening mental status examination were needed to deem a subject "mildly impaired" (25). Patients in that study with "mild impairment," a proportion of whom may have exhibited only age-related decline, represented 70% of the sample used in the prevalence estimate. Excluding these cases reveals a prevalence of 23% (25). Other studies have used similar definitions of mild impairment that did not require memory disturbance (16,19). Conversely, stringent criteria for a diagnosis of dementia based on formal neuropsychological test performance may lead investigators to underestimate the prevalence of PDD (26). More recent studies have adopted *Diagnostic and Statistical Manual of Mental Disorders* (DSM)-IIIR (27) criteria for the definition of dementia, with prevalence estimates ranging from 17.6% to 41.3% in community-based samples (28–32).

Several methods have been used to assess the degree of cognitive impairment among patients with PD in studies estimating prevalence. These methods have ranged from nonstandardized clinical examinations to screening tests, such as the Folstein Mini-Mental State Examination (MMSE) (33), to formal neuropsychological batteries. The effect of differing assessment methods on prevalence estimates was illustrated by Cummings (34), who demonstrated that studies using clinical examination alone estimated a lower prevalence of PDD (30%) than those using screening mental status examinations (40.5%) or formal neuropsychometric batteries (69.9%).

Sampling variability is a concern when estimating the prevalence of PDD, because data derived primarily from clinic-based or hospital-based populations may have limited applicability to the general population. Severity of disease, presence of atypical features, family history, age, race, education, and gender may differ between clinic and hospital patients and the general population. These differences may be especially likely in "institutionalized" samples (30). Community-based samples have been used in several studies in attempts to address this source of bias (13,19,29–32,35). Mayeux et al. (29) estimated, using strict criteria for a diagnosis of PD with dementia, a population-based prevalence ratio of PDD to be 41.3% in a multiethnic community, suggesting that previous studies may have underestimated prevalence. Notably, the prevalence ratio of PDD increased with age (68.7% for patients >80 y.o.). Therefore, limiting the study population to predominantly elderly patients may also lead researchers to estimate prevalence in the whole population inaccurately.

Although several earlier studies have not made comparisons with control samples when estimating prevalence (8,14,16,19–21), the choice of a control population may also influence prevalence ratio estimates. This potential effect is illustrated by a study by Mindham et al. (3), in which the use of a control group of age-matched and gender-matched psychiatric patients likely led the authors to underestimate the prevalence ratio. Their control group included patients with an organic etiology for their psychiatric problems, some of whom were given an initial psychiatric diagnosis of dementia. The control group also included several patients with depression and anxiety, which possibly affected neuropsychological test performance and contributed to the underestimate. Other studies have used external population controls (29,35), which may lead to bias in prevalence ratio estimates because of differing assessment and diagnostic methods, in addition to demographic differences among samples.

Estimating the prevalence of PDD may be a less desirable method of determining the frequency with which it occurs, even when methodologic problems are removed from consideration. A study by Marder et al. (4) showed that when age and disease duration are controlled for, PD patients with dementia have higher 5-year mortality rates than PD patients without dementia. Other studies have also demonstrated accelerated mortality with emergence of PDD (3,36–39). Prevalence is a function of both the incidence rate and disease duration. Therefore, if disease duration is shortened with the emergence of PDD, then the measurement of prevalence may underestimate the true frequency with which PDD occurs (4,40).

Incidence of PDD

The incidence of PDD has been measured using hospital-based (40–43) and community-based (31,44) samples, yielding incidence rates ranging from 42.6–112.5 per 1000 person-years (py) of observation. Notably, the two highest incidence rates of 95.3 per 1000 py (44) and 112.5/1.7 (31) were from community-based samples that used neuropsychological testing in diagnosing dementia. The relative risk (RR) adjusted for age, gender, and education differed between the two studies, reported as 5.9 and 1.7, respectively. This disparity likely resulted from a high rate of incident dementia in the control sample of one study (31). Other studies of hospital-based (45) and community-based (46) samples compared to controls without PD have reported RR of PDD of approximately 3 in those samples.

Incidence studies may be less susceptible to the effects of increased mortality in PDD. However, this difference is likely relative, not absolute. Aarsland et al. (44) estimated the incidence of PDD in a community-based prospective study with comparison to an external control group. In this study, 21% of patients with PD were lost to follow-up because they died during a 4-year interval between evaluations. Mortality associated with incident dementia between evaluations may have led these investigators to underestimate incidence. Choice of sampling interval length may affect estimates if incident dementia is associated with increased mortality. In addition, cognitive impairment may lead to increased subject attrition in longitudinal studies of PD, further contributing to the underestimation of dementia in incidence studies (47).

Risk Factors for PDD

Demographic risk factors reported in association with PDD include advanced age (29,31,40, 41,43,44,48,49), male gender (43,45,50–53), and lower educational attainment (52). Advanced age at onset of motor manifestations has been reported by some authors as a risk factor for PDD (49), but other authors have not found this association (31,43,44). Interestingly, age at baseline evaluation was not a significant predictor of dementia in these studies (31,43,44), suggesting that age alone may be the more significant risk factor. The association of male gender with PDD has been inconsistently reported and may reflect bias or an effect of confounding variables (43,51). Although lower educational attainment has been associated with increased risk of PDD (31,52), other studies have not found this association (31,42,44).

Several clinical features have been associated with increased risk of PDD. Severe extrapyramidal signs have been consistently reported as a risk factor for the development of PDD (6,31,37,43,48,54,55). Interestingly, signs that indicate predominantly nondopaminergic dysfunction (dysarthria, postural instability, gait disorder) (56–59) have been shown by some investigators (60–62) to be particularly associated with cognitive impairment in PD, in addition to bradykinesia in the dopaminergic spectrum (19,54,63–67). Levy et al. (60) studied the relationship between dopaminergic and nondopaminergic subscores of the Unified Parkinson Disease Rating Scale (UPDRS) (68) and incident dementia in a cohort of nondemented community-dwelling patients with PD who were followed prospectively. The subscore indicating predominantly nondopaminergic dysfunction, but not the subscore representing predominantly dopaminergic dysfunction, was significantly associated with increased risk of dementia. When the six domains of the UPDRS were entered into a Cox model, speech dysfunction and bradykinesia were significantly associated with incident dementia, whereas axial impairment approached significance. Data suggesting association between dysarthria, bradykinesia, and postural instability and the development of PDD complement the numerous reports of tremor predominance as a predictor of a benign clinical course (38,50,52, 62,69,70). Other investigators have demonstrated an association between incomplete or diminishing response to levodopa therapy and cognitive decline in PD (71–73), a finding that likewise favors a contribution of nondopaminergic mechanisms. Patients in the DATATOP cohort (74) with an older age at onset of PD (>57 y.o.) showed a more precipitous decline in mentation as measured by part I of the UPDRS than younger patients in that cohort did. Patients who had PD with postural instability and gait difficulty as predominant features were more likely than others to manifest cognitive decline in that study as well. Given the apparent effects of advanced age and severe extrapyramidal signs on cognition in PD, the interrelationship of age and extrapyramidal signs (EPS) to the risk of dementia was investigated. Levy et al. (53) studied the relationship of age and severity of EPS to incident dementia using a community-based prospective cohort design. Age and the UPDRS score at baseline were dichotomized at the median, and patients were followed prospectively in four groups (younger age/low EPS severity, younger age/high severity, older age/low severity, older age/high severity). Using younger age/low EPS severity as the reference group, the group with older age/high severity had a significantly increased risk of incident dementia (RR 9.7; 95% CI 3.9 to 24.4), whereas the younger age/high severity and older age/low severity groups did not. The authors interpreted this as reflective of a combined effect of aging and EPS severity on the risk of incident PDD rather than separate effects of either increasing age or EPS.

Bilateral onset of motor symptoms has been reported in one study to be associated with cognitive decline in PD (75). Bilateral onset of symptoms and incomplete response to levodopa should be interpreted cautiously as dementia risk factors, given the possibility that these events may represent clinical manifestations of an atypical or secondary parkinsonian syndrome (i.e., false positives) rather than idiopathic PD (26,76). Clinicopathologic studies have shown that the false positive rate for the diagnosis of PD is around 20% (76,77). In a study by Hughes et al. (76), adding asymmetric onset and no evidence of another etiology to the criterion of 2 of 3 cardinal features of PD increased diagnostic specificity (at the cost of decreasing sensitivity).

Some investigators have reported an association between depressive symptoms (31,78) or major depression (48,79) and the risk of cognitive decline or PDD. Other studies that used the Montgomery and Asberg Depression Rating Scale (80) longitudinally have not shown such an association (6,43). Several studies have reported an association of levodopa-induced psychosis and confusional states with cognitive decline in PD (48,50,55,81).

Neuropsychological testing may be helpful in predicting incident PDD. Mahieux et al. (42) reported that the picture completion subtest of the Weschler adult intelligence scale-revised (WAIS-R) (82), the interference section of the Stroop test (83), and a measurement of verbal fluency predicted dementia in nondemented patients with PD who were followed prospectively. Jacobs et al. (84) reported that baseline performance on two verbal fluency tasks (letter and category fluency) were independently associated with the development of dementia in a group of initially nondemented patients with PD in a longitudinal community-based epidemiologic study. In a reexamination of an expanded cohort with a longer duration of follow up (85), the same authors reported that poor performance on the total immediate recall and delayed recall portions of the Selective Reminding Test (86), as well as on the Identities and Oddities portion of the Mattis Dementia Rating Scale (87), were associated with incident PDD. Letter fluency performance also predicted PDD in the follow-up study. Therefore, measurements of verbal memory and executive functioning at baseline in nondemented patients with PD appear to predict incident dementia. The contribution of frontal lobe dysfunction to a preclinical state of PD dementia is illustrated by Piccirilli et al. (88), who showed that impairment on motor tasks sensitive to frontal lobe dysfunction may be detected years before the emergence of more generalized cognitive impairment in patients with PD.

Evaluations of environmental risk factors for PDD have been sparse. Pesticide exposure (51,52), chemical exposure (51), rural living (52), and well water exposure (52) have not been shown to increase risk of PDD. Cigarette smoking has been shown in two longitudinal studies (54,89) to be associated with an increased risk of PDD, the converse of what has been shown about smoking and the development of PD itself (90,91). Ebmeier et al. (54) reported a fourfold increase in risk of PDD among patients who were smoking, similar to the 4.5-fold increase reported by Levy et al. (89). Previous smoking was associated with a twofold increased risk in the Levy study as well. Two previous studies using a case-control design did not show such an association (51,52). Alcohol consumption and head injury have not been shown to increase risk of PDD (51,52).

Several gene alleles, such as apolipoprotein E epsilon 4 (APOE ε4), epsilon 2 (APOE ε2), cytochrome P450 mono-oxygenase (CYP2D6) and estrogen receptor 1 (ESR 1) and *Saitohin* gene polymorphisms, have been evaluated as potential risk factors for the development of PDD. Although one study reported an increase in APOE ε4 prevalence (92) in PDD patients, several other studies have not shown this result (93–96). Although the APOE ε4 allele has been shown to be common in patients with concomitant PD and Alzheimer's disease (AD) at autopsy (97), another study did not find this association (98), and speculation persists about the role of AD pathology in PD dementia. Therefore, the meaning of these findings remains uncertain (26). However, APOE ε2 has been shown to be associated with PDD in two population-based studies (99,100). CYP2D6 alleles have not been shown to be associated with increased risk of PDD (101). However, a gene-toxin interaction that increased the risk of PDD was reported by Hubble et al. (102). Patients with PD who had one copy of the cytochrome P450 allele CYP2D6 29B+ (associated with poor ability to metabolize debrisoquine) and who were exposed to pesticides had an 83% predicted probability of developing dementia, according to a logistic regression model. Marder et al. (103) reported an inverse association between estrogen replacement therapy and development of dementia in women with PD in a retrospective study. However, clinical trials in Alzheimer disease have not shown beneficial effects of estrogen replacement in prevention or treatment of the disease. The role of estrogen therapy in prevention or treatment of PDD has not been prospectively studied. The association of an estrogen receptor 1 gene polymorphism (ESR1 *Pvu*II) demonstrated in a Japanese population diagnosed clinically with PDD (104) could not be replicated in a Finnish study with neuropathologic correlation (105). The RR genotype of the *Saitohin* Q7R polymorphism within intron 9 of the tau gene was initially reported to be associated with late-onset AD (106), but this finding was not replicated in three subsequent studies (107–109). Clark et al.

(110) analyzed this polymorphism in a heterogenous population of patients with AD, PDD, and PD and found no significant differences in genotype or allele prevalences. Further, as had been previously reported (109), *Saitohin* Q and R alleles were in complete linkage disequilibrium with Tau H1 and H2 genotypes, respectively. A trend in white patients with PDD toward an increase in *Saitohin* QQ (Tau H1/H1) genotype was observed when these patients were compared to patients with PD and with controls, but this trend was not statistically significant.

Mutations in genes leading to Lewy body parkinsonism have been associated with concomitant dementia. Autosomal dominant Lewy body parkinsonism was identified in a large Italian family, with a causal mutation found at codon 53 (A53T) of the gene for alpha synuclein on chromosome 4q (111–113). Although most of the affected members of that kindred presented with PD with asymmetric tremor, rigidity, bradykinesia, and postural instability, one patient had clinically diagnosed and pathologically confirmed dementia with Lewy bodies (DLB) (114). Of the other families reported with the same mutation (115–117), one included family members with progressive cognitive impairment (116). A large American kindred has also been described in which a chromosome 4p haplotype cosegregates with the presence of early-onset PD. Members of this kindred have been clinically and pathologically diagnosed with DLB (118–122). Interestingly, recent evaluation has corrected previous interpretations to show linkage to chromosome 4q, leading to a reanalysis of the alpha-synuclein gene that revealed a heterozygous triplication of the whole gene. This triplication manifests as a twofold increase in alpha synuclein in platelets of affected relatives in that kindred (123).

Family history of dementia in first-degree relatives has been reported to be more common in patients with PDD (51). In addition, the possibility of familial aggregation of AD and PD with dementia was suggested by a study that showed a threefold increased risk of AD in siblings of demented patients with PD (124). When only siblings >65 years of age were considered in this study, the risk increased to fivefold. A study with only a small number of demented patients with PD did not find this association (125). The lack of association of AD in relatives of nondemented patients with PD has been recently confirmed (126).

CLINICAL AND NEUROPSYCHOLOGICAL FEATURES OF PDD

In general, the dementia associated with Parkinson's disease reflects predominant impairment of executive functions (concept formation, problem solving, set shifting and maintenance, difficulties with internally cued behavior), attention and concentration, "processing speed," and free recall with benefit from external cueing. Aside from verbal fluency, language is relatively preserved, as is limb praxis. Impaired visuospatial functioning may be observed. Personality change and various behavioral symptoms may contribute to the clinical picture.

Executive Functioning

The ability of patients with PDD to plan, organize, and regulate goal-directed behavior is impaired, constituting the central feature of PDD (127–129). In contrast to patients with frontal cortical dysfunction, patients with PD [and to a greater degree PDD (130)] have difficulties with shifting attention to novel stimuli, whereas perseverative errors are less frequently seen (127,131). In a study by Owen et al. (131), patients with PD treated with levodopa differed from untreated patients with PD, in that perseverative errors were more frequent in unmedicated patients engaged in an executive task; their performance more closely resembled that of a group of neurosurgical patients with frontal lobectomies. This finding suggests that levodopa therapy might have a beneficial effect on perseveration in patients with PD (131). Compared to patients with AD, demented patients with PD show more impairment on executive tasks and verbal fluency, with a lesser degree of semantic and episodic memory dysfunction (129,132). In contrast to memory function in patients with AD, memory function in patients with PDD has been shown to be associated with the degree of executive dysfunction (133). Speed of information processing has also been shown to differentiate PDD from AD (134).

Attention and Memory Functioning

Impaired attention, as measured by cognitive reaction time and vigilance, has been shown in patients with PDD (129). A recent study demonstrated a comparable degree of impaired reaction time, vigilance, and fluctuating attention in patients with PDD and those diagnosed clinically with DLB (135). Interestingly, patients with DLB who did not have evidence of parkinsonism exhibited a lesser degree of impairment on these measures. These data demonstrate overlap in cognitive performance between patients given clinical diagnoses of PDD and those diagnosed with DLB and question the arbitrary distinctions between the two disorders (135).

The profile of memory impairment in patients with PDD is one of impaired semantic and episodic memory with benefit from cueing (preserved recognition memory), which reflects a greater degree of retrieval failure than the encoding and retrieval impairment present in AD. Although acquisition of new information is impaired in PD, it is impaired to a lesser degree than that seen in AD (132,136,137). Patients with PDD differ from patients with AD (matched for dementia severity) in that they benefit more from controlled encoding situations, a difference that suggests that a distinction exists between the true amnestic syndrome of AD and the inefficient planning of encoding and retrieval in PDD. This aspect of PDD may represent the effects of striatofrontal dysfunction, whereas the sequelae of lesions of the hippocampus and temporal cortex are seen in AD (133).

Visuospatial Functioning

Visuospatial impairment in patients with PD has been reported by several authors (130,132,134, 136,138). When demented patients with PD have been compared to patients with AD matched for dementia severity, the patients with PDD have exhibited more severe impairment (132,134). Impairment in both visuoperceptual (130,139,140) and visuomotor (140) abilities has been reported in PD and PDD. These difficulties have been reported in some studies to be independent of degree of cognitive impairment (139,140). Stern et al. (141) demonstrated that patients with PD exhibit two distinct types of errors on tracing tasks: one arising primarily from motor dysfunction, and another related to higher-order control of sequential and predictive movements. The latter type of error correlated, in that study, with performance on constructional tasks and with general intellectual impairment. This finding suggests that visuospatial abilities in PD may be affected by the degree of executive dysfunction.

Language and Praxis

Although impaired verbal fluency has been reported to be more severe in PDD than in AD (132,134), language functioning in general is more severely affected in AD (134,142). Impaired naming and diminished content of spontaneous speech have been shown in PD, though it is less severe than in AD (142). Other studies have reported naming deficits (the "tip of the tongue" phenomenon) (143) and sentence comprehension difficulties (144,145), though these studies did not involve comparison to a control group or to AD patients. Patients with PD, compared with patients with AD, also exhibited decreased phrase length, impaired speech melody, dysarthria, and agraphia in a study by Cummings et al. (142), suggesting that patients with PD exhibit more prominent motor speech abnormalities, whereas AD patients experience more profound language dysfunction. The language deficits reported in PD may be more the result of impaired internally generated search strategies (dysexecutive syndrome) than true involvement of the language system (127,144).

Praxis is generally not impaired in patients with PDD, compared to patients with AD who have dementia of similar severity (134), although some authors have reported ideomotor apraxia in nondemented patients with PD compared with age-matched controls (146) and with a group of consecutively assessed control patients not matched for age or education (144). The authors of one study (146) suggested that defective encoding of visuospatial information (necessary for the memory of movements performed) and increased vulnerability to interference may account for apraxia in patients with PD. This suggests that the dysexecutive syndrome also has a deleterious effect on praxis in PD.

Psychiatric Symptoms

Depression in patients with PD has been reported to range from dysthymic disorder to major depression and an atypical depression with anxiety (147–150). Sano et al. (151), in a retrospective chart review of all patients with PD seen at an urban medical center over an 18-month period, found a prevalence of 5.4% for coincident depression and dementia. That study prospectively measured cerebrospinal fluid 5-hydroxyindoleacetic acid (5-HIAA) concentrations in patients with PD and showed decreased 5-HIAA levels in patients with dementia, depression, and dementia plus depression (lowest levels), a finding that suggests that the serotonergic system may play a role in depression and PDD. Other studies implicate the serotonergic system in PD-associated depression (147,148), although the level is not by itself a reliable marker of depression in PD (150). Neuropathologic (152,153) studies implicate dopaminergic and noradrenergic neurotransmitter systems in PD-associated depression, as well. Patients with PD who have concomitant depression have been shown to perform poorly on screening mental status examinations (148,154), frontal and frontal-subcortical tasks (155,156), and speed of processing (157). Although the effects of depression itself may be considered to account for these deficits, the possibility exists that a common frontal-subcortical system dysfunction may account for both the depression and the cognitive deficits in these patients (150).

Psychotic features have been reported in nondemented and demented patients with PD. In an outpatient clinic sample, 9% of patients with PD, 63% of whom were cognitively impaired, had experienced hallucinations(158), though the authors did not attempt to distinguish between drug-related and nondrug-related events. In another retrospective chart review of a clinic-based sample, Bell et al. (159) reported that 63% of incident cases with nondrug-related hallucinosis developed dementia during a nearly 5-year follow-up period. A study of 216 consecutive patients with PD showed that cognitive impairment was the main risk factor for formed visual hallucinations among patients receiving dopaminergic treatment (160). In a cross-sectional study of a population-based sample of patients with PDD and AD matched for age, gender, and MMSE score, hallucinations were more severe among the patients with PDD, and aberrant motor behavior, agitation, disinhibition, euphoria, and apathy were more severe among the patients with AD (161). Within the PDD group, apathy was more common in milder Hoehn and Yahr stages, and delusions increased with increasing severity of cognitive and motor dysfunction.

NEUROIMAGING IN PDD

Structural and functional imaging studies have been performed in patients with PDD. Results of these studies, although of interest, must be interpreted cautiously, because few studies have included neuropathologic correlation. Although one study reported no specific pattern of structural abnormalities in PDD by magnetic resonance imaging (MRI) (162), other studies have reported significant hippocampal atrophy (to an even greater degree than that seen in AD patients with mild to moderate dementia) (163) and atrophy of the substantia innominata comparable to that in patients with AD (164).

Single-photon emission computed tomography (SPECT) studies have commonly shown frontal hypoperfusion or bilateral temporal-parietal perfusion deficits similar to those in patients with AD (165–171). Positron emission tomography (PET) studies of PDD have shown a similar pattern of temporoparietal hypometabolism, superimposed on the milder global hypometabolism that is seen in nondemented patients with PD (172–174). PET studies of nondemented patients with PD have shown a positive correlation between frontal hypometabolism and working memory and executive functioning deficits (175,176). Interestingly, one study showed that, when compared to patients with AD who were matched for age, gender, and dementia severity, patients with PDD showed greater resting-state hypometabolism in the visual cortex and relatively preserved medial temporal metabolism (173). The pattern of temporal-parietal-occipital hypometabolism with relative medial temporal sparing has been described in patients with DLB (177,178). An abnormal resting state network of hypermetabolism in the medial and anterior temporal cortex, pons, and cerebellum, with hypometabolism in the parieto-occipital cortex, was reported in a recent PET study (179). The expression of this network was related to memory and visuospatial deficits. The authors of that study postulated that these changes were a marker of abnormal activation under increased task burden and reflected downstream effects of subcortical-cortical or cortico-cortical pathology.

PET activation studies focusing on executive functioning have demonstrated decreased pallidal blood flow during spatial planning stages, with a reduction in bilateral prefrontal and right caudate activation and increased hippocampal activation when levels of performance are more demanding (180–182). This hippocampal shift in activation has also been reported in normal controls performing tasks that encouraged declarative learning (183). In patients with PD, this shift may indicate a switch to declarative learning strategies in the presence of impaired striatum-mediated implicit learning (176). Studies by PET and functional MRI to investigate the effects of levodopa on these networks during executive and working memory tasks have generally shown that abnormal activation is reversed, without demonstrating that task performance is improved (184,185). Although these studies proposed to demonstrate that levodopa exerts a beneficial effect on mesocortical dopaminergic pathways, the lack of performance benefit suggests that either the mesocortical degeneration may not be the primary cause of cognitive deficits in PD or that the levodopa dose used was insufficient to reverse the cognitive deficits (176).

Imaging studies investigating abnormalities in neurotransmitter systems in PD and cognitive decline have been performed mostly on the dopaminergic system. In general, a decline in basal ganglia outflow, as measured by caudate dopamine transporter binding, has been observed in patients with mild-to-moderate-stage PD, whereas patients with later-stage PD have exhibited inappropriate dorsolateral prefrontal cortex activation of mesocortical dopaminergic origin (176,184–191). Cholinergic binding, assessed by SPECT using [123I] iodobenzovesamicol, an *in vivo* marker of the vesicular acetylcholine transporter, is reduced in parietal and occipital cortex in nondemented patients with PD, whereas in patients with PDD, the binding is more diffuse, similar to that seen in patients with early-onset AD (192). Tracers used to assess cholinergic, noradrenergic, and serotonergic systems are still in development but, once available, should contribute to understanding the role of these systems in PDD (176,193).

A recent proton magnetic resonance spectroscopy study (194) showed that patients with PDD, compared to controls and nondemented patients with PD, exhibited lower *N*-acetylaspartate (NAA) levels in the occipital cortex. The observed NAA levels correlated with the degree of cognitive impairment in that study. Notably, although patients with AD show decreased NAA values in the occipital region (suggesting neuronal dysfunction or loss), they also show an increase in myoinositol (MI), which indicates glial dysfunction (195–198). This increase in MI was not shown in the occipital cortex of PDD patients, suggesting a difference in underlying histopathologic changes between the two conditions (194).

NEUROPATHOLOGY OF PDD

Clinicopathologic studies of PDD can be divided into three main groups: those attributing PDD to (1) restricted subcortical pathology, (2) concomitant AD pathology, and (3) cortical Lewy bodies (127). Studies conducted before the advent of alpha-synuclein immunohistochemical staining emphasized the importance of restricted subcortical or AD pathology, whereas more recent studies using alpha-synuclein staining have reported the importance of Lewy body pathology.

Restricted Subcortical Pathology

Several reports have emphasized the role of subcortical pathologic changes in the brains of patients with PDD. Dopaminergic, noradrenergic, cholinergic, and serotonergic neurotransmitter systems have been implicated in the pathogenesis of PDD. Although pathology in the nigrostriatal dopaminergic pathway has been associated with subtle cognitive effects in some studies (199–201), the mesocorticolimbic dopaminergic system has been more consistently implicated in the pathogenesis of PDD. This system originates in the ventral tegmental area and the medial substantia nigra and projects to limbic and prefrontal areas and to the caudate nucleus (202–204).

Although patients with PD show considerable neuronal loss in the ventrolateral regions of the substantia nigra pars compacta, those with concomitant dementia have been reported to suffer more substantial neuronal loss from the medial region (203,205–208). This neuronal loss in the medial substantia nigra has been reported in demented patients with PD, with and without concomitant AD pathology. Others have failed to replicate the differential degeneration of the medial substantia nigra between demented and nondemented patients with PD (209). The ventral tegmental area has also been shown to suffer neuronal degeneration in demented patients with PD who do not have concurrent AD (207). Support for involvement of the mesocorticolimbic dopaminergic system in PD-associated dementia has been provided by the demonstration of dopamine loss in limbic and prefrontal cortex (56), monoamine terminal loss in prefrontal areas (detected by positron emission tomography) (210), and decreased tyrosine hydroxylase immunolabeling in the prefrontal cortex (211).

Involvement of the noradrenergic system in PD dementia is supported by neuropathologic studies reporting neuronal loss in the locus caeruleus (LC) in the brains of patients with PD who have cognitive impairment (152,207,212–214). Although neuronal loss in the locus caeruleus is established in PD (214,215), the extent of degeneration has been reported to be more severe in PDD (212,216). Other authors have failed to find an association between LC pathology and PDD (209,213,217). A clinicopathologic study (207) demonstrated that neuronal loss in the locus caeruleus was greater in patients with PDD (but without concurrent AD) than in patients with PD who are not demented. Locus caeruleus cell counts were not significantly different between PDD with and without concomitant AD in that study. Neuronal loss in the locus caeruleus was correlated with measures of neuronal loss within the ventral tegmental area (VTA), nucleus basalis of Meynert (NBM), medial substantia nigra pars compacta, and more Lewy bodies in the anterior cingulate gyrus. The authors speculated that PDD may stem from additive or even synergistic effect of pathology in multiple neuronal populations. Although AD pathology was found in 75% of demented patients with PD in one study (212), senile plaques and neurofibrillary tangles were not correlated with the degree of neuronal loss in the locus caeruleus or NBM or with choline acetyltransferase (ChAT) activity in the cortex, suggesting that intracortical pathology (as in AD) and damage to subcortical-cortical projections do not appear to evolve in parallel but may have an additive or complementary effect in the pathogenesis of PDD.

Although some studies report considerable cell loss in the NBM in nondemented patients with PD (209,212,218,219) and lack of difference in nucleolar volume between patients with PD and controls (218), other studies that report neuronal loss in the nucleus basalis of Meynert (203,220) support increased pathologic involvement of cholinergic systems in PDD. Lewy bodies were first described in the substantia innominata (medial septum/diagonal band of Broca and NBM) rather than the substantia nigra (221). Although neuronal loss in the NBM is present in patients with idiopathic PD (222,223), neuronal loss in the NBM and medial septum/diagonal band of Broca (DBB) was shown in a study by Whitehouse et al. to be more severe in demented patients with PD (220). The authors of that study hypothesized that dysfunction of the septal/DBB pathways to the hippocampus may be involved in memory loss in PD, whereas the loss of neurons from the NBM may play an important role in other cognitive deficits such as impaired processing speed (220). Perry et al. (224) demonstrated that demented patients with PD had extensive reduction of ChAT and less extensive reductions of acetylcholinesterase in all four cortical lobes. The reduction of ChAT in the temporal neocortex was found to correlate with the degree of cognitive impairment but not with the degree of AD pathology. The degeneration of neurons in the NBM of patients with PD may be a primary process (203,224), rather than a secondary degeneration of the NBM as seen in AD (225,226). In a comparative study of 50 autopsied PD cases (203), NBM cell loss ranging from 15% to 62% was not associated with dementia or substantial AD pathology, but neuronal loss of 64% to 90% was associated with dementia and frequently with severe cortical AD pathology. The author of that study postulated that degeneration of the ascending cholinergic system may precede the onset of cognitive impairment and that a critical threshold of 75% to 80% neuronal loss within the NBM must be reached before dementia becomes evident. This hypothesis is supported by the demonstration of frontal lobe cholinergic deficiency and NBM cell loss in patients with PD who do not have cognitive impairment (203,212).

Serotonergic involvement in PD has been suggested by studies that report neuronal loss in the dorsal raphe nuclei (DRN) (203,227). Increased neuronal loss in the DRN has been reported in patients with PDD, in whom it approaches the levels observed in patients with AD (203). Studies demonstrating the reduction of serotonin, serotonin metabolites, and receptors in the medial frontal cortex and striatum (56,228) and the relation of these observations to cognitive impairment in PD support a role for serotonergic pathology in PDD (203). However, some have suggested that DRN neuronal loss may be more associated with depression than with PDD (202).

Alzheimer Pathology

Differences exist in the intensity and distribution pattern of neuritic AD pathology (neurofibrillary tangles, neuritic plaques, and neuropil threads) between patients with PD and those with AD (203), but in general AD pathology is greater in demented patients with PD than in those with no or minimal cognitive impairment (202,203,209,229,230). Others have not found the same association between dementia and amyloid beta peptide deposition in patients with PD (231). Allocortical prealpha neurons of the entorhinal region (the axons of which constitute the perforant pathway) have been found to show severe neurofibrillary degeneration in demented patients with PD, with only mild to moderate neocortical AD pathology (232), whereas the same pathology in patients without PD has not been associated with cognitive impairment and presumably represents a very early stage of AD pathology (233). Although neuritic AD pathology in PD follows a pattern of progression similar to that found in early AD (spreading from allocortical areas to isocortex with early involvement of the entorhinal region of hippocampus) (230,234,235), involvement of isocortical regions corresponding to Braak and Braak stages V and VI occurs to a lesser degree (203), and neuritic AD pathology (as detected by tau immunostaining) may preferentially involve the frontal, temporal, and entorhinal cortices (236). This finding contrasts with the predominant involvement of primary sensory association areas seen in AD (203,237,238). Increasing stage of neuritic AD pathology has been shown to correlate with severity of dementia as measured by MMSE (33) in a comparative pathologic study of prospectively followed AD and age-matched patients with PD (203). In another clinicopathologic study, patients with PD who have moderate to severe dementia differed from mildly or nondemented patients with PD only in the degree of cortical AD lesions and not in degree of subcortical pathology in the substantia nigra (medial or lateral), LC, DRN, or NBM (202). PDD patients differed from nondemented patients with PD in that study by exhibiting more severe cortical AD lesions and higher neuronal loss in the medial substantia nigra.

Lewy Body Pathology

Three studies using alpha-synuclein immunohistochemical staining have emphasized the importance of Lewy body pathology in demented patients with PD. Two similar studies (239,240) that investigated the relationship of Lewy body and AD histopathologic changes to PDD have found that, by regression analysis, Lewy body changes in the cortex of demented patients correlated better than AD pathology with the presence of dementia. Apaydin et al. (241), in a retrospective clinicopathologic study, examined a subset of demented patients with PD who developed cognitive impairment at least 4 years after the onset of parkinsonism. Using modern immunohistochemical staining methods, 12 of the 13 patients in the study group exhibited evidence of diffuse or transitional Lewy body disease as the primary pathologic substrate for dementia, with mean and median Lewy body counts in neocortical and limbic areas increased nearly 10-fold versus a control group of patients with PD who were not demented. Alzheimer pathology in the study group was modest, with only one patient meeting the criteria of the National Institute on Aging and the Reagan Institute Working Group on the Diagnostic Criteria for the Neuropathologic Assessment of Alzheimer's Disease (242) for "intermediate probability of AD." Interestingly, neocortical Lewy body counts correlated with numbers of senile plaques and neurofibrillary tangles in this study, suggesting common origins or possible interaction between the two pathologies.

The possibility exists that dementia developing early in the course of PD may have an entirely different pathologic basis than dementia developing several years after the onset of parkinsonism (241). In addition, as noted by Apaydin et al. (241), patients included in many of the clinicopathologic studies were likely heterogeneous, with incomplete clinical information. The advent of modern immunohistochemical techniques shown to be more sensitive for detection of Lewy bodies (243,244), and use of more recent consensus criteria for the neuropathologic diagnosis of AD (242), may account for some of the discrepancies between early studies and those conducted more recently (241).

It therefore seems plausible that multiple underlying pathologic changes may account for the presence and degree of cognitive impairment in patients with PD, ranging from restricted disruption of subcortical-cortical projections to a combination of cortical (AD, Lewy body, or both) and subcortical pathology. Individual patients may exhibit pathologic involvement of these neuronal populations to varying degrees. As suggested by other authors (245,246), subcortical pathology in patients with PD may increase vulnerability to superimposed "early" AD pathology, at a stage when controls would appear cognitively normal. Alternatively, subcortical pathology may result in milder degrees of dementia, with increasing severity of dementia associated with superimposed cortical AD (202) or Lewy body pathology.

DIAGNOSIS OF PDD

Establishing a diagnosis of dementia in a patient with PD presents unique difficulties, mainly related to the co-occurrence of behavioral (i.e., depression) and motor dysfunction. Although PDD is included in the DSM IV (247) as a diagnostic entity, the criteria are relatively nonspecific, as it is included under the rubric of "other dementias" (127). Given the co-occurrence of behavioral or motor dysfunction or both in a patient with PD who presents with cognitive dysfunction, the utility of neuropsychological testing that is able to differentiate between the sequelae of these symptoms should be emphasized. Care must be taken to differentiate aspects of functional impairment caused by noncognitive symptoms. As with other dementing illnesses, a caregiver should preferentially be interviewed as well to assist in the assessment of cognitive, behavioral, and functional impairment.

The differential diagnosis of patients presenting with dementia and parkinsonism is broad and beyond the scope of this chapter. However, the main differential diagnostic considerations in a patient with known PD who develops cognitive impairment are domain-specific cognitive dysfunction not severe enough to qualify for dementia, depression (which may be of organic origin as outlined above), adverse effects of antiparkinsonian or other medication, and confusional states caused by metabolic or systemic disorders (127). DLB shares many features with PDD when fully developed, to the point that the two entities are clinically and pathologically indistinguishable (127). Currently, criteria for the diagnosis of DLB (248) require that motor symptoms not precede the development of cognitive impairment by more than 1 year, a guideline that is rather arbitrary and not based on objective data (127). The possibility exists that PDD and DLB lie along a clinical and pathologic spectrum, with motor-onset and cognitive-onset presentations, respectively. Further advances in neuroimaging and neuropathologic methods may contribute to our understanding of the relationships between the two disorders.

TREATMENT CONSIDERATIONS

Levodopa and Cognition in PD

Although no claims have been made of improved cognition in demented patients with PD (249), throughout the history of levodopa treatment for PD, improvement (250,251) and worsening (252–254) of specific domains of cognitive function have been reported. More recent studies have revealed that the effects of levodopa administration on cognition in PD are subtle and largely limited to beneficial effects on arousal and mood (127,255). An analysis of the DATATOP cohort (249) revealed subtle but significant improvements on neuropsychological tests that measured executive function in patients with PD who were treated with levodopa. No evidence of deleterious effect of levodopa on cognition was noted, and performance on most neuropsychological testing was unaffected by treatment. No conclusions about the effect of levodopa on cognition in PDD could be derived, given that the incidence of dementia in the cohort was low and that dementia was an initial exclusion criterion for enrollment. Concerns about adverse effects of long-term levodopa treatment on cognition in PD have not been substantiated (59,249,256,257).

Cholinesterase Inhibitors and Cognition in PD

Because the cholinergic neurotransmitter system has been shown to be involved in PDD (203, 220,224), and features of cognitive impairment (namely, attention and concentration) that may respond to enhanced cholinergic tone are frequently present, cholinesterase inhibitors could be useful in symptomatic treatment of PDD. However, theoretically this enhancement of cholinergic tone could also worsen extrapyramidal features of the disease (258). In mostly small, open studies, tacrine (259), donepezil (260–262), rivastigmine (263,264), and galantamine (265) have been reported to improve cognition in patients with PDD without significantly worsening extrapyramidal features. One study that showed cognitive benefit reported a significant worsening in motor symptoms with rivastigmine treatment, mainly manifesting as increased tremor (263). Smaller studies of donepezil (266–269), as well as a larger randomized double-blind placebo-controlled study of rivastigmine (270), have shown that cholinesterase inhibitors provide cognitive benefits in patients with DLB. Worsening of parkinsonism (mainly of tremor) was reported in one of the smaller studies of DLB patients (266).

Cholinesterase Inhibitors and Neuropsychiatric Features of PD

Several studies have reported beneficial effects of cholinesterase inhibitors on psychiatric symptoms in patients with PD. Psychosis has been reported to be ameliorated by cholinesterase inhibitors in PD without dementia (262), PDD (261,264) and DLB (266–270). One double-blind, randomized placebo-controlled study of donepezil in patients with PDD showed no benefit on psychiatric symptoms as a secondary outcome measured by the neuropsychiatric inventory (271), though only a small proportion of patients in that study manifested psychiatric features initially (260). A recent randomized controlled trial of rivastigmine in PPD (272) showed moderate improvements in cognition, activities of daily living, and psychiatric symptoms at the expense of increased tremor. Therefore, given concerns about use of neuroleptics in elderly patients with dementia or parkinsonism or both (273), cholinesterase inhibitors may be a reasonable therapeutic option, both for improving cognition and ameliorating psychosis in PDD, with careful attention to effects on extrapyramidal symptoms and signs.

Prophylaxis of PDD

Although no randomized prospective clinical trials have been performed with development of PDD as a primary end point, the DATATOP cohort was reported in a prospective study to show no benefit in cognitive test performance from selegeline, tocopherol, or a combination of the two (274).

SUMMARY

Dementia as a manifestation of idiopathic PD is an important feature of the disease in terms of QOL, prognosis, and clinical management. The pathophysiology of the disorder is likely a multifactorial process that encompasses derangement of multiple neuronal populations of both subcortical and cortical origin. This process results in a cognitive profile that largely reflects a dysexecutive syndrome. Currently, treatment of PDD is symptomatic. Further research is needed to elucidate the relationship of PDD to DLB and AD in hopes of developing and using appropriate therapeutic measures designed to address the underlying disease process.

REFERENCES

1. Parkinson J. An essay on the shaking palsy. London: Sherwood, Neely and Jones, 1817.
2. Ball B. De l'insanite dans la paralysie agitante. *Encephale* 1882;2:22–32.
3. Mindham RH, Ahmed SW, Clough CG. A controlled study of dementia in Parkinson's disease. *J Neurol Neurosurg Psychiatry* 1982;45(11):969–974.

4. Marder K, Leung D, Tang M, et al. Are demented patients with Parkinson's disease accurately reflected in prevalence surveys? A survival analysis. *Neurology* 1991;41(8):1240–1243.
5. Schrag A, Jahanshahi M, Quinn N. What contributes to quality of life in patients with Parkinson's disease? *J Neurol Neurosurg Psychiatry* 2000;69(3):308–312.
6. Aarsland D, Larsen JP, Tandberg E, et al. Predictors of nursing home placement in Parkinson's disease: a population-based, prospective study. *J Am Geriatr Soc* 2000;48(8):938–942.
7. Aarsland D, Larsen JP, Karlsen K, et al. Mental symptoms in Parkinson's disease are important contributors to caregiver distress. *Int J Geriatr Psychiatry* 1999; 14(10):866–874.
8. Oyebode JR, Barker WA, Blessed G, et al. Cognitive functioning in Parkinson's disease: in relation to prevalence of dementia and psychiatric diagnosis. *Br J Psychiatry* 1986;149:720–725.
9. Patrick H, Levy D. Parkinson's disease: a clinical study of 146 cases. *Arch Neurol Psychiatry* 1922;7:711–720.
10. de Smet Y, Ruberg M, Serdaru, et al. Confusion, dementia and anticholinergics in Parkinson's disease. *J Neurol Neurosurg Psychiatry* 1982;45(12):1161–1164.
11. Mindham RH. Psychiatric symptoms in Parkinsonism. *J Neurol Neurosurg Psychiatry* 1970;33(2):188–191.
12. Lewy F. Die Lehre von Tonus und der Bewegung Zugleich Systematiche Untersuchiner sur Klinik, Physiologie, Pathologie und Pathogenese der Paralysis Agitans. Berlin: Springer, 1923.
13. Mjones H. Paralysis agitans. *Acta Psychiat Neurol* 1949;54:1–195.
14. Pollock M, Hornabrook RW. The prevalence, natural history and dementia of Parkinson's disease. *Brain* 1966;89(3):429–448.
15. Sacks OW, Kohl MS, Messeloff CR, et al. Effects of levodopa in Parkinsonian patients with dementia. *Neurology* 1972;22(5):516–519.
16. Celesia GG, Wanamaker WM. Psychiatric disturbances in Parkinson's disease. *Dis Nerv Syst* 1972;33(9):577–583.
17. Martin WE, Loewenson RB, Resch JA, et al. Parkinson's disease. Clinical analysis of 100 patients. *Neurology* 1973;23(8):783–790.
18. Rajput AH, Rozdilsky B. Letter: Parkinsonism and dementia: effects of levodopa. *Lancet* 1975;1(7915):1084.
19. Martilla RJ, Rinne UK. Dementia in Parkinson's disease. *Acta Neurol Scand* 1976;54(5):431–441.
20. Sweet RD, McDowell FH, Feigenson JS, et al. Mental symptoms in Parkinson's disease during chronic treatment with levodopa. *Neurology* 1976;26(4):305–310.
21. Mindham RH, Marsden CD, Parkes JD. Psychiatric symptoms during l-dopa therapy for Parkinson's disease and their relationship to physical disability. *Psychol Med* 1976;6(1):23–33.
22. Lieberman A, Dziatolowski M, Kupersmith M, et al. Dementia in Parkinson disease. *Ann Neurol* 1979;6(4):355–359.
23. Sroka H, Elizan TS, Yahr MD, et al. Organic mental syndrome and confusional states in Parkinson's disease. Relationship to computerized tomographic signs of cerebral atrophy. *Arch Neurol* 1981;38(6):339–342.
24. Rajput AH, Offord K, Beard CM, et al. Epidemiological survey of dementia in parkinsonism and control population. *Adv Neurol* 1984;40:229–234.
25. Brown RG, Marsden CD. How common is dementia in Parkinson's disease? *Lancet* 1984;2(8414):1262–1265.
26. Levy G, Marder K. Prevalence, incidence and risk factors for dementia in Parkinson's disease. In: MA B, Agid Y, Choinard S et al., eds. Mental and behavioral dysfunction in movement disorders, Totowa, NJ: Humana Press, 2003:259–270.
27. Association AP. Diagnostic and statistical manual of mental disorders, 3rd ed. Revised. Washington DC: American Psychiatric Press, 1987.
28. Ebmeier KP, Calder SA, Crawford JR, et al. Dementia in idiopathic Parkinson's disease: prevalence and relationship with symptoms and signs of parkinsonism. *Psychol Med* 1991;21(1):69–76.
29. Mayeux R, Denaro J, Hemenegildo N, et al. A population-based investigation of Parkinson's disease with and without dementia. Relationship to age and gender. *Arch Neurol* 1992;49(5):492–497.
30. Tison F, Dartigues JF, Auriacombe S, et al. Dementia in Parkinson's disease: a population-based study in ambulatory and institutionalized individuals. *Neurology* 1995;45(4):705–708.
31. Marder K, Tang MX, Cote L, et al. The frequency and associated risk factors for dementia in patients with Parkinson's disease. *Arch Neurol* 1995;52(7):695–701.
32. Aarsland D, Tandberg E, Larsen JP, et al. Frequency of dementia in Parkinson disease. *Arch Neurol* 1996;53(6):538–542.
33. Folstein MF, Folstein SE, McHugh PR. "Mini-mental state." A practical method for grading the cognitive state of patients for the clinician. *J Psychiatr Res* 1975;12(3):189–198.
34. Cummings JL. Intellectual impairment in Parkinson's disease: clinical, pathologic, and biochemical correlates. *J Geriatr Psychiatry Neurol* 1988;1(1):24–36.
35. Aarsland D, Andersen K, Larsen JP, et al. Prevalence and characteristics of dementia in Parkinson disease: an 8-year prospective study. *Arch Neurol* 2003;60(3):387–392.
36. Ebmeier KP, Calder SA, Crawford JR, et al. Parkinson's disease in Aberdeen: survival after 3.5 years. *Acta Neurol Scand* 1990;81(4):294–299.
37. Piccirilli M, D'Alessandro P, Finali G, et al. Neuropsychological follow-up of parkinsonian patients with and without cognitive impairment. *Dementia* 1994;5(1):17–22.
38. Roos RA, Jongen JC, van der Velde EA. Clinical course of patients with idiopathic Parkinson's disease. *Mov Disord* 1996;11(3):236–242.
39. Louis ED, Marder K, Cote L, et al. Mortality from Parkinson disease. *Arch Neurol* 1997;54(3):260–264.
40. Mayeux R, Chen J, Mirabello E, et al. An estimate of the incidence of dementia in idiopathic Parkinson's disease. *Neurology* 1990;40(10):1513–1517.
41. Biggins CA, Boyd JL, Harrop FM, et al. A controlled, longitudinal study of dementia in Parkinson's disease. *J Neurol Neurosurg Psychiatry* 1992;55(7):566–571.
42. Mahieux F, Fenelon G, Flahault A, et al. Neuropsychological prediction of dementia in Parkinson's disease. *J Neurol Neurosurg Psychiatry* 1998;64(2):178–183.
43. Hughes TA, Ross HF, Musa S, et al. A 10-year study of the incidence of and factors predicting dementia in Parkinson's disease. *Neurology* 2000;54(8):1596–1602.
44. Aarsland D, Andersen K, Larsen JP, et al. Risk of dementia in Parkinson's disease: a community-based, prospective study. *Neurology* 2001;56(6):730–736.
45. Breteler MM, de Groot RR, van Romunde LK, et al. Risk of dementia in patients with Parkinson's disease, epilepsy, and severe head trauma: a register-based follow-up study. *Am J Epidemiol* 1995;142(12):1300–1305.

46. Rajput AH. Epidemiology of Parkinson's disease. *Can J Neurol Sci* 1984;11 (1 Suppl):156–159.
47. Levin BE, Katzen HL, Klein B, et al. Cognitive decline affects subject attrition in longitudinal research. *J Clin Exp Neuropsychol* 2000;22(5):580–586.
48. Stern Y, Marder K, Tang MX, et al. Antecedent clinical features associated with dementia in Parkinson's disease. *Neurology* 1993;43(9):1690–1692.
49. Hely MA, Morris JG, Reid WG, et al. Age at onset: the major determinant of outcome in Parkinson's disease. *Acta Neurol Scand* 1995;92(6):455–463.
50. Guillard A, Chastang C. [Long-term prognostic factors in Parkinson's disease (author's transl)]. *Rev Neurol (Paris* 1978;134(5):341–354.
51. Marder K, Flood P, Cote L, et al. A pilot study of risk factors for dementia in Parkinson's disease. *Mov Disord* 1990;5(2):156–161.
52. Glatt SL, Hubble JP, Lyons K, et al. Risk factors for dementia in Parkinson's disease: effect of education. *Neuroepidemiology* 1996;15(1):20–25.
53. Levy G, Schupf N, Tang MX, et al. Combined effect of age and severity on the risk of dementia in Parkinson's disease. *Ann Neurol* 2002;51(6):722–729.
54. Ebmeier KP, Calder SA, Crawford JR, et al. Clinical features predicting dementia in idiopathic Parkinson's disease: a follow-up study. *Neurology* 1990;40(8):1222–1224.
55. Elizan TS, Sroka H, Maker H, et al. Dementia in idiopathic Parkinson's disease. Variables associated with its occurrence in 203 patients. *J Neural Transm* 1986;65(3–4):285–302.
56. Agid Y, AM G, Ruberg M. The efficacy of levodopa treatment declines in the course of Parkinson's disease: do nondopaminergic lesions play a role? *Adv Neurol* 1990;53:83–100.
57. Bonnet AM, Loria Y, Saint-Hilaire MH, et al. Does long-term aggravation of Parkinson's disease result from nondopaminergic lesions? *Neurology* 1987;37(9):1539–1542.
58. Klawans HL. Individual manifestations of Parkinson's disease after ten or more years of levodopa. *Mov Disord* 1986;1(3):187–192.
59. Markham CH, Diamond SG. Long-term follow-up of early dopa treatment in Parkinson's disease. *Ann Neurol* 1986;19(4):365–372.
60. Levy G, Tang MX, Cote LJ, et al. Motor impairment in PD: relationship to incident dementia and age. *Neurology* 2000;55(4):539–544.
61. Pillon B, Dubois B, Cusimano G, et al. Does cognitive impairment in Parkinson's disease result from nondopaminergic lesions? *J Neurol Neurosurg Psychiatry* 1989;52(2):201–206.
62. Jankovic J, McDermott M, Carter J, et al. Variable expression of Parkinson's disease: a base-line analysis of the DATATOP cohort. The Parkinson Study Group. *Neurology* 1990;40(10):1529–1534.
63. Mortimer JA, Pirozzolo FJ, Hansch EC, et al. Relationship of motor symptoms to intellectual deficits in Parkinson disease. *Neurology* 1982;32(2):133–137.
64. Mayeux R, Stern Y. Intellectual dysfunction and dementia in Parkinson disease. *Adv Neurol* 1983;38:211–227.
65. Zetusky WJ, Jankovic J, Pirozzolo FJ. The heterogeneity of Parkinson's disease: clinical and prognostic implications. *Neurology* 1985;35(4):522–526.
66. Huber SJ, Paulson GW, Shuttleworth EC. Relationship of motor symptoms, intellectual impairment, and depression in Parkinson's disease. *J Neurol Neurosurg Psychiatry* 1988;51(6):855–858.
67. Marder K, Tang M, Hemenegildo N, et al. A factor analysis of extrapyramidal signs as risk factors for dementia in Parkinson's disease. *Mov Disord* 1993;8:409.
68. Stern M. The clinical characteristics of Parkinson's disease and parkinsonian syndromes: diagnosis and assessment. In Stern M, Murtig M, eds. *The comprehensive management of Parkinson's disease,* New York: PMA Publishing Corp, 1988:3–50.
69. Hoehn MM, Yahr MD. Parkinsonism: onset, progression and mortality. *Neurology* 1967;17(5):427–442.
70. Hershey LA, Feldman BJ, Kim KY, et al. Tremor at onset. Predictor of cognitive and motor outcome in Parkinson's disease? *Arch Neurol* 1991;48(10):1049–1051.
71. Piccirilli M, Piccinin GL, Agostini L. Characteristic clinical aspects of Parkinson patients with intellectual impairment. *Eur Neurol* 1984;23(1):44–50.
72. Portin R, Rinne UK. Predictive factors for cognitive deterioration and dementia in Parkinson's disease. *Adv Neurol* 1987;45:413–416.
73. Caparros-Lefebvre D, Pecheux N, Petit V, et al. Which factors predict cognitive decline in Parkinson's disease? *J Neurol Neurosurg Psychiatry* 1995;58(1):51–55.
74. Jankovic J, Kapadia AS. Functional decline in Parkinson disease. *Arch Neurol* 2001;58(10):1611–1615.
75. Viitanen M, Mortimer JA, Webster DD. Association between presenting motor symptoms and the risk of cognitive impairment in Parkinson's disease. *J Neurol Neurosurg Psychiatry* 1994;57(10):1203–1207.
76. Hughes AJ, Ben-Shlomo Y, Daniel SE, et al. What features improve the accuracy of clinical diagnosis in Parkinson's disease: a clinicopathologic study. *Neurology* 1992;42(6):1142–1146.
77. Hughes AJ, Daniel SE, Kilford L, et al. Accuracy of clinical diagnosis of idiopathic Parkinson's disease: a clinico-pathological study of 100 cases. *J Neurol Neurosurg Psychiatry* 1992;55(3):181–184.
78. Starkstein SE, Bolduc PL, Mayberg HS, et al. Cognitive impairments and depression in Parkinson's disease: a follow up study. *J Neurol Neurosurg Psychiatry* 1990;53(7):597–602.
79. Starkstein SE, Mayberg HS, Leiguarda R, et al. A prospective longitudinal study of depression, cognitive decline, and physical impairments in patients with Parkinson's disease. *J Neurol Neurosurg Psychiatry* 1992;55(5):377–382.
80. Montgomery SA, Asberg M. A new depression scale designed to be sensitive to change. *Br J Psychiatry* 1979;134:382–389.
81. Friedman A, Barcikowska M. Dementia in Parkinson's disease. *Dementia* 1994;5(1):12–16.
82. Weschler D. The Weschler adult intelligence scale-revised. San Antonio: Psychological Corporation, 1981.
83. Stroop J. Studies of interferences in serial verbal reactions. *J Exp Psychol* 1935;18:643–662.
84. Jacobs DM, Marder K, Cote LJ, et al. Neuropsychological characteristics of preclinical dementia in Parkinson's disease. *Neurology* 1995;45(9):1691–1696.
85. Levy G, Jacobs DM, Tang MX, et al. Memory and executive function impairment predict dementia in Parkinson's disease. *Mov Disord* 2002;17(6):1221–1226.
86. Buschke H, Fuld PA. Evaluating storage, retention, and retrieval in disordered memory and learning. *Neurology* 1974;24(11):1019–1025.
87. Mattis, S. Mental status examination for organic mental syndrome in the elderly patient. In Bellak L, Karasu T, eds. *Geriatric psychiatry*, New York: Grune & Stratton, 1976:77–121.

88. Piccirilli M, D'Alessandro P, Finali G, et al. Frontal lobe dysfunction in Parkinson's disease: prognostic value for dementia? *Eur Neurol* 1989;29(2):71–76.
89. Levy G, Tang MX, Cote LJ, et al. Do risk factors for Alzheimer's disease predict dementia in Parkinson's disease? An exploratory study. *Mov Disord* 2002;17(2):250–257.
90. Morens DM, Grandinetti A, Reed D, et al. Cigarette smoking and protection from Parkinson's disease: false association or etiologic clue? *Neurology* 1995;45(6):1041–1051.
91. Baron J. The epidemiology of cigarette smoking and Parkinson's disease. In: Clarke P, Quik M, Adlkofer F, et al., eds. *Effects of nicotine on biological systems II*. Basel: Birkhauser Verlag, 1995:313–319.
92. Arai H, Muramatsu T, Higuchi S, et al. Apolipoprotein E gene in Parkinson's disease with or without dementia. *Lancet* 1994;344(8926):889.
93. Marder K, Maestre G, Cote L, et al. The apolipoprotein epsilon 4 allele in Parkinson's disease with and without dementia. *Neurology* 1994;44(7):1330–1331.
94. Koller WC, Glatt SL, Hubble JP, et al. Apolipoprotein E genotypes in Parkinson's disease with and without dementia. *Ann Neurol* 1995;37(2):242–245.
95. Inzelberg R, Chapman J, Trevas TA, et al. Apolipoprotein E4 in Parkinson disease and dementia: new data and meta-analysis of published studies. *Alzheimer Dis Assoc Disord* 1998;12(1):45–48.
96. Whitehead AS, Bertrandy S, Finnan F, et al. Frequency of the apolipoprotein E epsilon 4 allele in a case-control study of early onset Parkinson's disease. *J Neurol Neurosurg Psychiatry* 1996;61(4):347–351.
97. Mattila PM, Koskela T, Roytta M, et al. Apolipoprotein E epsilon 4 allele frequency is increased in Parkinson's disease only with co-existing Alzheimer pathology. *Acta Neuropathol (Berl* 1998;96(4):417–420.
98. Egensperger R, Bancher C, Kosel S, et al. The apolipoprotein E epsilon 4 allele in Parkinson's disease with Alzheimer lesions. *Biochem Biophys Res Commun* 1996;224(2):484–486.
99. Harhangi BS, de Rijk MC, van Duijn CM, et al. APOE and the risk of PD with or without dementia in a population-based study. *Neurology* 2000;54(6):1272–1276.
100. Ramakrishnan R, Zareparsi S, Gancher S, et al. Risk factors for Parkinson's dementia: age, male gender, and apolipoprotein e2. *Neurology* 2001;56:A113.
101. Wilhelmsen K, Mirel D, Marder K, et al. Is there a genetic susceptibility locus for Parkinson's disease on chromosome 22q13? *Ann Neurol* 1997;41(6):813–817.
102. Hubble JP, Kurth JH, Glatt SL, et al. Gene-toxin interaction as a putative risk factor for Parkinson's disease with dementia. *Neuroepidemiology* 1998;17(2):96–104.
103. Marder K, Tang MX, Alfaro B, et al. Postmenopausal estrogen use and Parkinson's disease with and without dementia. *Neurology* 1998;50(4):1141–1143.
104. Isoe-Wada K, Maeda M, Yong J, et al. Positive association between an estrogen receptor gene polymorphism and Parkinson's disease with dementia. *Eur J Neurol* 1999;6(4):431–435.
105. Mattila KM, Rinne JO, Roytta M, et al. Lack of association between an estrogen receptor 1 gene polymorphism and Parkinson's disease with dementia. *Acta Neurol Scand* 2002;106(3):128–130.
106. Conrad C, Vianna C, Freeman M, et al. A polymorphic gene nested within an intron of the tau gene: implications for Alzheimer's disease. *Proc Natl Acad Sci USA* 2002;99(11):7751–7756.
107. Cook L, Brayne CE, Easton D, et al. No evidence for an association between Saitohin Q7R polymorphism and Alzheimer's disease. *Ann Neurol* 2002;52(5):690–691.
108. Streffer JR, Papassotiropoulos A, Kurosinki P, et al. Saitohin gene is not associated with Alzheimer's disease. *J Neurol Neurosurg Psychiatry* 2003;74(3):362–363.
109. Verpillat P, Ricard S, Hannequin D, et al. Is the saitohin gene involved in neurodegenerative diseases? *Ann Neurol* 2002;52(6):829–832.
110. Clark LN, Levy G, Tang MX, et al. The Saitohin 'Q7R' polymorphism and tau haplotype in multi-ethnic Alzheimer disease and Parkinson's disease cohorts. *Neurosci Lett* 2003;347(1):17–20.
111. Polymeropoulos MH, Higgins JJ, Golbe LI, et al. Mapping of a gene for Parkinson's disease to chromosome 4q21-q23. *Science* 1996;274(5290):1197–1199.
112. Polymeropoulos MH, Lavedan C, Leroy E, et al. Mutation in the alpha-synuclein gene identified in families with Parkinson's disease. *Science* 1997;276(5321):2045–2047.
113. Golbe LI, Di Iorio G, Sanges G, et al. Clinical genetic analysis of Parkinson's disease in the Contursi kindred. *Ann Neurol* 1996;40(5):767–775.
114. Langston JW, Sastry S, Chan P, et al. Novel alpha-synuclein-immunoreactive proteins in brain samples from the Contursi kindred, Parkinson's, and Alzheimer's disease. *Exp Neurol* 1998;154(2):684–690.
115. Papadimitriou A, Veletza V, Hadjigeorgiou GM, et al. Mutated alpha-synuclein gene in two Greek kindreds with familial PD: incomplete penetrance?. *Neurology* 1999;52(3):651–654.
116. Spira PJ, Sharpe DM, Halliday G, et al. Clinical and pathological features of a Parkinsonian syndrome in a family with an Ala53Thr alpha-synuclein mutation. *Ann Neurol* 2001;49(3):313–319.
117. Markopoulou K, Wszolek ZK, Pfeiffer RF, et al. Reduced expression of the G209A alpha-synuclein allele in familial Parkinsonism. *Ann Neurol* 1999;46(3):374–381.
118. Spellman G. Report of familial cases of parkinsonism. *JAMA* 1962;179:160–162.
119. Muenter MD, Forno LS, Hornykiewicz O, et al. Hereditary form of parkinsonism—dementia. *Ann Neurol* 1998;43(6):768–781.
120. Waters CH, Miller CA. Autosomal dominant Lewy body parkinsonism in a four-generation family. *Ann Neurol* 1994;35(1):59–64.
121. Farrer M, Gwinn-Hardy K, Muenter M, et al. A chromosome 4p haplotype segregating with Parkinson's disease and postural tremor. *Hum Mol Genet* 1999;8(1):81–85.
122. Gwinn-Hardy K, Mehta ND, Farrer M, et al. Distinctive neuropathology revealed by alpha-synuclein antibodies in hereditary parkinsonism and dementia linked to chromosome 4p. *Acta Neuropathol Berl* 2000;99(6):663–672.
123. Trojanowski JQ, Lee VM. Meeting summary—cell biology of Parkinson's disease and related neurodegenerative disorders. *Sci SAGE KE* 2003;2003(32):pe23.
124. Marder K, Tang MX, Alfaro B, et al. Risk of Alzheimer's disease in relatives of Parkinson's disease patients with and without dementia. *Neurology* 1999;52(4):719–724.
125. Mickel SF, Broste SK, Hiner BC. Lack of overlap in genetic risks for Alzheimer's and Parkinson's disease. *Neurology* 1997;48(4):942–949.
126. Levy G, Louis ED, Mejia-Santana H, et al. Lack of familial aggregation of Parkinson's disease and Alzheimer's disease. 2003, *Submitted*
127. Emre M. Dementia associated with Parkinson's disease. *Lancet Neurol* 2003;2(4):229–237.
128. Pillon B, Dubois B, Agid Y. Testing cognition may contribute to the diagnosis of movement disorders. *Neurology* 1996;46(2):329–334.

129. Litvan I, Mohr E, Williams J, et al. Differential memory and executive functions in demented patients with Parkinson's and Alzheimer's disease. *J Neurol Neurosurg Psychiatry* 1991;54(1):25–29.
130. Girotti F, Soliveri P, Carella F, et al. Dementia and cognitive impairment in Parkinson's disease. *J Neurol Neurosurg Psychiatry* 1988;51(12):1498–1502.
131. Owen AM, Roberts AC, Hodges JR, et al. Contrasting mechanisms of impaired attentional set-shifting in patients with frontal lobe damage or Parkinson's disease. *Brain* 1993;116(Pt 5):1159–1175.
132. Stern Y, Richards M, Sano M, et al. Comparison of cognitive changes in patients with Alzheimer's and Parkinson's disease. *Arch Neurol* 1993;50(10):1040–1045.
133. Pillon B, Deweer B, Agid Y, et al. Explicit memory in Alzheimer's, Huntington's, and Parkinson's diseases. *Arch Neurol* 1993;50(4):374–379.
134. Huber SJ, Shuttleworth EC, Freidenberg DL. Neuropsychological differences between the dementias of Alzheimer's and Parkinson's diseases. *Arch Neurol* 1989;46(12):1287–1291.
135. Ballard CG, Aarsland D, McKeith I, et al. Fluctuations in attention: PD dementia vs DLB with parkinsonism. *Neurology* 2002;59(11):1714–1720.
136. Pillon B, Dubois B, Ploska A, et al. Severity and specificity of cognitive impairment in Alzheimer's, Huntington's, and Parkinson's diseases and progressive supranuclear palsy. *Neurology* 1991;41(5):634–643.
137. Helkala EL, Laulumaa V, Soininen H, et al. Different error pattern of episodic and semantic memory in Alzheimer's disease and Parkinson's disease with dementia. *Neuropsychologia* 1989;27(10):1241–1248.
138. Levin BE, Llabre MM, Reisman S, et al. Visuospatial impairment in Parkinson's disease. *Neurology* 1991;41(3):365–369.
139. Villardita C, Smirni P, le Pira F, et al. Mental deterioration, visuoperceptive disabilities and constructional apraxia in Parkinson's disease. *Acta Neurol Scand* 1982;66(1):112–120.
140. Boller F, Passafiume D, Keefe NC, et al. Visuospatial impairment in Parkinson's disease. Role of perceptual and motor factors. *Arch Neurol* 1984;41(5):485–490.
141. Stern Y, Mayeux R, Rosen J, et al. Perceptual motor dysfunction in Parkinson's disease: a deficit in sequential and predictive voluntary movement. *J Neurol Neurosurg Psychiatry* 1983;46(2):145–151.
142. Cummings JL, Darkins A, Mendez M, et al. Alzheimer's disease and Parkinson's disease: comparison of speech and language alterations. *Neurology* 1988;38(5):680–684.
143. Matison R, Mayeux R, Rosen J, et al. "Tip-of-the-tongue" phenomenon in Parkinson disease. *Neurology* 1982;32(5):567–570.
144. Grossman M, Carvell S, Gollomp S, et al. Sentence comprehension and praxis deficits in Parkinson's disease. *Neurology* 1991;41(10):1620–1626.
145. Grossman M, Carvell S, Stern MB, et al. Sentence comprehension in Parkinson's disease: the role of attention and memory. *Brain Lang* 1992;42(4):347–384.
146. Goldenberg G, Wimmer A, Auff E, et al. Impairment of motor planning in patients with Parkinson's disease: evidence from ideomotor apraxia testing. *J Neurol Neurosurg Psychiatry* 1986;49(11):1266–1272.
147. Mayeux R, Stern Y, Cote L, et al. Altered serotonin metabolism in depressed patients with parkinson's disease. *Neurology* 1984;34(5):642–646.
148. Mayeux R, Stern Y, Williams JB, et al. Clinical and biochemical features of depression in Parkinson's disease. *Am J Psychiatry* 1986;143(6):756–759.
149. Schiffer RB, Kurlan R, Rubin A, et al. Evidence for atypical depression in Parkinson's disease. *Am J Psychiatry* 1988;145(8):1020–1022.
150. Cummings JL. Depression and Parkinson's disease: a review. *Am J Psychiatry* 1992;149(4):443–454.
151. Sano M, Stern Y, Williams J, et al. Coexisting dementia and depression in Parkinson's disease. *Arch Neurol* 1989;46(12):1284–1286.
152. Chan-Palay V. Depression and dementia in Parkinson's disease. Catecholamine changes in the locus ceruleus, a basis for therapy. *Adv Neurol* 1993;60:438–446.
153. Torack RM, Morris JC. The association of ventral tegmental area histopathology with adult dementia. *Arch Neurol* 1988;45(5):497–501.
154. Starkstein SE, Rabins PV, Berthier ML, et al. Dementia of depression among patients with neurological disorders and functional depression. *J Neuropsychiatry Clin Neurosci* 1989;1(3):263–268.
155. Taylor AE, Saint-Cyr JA, Lang AE, et al. Parkinson's disease and depression. A critical re-evaluation. *Brain* 1986;109(Pt 2):279–292.
156. Starkstein SE, Preziosi TJ, Berthier ML, et al. Depression and cognitive impairment in Parkinson's disease. *Brain* 1989;112(Pt 5):1141–1153.
157. Rogers D, Lees AJ, Smith E, et al. Bradyphrenia in Parkinson's disease and psychomotor retardation in depressive illness. An experimental study. *Brain* 1987;110(Pt 3):761–776.
158. Meco G, Bonifati V, Cusimano G, et al. Hallucinations in Parkinson disease: neuropsychological study. *Ital J Neurol Sci* 1990;11(4):373–379.
159. Bell K, Dooneief G, Marder K, et al. Non drug-induced psychosis in Parkinson's disease. *Neurology* 1991;41(Suppl 1):191.
160. Fenelon G, Mahieux F, Huon R, et al. Hallucinations in Parkinson's disease: prevalence, phenomenology and risk factors. *Brain* 2000;123(Pt 4):733–745.
161. Aarsland D, Cummings JL, Larsen JP. Neuropsychiatric differences between Parkinson's disease with dementia and Alzheimer's disease. *Int J Geriatr Psychiatry* 2001;16(2):184–191.
162. Huber SJ, Shuttleworth EC, Christy JA, et al. Magnetic resonance imaging in dementia of Parkinson's disease. *J Neurol Neurosurg Psychiatry* 1989;52(11):1221–1227.
163. Laakso MP, Partanen K, Riekkinen P, et al. Hippocampal volumes in Alzheimer's disease, Parkinson's disease with and without dementia, and in vascular dementia: An MRI study. *Neurology* 1996;46(3):678–681.
164. Hanyu H, Asano T, Sakurai H, et al. MR analysis of the substantia innominata in normal aging, Alzheimer disease, and other types of dementia. *AJNR Am J Neuroradiol* 2002;23(1):27–32.
165. Bissessur S, Tissingh G, Wolters EC, et al. rCBF SPECT in Parkinson's disease patients with mental dysfunction. *J Neural Transm Suppl* 1997;50:25–30.
166. Jagust WJ, Johnson KA, Holman BL. SPECT perfusion imaging in the diagnosis of dementia. *J Neuroimaging* 1995;5 (Suppl 1):S45–S52.
167. Tachibana H, Kawabata K, Tomino Y, et al. Brain perfusion imaging in Parkinson's disease and Alzheimer's disease demonstrated by three-dimensional surface display with 123I-iodoamphetamine.*Dementia* 1993;4(6):334–341.
168. Antonini A, De Notaris R, Benti R, et al. Perfusion ECD/SPECT in the characterization of cognitive deficits in Parkinson's disease. *Neurol Sci* 2001;22(1):45–46.
169. Sawada H, Udaka F, Kameyama M, et al. SPECT findings in Parkinson's disease associated with dementia. *J Neurol Neurosurg Psychiatry* 1992;55(10):960–963.

170. Kawabata K, Tachibana H, Sugita M. Cerebral blood flow and dementia in Parkinson's disease. *J Geriatr Psychiatry Neurol* 1991;4(4):194–203.
171. Spampinato U, Habert MO, Mas JL, et al. (99mTc)-HM-PAO SPECT and cognitive impairment in Parkinson's disease: a comparison with dementia of the Alzheimer type. *J Neurol Neurosurg Psychiatry* 1991;54(9):787–792.
172. Peppard RF, Martin WR, Carr GD, et al. Cerebral glucose metabolism in Parkinson's disease with and without dementia. *Arch Neurol* 1992;49(12):1262–1268.
173. Vander Borght T, Minoshima S, Giordani B, et al. Cerebral metabolic differences in Parkinson's and Alzheimer's diseases matched for dementia severity. *J Nucl Med* 1997;38(5):797–802.
174. Turjanski N, Brooks DJ. PET and the investigation of dementia in the parkinsonian patient. *J Neural Transm Suppl* 1997;51:37–48.
175. Marie RM, Rioux P, Eustache F, et al. Clues into the functional neuroanatomy of working memory: a PET study of resting brain glucose metabolism in Parkinson's disease. *Eur J Neurol* 1995;2:83–94.
176. Carbon M, Marie RM. Functional imaging of cognition in Parkinson's disease. *Curr Opin Neurol* 2003;16(4):475–480.
177. Minoshima S, Foster NL, Sima AA, et al. Alzheimer's disease versus dementia with Lewy bodies: cerebral metabolic distinction with autopsy confirmation. *Ann Neurol* 2001;50(3):358–365.
178. Higuchi M, Tashiro M, Arai H, et al. Glucose hypometabolism and neuropathological correlates in brains of dementia with Lewy bodies. *Exp Neurol* 2000;162(2):247–256.
179. Mentis MJ, McIntosh AR, Perrine K, et al. Relationships among the metabolic patterns that correlate with mnemonic, visuospatial, and mood symptoms in Parkinson's disease. *Am J Psychiatry* 2002;159(5):746–754.
180. Dagher A, Owen AM, Boecker H, et al. Mapping the network for planning: a correlational PET activation study with the Tower of London task. *Brain* 1999;122(Pt 10):1973–1987.
181. Owen AM, Doyon J. The cognitive neuropsychology of Parkinson's disease: a functional neuroimaging perspective. *Adv Neurol* 1999;80:49–56.
182. Dagher A, Owen AM, Boecker H, et al. The role of the striatum and hippocampus in planning: a PET activation study in Parkinson's disease. *Brain* 2001;124(Pt 5):1020–1032.
183. Poldrack RA, Clark J, Pare-Blagoev EJ, et al. Interactive memory systems in the human brain. *Nature* 2001;414(6863):546–550.
184. Cools R, Stefanova E, Barker RA, et al. Dopaminergic modulation of high-level cognition in Parkinson's disease: the role of the prefrontal cortex revealed by PET. *Brain* 2002;125(Pt 3):584–594.
185. Mattay VS, Tessitore A, Callicott JH, et al. Dopaminergic modulation of cortical function in patients with Parkinson's disease. *Ann Neurol* 2002;51(2):156–164.
186. Holthoff-Detto VA, Kessler J, Herholz K, et al. Functional effects of striatal dysfunction in Parkinson disease. *Arch Neurol* 1997;54(2):145–150.
187. Marie RM, Barre L, Dupuy B, et al. Relationships between striatal dopamine denervation and frontal executive tests in Parkinson's disease. *Neurosci Lett* 1999;260(2):77–80.
188. Rinne JO, Portin R, Ruottinen H, et al. Cognitive impairment and the brain dopaminergic system in Parkinson disease: [18F]fluorodopa positron emission tomographic study. *Arch Neurol* 2000;57(4):470–475.
189. Bruck A, Portin R, Lindell A, et al. Positron emission tomography shows that impaired frontal lobe functioning in Parkinson's disease is related to dopaminergic hypofunction in the caudate nucleus. *Neurosci Lett* 2001;311(2):81–84.
190. Muller U, Wachter T, Barthel H, et al. Striatal [123I]beta-CIT SPECT and prefrontal cognitive functions in Parkinson's disease. *J Neural Transm* 2000;107(3):303–319.
191. Ouchi Y, Yoshikawa E, Okada H, et al. Alterations in binding site density of dopamine transporter in the striatum, orbitofrontal cortex, and amygdala in early Parkinson's disease: compartment analysis for beta-CFT binding with positron emission tomography. *Ann Neurol* 1999;45(5):601–610.
192. Kuhl DE, Minoshima S, Fessler JA, et al. In vivo mapping of cholinergic terminals in normal aging, Alzheimer's disease, and Parkinson's disease. *Ann Neurol* 1996;40(3):399–410.
193. Grasby PM. Imaging the neurochemical brain in health and disease. *Clin Med* 2002;2(1):67–73.
194. Summerfield C, Gomez-Anson B, Tolosa E, et al. Dementia in Parkinson disease: a proton magnetic resonance spectroscopy study. *Arch Neurol* 2002;59(9):1415–1420.
195. Miller BL, Moats RA, Shonk T, et al. Alzheimer disease: depiction of increased cerebral myo-inositol with proton MR spectroscopy. *Radiology* 1993;187(2):433–437.
196. Shonk TK, Moats RA, Gifford P, et al. Probable Alzheimer disease: diagnosis with proton MR spectroscopy. *Radiology* 1995;195(1):65–72.
197. Jessen F, Block W, Traber F, et al. Proton MR spectroscopy detects a relative decrease of N-acetylaspartate in the medial temporal lobe of patients with AD. *Neurology* 2000;55(5):684–688.
198. Kantarci K, Jack CR, Jr., Xu YC, et al. Regional metabolic patterns in mild cognitive impairment and Alzheimer's disease: A 1H MRS study. *Neurology* 2000;55(2):210–217.
199. Dubois B, Boller F, Pillon B, et al. Cognitive deficits in Parkinson's disease. In: Boller F, Grafman J, eds. *Handbook of neuropsychology*, Amsterdam: Elsevier, 1991:195–240.
200. Pillon B, Deweer B, Michon A, et al. Are explicit memory disorders of progressive supranuclear palsy related to damage to striatofrontal circuits? Comparison with Alzheimer's, Parkinson's, and Huntington's diseases. *Neurology* 1994;44(7):1264–1270.
201. Rolls ET. Neurophysiology and cognitive functions of the striatum. *Rev Neurol (Paris)* 1994;150(8–9):648–660.
202. Paulus W, Jellinger K. The neuropathologic basis of different clinical subgroups of Parkinson's disease. *J Neuropathol Exp Neurol* 1991;50(6):743–755.
203. Jellinger KA. Morphological substrates of dementia in parkinsonism. A critical update. *J Neural Transm Suppl* 1997;51:57–82.
204. Parent A, Hazrati LN. Functional anatomy of the basal ganglia. I. The cortico-basal ganglia-thalamo-cortical loop. *Brain Res Brain Res Rev* 1995;20(1):91–127.
205. Jellinger KA, Paulus W. Clinico-pathological correlations in Parkinson's disease. *Clin Neurol Neurosurg* 1992;94 (Suppl):S86–S88.
206. Rinne JO, Rummukainen J, Paljarvi L, et al. Dementia in Parkinson's disease is related to neuronal loss in the medial substantia nigra. *Ann Neurol* 1989;26(1):47–50.

207. Zweig RM, Cardillo JE, Cohen M, et al. The locus ceruleus and dementia in Parkinson's disease. *Neurology* 1993;43(5):986–991.
208. Javoy-Agid F, Ruberg M, Taquet H, et al. Biochemical neuropathology of Parkinson's disease. In: Hassler R, Christ J, eds. *Parkinson specific motor and mental disorders.* New York: Raven Press, 1984:189–198.
209. Duyckaerts C, Gaspar P, Costa C, et al. Dementia in Parkinson's disease. Morphometric data. *Adv Neurol* 1993;60:447–455.
210. Marie RM, Barre L, Rioux P, et al. PET imaging of neocortical monoaminergic terminals in Parkinson's disease. *J Neural Transm Park Dis Dement Sect* 1995;9(1):55–71.
211. Gaspar P, Duyckaerts C, Alvarez C, et al. Alterations of dopaminergic and noradrenergic innervations in motor cortex in Parkinson's disease. *Ann Neurol* 1991;30(3):365–374.
212. Gaspar P, Gray F. Dementia in idiopathic Parkinson's disease. A neuropathological study of 32 cases. *Acta Neuropathol (Berl)* 1984;64(1):43–52.
213. Heilig CW, Knopman DS, Mastri, AR, et al. Dementia without Alzheimer pathology. *Neurology* 1985;35(5):762–765.
214. Mann DM, Yates PO. Pathological basis for neurotransmitter changes in Parkinson's disease. *Neuropathol Appl Neurobiol* 1983;9(1):3–19.
215. Greenfield J, Bosanquet F. The brainstem lesions in Parkinsonism. *J Neurol Neurosurg Psychiatry* 1953;16:213–226.
216. Chui HC, Mortimer JA, Slager U, et al. Pathologic correlates of dementia in Parkinson's disease. *Arch Neurol* 1986;43(10):991–995.
217. Boller F. Parkinson's disease and Alzheimer's disease. Are they associated? In: Hutton J, Kenny A, eds. *Senile dementia of the Alzheimer type.* New York: Liss, 1985.
218. Tagliavini F, Pilleri G, Bouras C, et al. The basal nucleus of Meynert in idiopathic Parkinson's disease. *Acta Neurol Scand* 1984;70(1):20–28.
219. Pendlebury W, Perl D. Nucleus basalis of Meynert. Severe loss in Parkinson's disease without dementia (Abstract). *Ann Neurol* 1984;16:129.
220. Whitehouse PJ, Hedreen JC, White CL, et al. Basal forebrain neurons in the dementia of Parkinson disease. *Ann Neurol* 1983;13(3):243–248.
221. Lewy F. Zur pathologischen Anatomie der Paralysis agitans. *Dtsch Z Nervenheilk* 1913;50:50–55.
222. Greenfield J. System degenerations of the cerebellum, brainstem and spinal cord. In: Blackwood W, McMenemey W, Meyer A, et al., eds. *Greenfield's neuropathology.* Baltimore: Williams & Wilkins, 1963:582–585.
223. Alvord EJ. The pathology of parkinsonism. In: Minckler J, ed. *Pathology of the nervous system.* New York: McGraw-Hill, 1968:1152–1161.
224. Perry EK, Curtis M, Dick DJ, et al. Cholinergic correlates of cognitive impairment in Parkinson's disease: comparisons with Alzheimer's disease. *J Neurol Neurosurg Psychiatry* 1985;48(5):413–421.
225. Saper CB, German DC, White CL, 3rd Neuronal pathology in the nucleus basalis and associated cell groups in senile dementia of the Alzheimer's type: possible role in cell loss. *Neurology* 1985;35(8):1089–1095.
226. Mufson EJ, Conner JM, Kordower JH. Nerve growth factor in Alzheimer's disease: defective retrograde transport to nucleus basalis. *Neuroreport* 1995;6(7):1063–1066.
227. Chan-Palay V, Hochli M, Jentsch B, et al. Raphe serotonin neurons in the human brain in normal controls and patients with senile dementia of the Alzheimer type and Parkinson's disease. *Dementia* 1992;3:253–259.
228. Ruberg M, Agid Y. Dementia in Parkinson's disease. In: Iversen L, Iversen S, Snyder S, eds. *Handbook of psychopharmacology,* volume 20. *Psychopharmacology of the aging nervous system.* New York: Plenum Press, 1988:157–206.
229. Braak H, Braak E. Neuropathological staging of Alzheimer-related changes. *Acta Neuropathol (Berl)* 1991;82(4):239–259.
230. Jellinger KA. Pathology of Parkinson's disease. Changes other than the nigrostriatal pathway. *Mol Chem Neuropathol* 1991;14(3):153–197.
231. Jendroska K, Lees AJ, Poewe W, et al. Amyloid beta-peptide and the dementia of Parkinson's disease. *Mov Disord* 1996;11(6):647–653.
232. Braak H, Braak E. Cognitive impairment in Parkinson's disease: amyloid plaques, neurofibrillary tangles, and neuropil threads in the cerebral cortex. *J Neural Transm Park Dis Dement Sect* 1990;2(1):45–57.
233. Dickson DW, Singer G, Davies P, et al. Regional immunocytochemical studies of brains of prospectively studied demented and nondemented normal elderly humans. In Nicolini M, Zatta P, Corain B, eds. *Alzheimer's disease and related disorders. Advances in the biosciences,* Volume 87. Oxford: Pergamon Press, 1993.
234. Arai H, Schmidt ML, Lee VM, et al. Epitope analysis of senile plaque components in the hippocampus of patients with Parkinson's disease. *Neurology* 1992;42(7):1315–1322.
235. Bancher C, Jellinger K, Lassmann H, et al. Correlations between mental state and quantitative neuropathology in the Vienna Longitudinal Study on Dementia. *Eur Arch Psychiatry Clin Neurosci* 1996;246(3):137–146.
236. Vermersch P, Delacourte A, Javoy-Agid F, et al. Dementia in Parkinson's disease: biochemical evidence for cortical involvement using the immunodetection of abnormal Tau proteins. *Ann Neurol* 1993;33(5):445–450.
237. Vermersch P, Frigard B, Delacourte A. Mapping of neurofibrillary degeneration in Alzheimer's disease: evaluation of heterogeneity using the quantification of abnormal tau proteins. *Acta Neuropathol (Berl)* 1992;85(1):48–54.
238. Hof P, Morrison J. The cellular basis of cortical disconnection in Alzheimer disease and related dementing conditions. In Terry R, Katzmann R, Bick K, eds. *Alzheimer disease.* New York: Raven Press, 1994:197–229.
239. Mattila KM, Rinne JO, Roytta M, et al. Dipeptidyl carboxypeptidase 1 (DCP1) and butyrylcholinesterase (BCHE) gene interactions with the apolipoprotein E epsilon4 allele as risk factors in Alzheimer's disease and in Parkinson's disease with coexisting Alzheimer pathology. *J Med Genet* 2000;37(10):766–770.
240. Hurtig HI, Trojanowski JQ, Galvin J, et al. Alpha-synuclein cortical Lewy bodies correlate with dementia in Parkinson's disease. *Neurology* 2000;54(10):1916–1921.
241. Apaydin H, Ahlskog JE, Parisi JE, et al. Parkinson disease neuropathology: later-developing dementia and loss of the levodopa response. *Arch Neurol* 2002;59(1):102–112.

242. Consensus recommendations for the postmortem diagnosis of Alzheimer's disease. The National Institute on Aging, and Reagan Institute Working Group on Diagnostic Criteria for the Neuropathological Assessment of Alzheimer's Disease. *Neurobiol Aging*, 1997;18 (4 Suppl): p. S1–S2.
243. Baba M, Nakajo S, Tu PH, et al. Aggregation of alpha-synuclein in Lewy bodies of sporadic Parkinson's disease and dementia with Lewy bodies. *Am J Pathol* 1998;152(4):879–884.
244. Spillantini MG, Crowther RA, Jakes R, et al. Alpha-synuclein in filamentous inclusions of Lewy bodies from Parkinson's disease and dementia with Lewy bodies. *Proc Natl Acad Sci USA* 1998;95(11):6469–6473.
245. Quinn NP, Rossor MN, Marsden CD. Dementia and Parkinson's disease—pathological and neurochemical considerations. *Br Med Bull* 1986;42(1):86–90.
246. Jendroska K. The relationship of Alzheimer-type pathology to dementia in Parkinson's disease. *J Neural Transm Suppl* 1997;49:23–31.
247. Association AP. Diagnostic and statistical manual of mental disorders, 4th ed. Washington: American Psychological Association, 2000.
248. McKeith IG, Galasko D, Kosaka K, et al. Consensus guidelines for the clinical and pathologic diagnosis of dementia with Lewy bodies (DLB): report of the consortium on DLB international workshop. *Neurology* 1996;47(5):1113–1124.
249. Growdon JH, Kieburtz K, McDermott MP, et al. Levodopa improves motor function without impairing cognition in mild non-demented Parkinson's disease patients. Parkinson Study Group. *Neurology* 1998; 50(5):1327–1331.
250. Beardsley JV, Puletti F. Personality (MMPI) and cognitive (WAIS) changes after levodopa treatment. *Arch Neurol* 1971;25(2):145–150.
251. Loranger AW, Goodell H, Lee JE, et al. Levodopa treatment of Parkinson's syndrome. Improved intellectual functioning. *Arch Gen Psychiatry* 1972;26(2):163–168.
252. Huber SJ, Shulman HG, Paulson GW, et al. Dose-dependent memory impairment in Parkinson's disease. *Neurology* 1989;39(3):438–440.
253. Poewe W, Berger W, Benke T, et al. High-speed memory scanning in Parkinson's disease: adverse effects of levodopa. *Ann Neurol* 1991;29(6):670–673.
254. Prasher D, Findley L. Dopaminergic induced changes in cognitive and motor processing in Parkinson's disease: an electrophysiological investigation. *J Neurol Neurosurg Psychiatry* 1991;54(7):603–609.
255. Saint-Cyr JA, Taylor AE, Lang AE. Neuropsychological and psychiatric side effects in the treatment of Parkinson's disease. *Neurology* 1993;43 (12 Suppl 6): S47–S52.
256. Hietanen M, Teravainen H. Dementia and treatment with L-dopa in Parkinson's disease. *Mov Disord* 1988; 3(3):263–270.
257. Cedarbaum JM, Gandy SE, McDowell FH. "Early" initiation of levodopa treatment does not promote the development of motor response fluctuations, dyskinesias, or dementia in Parkinson's disease. *Neurology* 1991; 41(5):622–629.
258. Duvoisin RC. Cholinergic-anticholinergic antagonism in parkinsonism. *Arch Neurol* 1967;17(2):124–136.
259. Hutchinson M, Fazzini E. Cholinesterase inhibition in Parkinson's disease. *J Neurol Neurosurg Psychiatry* 1996;61(3):324–325.
260. Aarsland D, Laake K, Larsen JP, et al. Donepezil for cognitive impairment in Parkinson's disease: a randomised controlled study. *J Neurol Neurosurg Psychiatry* 2002;72(6):708–712.
261. Bergman J, Lerner V. Successful use of donepezil for the treatment of psychotic symptoms in patients with Parkinson's disease. *Clin Neuropharmacol* 2002;25(2): 107–110.
262. Fabbrini G, Barbanti P, Aurilia C, et al. Donepezil in the treatment of hallucinations and delusions in Parkinson's disease. *Neurol Sci* 2002;23(1):41–43.
263. Korczyn AD, Giladi N. Acetylcholinesterase inhibitors in the treatment of dementia in Parkinson's disease. In: Bedard M-A, Agid Y, Chouinard S et al., eds. *Mental and behavioral dysfunction in movement disorders*. Totowa, NJ: Humana Press, 2003:295–301.
264. Reading PJ, Luce AK, McKeith IG. Rivastigmine in the treatment of parkinsonian psychosis and cognitive impairment: preliminary findings from an open trial. *Mov Disord* 2001;16(6):1171–1174.
265. Aarsland D, Hutchinson M. Galantamine for Parkinson's disease with dementia. *Eur Neuropsychopharm* 2002;12 (Suppl 12):S378–S379.
266. Shea C, MacKnight C, Rockwood K. Donepezil for treatment of dementia with Lewy bodies: a case series of nine patients. *Int Psychogeriatr* 1998;10(3):229–238.
267. Kaufer DI, Catt KE, Lopez OL, et al. Dementia with Lewy bodies: response of delirium-like features to donepezil. *Neurology* 1998;51(5):1512.
268. Fergusson E, Howard R. Donepezil for the treatment of psychosis in dementia with Lewy bodies. *Int J Geriatr Psychiatry* 2000;15(3):280–281.
269. Samuel W, Caligiuri M, Galasko D, et al. Better cognitive and psychopathologic response to donepezil in patients prospectively diagnosed as dementia with Lewy bodies: a preliminary study. *Int J Geriatr Psychiatry* 2000;15(9):794–802.
270. McKeith I, Del Ser T, Spano P, et al. Efficacy of rivastigmine in dementia with Lewy bodies: a randomised, double-blind, placebo-controlled international study. *Lancet* 2000;356(9247):2031–2036.
271. Cummings JL, Mega M, Gray K, et al. The Neuropsychiatric Inventory: comprehensive assessment of psychopathology in dementia. *Neurology* 1994;44(12): 2308–2314.
272. Emre M, Aarsland D, Albanese A, et al. Rivastigmine for dementia associated with Parkinson's disease. *N Engl J Med* 2004;351(24):2509–2518.
273. McKeith I, Fairbairn A, Perry R, et al. Neuroleptic sensitivity in patients with senile dementia of Lewy body type. *BMJ* 1992;305(6855):673–678.
274. Kieburtz K, McDermott M, Como P, et al. The effect of deprenyl and tocopherol on cognitive performance in early untreated Parkinson's disease. Parkinson Study Group. *Neurology* 1994;44(9):1756–1759.

9
Behavioral Changes as Side Effects of Medication Treatment for Parkinson's Disease

Jennifer S. Hui, Gail A. Murdock, Joseph S. Chung, and Mark F. Lew

Keck/University of Southern California School of Medicine, Los Angeles, California

Since the introduction of levodopa in 1967 (1) for the treatment of Parkinson's disease (PD), a complex constellation of behavioral abnormalities has been observed in treated patients. The effects of exogenous dopaminergic agents (L-dopa and dopamine agonists) on the mesolimbic system have been implicated as the primary cause. However, recent epidemiologic and experimental data suggest that although medication plays an integral role in the expression of abnormal behaviors, other factors such as duration of disease, cognitive status, and age may contribute (2–4).

The scope of behaviors associated with antiparkinsonian medication has expanded in the last five years, with examples of compulsive and addictive behavior becoming increasingly prominent (5). In the same time frame, methods of pharmacologic treatment for patients with PD have changed demonstrably with the release and availability of new-generation, non–ergot-derived dopamine agonists. Long-term data demonstrating diminished motor fluctuations with dopamine agonist therapy has led to more extensive use of these medications, resulting in an increase of pathologic behavioral sequelae not previously seen in routine clinical practice.

This chapter focuses on the clinical features, mechanisms, and treatment of two emerging categories of behavior associated with antiparkinsonian medication: psychotic symptoms and reward-based behaviors. Each category is illustrated with actual patient cases.

PSYCHOTIC SYMPTOMS

Case History

A 75-year-old Asian male with a nine-year history of PD and two years of progressive dementia presented to the office with complaints of "seeing little people" in the house. According to his wife, this symptom started approximately two months earlier, after he had a urinary tract infection. He frequently saw bugs crawling on the walls and would often converse with his sister, who had passed away. After two weeks of treatment with antibiotics, his wife stated, most of his hallucinations resolved, with the exception of the "little people." The patient was extremely bothered by seeing these people in the house, because he felt that they frequently chided him, especially at night.

His current regimen included carbidopa/levodopa (CD/LD) 25/100 mg, 1.5 tablets 4 times daily and 1 tablet at bedtime. Higher or more frequent doses of CD/LD caused excessive daytime sleepiness. The presence of relatively severe rigidity made it impractical to reduce his medication. Quetiapine in escalating doses up to 75 mg at bedtime was added to his regimen. He slept well, with no additional daytime sleepiness. The hallucinations resolved completely.

Epidemiology

Psychotic symptoms, such as hallucinations and delusions, are one of the most commonly reported behavioral side effects of antiparkinsonian therapy.

Psychosis in patients with PD rarely occurred before the introduction of levodopa (6). Current estimates of the prevalence of hallucinations and delusions in patients with PD vary, ranging from 10% to 39%, because of differences in patient selection (hospital or community-based), survey methodology, and lack of prospective studies.

In one of the few publications that specifically examines drug-induced complications, Cummings performed a literature review in which behavioral disturbances were included only if they appeared for the first time soon after antiparkinsonian treatment was initiated or after the dosage was increased, and if the behavior improved after discontinuing or decreasing the dosage (7). Drug-induced hallucinations, mostly visual, were found in 6% to 38% of patients taking dopaminergic medication. Delusions were reported in 3% to 17% of patients given levodopa, bromocriptine, or pergolide, but markedly higher (30%–83%) in those treated with lisuride infusions. These variable and wide ranges testify to the lack of uniformity in study designs included in this review, most of which did not examine prevalence but reported psychotic symptoms merely as side effects.

A number of prospective epidemiologic studies have more clearly identified the prevalence of psychosis in certain populations. Fenelon et al. derived a high estimate of prevalence in a population of 216 patients by including minor forms of hallucinations, such as the feeling of a presence in the room (presence hallucinations), or brief passing visions of a person or animal (passage hallucinations). The overall prevalence of hallucinations was reported as 39.8%. Formed visual hallucinations occurred in 22.2% of patients, and auditory hallucinations in 9.7% (3). Adopting a more conservative approach, Aarsland et al. conducted a community-based prospective study of 245 patients using the thought disorder subscale of the Unified Parkinson's Disease Rating Scale (UPDRS) (8). The overall prevalence of hallucinations was 16%, with 10% of patients reporting retained insight (9).

Several studies have shown that both hallucinations and delusions are more common in patients with PD associated with dementia than in nondemented patients with PD (10,11); delusions were reported in as many as 29% of demented patients with PD, compared to 7% of nondemented patients with PD (10). Hallucinations and side effects also appear more commonly in patients receiving polypharmacy (12–15) or in patients treated with dopamine agonists than in those exposed to levodopa monotherapy (16–18). In a study in which pramipexole was supplemented with levodopa in patients with advanced PD, 21% of the subjects who were given both medications experienced hallucinations compared to 6% of subjects given levodopa alone (13).

Finally, elderly patients are often perceived as being more susceptible than others to the behavioral side effects of antiparkinsonian medication. Although few studies have addressed this issue, a recent chart review of elderly patients (age >80 years) revealed a tolerability rate of 55/120 (46%) of dopamine agonist trials in a population of 69 patients; however, participants were carefully selected as appropriate medication candidates (19). Overall, despite large variation in the methods used to assess psychotic symptoms in patients with PD, these and other epidemiologic surveys have generally documented a prevalence of between 20% and 30% (17,20).

Clinical Features

Psychosis is an impaired perception of reality, often involving hallucinations, delusions, confusion, and delirium (21). The psychotic symptoms of patients with PD, however, are unique in that they occur in the context of a clear sensorium, often with preserved insight. Virtually all antiparkinsonian medication can induce psychosis in susceptible individuals, with anticholinergics carrying a greater risk than dopaminergic therapies of inducing a confusional state or delirium. The most common symptoms are visual hallucinations consisting of familiar or unfamiliar people, animals, or objects. They are typically vivid, nonfrightening, occasionally bizarre or miniaturized, and they occur more frequently at night. They can be recurrent and appear real enough for the patient to attempt interaction with them, which often causes the hallucinations to disappear.

In a study of 216 patients, 55 (25.5%) experienced minor hallucinations, the most frequent type being "presence" hallucinations in which patients felt that a person was in the room or behind them but could not be seen (3). Most often, the hallucination was a strong perception, with patients stating "the image is behind me, but when I turn around, it isn't there." In seven cases, the presence was a relative of the patient. "Passage" hallucinations were second in frequency and consisted of a person or an identifiable animal, usually a cat or dog, passing briefly off to the side. All patients with minor hallucinations except one were on antiparkinsonian medication. Formed visual hallucinations occurred in 48 (22.2%) subjects, usually consisting of persons (73%) or animals (33%). Deceased relatives were seen by 19% of patients. All patients were being treated with antiparkinsonian medication.

Holroyd et al., in a prospective study of 98 patients, identified 30 (29.4%) patients with visual hallucinations (2). Visions of persons were most common (57.7%), followed by objects (30.8%) and animals (26.9%), but often with overlapping content. Most hallucinations were stationary (65.4%) but some were kinetic (26.9%). Miniaturized visions were also common (34.6%), though not as common as hallucinations of normal-sized figures (46.2%). The tendency for hallucinations to occur in the evening was illustrated in a questionnaire completed by 21 hallucinating patients, which showed that most (52.4%) of the patients only saw images in dim ambient lighting (22). Several examples of visual hallucinations encountered in these studies and in our experience include "running black horses," "cats everywhere," "strange people," and "small devils."

Although less common, auditory hallucinations are experienced by patients with PD, usually in conjunction with visual hallucinations. Of 216 patients with PD, 21 (9.7%) experienced auditory hallucinations. In seven patients, the sounds or voices accompanied a simultaneous visual scene. Only five patients (2.3%) did not have a history of visual hallucinations (3). In a separate cohort of 121 patients with PD, Inzelberg et al. found that 10 patients (8%) experienced auditory hallucinations, all of whom also had a history of visual hallucinations. The content was incomprehensible in five, and typically, the auditory hallucinations were voices. The voices were of neutral effect and discussed various topics, and in two patients, the voices seemed familiar (a late husband). In this series, auditory and visual hallucinations were never related in content and would occur at separate times in the same individual (23). All patients were being treated with CD/LD. Tactile, gustatory, and olfactory hallucinations have been described in patients with PD (2,24).

Our experience indicates that delusions in patients with PD are typically of a persecutory nature involving marital or financial infidelity. These delusions are frequently associated with an otherwise clear sensorium and intact perception of reality in other domains, although delirium may be present. Only a few systematic studies exist of delusions independent of hallucinations in patients with PD. A recent review of psychiatric symptoms in patients with PD and in dementia with Lewy bodies (DLB) documented delusions in 20 of 131 patients with PD (15.3%), including those with dementia (10). In patients with PD, paranoid ideation was most common (9.2%), followed by delusions of boarding an uninvited houseguest (8.4%), characters from television in the room (4.6%), and spouse infidelity (3%). These false beliefs, particularly those involving spousal infidelity, can be pervasive and extremely disruptive to quality of life among family and caretakers.

Case History

A 67-year-old white man, brought to the office by his two daughters, insisted that the neighbors were crawling under his house to kill him with poisonous gas. The patient was enrolled in a clinical trial for a new dopamine agonist and was at the time receiving the highest dose of the new medication in an open-label trial.

The patient maintained that his neighbor was "out to get him," and he called the police because he heard someone crawling underneath his home. When the police arrived, they were unable to find anyone, but the patient maintained that they found a piece of tubing in the crawlspace that was not his. The daughters confirmed that the patient proceeded to spend the remainder of the evening pacing in his living room watching out of the window for his neighbor. The patient had a well-stocked gun closet in his home and had a shotgun with him as he stood vigil all night.

The patient was removed from the trial and preferred to remain off PD medication for several months. He moved in with his daughters for three weeks, and all firearms were removed from his home. His delusions and paranoia cleared completely in less than a week, once he was weaned off his dopamine agonist therapy.

Associated Risk Factors and Pathophysiology

Although antiparkinsonian medication was originally implicated as the major cause of psychotic symptoms in patients with PD (25), few studies have found a definite correlation between psychotic symptoms and the dosage or duration of dopaminergic medications. Even the number of medications has not been consistently shown to predict psychotic symptoms (10,17). Furthermore, Goetz et al. found that high-dose IV (intravenous) infusions of levodopa in five PD subjects who experienced hallucinations daily did not induce any visual symptoms; this finding demonstrates that rapidly escalating or high levels of dopaminergic stimulation do not necessarily induce psychotic side effects (26). Conversely, epidemiologic studies have consistently identified age, cognitive decline, sleep disturbance, and duration and severity of extra-pyramidal disease as risk factors for psychosis in patients with PD, thus raising the possibility of other pathophysiologic mechanisms (2,3,9,10,17,22,27). However, given that reduction or withdrawal of antiparkinsonian therapy remains an effective treatment for psychosis in patients with PD, medication clearly can induce or worsen psychotic symptoms in susceptible individuals.

The mechanism for drug-induced symptoms remains poorly understood. The continuum from vivid dreams to hallucinations to confusional states has long been proposed as a dopaminergic 'kindling' phenomenon, with increasing receptor supersensitivity in the mesolimbic system as a possible mechanism (28). More recently, Graham et al. invoked this concept to explain the higher propensity for dopamine agonists to cause hallucinations (17). They hypothesized that the mesolimbic dopamine neurons degenerate faster than the postsynaptic nigrostriatal neurons. Exposure to dopamine agonist therapy would preferentially stimulate the supersensitive receptors of the mesolimbic system, causing behavioral side effects. Psychotic patients with PD have greater numbers of striatal dopamine receptors than those without psychosis (7). Alternatively, phenotypic variations in dopamine receptor subtypes may cause certain patients to be more susceptible to exogenous dopamine; some authors suggest that particular existing receptors may be "presensitized" (17,26). Cummings suggested that the D2 receptors may be the responsible subtype, because most dopaminergic agents exhibit D2 effects (7).

Most studies indicate that certain individuals are predisposed to experiencing medication-induced side effects, regardless of the dosage. Evidence for this concept of a pharmacologically vulnerable population is the observation that levodopa can greatly exacerbate psychosis when given to patients with a preexisting diagnosis of schizophrenia (29). A study that compared the natural history of hallucinations among patients with early or late hallucination onset and an initial diagnosis of PD confirmed this observation (4). Of the 12 patients with PD who developed early hallucinations (within three months of starting dopaminergic therapy), all had either progressed to alternate diagnoses within five years (five with Alzheimer's disease, two with DLB, and one with postencephalitic parkinsonism) or had major preexisting psychiatric diagnoses that preceded their extra-pyramidal symptoms by decades (four subjects). The diagnosis of PD changed in only 8 of the 58 subjects who developed hallucinations after one year of dopaminergic therapy. In addition, the mean dose of levodopa among the early hallucinators (142 mg) was significantly lower than that among the late hallucinators (794 mg), suggesting causative factors other than medication dosage.

Cognition and Dementia

Cognitive impairment has been uniformly identified as a risk factor for developing psychotic symptoms in patients with PD (2,3,9,10,22,27); one study, however, demonstrated an associated decline in symptoms during the Mini-Mental State Examination (MMSE), with successive PD populations showing no symptoms (mean score = 26), hallucinations with insight (mean score = 18.1), and confusional states (mean score = 13.5) (9). The role of cognition in hallucinosis is most likely multifactorial, starting with impaired processing of visuospatial stimuli, which results in visual misinterpretation. Hallucinations have been shown to occur more frequently in patients with PD whose visual acuity is impaired (2). Deficits in both basic electrophysiologic measures and higher cortical processing of visual information have been demonstrated in patients with PD, with occipital lobe metabolism particularly affected in DLB (30,31). Eye movement abnormalities in patients with PD have additionally been associated with impaired spatial working memory (30).

Disturbance of cholinergic pathways in PD with dementia has been implicated in the development of psychotic symptoms. Loss of neurons from the basal nucleus of Meynert may indirectly influence function of the brainstem reticular formation responsible for arousal and sleep (32). As a result, cholinesterase inhibitors are being investigated as treatment for psychotic symptoms (33–35). An alternative hypothesis invokes disruption in the acetylcholine:serotonin ratio, which causes behavioral side effects through greater serotonergic effects on the limbic system. Odansetron, a 5-HT3 (5-hydroxytryptamine) antagonist, has been reported to lessen levodopa-induced hallucinations (36). Others have proposed that paralimbic Lewy bodies and Alzheimer-type pathology may lower the threshold for psychotic symptoms (9). Once cognitive dysfunction occurs, impaired judgment can further amplify medication-induced behavioral changes. The presence of hallucinations and delusions in patients with PD is a risk factor for nursing home placement and subsequent mortality (36,37). This association illustrates the importance of identifying this cohort of patients promptly and pursuing aggressive antipsychotic therapy.

Sleep Disorders

The pharmacology and the role of dopaminergic medication in the development of complex visual hallucinations has been reviewed (32). Similarities have been noted among the visual symptoms of patients with PD, hypnagogic hallucinations in narcolepsy, and peduncular hallucinosis, all of which involve lesions of the pons and midbrain (24,37). Brainstem control of sleep and arousal has been linked to hallucinosis in patients with PD by numerous studies demonstrating sleep disturbances in patients with PD, although no unifying explanation remains (3,27,38,39). Pappert et al. demonstrated an important interaction between altered dream phenomena [vivid dreams, rapid eye movement (REM) behavior disorder] and hallucinosis in patients with PD, which suggests a common underlying mechanism (38). A separate study of 10 patients with PD (5 hallucinators) showed substantially decreased sleep efficiency and reduced REM percentage in hallucinators (mean, 5%) compared to nonhallucinators (mean, 20%) (39). These researchers hypothesized that reductions in REM sleep can lead to hallucinations in patients with PD. Manford and Andermann suggest that levodopa further reduces REM sleep, thereby increasing the propensity for hallucinosis in patients with PD who have preexisting sleep disruption (32).

Arnulf et al. proposed, in a controversial hypothesis, that psychosis in patients with PD reflects a narcolepsy-like REM sleep disorder, with hallucinations being analogous to daytime REM intrusions (37). He documented the presence of REM behavior disorder in 10 of 10 patients with PD who experienced hallucinations and delusions, compared to 6 of 10 without hallucinations and delusions. Hallucinators tended to be drowsier during the day, had sleep-onset REM during daytime naps, and demonstrated post-REM delusions in the awake but drowsy state.

Other Risk Factors

From the numerous studies conducted since the dopamine "kindling" hypothesis was first proposed, it appears likely that multiple neurotransmitters other than the mesolimbic circuit are involved in the development of psychotic symptoms. A history of depression has been mentioned as a potential risk factor, suggesting the involvement of both serotonin and dopamine; some studies even raise the possibility of psychotic depression in patients with PD (2,27,40,41).

Finally, duration and severity of extra-pyramidal disease, together with cognitive decline, have been associated in almost all epidemiologic studies with increased susceptibility to medication-induced side effects (2,3,17,27,41). In one study, severe cognitive disorder (<24/32 on the Mini-Mental Parkinson test) and duration of disease (>8 years) both predicted visual hallucinations (3). These risk factors are likely markers for advancing global neurodegeneration, with accompanying receptor hypersensitivity and reduced capacity for neurochemical compensation.

Anxiety and Affective Symptoms

Early reports of levodopa-induced "mental disorders" documented episodes of mania, depression, and anxiety associated with increasing doses of medication. Although depression clearly occurs more commonly in patients with PD, it remains doubtful whether depression can be induced by dopaminergic therapy. A small number of authors have reported an increased incidence of depression in patients taking high doses of levodopa for a long duration, although these studies are likely confounded by disease severity and duration and the high baseline prevalence of depression in patients with PD (42,43). Levodopa-induced elevated mood and mania, on the other hand, have been documented more consistently in case reports substantiated by double-blind, controlled trials (44). The reported cases of mania include dose-related characteristics of euphoria, grandiosity, pressured speech, and impulsivity (45,46).

We have recently become more aware of anxiety as a levodopa-responsive behavioral trait. Anxiety, like depression, is highly prevalent in patients with PD, and the two are often seen concurrently (47). Several reports suggest an improvement in anxious symptoms with levodopa administration. Maricle et al. conducted a double-blind, placebo-controlled trial of the effect of levodopa infusions on mood and anxiety (44). Anxiety reduction and mood elevation of greater than 20% on a visual analog scale were seen in most patients, although anxiety measures were not statistically significant in this population of eight patients. The effects were dose-dependent, and visual analog results were discordant with tapping speed measures, arguing against the proposed idea that improvement in mood is a direct result of motor improvement.

Vazquez, in a study of the frequency of panic attacks in patients with PD, found that most panic attacks (90.3%) occurred during the "off" period (48). In addition, patients with PD who experienced panic attacks were treated for a longer duration and with higher doses of levodopa (842 mg/d) than patients with PD who did not have panic attacks (570 mg/d). Patients who experienced panic attacks had significantly more dyskinesias and motor fluctuations than those who did not, and levodopa was "of greater benefit" to those with panic attacks, although whether the benefit was motor or behavioral was not reported.

General Treatment of Drug-Induced Abnormal Behaviors in PD

The management of patients with PD who experience treatment-induced psychoses and other behavioral disorders depends on the specific presentation and severity of symptoms. The first challenge for the treating physician is determining the presence of these symptoms. Patients may be concerned that by reporting hallucinations they will be labeled as "crazy." By explaining that such symptoms are known side effects of the patient's medication, the physician can explore possible environmental triggers, such as sensory deprivation or overload. Often, the abnormal behaviors may not disrupt the patient or the caregiver's daily activities, and treatment may not be necessary. The patient may present as being unconcerned about the hallucinations or as accepting the psychotic symptoms, and in such cases, treatment is indicated to assist with reality testing and healthy mental functioning.

Frequently, the physician may not specifically question the patient, caregiver, or both regarding the presence of psychotic symptoms, and the information may not be volunteered. It is of the utmost importance for the examining neurologist to routinely include several questions specifically about the patient's psychiatric status to ascertain whether hallucinations or delusions are present.

When psychoses pervade the patient's daily routine and interrupt function, altering the medication regimen by diminishing or removing the most likely culprits is routine. Systematically removing the adjunctive therapies before adjusting the levodopa dosage can be effective in alleviating problematic behavior without substantially diminishing treatment benefit. We discontinue anticholinergics, amantadine, selegiline, dopamine agonists, catechol-O-methyltransferase (COMT) inhibitors, and finally, levodopa.

Unfortunately, dose reduction commonly leads to intolerable worsening of motor function. When this is the case, the use of an atypical neuroleptic is warranted to effectively treat the behavioral-psychiatric syndrome while maintaining adequate control of PD. These medications include clozapine, quetiapine, olanzapine, risperidone, ziprasidone, and aripiprazole. Other therapies for treatment-related psychoses and psychiatric disorders such as aggressive, inappropriate behavior, agitation, and anxiety include odansetron, cholinesterase inhibitors, and electroconvulsive therapy (ECT) (49–51).

Atypical Neuroleptics

Atypical neuroleptics must be used in the place of conventional neuroleptics because of their reduced propensity to worsen the motor aspect of parkinsonism. An atypical neuroleptic is defined pharmacologically by a decreased tendency to induce elevated levels of serum prolactin (except risperidone) and extra-pyramidal signs (52,53). Antagonism of 5HT2 receptors and decreased inhibition of D2 receptors were initially thought to be the mechanism responsible for the induction of prolactin and extra-pyramidal symptoms (54). Loose and fast dissociation of the dopamine D2 receptor is another popular hypothesis. The loose binding allows endogenous dopamine to displace the loosely bound antipsychotic, and the rapid dissociation does not allow for induction of prolactin production or extra-pyramidal symptoms (EPS) (55). The loose binding mechanism may explain why lower doses of the atypical neuroleptics adequately treat L-dopa-induced psychoses, whereas large doses must be administered to ameliorate psychoses in schizophrenia. Side effects commonly seen with atypical neuroleptics include sedation, weight gain, prolonged QT interval, and abnormalities in glucose and lipid levels (56). When atypical neuroleptic treatment is indicated, a low dosage is started at bedtime and increased slowly every 3 to 7 days until a minimally effective dosage is identified (57).

Clozapine (Clozaril®)

In 1989, Clozapine was introduced in the United States as the first atypical antipsychotic medication (58). It controlled both the positive and negative symptoms of psychoses in schizophrenia to a greater extent than the typical neuroleptics. It remains a powerful and effective therapy for schizophrenia refractory to treatment with routine dopamine receptor blocking agents. Doses used to treat drug-induced psychoses of Parkinson's disease are much lower (6.25–100 mg) than those for schizophrenia (300–900 mg). The reported mechanism of action of clozapine includes blockade of D1, D2, D3, and D5 receptors and a high affinity for the D4 receptor. This finding is consistent with the fact that clozapine is more active at limbic than at striatal dopamine receptors and does not cause extra-pyramidal adverse reactions. Additionally, clozapine has antagonist activity at cholinergic, serotonergic, adrenergic, and histaminergic receptors.

Clozapine is the only atypical neuroleptic that has been shown in multiple placebo-controlled trials to eliminate dopamine-induced psychosis in a robust, reliable fashion and not to worsen the extra-pyramidal state. This finding was elaborated in two double-blind trials performed by the Parkinson Study Group and the French Clozapine Study Group in 1999 (59,60). Both studies included 60 patients with PD and drug-induced psychosis. Importantly, these studies precluded any change in baseline PD medications during the study period. This study design enabled a more meaningful interpretation of clozapine's role in worsening parkinsonism. Significant improvement in both primary and secondary variables was seen with no significant worsening of the UPDRS motor scores observed in both studies. Clozapine dosing ranged from 6.25 mg to 50 mg per day.

Clozapine is unique among the other atypical neuroleptics in that it has been shown to control tremor to the same degree as tremor-specific medications, the anticholinergics. Clozapine was compared with benztropine in a 24-patient double-blind crossover trial. Clozapine at mean doses of 39 mg controlled tremor as effectively as 3.0 mg of benztropine (61). This effectiveness may be attributable to clozapine's very substantial anticholinergic profile (62). This quality may also confer an additional anti-EPS mechanism. Ironically, sialorrhea is seen frequently with clozapine rather than dry mouth, a common side effect of anticholinergics. The mechanism is unknown and may be a reason for poor tolerance.

Clozapine labeling carries "black box" warnings for agranulocytosis, seizures, myocarditis, and orthostatic hypotension with other potential cardiovascular or respiratory effects. Despite these warnings, it remains the gold standard for treatment of psychoses in patients with PD. The most worrisome side effect of clozapine use is idiosyncratic agranulocytosis. This finding led to the formation of the Clozaril National Registry, which oversees the dispensing of clozapine in the United States. Their database of 99,502 patients with schizophrenia who received clozapine over a period of five years (from 1990 to 1994) was reviewed in 1998. The rate of agranulocytosis was 0.38% (382 cases), with only 12 deaths attributed to agranulocytosis (63). The dispensing of clozapine requires weekly complete blood counts. After six months, WBC (white blood cell) monitoring may take place every 2 weeks. Typically, neutropenia has no correlation to dose but nearly all risk occurs during the first 3 months of treatment. In our experience, if a patient has a drop in WBC to <3000 or an Absolute Neutrophil Count (ANC) <1500, we temporarily hold the dosing for 3 to 7 days and rechallenge the patient once WBC normalizes.

Other problematic side effects of clozapine therapy include confusion, tachycardia, orthostasis, and weight gain. A recent task force formed by the Movement Disorders Society (MDS) for an evidence-based review of clozapine use in Parkinson's disease with drug-induced psychosis (DIP) concluded in 2002 that "Clozapine was clinically useful for the short-term (4 weeks) management of DIP in PD. It is also possibly useful for the long-term management of some patients" (64). The following case scenario illustrates the powerful therapeutic effects of clozapine in treating psychosis in patients with PD.

Case History

A 68-year-old-woman with a 7-year history of PD requested to speak to her physician privately, without her family. She proceeded to detail that her husband was having an affair with the caregiver the family had hired to help the patient. She noted that she heard her husband leave their bedroom late at night to be with the caregiver. The family reported that the patient insisted that several bedrooms be bolted shut so that these rooms could not be used for these late-night rendezvous. Additionally, the family confirmed that a caregiver did work with the patient but that she worked days only (from 9 AM to 5 PM) and that no relationship was present between the caregiver and the patient's husband.

The patient was taking 50/200 mg CR CD/LD (carbidopa/levodopa) plus a 25/100 mg CD/LD tablet four times daily with entacapone. Entacapone was discontinued, and "off" time worsened considerably, with no resolution of the patient's delusions and paranoia. Quetiapine 75 mg qhs and 25 mg b.i.d. caused substantial sedation, with little improvement in the patient's delusional state. Quetiapine was discontinued, and clozapine therapy was initiated at 6.25 mg HS after a baseline normal complete blood count (CBC) was drawn. After 3 days, the dosage was escalated to 25 mg of clozapine HS, and the patient's delusional state waned dramatically.

Quetiapine (Seroquel®)

This drug, next to clozapine, may have the lowest EPS profile of the atypical neuroleptics currently available (65). No controlled studies have been performed of quetiapine for the treatment of PD with DIP. In one open-label report of 69 patients with PD and DIP, 44 of whom were neuroleptic naive, 18% experienced deterioration of motor function (66). Other reports suggest that this medication is well tolerated, is slightly less effective than clozapine in relieving psychoses, and may have a slightly higher propensity to produce mild deterioration in motor function than clozapine (67). Typical effective doses are from 75 mg to 100 mg per day.

In one report, higher doses (200 mg to 400 mg/day) were tolerated in two patients whose doses were titrated over a period of 12 to 16 weeks (68). The Movement Disorders Society evidence-based review of treatment in Parkinson's disease with drug-induced psychosis concluded that because of the lack of controlled studies, the use of quetiapine is "considered investigational" (64). Of the available atypical neuroleptics, quetiapine is the least likely to worsen motor function, with the exception of clozapine. Quetiapine is easier to use than clozapine, which makes quetiapine our first choice among the atypical neuroleptics for treating PD with DIP. We have also used quetiapine successfully to treat other behavioral problems such as anxiety, agitation, insomnia, and depression. If the treatment is not effective after increasing the dosage of quetiapine up to 200 mg qhs as tolerated, we switch the patient to clozapine to control psychotic symptoms and other syndromes.

Olanzapine (Zyprexa®)

The EPS profile of olanzapine is thought to be less prominent than that of risperidone and more prominent than that of clozapine and quetiapine (69). Olanzapine is the most commonly prescribed antipsychotic in the United States. Only one double-blind trial has been performed to evaluate the efficacy and safety of olanzapine in Parkinson's disease. A trial comparing clozapine use to olanzapine use in 28 patients had to be stopped prematurely because of "safety stopping rules." The group that was treated with olanzapine experienced a significant worsening of motor function (70). In addition, no improvement was seen in the primary outcome measure for psychosis. The dosage of olanzapine used was between 2.5 mg and 15 mg. The Movement Disorders Society evidence-based review of treatment in Parkinson's disease with drug-induced psychosis concluded that "there is insufficient evidence to demonstrate efficacy of olanzapine," and at low conventional doses it carries an unacceptable risk of motor deterioration (64).

Risperidone (Risperdal®)

Risperidone is considered the least "atypical" of the atypical neuroleptics. Some have argued that it should not be in the category of atypicals (71). It has an EPS profile similar to that of haloperidol (72). It has been shown to cause increased prolactin secretion and tardive dyskinesias in neuroleptic-naive patients. No controlled studies have been conducted of risperidone for treatment of PD with DIP. Open-label reports are conflicting as to the propensity of this medication to worsen motor function in PD patients (73). A meta-analysis of 82 patients with Parkinson's disease treated with risperidone showed that 23 patients experienced deterioration of motor function (53). In clinical practice, this medication routinely causes motor deterioration in PD to a degree similar to that caused by the typical neuroleptics (72). Even the low dosages should be used cautiously, if at all, in PD patients, especially in doses over 1 mg (74).

Ziprasidone (Geodon®) and Aripiprazole (Abilify®)

Ziprasidone and aripiprazole are the newest atypical neuroleptics available in the United States to treat schizophrenia. No reports have been published of their use in PD with DIP. Ziprasidone and risperidone have shown the ability to prolong the QT interval, which raises concern about serious cardiac events like torsade de pointes and sudden death (75). In regard to ziprasidone's EPS profile, a report in 2002 ranked ziprasidone equal to olanzapine (76). This profile suggests that ziprasidone would not be an effective neuroleptic for patients with baseline extra-pyramidal syndromes.

Aripiprazole is unique in that it has partial agonist activity at the dopamine D2 receptors. Because of this mechanism, it should be in a category separate from the atypicals. In hypodopaminergic states, aripiprazole acts as a D2 agonist, and in hyperdopaminergic states, it acts as a D2 antagonist (77). A study of 932 schizophrenics in a short-term (4- to 6-week) double-blind trial showed an EPS profile similar to that of placebo on multiple scales (56). In addition to its low potential for EPS, aripiprazole has also demonstrated a low potential for sedation, weight gain, QT prolongation, and changes in glucose and cholesterol levels, unlike many of the other atypical neuroleptics. On the basis of this favorable profile, this medication may be worthy of trials in treatment for PD with DIP.

Other Therapeutic Interventions

Cholinesterase inhibitors, serotonin antagonists, and electroconvulsive therapy are other methods available for treating medication-induced psychoses in Parkinson's disease. Several small open-label studies with donepezil and rivastigmine suggest that this group of agents may be beneficial (35,49,78). The mechanism may be by alleviating the decrease in cholinergic tone caused by loss of neurons in the nucleus of Meynert, which is seen in both patients with PD and patients with Alzheimer's disease (79). This loss of cholinergic tone observed in patients with Parkinson's disease may lead to the "cerebral conditions required for the emergence of psychosis (80)."

The serotonin antagonist odansetron is an expensive antiemetic and selective 5HT3 receptor antagonist. A few conflicting small open-label reports have been published concerning its benefit in treating PD and DIP (50,81). Finally, case reports suggest ECT may be beneficial in PD with drug-induced psychosis. Because initial frequent sessions of ECT require hospitalization and may induce delirium, it should be used only as a last resort, after drug manipulations have failed (51).

SIDE EFFECTS OF PD TREATMENT THAT RESULT IN LOSS OF IMPULSE CONTROL

(Pathological gambling, hypersexuality, and other forms of disinhibition)

Reward-Based Behaviors

Case History

A 45-year-old man with a 5-year history of PD presented while taking a dose of 4 mg pramipexole t.i.d. to treat severe limb dystonia. He found the treatment to be extremely effective in alleviating rigidity, spasm, and dystonic posturing of the right arm and hand. He was accompanied by an older sister who detailed that the patient was spending thousands of dollars weekly on Internet pornography sites, visits to prostitutes, and in strip joints. This behavior started 6 months after he initiated therapy with a dopamine agonist. Advertisements were placed in a local paper by the patient to offer his services as a "go-go dancer" at sororities. Several altercations ensued, related to the patient's failure to pay for services, and he was eventually evicted from his apartment complex. The patient described a sensation of "being out of control." Dopamine agonist therapy was terminated. Initiation of levodopa and atypical neuroleptics eliminated the patient's compulsive and disinhibited behaviors within 2 weeks.

Case History

A 54-year-old man with a 3-year history of PD was started on an escalating dose of ropinerole up to 4 mg t.i.d. He presented to his visit extremely distraught after an acute separation from his wife. For several months before presentation, he had been spending several hundred dollars weekly on lottery ticket "scratchers." Being a grocery store clerk, he lived on a strict budget, and his wife apparently noticed several checks made by him for $200. The patient described being unable to drive past the local convenience store without stopping to buy scratchers. This behavior culminated in a trip to Las Vegas, where he spent several hundred more dollars. He temporarily separated from his wife. Agonist therapy was discontinued, and L-dopa treatment was initiated. Within several weeks, the patient described that he was "back to normal" and "in control" again. He reconciled with his wife and was able to completely discontinue his habit of buying lottery tickets.

Background

For 30 years, levodopa therapy has been the treatment of choice for idiopathic Parkinson's disease (PD). Levodopa is beneficial because it partially replaces deficient nigrostriatal dopamine stores (82). Most patients with PD respond favorably to levodopa, especially those experiencing bradykinesia and rigidity. After an initial positive response to CD/LD, the "honeymoon period," more than 50% of patients will experience considerable side effects within 5 years (83). A follow up study of 370 original participants in DATATOP showed that problems from long-term levodopa therapy developed after a mean duration of 18 months of treatment with CD/LD; the problems included motor fluctuations (wearing off and freezing), dyskinesias, and mental status changes (84). Despite the development of these adverse conditions, most patients remain dependent on CD/LD treatment in order to function.

In an effort to find new ways to treat motor fluctuations resulting from long-term levodopa use, a number of dopamine agonists (DA) have been investigated, and some have demonstrated remarkable promise. Because DA stimulate the postsynaptic receptors and have a longer half-life than CD/LD, they are useful when combined with CD/LD treatment (85). Treatment with DA results in fewer dyskinesias and other motor complications than treatment with CD/LD (14) but is not as effective in treating the motor symptoms of PD. Whether newly diagnosed PD patients should start monotherapy with DA or CD/LD in order to capitalize on the potential antioxidant properties remains controversial (86). However, the neurobehavioral side effects of DA used in the treatment of PD have manifested more prominently to researchers and clinicians.

Case History

A 72-year-old widowed Asian man with a 12-year history of PD was started on pramipexole monotherapy eight years earlier. He presented to his internist for a general physical exam dressed in "full drag," wearing a dress, stockings, high-heeled shoes, and extensive makeup and lipstick. He was taking pramipexole 1 mg t.i.d. and CD/LD 25/100 mg 1 tab q.i.d.

After the appointment, his internist referred him to his neurologist for evaluation. The patient stated that he had been dressing in women's clothes for several years, "for fun." He was weaned off his dopamine agonist and his CD/LD dosage was increased to 1.5 tabs q.i.d. His caregiver reported that no further cases of cross-dressing occurred.

Case History

A 54-year-old white male with a four-year history of PD was receiving agonist monotherapy, taking ropinerole 6 mg t.i.d. His partner of 10 plus years called the office to report that the patient was "engaging in dangerous and risky behaviors" and insisted the patient be seen urgently. He also stated that this behavior was "totally out of character" for the patient. The patient described that he felt "totally out of control." He had been meeting men on the Internet and traveling throughout the country to "see them." We gradually discontinued his agonist therapy over two weeks and started CD/LD. When seen in the office six weeks later, the patient described that he felt he was "back to his normal self."

Behavioral problems in Parkinson's disease have been associated with the side effects of LD/CD therapy (hallucinations, delusions) and with impulse-control issues (physical and verbal abusiveness, wandering, socially inappropriate behaviors) related to advanced PD and declining cognitive abilities (87). Since the introduction of dopamine agonists, new behavioral problems have been presenting in the PD population. Case reports identifying disorders of impulse control and increased risk-taking behavior have emerged. These behaviors, which range from pathologic gambling to hypersexuality and hypomania, are not behaviors typically seen in PD.

Even when focusing on the neuropsychiatric problems of patients with PD, Aarsland et al. reported that the most common psychiatric symptoms observed were depression (38%) and hallucinations (27%). In their population, euphoria and disinhibition were the least common psychiatric symptoms observed (41). With the increased use of new dopaminergic treatments, clinicians are reporting improvements in motor problems (i.e. reduced dyskinesias) along with the development of neurobehavioral symptoms in their PD patients, including disinhibition, impaired judgment, emotional lability, hypersexuality, anger and irritability, mania, and lack of awareness of changes in behavior (88).

Over the past few years, as movement disorder specialists have begun to question patients, spouses, and families about risk-taking, compulsions, and impulsive behaviors, awareness of these unusual activities has increased. This increased awareness indicates that clinicians have developed the ability to elicit responses to unusual questions; however, this approach has also resulted in the initiation of a more thorough, systematic screening for disinhibition, impulsiveness, and addictive behaviors [for example, the Shorter PROMIS Questionnaire for assessing multiple addictive and impulsive behaviors (89) or the Minnesota Multiphasic Personality Inventory-2 (90)].

We identified the following risk-taking, impulsive behaviors: promiscuity (through access to prostitutes), hypersexuality, gambling (casino and on-line), fast driving, stalking (of spouse or partner), shopping, and cross-dressing. Consistently, these behaviors started after the onset of dopaminergic agonist treatment (with or without CD/LD) and were reported to cease upon termination of agonist treatment. Most of the patients, or their family members, reported that they were distressed or worried about the occurrence of these behaviors, and they reported that these behaviors had a negative effect on the patient's social and occupational functioning or both.

Impulse-control disorders in the DSM-IV (*The Diagnostic and Statistical Manual of Mental Disorders*, 4th edition) include pathologic gambling. The hallmark of these disorders is the failure to resist an impulse or temptation. These impulses are preceded by increasing tension or arousal, and when the act is completed, the individual tends to experience a sense of gratification or release (21).

Although these behaviors may hold a social stigma, a mechanism within the individual seems to inspire a stronger, more rewarding incentive. Whether this process is considered an addiction, compulsion, or drive, a reward mechanism seems to be in place, which propels the individual to follow through with the behavior, which brings a corresponding release or sense of relief.

A number of cases have been reported in which an impulse-control disorder started after the onset of treatment with dopaminergic agents (including dopamine agonists, amantadine, and monoamine oxidase inhibitors). These findings correlate with our experience. The behaviors include pathologic gambling (91,92), transvestic fetishism (93), hypersexuality (94,95), sexual deviation (96), zoophilia (97), and increased libido (98). These impulsive behaviors ceased when the dopaminergic agent was stopped; however, the symptoms of Parkinson's disease worsened, resulting in a challenging clinical picture. In our population, all patients exhibiting this genre of behavioral abnormality have been taking a dopamine agonist.

In 2000, Molina et al. studied 12 patients who presented with pathologic gambling (99). Of these 12 patients, nine began gambling after starting CD/LD therapy. The two patients who were gamblers before PD was diagnosed reported a substantial increase in their gambling behavior after the initiation of CD/LD therapy. Most of these patients reported that the gambling behavior occurred almost exclusively during their "on" periods. Interestingly, almost 50% of this group of patients also reported an increase in alcohol abuse and dependence, which presented after their diagnosis of PD.

Individuals with Parkinson's disease who develop impulsivity, disinhibition, and compulsions after the onset of dopaminergic treatment should be evaluated more thoroughly to determine if they possessed any unique, risk-taking, addictive behaviors before PD was diagnosed. We found that patients often denied the presence of impulsive or compulsive behaviors and other psychiatric problems before their treatment for PD.

Perhaps one of the most surprising aspects of the current studies is that researchers have historically reported a lifelong or "premorbid" Parkinson's personality type. This distinctive personality profile has been characterized as inflexible, introverted, harm avoidant, low novelty seeking, stoic, and over controlled (100,101). Recent developments in neuroimaging have provided the means to determine if a connection exists between dopaminergic systems and the presenting personality changes. By use of positron emission tomography and functional MRI (magnetic resonance imaging), researchers are determining that the relationship of dopamine to Parkinson's personality is complex and controversial. A study by Kaasinen and colleagues confirmed that individuals with Parkinson's disease show low–novelty-seeking behavior; however, they observed in their study that this trait did not appear to be dopamine dependent (102).

Animal research has indicated that dopamine systems are directly involved in the processing of reward mechanisms (103). Such studies have shown that impairment in dopamine transmission results in deficits in the perception of rewards. In humans, the dopamine D2 receptor has been implicated in brain reward systems and is considered to be involved in alcohol and drug dependency (91).

The dopaminergic system may be involved in the internal reward mechanism such that abnormal risk-seeking or addictivelike behaviors could be the result of impairment in dopamine receptor genes (99). To compensate for the lack of dopamine in the nigrostriatal structures, CD/LD, dopamine agonists, or both are administered to ameliorate motor difficulties and behavioral features, including loss of initiative and motivation (92). The concurrent increase in dopamine in the mesocorticolimbic dopaminergic system may exceed what is required, resulting in relative overstimulation. Overstimulation may lead to enhanced reward-seeking and thrill-seeking behaviors, impulse-control problems, or both in a certain population of patients with PD. This over-stimulation of the central mesolimbic dopamine system has been implicated in cases where patients with PD have demonstrated possible addiction to dopaminergic treatment (104). Cases of misuse and abuse of dopamine agonists, termed "hedonistic homeostatic dysregulation," have been observed in some patients with PD, resulting in compulsive medication use, hoarding behaviors, and bingeing. Additionally, these patients continue in their pathologic use of the dopamine agonist in an attempt to avoid the effects of withdrawing from the medication (105). The influence of dopamine on systems involved in addiction, thrill-seeking, and reward-seeking behaviors only further complicates the management of the disease process in PD.

Treatment

The treating physician must navigate between severe motor symptoms and inappropriate, impulsive behavior. Our own practice in cases of impulsive, obsessive, disinhibited behavior including self mutilation, gambling, stalking, cross-dressing, hypersexuality, inappropriate sexual behavior, and inappropriate spending has been to discontinue or radically minimize treatment with dopamine agonists. These behavioral issues have resolved when use of dopamine agonists has stopped. Other approaches include maintaining dopaminergic therapy but adding an atypical neuroleptic.

The complexity this clinical dilemma presents is the issue of how to treat worsening motor status. Most patients tolerate either initiation of CD/LD therapy or modest increase of CD/LD doses to replace dopaminergic benefit lost by discontinuing the agonist. In rare cases when complete cessation of the agonist has been poorly tolerated, small doses of agonist were restarted very conservatively and judiciously to address severe motor complications that were not tolerated.

We have not seen these behaviors in patients taking any formulation of CD/LD or any other PD medicines without simultaneous use of an agonist, including pergolide, pramipexole, or ropinerole. Although we have not seen these behaviors in patients on bromocriptine, this fact most likely reflects the fact that this agonist has rarely been used in the past 13 years since the advent of newer agonists. Bromocriptine has been reported to induce similar side effects, such as gambling (106).

Further research is needed to identify, in a prospective fashion, the growing spectrum and prevalence of behavioral abnormalities in patients with PD patients who are taking dopamine agonist therapy. This research can be accomplished only by large multicenter prospective trials to evaluate these issues.

REFERENCES

1. Cotzias GC, Van Woert MH, Schiffer LM. Aromatic amino acids and modification of parkinsonism. *N Engl J Med* 1967;276(7):374–379.
2. Holroyd S, Currie L, Wooten GF. Prospective study of hallucinations and delusions in Parkinson's disease. *J Neurol Neurosurg Psychiatry* 2001;70(6):734–738.
3. Fenelon G, Mahieux F, Huon R, et al. Hallucinations in Parkinson's disease: prevalence, phenomenology and risk factors. *Brain* 2000;123(Pt 4):733–745.
4. Goetz CG, Vogel C, Tanner CM, et al. Early dopaminergic drug-induced hallucinations in parkinsonian patients. *Neurology* 1998;51(3):811–814.
5. Driver-Dunckley E, Samanta J, Stacy M. Pathological gambling associated with dopamine agonist therapy in Parkinson's disease. *Neurology* 2003;61(3):422–423.
6. Factor SA, Molho ES, Podskalny GD, et al. Parkinson's disease: drug-induced psychiatric states. *Adv Neurol* 1995;65:115–138.
7. Cummings JL. Behavioral complications of drug treatment of Parkinson's disease. *J Am Geriatr Soc* 1991;39(7):708–716.
8. Fahn S, Elton R, Members of the UPDRS Development Committee. Unified Parkinson's disease rating scale. *Recent developments in Parkinson's disease.* Florham Park, NJ: MacMillan Healthcare Information, 1987:153–163.
9. Aarsland D, Larsen JP, Cummins JL, et al. Prevalence and clinical correlates of psychotic symptoms in Parkinson disease: a community-based study. *Arch Neurol* 1999;56(5):595–601.
10. Aarsland D, Cummings JL, Larsen JP. Neuropsychiatric differences between Parkinson's disease with dementia and Alzheimer's disease. *Int J Geriatr Psychiatry* 2001;16(2):184–191.
11. Naimark D, Jackson E, Rockwell E, et al. Psychotic symptoms in Parkinson's disease patients with dementia. *J Am Geriatr Soc* 1996;44(3):296–299.
12. Parkinson Study Group. Entacapone improves motor fluctuations in levodopa-treated Parkinson's disease patients. *Ann Neurol* 1997;42(5):747–755.
13. Lieberman A, Ranhosky A, Korts D. Clinical evaluation of pramipexole in advanced Parkinson's disease: results of a double-blind, placebo-controlled, parallel-group study. *Neurology* 1997;49(1):162–168.
14. Bennett JP, Piercey MF. Jr., Pramipexole—a new dopamine agonist for the treatment of Parkinson's disease. *J Neurol Sci* 1999;163(1):25–31.
15. Tanner CM. Loss of nLC neurons. *Neurology* 1983;33(4):524.
16. Parkinson Study Group. Pramipexole vs levodopa as initial treatment for Parkinson disease: a randomized controlled trial. *JAMA* 2000;284(15):1931–1938.
17. Graham JM, Grunewald RA, Sagar HJ. Hallucinosis in idiopathic Parkinson's disease. *J Neurol Neurosurg Psychiatry* 1997;63(4):434–440.
18. Boyd A. Bromocriptine and psychosis: a literature review. *Psychiatr Q* 1995;66(1):87–95.
19. Shulman LM, Minagar A, Rabinstein A, et al. The use of dopamine agonists in very elderly patients with Parkinson's disease. *Mov Disord* 2000;15(4):664–668.
20. Friedman A, Sienkiewicz J. Psychotic complications of long-term levodopa treatment of Parkinson's disease. *Acta Neurol Scand* 1991;84(2):111–113.
21. *Task Force on the DSM-IV. Diagnostic and Statistical Manual of Mental Disorders*, 4th ed. Washington, DC: American Psychiatric Association, 1994.
22. Barnes J, David AS. Visual hallucinations in Parkinson's disease: a review and phenomenological survey. *J Neurol Neurosurg Psychiatry* 2001;70(6):727–733.
23. Inzelberg R, Kipervasser S, Korczyn AD. Auditory hallucinations in Parkinson's disease. *J Neurol Neurosurg Psychiatry* 1998;64(4):533–535.
24. Poewe W. Psychosis in Parkinson's disease. *Mov Disord* 2003;18 (Suppl. 6):S80–S87.
25. Goodwin FK. Psychiatric side effects of levodopa in man. *JAMA* 1971;218(13):1915–1920.
26. Goetz CG, Pappert EJ, Blasucci LM, et al. Intravenous levodopa in hallucinating Parkinson's disease patients: high-dose challenge does not precipitate hallucinations. *Neurology* 1998;50(2):515–517.
27. Sanchez-Ramos JR, Ortoll R, Paulson GW. Visual hallucinations associated with Parkinson disease. *Arch Neurol* 1996;53(12):1265–1268.
28. Moskovitz C, Moses H, Klawans HL III. Levodopa-induced psychosis: a kindling phenomenon. *Am J Psychiatry* 1978;135(6):669–675.
29. Klawans HL. Psychiatric side effects during the treatment of Parkinson's disease. *J Neural Transm Suppl* 1988;27:117–122.
30. Bodis-Wollner I. Neuropsychological and perceptual defects in Parkinson's disease. *Parkinsonism Relat Disord* 2003;9 (Suppl. 2):S83–S89.
31. Albin RL, Minoshima S, D'Amato CJ, et al. Fluorodeoxyglucose positron emission tomography in diffuse Lewy body disease. *Neurology* 1996;47(2):462–466.
32. Manford M, Andermann F. Complex visual hallucinations. Clinical and neurobiological insights. *Brain* 1998;121(Pt 10):1819–1840.
33. McKeith I, Del Ser T, Spano P, et al. Efficacy of rivastigmine in dementia with Lewy bodies: a randomized, double-blind, placebo-controlled international study. *Lancet* 2000;356(9247):2031–2036.
34. Minett TS, Thomas A, Wilkinson LM, et al. What happens when donepezil is suddenly withdrawn? An open label trial in dementia with Lewy bodies and Parkinson's disease with dementia. *Int J Geriatr Psychiatry* 2003;18(11):988–993.
35. Bergman J, Lerner V. Successful use of donepezil for the treatment of psychotic symptoms in patients with Parkinson's disease. *Clin Neuropharmacol* 2002;25(2):107–110.
36. Zoldan J, Friedberg G, Goldberg-Stern H, et al. Ondansetron for hallucinosis in advanced Parkinson's disease. *Lancet* 1993;341(8844):562–563.
37. Arnulf I, Bonnet AM, Damier P, et al. Hallucinations, REM sleep, and Parkinson's disease: a medical hypothesis. *Neurology* 2000;55(2):281–288.
38. Pappert EJ, Goetz CG, Niederman FG, et al. Hallucinations, sleep fragmentation, and altered dream phenomena in Parkinson's disease. *Mov Disord* 1999;14(1):117–121.
39. Comella CL, Tanner CM, Ristanovic RK. Polysomnographic sleep measures in Parkinson's disease patients with treatment-induced hallucinations. *Ann Neurol* 1993;34(5):710–714.
40. Giladi N, Treves TA, Paleacu D, et al. Risk factors for dementia, depression and psychosis in long-standing Parkinson's disease. *J Neural Transm* 2000;107(1):59–71.

41. Aarsland D, Larsen JP, Lim NG, et al. Range of neuropsychiatric disturbances in patients with Parkinson's disease. *J Neurol Neurosurg Psychiatry* 1999;67(4): 492–496.
42. Huber SJ, Paulson GW, Shuttleworth EC. Relationship of motor symptoms, intellectual impairment, and depression in Parkinson's disease. *J Neurol Neurosurg Psychiatry* 1988;51(6):855–858.
43. Mindham RH. Psychiatric symptoms in Parkinsonism. *J Neurol Neurosurg Psychiatry* 1970;33(2):188–191.
44. Maricle RA, Nutt JG, Valentine RJ, et al. Dose-response relationship of levodopa with mood and anxiety in fluctuating Parkinson's disease: a double-blind, placebo-controlled study. *Neurology* 1995;45(9):1757–1760.
45. O'Brien CP, DiGiacomo JN, Fahn S, et al. Mental effects of high-dosage levodopa. *Arch Gen Psychiatry* 1971;24(1):61–64.
46. Ryback RS, Schwab RS. Manic response to levodopa therapy. Report of a case. *N Engl J Med* 1971;285(14): 788–789.
47. Menza MA, Robertson-Hoffman DE, Bonapace AS. Parkinson's disease and anxiety: co morbidity with depression. *Biol Psychiatry* 1993;34(7):465–470.
48. Vazquez A, Jimenez-Jimenez FJ, Garcia-Ruiz P, et al. "Panic attacks" in Parkinson's disease. A long-term complication of levodopa therapy. *Acta Neurol Scand* 1993;87(1):14–18.
49. Fabbrini G, Barbanti P, Aurilia C, et al. Donepezil in the treatment of hallucinations and delusions in Parkinson's disease. *Neurol Sci* 2002;23(1):41–43.
50. Zoldan J, Friedberg G, Livneh M, et al. Psychosis in advanced Parkinson's disease: treatment with ondansetron, a 5-HT3 receptor antagonist. *Neurology* 1995;45(7):1305–1308.
51. Kennedy R, Mittal D, O'Jile J. Electroconvulsive therapy in movement disorders: an update. *J Neuropsychiatry Clin Neurosci* 2003;15(4):407–421.
52. D'Souza C, Gupta A, Alldrick MD, et al. Management of psychosis in Parkinson's disease. *Int J Clin Pract* 2003;57(4):295–300.
53. Factor SA, Friedman JH, Lannon MC, et al. Clozapine for the treatment of drug-induced psychosis in Parkinson's disease: results of the 12 week open label extension in the PSYCLOPS trial. *Mov Disord* 2001;16(1): 135–139.
54. Meltzer HY, Matsubara S, Lee JC. The ratios of serotonin2 and dopamine2 affinities differentiate atypical and typical antipsychotic drugs. *Psychopharmacol Bull* 1989;25(3):390–392.
55. Seeman P. Atypical antipsychotics: mechanism of action. *Can J Psychiatry* 2002;47(1):27–38.
56. Marder SR, McQuade RD, Stock E, et al. Aripiprazole in the treatment of schizophrenia: safety and tolerability in short-term, placebo-controlled trials. *Schizophr Res* 2003;61(2-3):123–136.
57. Olanow CW, Watts RL, Koller WC. An algorithm (decision tree) for the management of Parkinson's disease (2001): treatment guidelines. *Neurology* 2001; 56 (11 Suppl 5): S1–S88.
58. FDA approves clozapine for treatment of schizophrenia; careful monitoring required. *Hosp Community Psychiatry* 1989; 40(12): 1310.
59. The French Clozapine Parkinson Study Group. Clozapine in drug-induced psychosis in Parkinson's disease. *Lancet* 1999;353(9169):2041–2042.
60. The Parkinson Study Group. Low-dose clozapine for the treatment of drug-induced psychosis in Parkinson's disease. *N Engl J Med* 1999;340(10):757–763.
61. Friedman JH, Koller WC, Lannon MC, et al. Benztropine versus clozapine for the treatment of tremor in Parkinson's disease. *Neurology* 1997;48(4):1077–1081.
62. Meltzer HY. Role of serotonin in the action of atypical antipsychotic drugs. *Clin Neurosci* 1995;3(2):64–75.
63. Honigfeld G, Arellano F, Sethi J, et al. Reducing clozapine-related morbidity and mortality: 5 years of experience with the Clozaril National Registry. *J Clin Psychiatry* 1998;59 (Suppl. 3):3–7.
64. Drugs to treat dementia and psychosis: management of Parkinson's disease. *Mov Disord* 2002;17 (Suppl. 4): S120–S127.
65. Saller CF, Salama AI. Seroquel: biochemical profile of a potential atypical antipsychotic. *Psychopharmacology (Berl)* 1993;112(2-3):285–292.
66. Fernandez HH. Quetiapine for l-dopa-induced psychosis in PD. *Neurology* 2000;55(6):899.
67. Fernandez HH, Trieschmann ME, Friedman JH. Treatment of psychosis in Parkinson's disease: safety considerations. *Drug Saf* 2003;26(9):643–659.
68. Parsa MA, Bastani B. Quetiapine (Seroquel) in the treatment of psychosis in patients with Parkinson's disease. *J Neuropsychiatry Clin Neurosci* 1998;10(2): 216–219.
69. Carlson CD, Cavazzoni PA, Berg PH, et al. An integrated analysis of acute treatment-emergent extrapyramidal syndrome in patients with schizophrenia during olanzapine clinical trials: comparisons with placebo, haloperidol, risperidone, or clozapine. *J Clin Psychiatry* 2003;64(8):898–906.
70. Goetz CG, Blasucci LM, Leurgans S, et al. Olanzapine and clozapine: comparative effects on motor function in hallucinating PD patients. *Neurology* 2000;55(6): 789–794.
71. Friedman JH, Factor SA. Atypical antipsychotics in the treatment of drug-induced psychosis in Parkinson's disease. *Mov Disord* 2000;15(2):201–211.
72. Rosebush PI, Mazurek MF. Neurologic side effects in neuroleptic-naive patients treated with haloperidol or risperidone. *Neurology* 1999;52(4):782–785.
73. Mohr E, Mendis T, Hildebrand K, et al. Risperidone in the treatment of dopamine-induced psychosis in Parkinson's disease: an open pilot trial. *Mov Disord* 2000;15(6):1230–1237.
74. Wolters EC, Berendse HW. Management of psychosis in Parkinson's disease. *Curr Opin Neurol* 2001;14(4): 499–504.
75. Gury C, Canceil O, Iaria P. Antipsychotic drugs and cardiovascular safety: current studies of prolonged QT interval and risk of ventricular arrhythmia. *Encephale* 2000;26(6):62–72.
76. Tarsy D, Baldessarini RJ, Tarazi FI. Effects of newer antipsychotics on extrapyramidal function. *CNS Drugs* 2002;16(1):23–45.
77. Stahl SM. Dopamine system stabilizers, aripiprazole, and the next generation of antipsychotics, part 2: illustrating their mechanism of action. *J Clin Psychiatry* 2001;62(12):923–924.
78. Reading PJ, Luce AK, McKeith IG. Rivastigmine in the treatment of parkinsonian psychosis and cognitive impairment: preliminary findings from an open trial. *Mov Disord* 2001;16(6):1171–1174.

79. Whitehouse PJ, Martino AM, Marcus KA, et al. Reductions in acetylcholine and nicotine binding in several degenerative diseases. *Arch Neurol* 1988; 45(7):722–724.
80. Cummings JL. Managing psychosis in patients with Parkinson's disease. *N Engl J Med* 1999;340(10): 801–803.
81. Eichhorn TE, Brunt E, Oertel WH. Ondansetron treatment of L-dopa-induced psychosis. *Neurology* 1996; 47(6):1608–1609.
82. Marsden CD. Parkinson's disease. *J Neurol Neurosurg Psychiatry* 1994;57(6):672–681.
83. Marsden CD. Problems with long-term levodopa therapy for Parkinson's disease. *Clin Neuropharmacol* 1994;17 (Suppl. 2):S32–S44.
84. Parkinson Study Group. Impact of deprenyl and tocopherol treatment on Parkinson's disease in DATATOP patients requiring levodopa. *Ann Neurol* 1996;39(1):37–45.
85. Djaldetti R, Melamed E. Management of response fluctuations: practical guidelines. *Neurology* 1998;51 (2 Suppl 2): S36–S40.
86. Montastruc JL, Rascol O, Senard JM. Current status of dopamine agonists in Parkinson's disease management. *Drugs* 1993;46(3):384–393.
87. Fernandez HH, Lapane KL, Ott BR et al., SAGE Study Group. Gender differences in the frequency and treatment of behavior problems in Parkinson's disease. Systematic assessment and geriatric drug use via epidemiology. *Mov Disord* 2000;15(3):490–496.
88. Roane DM, Yu M, Feinberg TE, et al. Hypersexuality after pallidal surgery in Parkinson disease. *Neuropsychiatry Neuropsychol Behav Neurol* 2002;15(4):247–251.
89. Christo G, Jones SL, Haylett S, et al. The shorter PROMIS questionnaire: further validation of a tool for simultaneous assessment of multiple addictive behaviors. *Addict Behav* 2003;28(2):225–248.
90. Hathaway SR, McKinley JC. *Minnesota Multiphasic Personality Inventory - 2*. Minneapolis, MN: The University of Minnesota Press, 1989.
91. Seedat S, Kesler S, Niehaus DJ, et al. Pathological gambling behavior: emergence secondary to treatment of Parkinson's disease with dopaminergic agents. *Depress Anxiety* 2000;11(4):185–186.
92. Gschwandtner U, Aston J, Renaud S, et al. Pathologic gambling in patients with Parkinson's disease. *Clin Neuropharmacol* 2001;24(3):170–172.
93. Riley DE. Reversible transvestic fetishism in a man with Parkinson's disease treated with selegiline. *Clin Neuropharmacol* 2002;25(4):234–237.
94. Vogel HP, Schiffter R. Hypersexuality—a complication of dopaminergic therapy in Parkinson's disease. *Pharmacopsychiatria* 1983;16(4):107–110.
95. Uitti RJ, Tanner CM, Rajput AH, et al. Hypersexuality with antiparkinsonian therapy. *Clin Neuropharmacol* 1989;12(5):375–383.
96. Quinn NP, Toone B, Lang AE, et al. Dopa dose-dependent sexual deviation. *Br J Psychiatry* 1983;142: 296–298.
97. Jimenez-Jimenez FJ, Sayed Y, Garcia-Soldevilla MA, et al. Possible zoophilia associated with dopaminergic therapy in Parkinson disease. *Ann Pharmacother* 2002; 36(7-8):1178–1179.
98. Wittstock M, Benecke R, Dressler D. Cabergoline can increase penile erections and libido. *Neurology* 2002; 58(5):831.
99. Molina JA, Sainz-Artiga MJ, Fraile A, et al. Pathologic gambling in Parkinson's disease: a behavioral manifestation of pharmacologic treatment? *Mov Disord* 2000;15(5):869–872.
100. Menza MA, Golbe LI, Cody RA, et al. Dopamine-related personality traits in Parkinson's disease. *Neurology* 1993;43(3 Pt 1):505–508.
101. Heberlein I, Ludin HP, Scholz J, et al. Personality, depression, and premorbid lifestyle in twin pairs discordant for Parkinson's disease. *J Neurol Neurosurg Psychiatry* 1998;64(2):262–266.
102. Kaasinen V, Nurmi E, Bergman J, et al. Personality traits and brain dopaminergic function in Parkinson's disease. *Proc Natl Acad Sci U S A* 2001;98(23):13272–13277.
103. Schultz W. Dopamine neurons and their role in reward mechanisms. *Curr Opin Neurobiol* 1997;7(2):191–197.
104. Merims D, Galili-Mosberg R, Melamed E. Is there addiction to levodopa in patients with Parkinson's disease? *Mov Disord* 2000;15(5):1014–1016.
105. Giovannoni G, O'Sullivan JD, Turner K, et al. Hedonistic homeostatic dysregulation in patients with Parkinson's disease on dopamine replacement therapies. *J Neurol Neurosurg Psychiatry* 2000;68(4):423–428.
106. Montastruc JL, Schmitt L, Bagheri H. Pathological gambling behavior in a patient with Parkinson's disease treated with levodopa and bromocriptine. *Rev Neurol (Paris)* 2003;159(4):441–443.

10

Psychiatric Symptoms Following Surgery for Parkinson's Disease with an Emphasis on Subthalamic Stimulation

Valerie Voon,[1] Elena Moro,[2] Jean A. Saint-Cyr,[3] Andres M. Lozano,[4] and Anthony E. Lang[2]

[1]*Department of Psychiatry;* [2]*Department of Medicine, Division of Neurology;*
[3]*Department of Surgery, Division of Neurosurgery, Neuropsychology Clinic;*
[4]*Department of Surgery, Division of Neurosurgery, Toronto Western Hospital,
UHN, Toronto, Canada*

Parkinson's disease (PD) is a neurodegenerative disorder characterized by motor, psychiatric, and cognitive symptoms, the management of which includes medical and neurosurgical therapies. Deep brain stimulation (DBS) is a neurosurgical procedure that uses long-term high-frequency electric stimulation delivered through implanted quadripolar electrodes applied to specific targets of interest. Both bilateral globus pallidus interna (GPi) and subthalamic nucleus (STN) DBS substantially improve motor disability, motor fluctuations, and levodopa-induced dyskinesias (1,2). The STN procedure also enables a considerable reduction in antiparkinsonian medications (3).

A variety of psychiatric symptoms have been reported to follow subthalamic stimulation for PD. Authors of a recent two-year prospective study of 48 patients who had undergone bilateral STN DBS reported that "transient psychiatric symptoms were the most commonly noted therapy-related side effects" (4).

The causes of psychiatric symptoms following subthalamic stimulation in patients with PD can be separated into five categories: preoperative factors (including premorbid psychiatric vulnerabilities) (5); surgical factors (including the duration of the surgical procedure and the number of electrode passes) (6); STN stimulation factors; postoperative factors (including the changes in antiparkinsonian drugs) (7,8); and factors related to psychosocial adjustment (including psychological "reactive" changes in response to motor and functional changes, unrealistic expectations, limited social support, changes in identity or interpersonal relationships, or the loss of the "sick role" of the patient within the family) (9).

Parkinson's disease is a disorder associated with high psychiatric comorbidity. In clinical practice, the issue of preoperative psychiatric vulnerability, as with that of preoperative cognitive status, takes on an important role. Psychiatric symptoms, unlike cognitive symptoms, are potentially modifiable and treatable. Beyond the focus on symptoms, the relevant clinical outcomes following subthalamic stimulation extend to the factors involved in quality of life (QOL) and social and occupational functioning.

The functional neuroanatomy of the STN and cortical, brainstem, and thalamic regions implicated in the psychiatric symptoms associated with STN stimulation are summarized in Table 10-1. For the purposes of comparison, the literature on unilateral pallidotomy and bilateral GPi stimulation are summarized in Tables 10-2 and 10-3. The literature on psychiatric symptoms and STN stimulation are reviewed, and issues in the psychiatric preoperative assessment and postoperative management are also discussed.

TABLE 10-1. *Functional neuroanatomy of the subthalamic nucleus projections and psychiatric relevance*

Neuroanatomic regions	Relationship to subthalamic nucleus (STN)
Anterior cingulate (AC), orbitofrontal cortex, hippocampus, amygdala	Connection to medial limbic STN via "indirect" pathway and connections of basal ganglia circuitry (10a,11) Activation of AC on STN stimulation neuroimaging (12)
Lateral hypothalamus (LH), ventral tegmental area (VTA)	Projection from medial limbic STN to LH and VTA (11,13) Implicated in psychiatric symptoms of STN stimulation (14) Implicated in reward mechanisms (15)
Substantia nigra (SN)	Projection to SN via basal ganglia circuitry (11) Stimulation associated with acute depressive symptoms (16)
Pedunculopontine nucleus (PPN)	Reciprocal projections of PPN to STN (11,17) Implicated in STN hyperactivity in PD animal model (17) Proposed mediator of reward effects of VTA (18,19) Reward effects of opiates, amphetamines, food, sex, and nicotine blocked in animal studies with PPN lesions (18,19)
Dorsal raphe nucleus	Projection of serotonergic fibers to STN (11)
Prelimbic/medial orbitofrontal cortex (PL/MO)	Direct projection from limbic cortical region PL/MO to medial limbic STN in rodents (20,21)
Area TE of inferotemporal cortex	Cortico-striato-thalamo-cortical loop originating in Area TE (22) Implicated in visual hallucinations in PD (22)
Fiber bundles	Stimulation more likely to affect large myelinated axons than cell bodies (23) Most effective site of stimulation at anterodorsal border of sensorimotor STN with current diffusion to fiber bundles (24,25) Neuroanatomical regions implicated: zona incerta, fields of Forel (pallidothalamic fibers), pallidosubthalamic fibers (26,27), medial forebrain bundle (SN and VTA fibers) (28), ascending serotonergic fibers
Thalamic nuclei	Projection of parafascicular (PF) thalamic nuclei to STN implicated in STN hyperactivity in PD animal models (17) PF nuclei project to limbic and cognitive STN regions (11)

STN, subthalamic; LH, Lateral hypothalamus.

TABLE 10-2. *Psychiatric symptoms in patients with Parkinson's disease following unilateral pallidotomy*

Study (Other studies of same cohort)	Study design/number of patients	Symptom/Scale	Time of assessment after surgery	Conclusions and limitations of study
Alegret, 2003 (29) [Junque, 1999] (30)	Prospective uncontrolled 3 mo (n = 15) 4 y (n = 11)	Obsessive–compulsive symptoms; Mood MOCI BDI	3 mo 4 y	Improvement of MOCI at 3 months (4/15 to 1/15 pts) not sustained at 4 years. Mean BDI scores high and association with elevated MOCI pts unknown. No change BDI.
Baron, 2000 (31) [Baron, 1996] (32)	Prospective uncontrolled 1 y (n = 10) 4 y (n = 10)	Depression Anxiety HDRS HADS	1 y 4 y	Postoperative depression (6/10 pts over 4 yrs) related to past history of depression. Improvements in HDRS and HARS not sustained after one year.

(continues)

TABLE 10-2. *Continued*

Study (Other studies of same cohort)	Study design/number of patients	Symptom/Scale	Time of assessment after surgery	Conclusions and limitations of study
Bezarra, 1999 (33)	Case series 17 left PVP 13 right PVP	Depression DSM-IV	Unknown	Observational study: MDE associated with right PVP (5/17 pts) vs. left PVP (0/11 pts). However, past history of depression unknown.
Higginson, 2001 (34)	Prospective comparison group PVP (n = 24) Unilat GPi stim (n = 10)	Anxiety DSM-IV BAI	4 mo	Anxiety diagnoses decreased from 72% to 49%. Both symptoms of anxiety which are distinct (subjective) and overlapping (total, autonomic, neurophysiologic) with PD improved, suggesting true reduction in anxiety. Panic did not improve.
Lombardi, 2000 (35)	Prospective uncontrolled (n = 26)	Depression GDI	3 mo 6 mo	Improvement in GDI. No association with laterality.
Mendez, 2004 (36)	Case report (n = 1)	Hypersexuality and atypical sexual behaviors	"immediately"	Case report: Hypersexuality related to possible interaction of lesion in anterolateral GPi (with internal capsule involvement) with dopaminergic medications. However, insufficient reporting of frontal cognitive status.
Okun, 2003 (37)	Case report (n = 2)	Mania	"immediately"	Case report: Lesions within anteromedial GPi (R or L) may be associated with transient mania.
Perrine, 1998 (38) [Dogali, 1995] (39)	Prospective nonrandom wait list control PVP (n = 28) Control (n = 10)	Depression BDI	Mean 8.3 mo	No difference in BDI between surgical and control group. Reported incidence of depression 38.2% based on BDI scores. However, BDI cutoffs for diagnosis not valid in PD [1/18 transient hypersexuality; manic symptoms unknown (40)].
Rettig, 2000 (41)	Prospective uncontrolled (n = 42)	Depression BDI	3 mo 12 mo	Improvement in BDI. No association with laterality.
Trepanier, 2000 (42) [Trepanier, 1998] (43)	Prospective comparison PVP (n = 42) bilateral PVP (n = 3) bilateral GPi DBS (n = 4)	Behavioral symptoms FLOPS	3 to 6 mo	Differences between patient and caregiver reports suggest limited insight into behavioral symptoms. Poor insight into deficits, lability, impulsiveness.

(continues)

TABLE 10-2. *Continued*

Study (Other studies of same cohort)	Study design/number of patients	Symptom/Scale	Time of assessment after surgery	Conclusions and limitations of study
Vitek, 2003 (44) [Green, 2000] (45)	Prospective randomized wait-list control PVP (n = 17) Control (n = 16)	Depression Anxiety DSM-III R HDRS (inclusion/ exclusion); GDI HARS STAI, SSAI	3 mo 6 mo	Postoperative depression related to past history of depression irrespective of surgical procedure (2/17 surgical vs. 5/16 control pts developed MDE; 6/7 had past history of MDE). No relationship with laterality. No change HDRS, GDI, HARS. Following exclusionary analysis, improvement of trait anxiety but not state anxiety. No association with laterality.

mo, months; y, years; MOCI, Maudsley Obsessive Compulsive Inventory; BDI, Beck Depression Inventory; HDRS, Hamilton Depression Rating Scale; HARS, Hamilton Anxiety Rating Scale; BDI, Beck Depression Inventory; PVP, Posteroventral pallidotomy; DSM-IV, Diagnostic and Statistical Manual of Mental Disorders, Version IV; BAI, Beck Anxiety Inventory; PD, Parkinson's disease; GDI, Geriatric Depression Inventory; GPi, globus pallidus interna; FLOPS, Frontal Lobe Personality Scale; DBS, deep brain stimulation; SSAI/STAI, Speilberger State and Trait Anxiety Inventory.

TABLE 10-3. *Psychiatric symptoms in patients with Parkinson's disease following pallidal stimulation*

Study (Other studies of same cohort)	Study design	Number of patients	Symptom/Scale	Time of assessment after surgery	Conclusions and limitations of study
Ardouin, 1999 (46) [Pillon, 2000] (47)	Prospective comparison bilateral	STN: 49 GPi: 13	Depression BDI	3 to 6 mo	Improvement of BDI with bilateral STN and GPi stimulation.
Fields, 1999 (48)	Prospective uncontrolled bilateral	6	Depression BDI	3 mo	No change in BDI with bilateral GPi stimulation.
Krause, 2001 (49)	Prospective comparison bilateral	STN: 12 GPi: 6	Increased libido	Unknown	2/16 GPi and 1/12 STN developed increased libido. Unclear if mania ruled out.
Miyawaki, 2000 (50)	Case report bilateral	1	Mania		Case report: recurrent mania following Rt, Lt, and bilateral GPi stimulation.
Roane, 2002 (51)	Case report unilateral		Hypersexuality		Case report: Hypersexuality after Lt GPi stimulation with previous Rt PVP. However, hypersexuality in context of mixed manic symptoms.

(continues)

TABLE 10-3. *Continued*

Study (Other studies of same cohort)	Study design	Number of pts	Symptom/ Scale	Time of assessment after surgery	Conclusions and limitations of study
Troster, 1997 (52)	Prospective uncontrolled unilateral	9	Depression		No change in BDI after unilateral GPi stimulation.
			Anxiety		Improvement in BAI after unilateral GPi stimulation.
Volkmann, 2001 (8)	Prospective comparison bilateral	GPi: 11	BDI BAI Depression	6 and 12 mo	Bilateral STN (3/16) associated with more postoperative depression than bilateral GPi (0/11) (excluding dopaminergic withdrawal symptoms: 6/18 in STN).
		STN: 16	Anxiety HDRS STAI		Improvement in HDRS following bilateral GPi and STN stimulation.
Vingerhoets, 1999 (52)	Prospective uncontrolled unilateral	20	Depression BDI	3 mo	No change in BDI with unilateral GPi stimulation (excluding items secondary to parkinsonism).

STN, subthalamic nucleus; GPi, globus pallidus interna; BDI, Beck Depression Inventory; mo, months; Rt, right; Lt, left; BAI, Beck Anxiety Inventory; HDRS, Hamilton Depression Rating Scale; STAI, Speilberger Trait Anxiety Inventory.

PSYCHIATRIC SYMPTOMS FOLLOWING SUBTHALAMIC STIMULATION

Depression

Depression is the most commonly reported psychiatric symptom following STN stimulation and has thus received the most study. Prospective studies have reported postoperative depression rates of 1.5% to 25% (4,5,8,53–58). Two of these studies, designed specifically to examine postoperative psychiatric symptoms using diagnostic criteria, reported rates of 21% and 25%, with onset primarily within the first two postoperative months (5,54). A third study that distinguished between patients with depression who required antidepressants and patients with "transient depression" secondary to changes in dopaminergic medications reported rates of 18% and 38%, respectively (8). In a 5-year prospective study by Krack et al., only one of 49 patients (2%) was depressed within the first 3 postoperative months, with seven of 49 patients (17%) developing transient depressive episodes in the long term (53). These rates vary across sites for a variety of reasons: differences in the inclusion criteria of patients with preoperative psychiatric vulnerabilities, group versus individual differences, differences in measurement scales, and the involvement of psychiatric assessments.

The pallidotomy literature can provide some insights into the methodologic issues in the STN stimulation literature (Table 10-1). For instance, despite uncontrolled studies that suggest an elevated incidence of postoperative depression, no evidence was seen in studies using a wait-list control group that unilateral pallidotomy increased the individual risk of developing postoperative depression (45,58). The greatest risk associated with the development of postoperative depression in both the unilateral pallidotomy and the wait-list control groups was a prior history of depression (44,45).

A range of etiologies for postoperative depression has been suggested, including preoperative vulnerabilities (5), dopaminergic medication changes (7,8), psychosocial changes (5,9), and stimulation effects (16,59).

Depression Etiology: the Natural Course of Depression

Depression is found in as many as 40% to 50% of all patients with PD and has been extensively reviewed in the literature (60). In one retrospective study, the incidence rate of depression in patients with PD was reported to be 1.86% per year, suggesting that the natural course of depression in patients with PD is insufficient to account for the incidence rates of postoperative depression (61).

Depression Etiology: Preoperative Vulnerabilities

Houeto et al. examined the role of preoperative vulnerabilities in a retrospective review (5). Five of 24 patients with PD (21%) developed depression within the first 2 months following STN stimulation surgery. Four of the five patients who developed postoperative depression had a history of preoperative depression. Further examination revealed that 12 of the 24 patients (50%) had a history of preoperative depression; however, 8 of these 12 patients (66%) who had preoperative depression did not develop postoperative depression. This finding suggests that a history of preoperative depression may act as a risk factor, rather than a necessary outcome.

In contrast to this finding, in a well-designed prospective study that focused on risk factors for depressive symptoms in patients with PD who underwent STN DBS, Berney et al. reported that a personal history of depression, a family psychiatric history, and a preoperative depression score did not differ between the postoperatively depressed (25%) and nondepressed groups (54). These authors concluded that the postoperative depression could be a result of the surgery, stimulation, an unrecognized vulnerability, or other potential psychological mood changes, such as adaptation to sudden improvements in disability.

Depression Etiology: Dopaminergic Medication Withdrawal

The reduction of dopaminergic medications following STN stimulation has been associated with depressive symptoms (7,8). Volkmann et al. described a "transient depressive state" in 6 of 16 patients (38%) resulting from decreases in dopaminergic medications (8). The "transient depressive state" resolved in the six patients after dopaminergic medications were increased. An additional 3 of 16 patients (19%) developed depression that required antidepressant intervention. The criteria for both "transient depressive state" and depression were not defined.

The affective and behavioral effects of levodopa abuse have been compared to psychostimulant abuse; because these drugs increase catecholaminergic activity, similar underlying neural substrates may be involved (62–64). D2 receptor antagonists and lesions selectively applied to dopaminergic neurons projecting to the nucleus accumbens from the ventral tegmental area result in a decrease in reinforcing properties of psychostimulants in animal studies. These dopaminergic mesolimbic projections are implicated in the reinforcement leading to abuse (15,65). The nucleus accumbens is postulated to be crucial to the positive reinforcing effects of all drugs of abuse (15,65).

Postoperative "depression" or dysphoria can be partly attributed to a withdrawal symptom caused by the decrease in dopaminergic medications. The diagnostic criteria for withdrawal syndromes following chronic psychostimulant abuse are characterized by dysphoria and anhedonia and at least two additional symptoms of vivid, unpleasant dreams, insomnia or hypersomnia, increased appetite, or psychomotor retardation or agitation (65).

Depression Etiology: Stimulation-Related Symptoms

Reports of depressive states with onset time-locked to stimulation are rare, but such reports help delineate a direct association with stimulation. Bejjani et al. reported a woman with PD with no known premorbid psychiatric history who developed a profound depressive state fulfilling *Diagnostic and Statistical Manual of Mental Disorders,* 4th edition (DSM-IV) criteria with stimulation of the contact located within the left central substantia nigra (SN) pars reticulata (16). Functional neuroimaging demonstrated a substantial increase in blood flow in the left orbitofrontal cortex, globus pallidus, amygdala, anterior thalamus, and right parietal lobe, associated with the experience of acute sadness. The authors suggest that the depression was secondary to either excitation or inhibition of fibers within the SN or by stimulation of nigrothalamic neurons with subsequent projections to the prefrontal cortex and amygdala.

Stefurak et al. reported on a woman with PD and a premorbid history of recurrent depression who developed an acute depressive state with stimulation of the contact located within the right zona incerta and fields of Forel (59). The depressive state was characterized by symptoms of subjective apathy, dysphoria, anhedonia, and blunted affect, which resolved immediately when the stimulation was stopped. Functional MRI demonstrated right-sided BOLD signal increases in the superior prefrontal cortex, anterior cingulate, anterior thalamus, caudate, and brainstem, and decreases in medial prefrontal cortex. These increases were similar to positron emission tomography (PET) changes seen in mood-induction paradigms in subjects with remitted depression. These authors suggest that afferent or efferent connections adjacent to the STN within the zona incerta and fields of Forel, including reciprocal connections to the SN or to the PPN (pedunculopontine nucleus) nuclei, may have been involved.

Doshi et al. reported on 2 of 31 patients who experienced an acute transient depressive state, marked by easy tearfulness with provocation, that was associated with changes in stimulation contacts (66). The depressive states were described as qualitatively different from the patients' premorbid histories of depression. Unfortunately, the anatomic localization of the contacts was not confirmed in the paper.

Kumar et al. reported a similar patient who developed acute sadness secondary to a unilateral increase in stimulation parameters at a previously therapeutic contact (67). Again, anatomic localization was not provided in the paper; however, the therapeutic motor efficacy of the contact suggests localization within the STN.

Immediate mood changes following randomized changes in stimulation contacts in patients who underwent unilateral STN and GPi were recently studied by Okun et al., using a Visual Analogue Mood Scale (68). Stimulation at optimally placed contacts was associated with greater improvement of mood in both STN and GPi stimulation, compared with no stimulation. Stimulation in contacts dorsal and ventral to the optimal contact was associated with slightly greater worsening of mood symptoms for the STN group than for the GPi group. The authors suggest that changes in mood and cognition may more likely be associated with STN stimulation than with GPi, given differences in the sizes of the nuclei, and thus greater propensity for current spread to the nonmotor regions of the STN and the adjacent fiber pathways.

The cases differ with respect to the phenomenologic descriptions of the depressive states. Preliminary observations suggest that stimulation of the STN (although definitive localization was not established in the reports), if associated with decreases in mood, results in sadness or easy tearfulness that may be qualitatively different from a major depressive episode. Stimulation of limbic areas outside the STN, such as the SN, the zona incerta, or the fields of Forel, may be more closely associated with the cognitive, affective, and behavioral states of major depression. These findings are in keeping with the report by Okun et al. that differentiates between acute mood symptoms with stimulation of optimal contacts symptoms associated with stimulation dorsal or ventral to the optimal contact (68). Clearly, additional well-described and carefully evaluated cases are required to refine these initial postulates.

These case reports suggest the role of stimulation in inducing acute changes in mood, although no evidence demonstrates that these acute symptoms persist. Notably, three of these five cases with acute stimulation-induced depressive symptoms had a premorbid history of depression, which suggests an interaction between an underlying vulnerability and the site of stimulation (59,66).

Mania and Other Symptoms of Mood Elevation

In Krack et al.'s 5-year prospective study of 49 STN DBS patients, 5 (10%) developed postoperative hypomania within the first 3 postoperative months (53). Incidence rates reported in the literature of either postoperative hypomanic or manic symptoms range from 6% to 15% (4,5,69).

Both euphoria and the improvement of depression scores have been conceptually linked with the continuum of postoperative symptoms characterized by mood elevation (14,70). Euphoria is a common transient state noted in 75% of post STN stimulation patients (5). A feeling of well being is reported after surgery (71). Multiple prospective studies following STN DBS surgery have reported statistically significant improvements in mean depression scores at 3 and 12 months after surgery, compared with preoperative scores (8,46,47,55,72). However, the studies do not differentiate between the items in the depression scales, which may be etiologically related to improvement of motor symptoms. These methodologic issues are relevant in the pallidotomy literature (Table 10-1). For instance, in comparison to uncontrolled studies, two well-designed studies that used wait-list controls did not document any changes in depression scores following unilateral pallidotomy (38,44,45). Furthermore, one of the studies documented an improvement in "inclusive" (those that included all positive items, regardless of etiology) but not "etiologic" (those that excluded items more likely related to PD than to depression) scores on a depression rating scale, a finding that suggests that the improvement was related to improvement in motor functioning following pallidotomy (44,45).

The etiology of hypomania and mania has been postulated to be related to surgical insertional effects (69), stimulation (69,70), synergy between dopaminergic medications and stimulation (14,69), underlying vulnerabilities (73), and psychological "reactivity."

Hypomania Etiology: Surgical and Stimulation Effects

Romito et al. reported the onset of hypomania in one patient preceding the onset of STN stimulation, suggesting that electrode insertion plays an etiologic role that results in localized edema or microlesioning affecting the STN-limbic region (69).

The demonstration of acute symptoms time-locked to stimulation enables insight into the role of stimulation in the pathophysiology of chronic mood symptoms. A relationship has been hypothesized between symptoms characterized by mood elevation, including acute mirthful laughter, and the mood-enhancing effects of stimulation, with intermediate symptoms of euphoria, hypomania, and mania, and long-term improvements in depression rating scores (14,70). Krack et al. first proposed that chronic stimulation of the STN and limbic system, particularly that portion involving the lateral hypothalamus and ventral tegmental area (VTA), could play a role in euphoria and hypomania, separate and distinct from their shared correlation with psychological "reactivity." The authors describe two PD patients in whom high stimulation parameters of previous therapeutically beneficial contacts located within the STN resulted in acute mirthful laughter (70).

Herzog et al. described a patient whose manic symptoms, temporally linked to STN stimulation, did not improve when the stimulation was stopped, whereas the parkinsonian symptoms worsened. This observation supports a dissociation between motor and limbic circuits (73). Decreases in stimulation resulted in the rapid appearance of a mixed affective picture with concurrent anhedonic symptoms and unabated manic symptoms, suggesting that the postoperative manic and depressive symptoms had different underlying pathophysiologies.

Stimulation of the limbic system outside the STN has also been associated with manic symptoms. Kulisevsky et al. reported manic symptoms developing in three patients with bilateral stimulation of contacts within the midbrain caudal to the SN (40). Proposed etiologies include dopamine release from the VTA projections, midbrain projections to the orbitofrontal cortex (OFC), anterior cingulate, or other nondopaminergic nuclei.

Finally, with respect to laterality, case reports revealed one patient with manic symptoms and one with mirthful laughter associated with right-sided stimulation. Although limited conclusions can be drawn from a single case, this finding is in keeping with the literature on the association of manic symptoms with right hemispheric lesions (74).

Hypomania Etiology: Synergy with Dopaminergic Medication

A synergistic effect of stimulation and dopaminergic medications has been suggested on the basis of observations that mania has improved either with a decrease in stimulation or with a decrease in dopaminergic medications (14,69). Mania, hypomania, and euphoria have all been associated with dopaminergic medications. Funkiewiez et al. demonstrated parallels between the mood-enhancing effects of levodopa and those of STN stimulation (62). Using systematic questionnaires, the authors investigated the perception of euphoria, motivation, fatigue, anxiety, and tension. Patients both in the on-stimulation state and those taking levodopa perceived a greater improvement of these features than the groups of patients in the off-stimulation state and those not taking levodopa. Funkiewiez et al. postulated that the mood-elevating properties of both STN stimulation and levodopa, given their similarities, might be mediated by the STN-limbic system.

The mechanism of the synergy between stimulation effects and dopaminergic medications has not yet been determined. On the basis of two studies that used [^{11}C] raclopride PET imaging, the release of endogenous dopamine from the nigrostriatal system does not mediate the motor effects of STN stimulation (75,76). Similar studies may be useful to clarify the role of the dopaminergic VTA projections in the psychiatric symptoms associated with STN stimulation.

Hypomania Etiology: Psychological "Reactivity"

Euphoria and the overall improvements in depression rating scores have been conceptually linked within the continuum of postoperative symptoms characterized by mood elevation. Biological factors have been postulated to play an etiological role separate from the role of psychological "reactivity" (14,70). However, the fact that euphoria is common in the postoperative period in patients who have undergone organ transplant surgery, independent of corticosteroid use, suggests that this symptom may be more related to psychological "reactive" improvements in mood, in response to dramatic functional changes, than to a biological etiology (77).

Hypomania Etiology: Premorbid Vulnerabilities

In case reports, some patients who exhibited manic symptoms had either an individual history of premorbid depression or emotional lability, or a family history of bipolar disorder, suggesting the potential role of premorbid vulnerability (69,70,73). However, the underlying association is not clear, given the nature of these studies as case reports.

Visual Hallucinations

Visual hallucinations were not reported in the first 3 postoperative months in Krack et al.'s 5-year follow-up study of 49 patients who underwent STN stimulation, although the extent of systematic assessment was not reported (53). Hallucinations developed in 5 of the 49 patients (10%) during long-term follow up, 3 of whom had persistent cognitive deficits. Herzog et al. reported that three of 48 patients (6%) developed visual hallucinations or psychotic symptoms, although the temporal association with surgery or stimulation was not clear (4). Onset of hallucination, which was either time-locked to stimulation or which occured within the first 3 postoperative months, reflects stimulation or medication effects, whereas onset after the first 3 postoperative months is more likely to be related to the disease process itself or to the eventual increases in dopaminergic medications.

Diederich et al. reported the new onset of visual hallucinations (VH) in a patient with PD after STN DBS (78); the hallucinations responded to discontinuation of levodopa. Three years later, with a third electrode inserted within the zona incerta, VH recurred time-locked with stimulation in that patient. The patient responded to clozapine, allowing stimulation to continue. The phenomenology of the stimulation-induced VH was identical to that of VH in PD, suggesting similarities in pathophysiology. Potential etiologies include activation of the medial limbic-STN or activation of projections to the VTA-mesolimbic system. Activation of the ascending serotonergic fibers crossing the zona incerta could have caused increased serotonergic activity, which some researchers have suggested is related to VH. Inhibition of these fibers could also have altered the dopamine-serotonin balance, resulting in a relative increase in dopaminergic activity.

Alternatively, the cortico-striato-thalamo-cortical loop involving Area TE of the inferotemporal cortex has been proposed by Middleton and Strick to play a pathophysiologic role in the visual hallucinations in patients with PD (22). STN stimulation affecting this circuit could potentially mediate the visual hallucinations.

PREOPERATIVE ASSESSMENT

The assessment for psychiatric risk should be individualized and is multifactorial in nature. The following recommendations are made on the basis of clinical experience; the literature is insufficient to guide the management of these patients. Nonmotor factors to be considered in assessing risk include the severity of the preoperative psychiatric symptoms (hospitalization, need for or response to treatment, insight, behavioral disturbances, self-harm behavior), adequacy of current psychiatric interventions (untreated, partially treated, or remitted), family psychiatric history, age, cognitive reserves, adherence to follow-up and medications, coping skills, expectations, and adequacy of social supports. The adequacy of long-term follow up and access to psychiatric resources should be considered, particularly for those considered to be at elevated psychiatric risk.

Psychosocial factors play a role in a multifactorial risk assessment. Parallels can be drawn from the literature on epilepsy, a chronic disease with a similar dramatic postsurgical outcome. However, the onset of epilepsy and the subsequent surgery occur at a much earlier age, thus presenting a differing set of psychosocial difficulties. Factors that predict a good QOL and positive surgical outcomes following surgery for epilepsy include good psychological adjustment, good self-perceived QOL, low neuroticism (trait anxiety), learned resourcefulness (taking active responsibility for one's circumstances), and having adequate social supports (79). Factors associated with poor outcome include substantial psychological distress, high neuroticism, low learned resourcefulness, unrealistic expectations, and poor interpersonal interactions with the physician (79). These factors could potentially play a role in the outcome following surgery for PD and would benefit from being studied in a prospective manner in patients with PD.

Given the high comorbidity of psychiatric disorders in the general population of patients with PD, a preoperative assessment enables the clinician to identify those patients who are at elevated postoperative psychiatric risk. Psychiatric management before surgery, psychoeducation of the patient and caregiver, and close psychiatric follow-up to facilitate early intervention may modify the psychiatric risk. Areas to be assessed include mood, psychotic symptoms, anxiety, levodopa abuse, and suicidal ideation.

Absolute Contraindications

Absolute or nonmodifiable psychiatric contraindications to STN stimulation surgery include diagnoses of primary psychiatric disorders, including psychotic disorders, unremitting substance dependence, treatment-refractory bipolar disorder, and treatment-refractory depression. These primary psychiatric disorders should be distinguished from medication-induced symptoms. Severe personality disorders with a demonstrated history of adherence difficulties can be considered an absolute contraindication. No literature is available on patients with such comorbid disorders undergoing STN DBS surgery. However, given the potential postoperative psychiatric complications and the intensive nature of the procedure and subsequent follow up, the patient's ability to tolerate the procedure and subsequent adherence would likely be impaired.

Preoperative Depression

The prevalence of depression in the general population of patients with PD is reported to be 40% to 50% (80). The only psychiatric contraindication in the Core Assessment Program for Surgical Intervention Therapies in Parkinson's Disease (CAPSIT-PD) criteria is the presence of current depression of moderate severity with a Montgomery Asberg Depression Rating Scale (MADRS) score of greater than 19 (81). Several issues arise in interpreting this criterion.

First, psychiatric rating scales document a cross-sectional measure of depression severity in a disorder known to be episodic and fluctuating in nature. As we have mentioned, psychiatric assessment should be multifactorial and should address further qualifying information. For instance, a patient with moderate untreated depression differs considerably from one with a history of depression with multiple psychiatric admissions and poor support.

Second, the selection of depression rating scales has not been adequately studied in these patients. The CAPSIT-PD uses the clinician-rated MADRS. Several other studies have used the clinician-rated Hamilton Depression Rating Scale (HDRS) and the patient-rated Beck Depression Inventory (BDI), Geriatric Depression Inventory (GDI), and Zung Depression Rating Scale. The MADRS, HDRS and BDI have been validated in patients with PD (82). Screening and diagnostic cutoffs have been noted to differ from that of the general population (82,83). The reliability of patient-rated instruments in the context of patients who may be concerned about exclusion from surgery for psychiatric reasons may also be an issue.

Whether a preoperative history of depression is a risk factor for postoperative depression is not clear from the literature; at the very least, it has been shown to be insufficient on its own to predict a postoperative depression (5,54). Given the heterogeneity of preoperative depression, the literature is not sufficiently refined to determine whether severity, adequacy of preoperative psychiatric interventions (untreated, partially treated or remitted), or a potential interaction of this vulnerability with the site of stimulation or dopaminergic medication withdrawal may play a role in etiology.

Psychiatric symptoms are potentially treatable and reversible during both the preoperative and postoperative period. The presence of moderate or severe depression should be treated before surgery. Whether effective treatment of preoperative depression changes the postoperative risk is not known. On the basis of clinical experience, the risks with treated depression or prophylaxis for depression may be lower, although further trials are necessary to support this observation. Actively managing preoperative depression, identifying patients who require particularly close psychiatric follow up, suggesting a gradual decrease in dopaminergic medications to prevent withdrawal syndromes, and providing psychoeducation for the patient and family may further ameliorate the risk.

Preoperative Medication-Induced Mania or Visual Hallucinations

The prevalence of medication-induced mania in the general population of patients with PD has been reported at 1.5% (84), and that of medication-induced hallucinations reaches 25% to 30% (84). These symptoms can limit optimal dosing of dopaminergic medications, whereas subthalamic stimulation can potentially enable a considerable reduction in levodopa dosage equivalents (3). However, patients with a history of preoperative medication-induced hypomania or mania are theoretically at greater risk of short-term postoperative hypomania, given their underlying vulnerabilities and the synergistic effects observed between STN stimulation and dopaminergic medications. Whether patients with a premorbid history of medication-induced mania or hallucinations are reasonable candidates for surgery is a question that has not yet been answered. The outcomes for these patients have not been reported in the literature.

We have had experience with two patients who had histories of medication-induced mania of moderate severity that lasted longer than a year. Following psychiatric stabilization, STN stimulation surgery and decreases in their dopaminergic medications resulted in substantial improvements in motor functioning and QOL. One patient had postoperative manic symptoms that were reversible with decreased stimulation parameters.

A careful assessment is necessary to distinguish between primary disorders and medication-induced disorders. Primary disorders may be a relative contraindication for surgery, whereas medication-induced disorders may be a supportive indication for surgery, pending further studies (85).

Preoperative hypomanic or manic symptoms and hallucinations should be actively treated before surgery. Although the literature contains no data to support this recommendation, minimizing any intraoperative or early postoperative exacerbation of symptoms would be prudent.

POSTOPERATIVE MANAGEMENT

Depression

A robust association between depression and QOL scores has been demonstrated in the PD literature (86). Similarly, the improvement in QOL scores 3 months after STN stimulation surgery was found to have a greater association with improvements in depression scores than with improvements in motor scores (87). These findings indirectly suggest that postoperative depression should be actively identified and treated. The following discussion is based on expert opinion and clinical experience, because the literature on postoperative depression is otherwise very limited.

As we have explained, the dopaminergic medication withdrawal syndrome may overlap considerably with psychostimulant withdrawal. The symptoms of psychostimulant withdrawal can be difficult to distinguish from depression. From the psychiatric literature on psychostimulant withdrawal and depression, the following points can be concluded.

Postoperative withdrawal dysphoria caused by changes in dopaminergic medication could potentially be distinguished from a major depressive episode by its temporal onset in relation to the medication change, the response to increasing dopaminergic medications, or the expected natural course of gradual improvement over weeks (65). Symptoms lasting longer than 3 weeks following changes in dopaminergic medications suggest an underlying primary depression. The symptoms may overlap with those of a major depressive episode, exacerbating or unmasking a depressive episode in patients with underlying vulnerabilities (65). In such potentially predisposed individuals, a gradual reduction in dopaminergic medication dosages may prevent withdrawal syndromes. Severe symptoms, suicidal ideation, and a premorbid history of depression may justify early referrals for psychiatric management.

The current clinical management of depressive symptoms is in keeping with the psychiatric literature on psychostimulant withdrawal and depression. Volkmann et al. described the "transient depressive state" resolving in 6 of 16 patients after dopaminergic medication dosages were increased, with an additional three patients requiring antidepressant intervention (who presumably did not respond to changes in their dopaminergic doses) (8).

Following an increase in levodopa dose, should a dopamine agonist be required, pramipexole may exert additional antidepressant effects, as demonstrated in a recent randomized pramipexole, pergolide, and placebo-controlled study on depression in PD (88). Antidepressants can be considered in patients who have not responded to changes in dopaminergic medications.

Psychotherapy should address any specific identity issues, relationship issues, or losses that may arise, and adequate support should be provided.

Mania or Hallucinations

Hypomanic symptoms occur primarily during the first 3 postoperative months, and most episodes are time limited (53,69). Psychoeducation of patients and particularly of caregivers, given the often limited insight into symptoms, is essential for early identification and intervention. Because the symptoms are transient, the need for treatment depends on the severity of symptoms and the adequacy of support and follow up. The potential risk of harm to self or others, risk-taking behaviors (driving, spending, gambling, sexual activity), and caregiver burden should be assessed. On the basis of expert opinion, first-line treatment options, in conjunction with managing motor symptoms, include decreasing dopaminergic medication dosage or changing stimulation parameters (7,69) and discontinuing medications, such as antidepressants, that may be contributing to the induction of mania. Should this intervention be insufficient, either an atypical antipsychotic (quetiapine or clozapine) or a mood stabilizer, such as valproic acid, might be added; both have been used in managing medication-induced mania in patients with PD (84). Carbamezapine and clozapine have been reported to be useful in the management of one patient with manic and psychotic symptoms following STN stimulation (73).

The use of clozapine or a change in stimulation parameters has been reported to be effective in treating postoperative visual hallucinations (73,78).

Apathy

Apathy, a syndrome defined as a lack of interest, emotion, and motivation, has been reported in the postoperative period (7,53). Apathy can occur during the early postoperative period, secondary to dopaminergic withdrawal, and responds to increases in dopaminergic treatment (7,53). The etiology of postoperative apathy is in part mediated by postoperative decreases in dopaminergic medications but may also be intrinsic to the underlying effects of PD. Krack et al. report the prevalence of long-term apathy in 42 patients during the third postoperative year to be 12% (5 patients); in this study, apathy paralleled a decrease in frontal cognitive function (53).

The prevalence of apathy in the general population of patients with PD has been reported to be between 16.5% to 42% (89,90). Apathy, understood as a distinct clinical syndrome, also has conceptual and clinical overlaps with depression, hedonic tone, personality traits, and cognitive function. In the patients with PD, apathy has been reported to be most prominently associated with cognitive and, particularly, executive dysfunction, rather than with depressive symptoms (89).

The assessment of apathy should include caregiver assessments, because insight with respect to this symptom is often poor. We have had the experience of improvement in postoperative long-term apathy in one patient following antidepressant management of subsyndromal depression (depression that does not fulfill diagnostic criteria) and in another with cholinesterase inhibitors in the context of dementia. The caregiver should be educated regarding the causes of and limitations imposed by this behavioral symptom.

Levodopa Use for Nonmotor Effects

The ongoing use of levodopa for its subjective euphorigenic effects, rather than its motor effects, has been reported in the postoperative period (7). Two of 24 patients reported in the retrospective study by Houeto et al. developed postoperative levodopa-addictive behaviors, both of whom had preoperative histories of such behaviors (5). Potential vulnerabilities include patients with a history of hedonistic homeostatic dysregulation as described by Giovannoni et al. (addiction, novelty-seeking behaviors, hypomania) (5,63) or a predisposition to addiction (63).

Anxiety

Generalized anxiety disorder (GAD) was diagnosed retrospectively in 18 of 24 patients with PD (75%) following STN DBS, 17 of whom had a preoperative history of GAD. Ten patients (42%) had a specific fear that the stimulator would suddenly fail (5). The DSM-IV criteria for GAD has limited interrater reliability, and the extent to which these symptoms overlap with those of other comorbid psychiatric disorders is not known. However, overall group anxiety rating scores have been reported in some studies to significantly improve on anxiety measurements (56,72), although specificity of the symptoms was not reported.

The symptom of fear that the stimulator will fail may respond to interventions for anxiety or phobias. The duration of this specific symptom is not known; it may respond to time, cognitive-behavioral interventions, or both. We have also had the experience that this phobic symptom resolved with antidepressant therapy in two patients with mild comorbid depression, one in the first 3 postoperative months, and the second 2 years following surgery.

Emotional Reactivity

Emotional reactivity, defined as excessive mood-congruent emotional responses to minor triggers, was identified in 75% of patients who underwent STN stimulation (5). The symptom can also be seen in comorbid states, such as depression or anxiety, and its prevalence in the general PD population is not known.

Schneider et al. studied emotional processing during STN stimulation, using a mood-induction paradigm of exposure to slides with differing facial expressions (71). Consistent with the observation of increased emotional reactivity, the on-stimulation state was associated with better emotional experience and recall of emotionally valenced memory (in immediate but not delayed recall) than the off-stimulation state was.

Suicidal Ideation

A multicenter retrospective study of completed and attempted suicides was recently initiated by our center. A total of 16 centers worldwide were surveyed, with a 50% response rate and a reported total of 406 patients who had undergone surgery. Two completed suicides (0.5%, 3 months, and 3 years after surgery) and seven suicide attempts (1.7%, average 11.4 months after surgery) occurred. Three patients attempted suicide within the first 2 postoperative months, and four patients attempted suicide 6 to 24 months after surgery. Four patients who attempted suicide used means associated with high lethality. The literature revealed an additional two completed suicides among 73 STN DBS patients (2.7%) (5,53) from centers not included within this survey and an additional four of 80 patients (5.0%) who attempted suicide between 3 months and 5 years after surgery (53,66).

These results are in contrast to the low baseline rates of completed suicides in the general population of patients with PD, despite the fact that PD is a progressive medical illness with a considerable health burden, which is highly comorbid with depression and anxiety. The rate of completed suicides in elderly patients with PD has been recently reported to be 10 times lower than that in the general population (one-year incidence rates of 0.016% and 0.16%, respectively, controlled for age and gender) (91). However, the risk of suicide in the young PD population with advanced disease presenting for surgery is likely higher than this baseline.

Patients should be carefully assessed for any premorbid history of suicidal ideation or attempts. Patients and caregivers should be forewarned about potential psychiatric complications, including suicidal ideation, with emphasis placed on the importance of adequate monitoring and communication and on the reversibility of the symptoms with active management. Patients with postoperative suicidal ideation should be referred for psychiatric management.

Social Outcome

Clinically relevant outcomes include factors such as QOL, functioning, and social outcomes. In a retrospective short-term study that used the Social Adjustment Scale, late age of onset was associated with poor global social adjustment (5). Poor adjustment in social life, leisure, and social adaptation was associated with persistence of levodopa-induced motor symptoms. Despite motor improvements, marital relations of 25% of patients deteriorated, an effect hypothesized to be related to changes in autonomy and roles (5). Individual or couples therapy may be necessary to address such issues.

In attempting to understand these relationship impairments from a social-cognition perspective, two recent intriguing studies found postoperative impairments in nonverbal emotional processing, documented as a selective decrease in the ability to recognize or decode negative facial expressions, such as anger or sadness (92,93). The authors postulate that these observed deficits in the recognition of social cues may be related to downstream effects from STN stimulation on the medial prefrontal cortex.

Obsessive–Compulsive Symptoms

STN stimulation localized within the anteromedial STN and zona incerta has been associated with the improvement of comorbid obsessive–compulsive disorder in two patients with PD (80). The implications of this report have been extensively discussed elsewhere (94). Obsessive–compulsive symptom scores as measured on the Maudsley Obsessive Compulsive Inventory scale have been reported to improve in patients with PD following STN stimulation (95). However, depression scores were not reported, which represents a potential confounder.

Cognitive Symptoms

The literature on the effect of STN stimulation on cognitive symptoms has been more extensively studied and reviewed elsewhere and will be summarized here (for reviews, see Woods et al.) (96). Most studies documented minimal, transient, or no postoperative cognitive effects. A decline in verbal fluency following STN stimulation has been the most consistently documented finding (6,19,22). Several studies have shown postoperative improvements in measures of information processing speed and working memory (46,47,97). The effect of STN stimulation on cognitive function has been postulated to be related to stimulation affecting the nonmotor cognitive loops.

Some evidence exists that patients with either preexisting cognitive deficits or dementia (6,98) and patients older than 69 at the time of surgery (6) could have postoperative worsening of cognitive outcomes. These subsets of patients were considered at risk because of the vulnerability of their underlying limited cognitive reserves. Despite limitations in the evidence, a pragmatic approach supports preexisting dementia as a contraindication for STN.

In the five-year prospective study by Krack et al., dementia developed in 6% of the patients in long-term follow up, a finding that the authors suggest reflects the underlying disease process (7). Dementia is a common late complication of PD, reported in approximately 40% of patients, with a recent study documenting an 8-year prevalence rate of 78% in older patients with PD (mean age 72 years) (10b). As in the general population of patients with PD, the appearance of behavioral symptoms of apathy and hallucinations paralleled the cognitive decline in the postoperative population (7).

Given the likely underlying relationship of postoperative dementia to the process of neurodegeneration in patients with PD, the literature on dementia in PD and on cholinesterase inhibitors can be used to guide management of postoperative dementia. Aside from medications, a multidisciplinary approach should be used to manage dementia.

SUMMARY

Bilateral subthalamic stimulation is a very effective neurosurgical treatment for advanced Parkinson's disease. Despite the range and frequency of psychiatric symptoms occurring in the postoperative state, most of these symptoms are transient and manageable. In clinical practice, preoperative psychiatric vulnerability, as with that of preoperative cognitive status, takes on an important role. Psychiatric assessment and active preoperative and postoperative intervention can potentially modify psychiatric outcomes. These psychiatric and psychological issues will take on greater importance, particularly with the rapid expansion of the number of neurosurgical sites and the need for adequate assessment and optimal management of patients. The paucity of the literature underscores the need for well-designed studies on psychiatric issues investigating both pathophysiology and clinical outcomes.

REFERENCES

1. Limousin P, Pollak P, Benazzouz A, et al. Effect on parkinsonian signs and symptoms of bilateral subthalamic nucleus stimulation. *Lancet* 1995;345:91–95.
2. The Deep-Brain Stimulation for Parkinson's Disease Study Group. Deep-brain stimulation of the subthalamic nucleus or the pars interna of the globus pallidus in Parkinson's disease. *N Engl J Med* 2001;345:956–963.

3. Moro E, Scerrati M, Romito LM, et al. Chronic subthalamic nucleus stimulation reduces medication requirements in Parkinson's disease. *Neurology* 1999;53:85–90.
4. Herzog J, Volkmann J, Krack P, et al. Two-year follow up of subthalamic deep brain stimulation in Parkinson's disease. *Mov Disord* 2003;18:1332–1337.
5. Houeto JL, Mesnage V, Mallet L, et al. Behavioral disorders, Parkinson's disease and subthalamic stimulation. *J Neurol Neurosurg Psychiatry* 2002;72:701–705.
6. Saint-Cyr JA, Trepanier LL, Kumar R, et al. Neuropsychological consequences of chronic bilateral stimulation of the subthalamic nucleus in Parkinson's disease. *Brain* 2000;123:2091–2108.
7. Krack P, Fraix V, Mendes A, et al. Postoperative management of subthalamic nucleus stimulation for Parkinson's disease. *Mov Disord* 2002;17(Suppl. 3): S188–S197.
8. Volkmann J, Allert N, Voges J, et al. Safety and efficacy of pallidal or subthalamic nucleus stimulation in advanced PD. *Neurology* 2001;56:548–551.
9. Brown RG. Behavioral disorders, Parkinson's disease and subthalamic stimulation. [Letter to editor] *J Neurol Neurosurg Psychiatry* 2002;72:689.
10a. Alexander GE, DeLong MR, Strick PL. Parallel organization of functionally segregated circuits linking basal ganglia and cortex. *Annu Rev Neurobiol* 1986;9: 357–381.
10b. Aarsland D, Andersen K, Larsen JP, et al. Prevalence and characteristics of dementia in Parkinson disease: an 8-year prospective study. *Arch Neurol* 2003;60:387–392.
11. Parent A, Hazrati LN. Functional anatomy of the basal ganglia. II. The place of the subthalamic nucleus and external pallidum in basal ganglia circuitry. *Brain Res Rev* 1995;20:128–154.
12. Hilker R, Voges J, Weisenbach S, et al. Subthalamic nucleus stimulation restores glucose metabolism in associative and limbic cortices and in cerebellum: evidence from a FDG-PET study in advanced Parkinson's disease. *J Cereb Blood Flow Metab* 2004;24:7–16.
13. Groenewegen HJ, Berendse HW. Connections of the subthalamic nucleus with ventral striatopallidal parts of the basal ganglia in the rat. *J Comp Neurol* 1990; 294:607–622.
14. Krack P, Ardouin C, Funkiewiez A, et al. What is the influence of STN stimulation on the limbic loop? In: Kultas-Ilinsky K, Ilinsky IA, eds. *Basal ganglia and thalamus in health and movement disorders*. New York: Kluwer Academic/Plenum Publishers, 2001.
15. Koob GF, Nestler EJ. The neurobiology of drug addiction. In: Salloway S, Malloy P, Cummings JL, eds. *The neuropsychiatry of limbic and subcortical disorders*. Washington, DC: American Psychiatric Press, 1997.
16. Bejjani BP, Damier P, Arnulf I, et al. Transient acute depression induced by high-frequency deep brain stimulation. *N Engl J Med* 1999;340:1476–1480.
17. Orieux G, Francois C, Feger J, et al. Metabolic activity of excitatory parafascicular and pedunculopontine inputs to the subthalamic nucleus in a rat model of Parkinson's disease. *Neuroscience* 2000;97:79–88.
18. Nader K, van der Kooy D. Deprivation state switches the neurobiological substrates mediating opiate reward in the ventral tegmental area. *J Neurosci* 1997;17:383–390.
19. Laviolette SR, Alexson TO, van der Kooy D. Lesions of the tegmental pedunculopontine nucleus block the rewarding effects and reveal the aversive effects of nicotine in the ventral tegmental area. *J Neurosci* 2002;22:8653–8660.
20. Orieux G, Francois C, Feger J, et al. Consequences of dopaminergic denervation on the metabolic activity of the cortical neurons projecting to the subthalamic nucleus in the rat. *J Neurosci* 2002;22:8762–8770.
21. Maurice N, Deniau JM, Menetrey A, et al. Prefrontal cortex-basal ganglia circuits in the rat: involvement of ventral pallidum and subthalamic nucleus. *Synapse* 1998;29:363–370.
22. Middleton FA, Strick PL. The temporal lobe is a target of output from the basal ganglia. *Proc Natl Acad Sci* 1996;93:8683–8687.
23. Ashby P, Kim YJ, Kumar R, et al. Neurophysiological effects of stimulation through electrodes in the human subthalamic nucleus. *Brain* 1999;122:1919–1931.
24. Voges J, Volkmann J, Allert N, et al. Bilateral high-frequency stimulation in the subthalamic nucleus for the treatment of Parkinson's disease: correlation of therapeutic effect with anatomical electrode position. *J Neurosurg* 2002;96:269–279.
25. Saint-Cyr JA, Hoque T, Pereira LC, et al. Localization of clinically effective stimulating electrodes in the human subthalamic nucleus on magnetic resonance imaging. *J Neurosurg* 2002;97:1152–1166.
26. Parent A, Cossete M, Levesque M. Anatomical considerations in basal ganglia surgery. In: Lozano AM, ed. *Movement disorder surgery. Progress in neurological surgery*. Basel: Karger, 2000:21–30.
27. Hamani C, Saint-Cyr JA, Fraser J, et al. The subthalamic nucleus in the context of movement disorders. *Brain* 2003;127:4–20.
28. Cossette M, Levesque M, Parent A. Extrastriatal dopaminergic innervation of human basal ganglia. *Neurosci Res* 1999;34:51–54.
29. Alegret M, Valldeoriola F, Tolosa E, et al. Cognitive effects of unilateral posteroventral pallidotomy: a 4 year follow-up study. *Mov Disord* 2003;18:323–328.
30. Junque C, Alegret M, Nobbe FA, et al. Cognitive and behavioral changes after unilateral posteroventral pallidotomy: relationship with lesional data from MRI. *Mov Disord* 1999;14:780–789.
31. Baron MS, Vitek JL, Bakay RA, et al. Treatment of advanced Parkinson's disease by unilateral posterior GPi pallidotomy: 4-year results of a pilot study. *Mov Disord* 2000;15:233–237.
32. Baron MS, Vitek JL, Bakay RA, et al. Treatment of advanced Parkinson's disease by posterior GPi pallidotomy: 1-year results of a pilot study. *Ann Neurol* 1996;40: 355–366.
33. Bezerra ML, Martinez JV, Nasser JA. Transient acute depression induced by high-frequency deep-brain stimulation. *N Engl J Med* 1999;341:1003.
34. Higginson CI, Fields JA, Troster AI. Which symptoms of anxiety diminish after surgical interventions for Parkinson disease? *Neuropsychiatry Neuropsychol Behav Neurol* 2001;14:117–121.
35. Lombardi WJ, Gross RE, Trepanier LL, et al. Relationship of lesion location to cognitive outcome following microelectrode-guided pallidotomy for Parkinson's disease: support for the existence of cognitive circuits in the human pallidum. *Brain* 2000;123:746–758.
36. Mendez MF, O'Connor SM, Lim GT. Hypersexuality after right pallidotomy for Parkinson's disease. *J Neuropsychiatry Clin Neurosci* 2004;16:37–40.
37. Okun MS, Bakay RA, DeLong MR, et al. Transient manic behavior after pallidotomy. *Brain Cogn* 2003; 52:281–283.

38. Perrine K, Dogali M, Fazzini E, et al. Cognitive functioning after pallidotomy for refractory Parkinson's disease. *J Neurol Neurosurg Psychiatry* 1998; 65:150–154.
39. Dogali M, Fazzini E, Kolodny E, et al. Stereotactic ventral pallidotomy for Parkinson's disease. *Neurology* 1995;45:753–761.
40. Kulisevsky J, Berthier ML, Gironell A, et al. Mania following deep brain stimulation for Parkinson's disease. *Neurology* 2002;59:1421–1424.
41. Rettig GM, York MK, Lai EC, et al. Neuropsychological outcome after unilateral pallidotomy for the treatment of Parkinson's disease. *J Neurol Neurosurg Psychiatry* 2000;69:326–336.
42. Trepanier LL, Kumar R, Lozano AM, et al. Neuropsychological outcome of GPi pallidotomy and GPi or STN deep brain stimulation in Parkinson's disease. *Brain Cogn* 2000;42:324–347.
43. Trepanier LL, Saint-Cyr JA, Lozano AM, et al. Neuropsychological consequences of posteroventral pallidotomy for the treatment of Parkinson's disease. *Neurology* 1998;51:207–215.
44. Vitek JL, Bakay RA, Freeman A, et al. Randomized trial of pallidotomy versus medical therapy for Parkinson's disease. *Ann Neurol* 2003;53:558–569.
45. Green J, McDonald WM, Vitek JL, et al. Neuropsychological and psychiatric sequelae of pallidotomy for PD: clinical trial findings. *Neurology* 2002;58:858–865.
46. Ardouin C, Pillon B, Peiffer E, et al. Bilateral subthalamic or pallidal stimulation for Parkinson's disease affects neither memory nor executive functions: a consecutive series of 62 patients. *Ann Neurol* 1999; 46:217–223.
47. Pillon B, Ardouin C, Damier P, et al. Neuropsychological changes between "off" and "on" STN or GPi stimulation in Parkinson's disease. *Neurology* 2000; 55:411–418.
48. Fields JA, Troster AI, Wilkinson SB, et al. Cognitive outcome following staged bilateral pallidal stimulation for the treatment of Parkinson's disease. *Clin Neurol Neurosurg* 1999;101:182–188.
49. Krause M, Fogel W, Heck A, et al. Deep brain stimulation for the treatment of Parkinson's disease: subthalamic nucleus versus globus pallidus internus. *J Neurol Neurosurg Psychiatry* 2001;70:464–470.
50. Miyawaki E, Perlmutter JS, Troster AI, et al. The behavioral complications of pallidal stimulation: a case report. *Brain Cogn* 2000;42:417–434.
51. Roane DM, Yu M, Feinberg TE, et al. Hypersexuality after pallidal surgery in Parkinson's disease. *Neuropsychiatry Neuropsychol Behav Neurol* 2002;15:247–251.
52. Troster AI, Fields JA, Wilkinson SB, et al. Unilateral pallidal stimulation for Parkinson's disease: neurobehavioral functioning before and 3 months after electrode implantation. *Neurology* 1997;49:1078–1083.
53. Krack P, Batir A, Van Blercom N, et al. Five-year follow-up of bilateral stimulation of the subthalamic nucleus in advanced Parkinson's disease. *N Eng J Med* 2003;349: 1925–1934.
54. Berney A, Vingerhoets F, Perrin A, et al. Effect on mood of subthalamic DBS for Parkinson's disease: a consecutive series of 24 patients. *Neurology* 2002;59: 1427–1429.
55. Martinez-Martin P, Valldeoriola F, Tolosa E, et al. Bilateral subthalamic nucleus stimulation and quality of life in advanced Parkinson's disease. *Mov Disord* 2002;17:372–377.
56. Dujardin K, Defebvre L, Krystkowiak P, et al. Influence of chronic bilateral stimulation of the subthalamic nucleus on cognitive function in Parkinson's disease. *J Neurol* 2001;248:603–611.
57. Ostergaard K, Sunde N, Dupont E. Effects of bilateral stimulation of the subthalamic nucleus in patients with severe Parkinson's disease and motor fluctuations. *Mov Disord* 2002;17:693–700.
58. Vingerhoets FJG, Villemure JG, Temperli P, et al. Subthalamic DBS replaces levodopa in Parkinson's disease: two-year follow up. *Neurology* 2002;58:396–401.
59. Stefurak T, Mayberg H, Mikulis D, et al. Deep brain stimulation for PD dissociates mood and motor circuits: an fMRI case study. *Mov Disord* 2003;18:1508–1516.
60. Burn DJ. Beyond the iron mask: towards better recognition and treatment of depression associated with Parkinson's disease. *Mov Disord* 2002;17:445–454.
61. Doonief G, Mirabello E, Bell K, et al. An estimate of the incidence of depression in idiopathic Parkinson's disease. *Arch Neurol* 1992;49:305–307.
62. Funkiewiez A, Ardouin C, Krack P, et al. Acute psychotropic effects of bilateral subthalamic nucleus stimulation and levodopa in Parkinson's disease. *Mov Disord* 2003;18:524–530.
63. Giovannoni G, O'Sullivan JD, Turner K, et al. Hedonistic homeostatic dysregulation in patients with Parkinson's disease on dopamine replacement therapies. *J Neurol Neurosurg Psychiatry* 2000;68:423–428.
64. Lawrence AD, Evans AH, Lees AJ. Compulsive use of dopamine replacement therapy in Parkinson's disease: reward systems gone awry? *Lancet Neurol* 2003;2: 595–604.
65. Gold MS, Miller NS. Cocaine (and crack): neurobiology. In: Lowinson JH, Ruiz P, Millman RB et al., eds. *Substance abuse: a comprehensive textbook*. Baltimore, MD: Williams & Wilkins, 1997.
66. Doshi PK, Chhaya N, Bhatt MH. Depression leading to attempted suicide after bilateral subthalamic nucleus stimulation for Parkinson's disease. *Mov Disord* 2002;17:1084–1085.
67. Kumar R, Lozano AM, Sime E, et al. Comparative effects of unilateral and bilateral subthalamic nucleus deep brain stimulation. *Neurology* 1999;53:561–566.
68. Okun MS, Green J, Saben R, et al. Mood changes with deep brain stimulation of STN and GPi: results of a pilot study. *J Neurol Neurosurg Psychiatry* 2003;74: 1584–1586.
69. Romito LM, Raja M, Daniele A, et al. Transient mania with hypersexuality after surgery for high frequency stimulation of the subthalamic nucleus in Parkinson's disease. *Mov Disord* 2002;17:1371–1374.
70. Krack P, Kumar R, Ardouin C, et al. Mirthful laughter induced by subthalamic nucleus stimulation. *Mov Disord* 2001; 16:867–875.
71. Schneider F, Habel U, Volkmann J, et al. Deep brain stimulation of the subthalamic nucleus enhances emotional processing in Parkinson disease. *Arch Gen Psychiatry* 2003;60:296–302.
72. Daniele A, Albanese A, Contarino P, et al. Cognitive and behavioral effects of chronic stimulation of the subthalamic nucleus in patients with Parkinson's disease. *J Neurol Neurosurg Psychiatry* 2003;74: 175–182.
73. Herzog J, Reiff J, Krack P, et al. Manic episode with psychotic symptoms induced by subthalamic nucleus stimulation in a patient with Parkinson's disease. *Mov Disord* 2003;18:1382–1384.

74. Shulman KI. Disinhibition syndromes, secondary mania and bipolar disorder in old age. *J Affect Disord* 1997;46:175–182.
75. Abosch A, Kapur S, Lang AE, et al. Stimulation of the subthalamic nucleus in Parkinson's disease does not produce striatal dopamine release. *Neurosurgery* 2003; 53:1095–1105.
76. Strafella AP, Sadikot Af, Dagher A. Subthalamic deep brain stimulation does not induce striatal dopamine release in Parkinson's disease. *NeuroReport* 2003;14: 1287–1289.
77. Olbrisch ME, Levenson JL. Psychosocial assessment of organ transplant candidates. *Psychosomatics* 1995; 36:263–243.
78. Diederich NJ, Alesch F, Goetz C. Visual hallucinations induced by deep brain stimulation in Parkinson's disease. *Clin Neuropharmacol* 2000;23:287–289.
79. Derry PA, Wiebe S. Psychological adjustment to success and to failure following epilepsy surgery. *Can J Neurol Sci* 2000;27(Suppl. 1):S116–S120.
80. Mallet L, Mesnage V, Houeto JL, et al. Compulsions, Parkinson's disease and stimulation. *Lancet* 2002;360: 1302–1304.
81. Defer GL, Widner H, Marie RM. Core assessment program for surgical interventional therapies in Parkinson's disease (CAPSIT-PD). *Mov Disord* 1999;14:145–152.
82. Leentjens AF, Verhey FR, Lousberg R. The validity of the Hamilton and Montgomery-Asberg depression rating scales as screening and diagnostic tools for depression in Parkinson's disease. *Int J Geriatr Psychiatry* 2000;15:644–649.
83. Leentjens AF, Verhey FR, Luijckx GJ. The validity of the Beck Depression Inventory as a screening and diagnostic instrument for depression in patients with Parkinson's disease. *Mov Disord* 2000;15:1221–1224.
84. Molho ES. Psychosis and related problems. In: Factor SA, Weiner WJ, eds. *Parkinson's disease: diagnosis and clinical management.* New York: Demos Medical Publishing, 2002:465–480.
85. Lang AE, Widner H. Deep brain stimulation for Parkinson's disease: patient selection and evaluation. *Mov Disord* 2002;17(Suppl. 3):S94–S101.
86. Schrag A, Jahanshahi M, Quinn N. What contributes to quality of life in patients with Parkinson's disease? *J Neurol Neurosurg Psychiatry* 2000;69:308–312.
87. Troster AI, Fields JA, Wilkinson S, et al. Effect of motor improvement on quality of life following subthalamic stimulation is mediated by changes in depressive symptomatology. *Stereotact Funct Neurosurg* 2003;80:43–47.
88. Rektorova I, Rektor I, Bares M, et al. Pramipexole and pergolide in the treatment of depression in Parkinson's disease: a national multicentre prospective randomized study. *Eur J Neurol* 2003;10:399–406.
89. Pluck GC, Brown RG. Apathy in Parkinson's disease. *J Neurol Neurosurg Psychiatry* 2002;73:636–642.
90. Aarsland D, Larsen JP, Lim NG, et al. Range of neuropsychiatric disturbances in patients with Parkinson's disease. *J Neurol Neurosurg Psychiatry* 1999; 67:492–496.
91. Myslobodsky M, Lalonde FM, Hicks L. Are patients with Parkinson's disease suicidal? *J Geriatr Psychiatry Neurol* 2001;14:120–124.
92. Schroeder U, Kuehler A, Hennenlotter A, et al. Facial expression recognition and subthalamic nucleus stimulation. *J Neurol Neurosurg Psychiatry* 2004;75: 648–650.
93. Dujardin K, Blairy S, Defebvre L, et al. Subthalamic stimulation induces deficits in decoding emotional facial expressions in Parkinson's disease. *J Neurol Neurosurg Psychiatry* 2004;75:202–208.
94. Voon V. Repetition, repetition, repetition: compulsive and punding behaviors in Parkinson's disease. [Editorial] *Mov Disord* 2004;19:367–370.
95. Alegret M, Junque C, Valldeoriola F, et al. Effects of bilateral subthalamic stimulation on cognitive function in Parkinson's disease. *Arch Neurol* 2001;58: 1223–1227.
96. Woods SP, Fields JA, Troster AI. Neuropsychological sequelae of subthalamic nucleus deep brain stimulation in Parkinson's disease: a critical review. *Neuropsychol Rev* 2002;12:111–126.
97. Jahanshahi M, Ardouin CMA, Brown RG, et al. The impact of deep brain stimulation on executive function in Parkinson's disease. *Brain* 2000;123:1142–1154.
98. Fields JA, Troster AI. Cognitive outcomes after deep brain stimulation for Parkinson's disease: a review of initial studies and recommendations for future research. *Brain Cogn* 2000;42:268–293.

11

Neurodegenerative Disorders with Diffuse Cortical Lewy Bodies

Adam S. Fleisher and John M. Olichney

*Department of Neuroscience, UCSD Department of Neurosciences,
University of California, San Diego, La Jolla, California*

HISTORIC OVERVIEW

In 1912, Frederic Lewy described eosinophilic neuronal inclusion bodies in cases of "paralysis agitans" or idiopathic Parkinson's disease (PD) (1). Lewy bodies (LBs) were initially found in a restricted distribution that primarily involved the substantia nigra, locus ceruleus, dorsal vagus motor nucleus, and substantia innominata. At that time, it was generally thought that in "shaking palsy," as James Parkinson himself said, "the senses and intellects are uninjured" (2). Later advances have shown that neocortical LBs and Lewy neurites (LNs) are seen in PD and in other neurological disorders associated with cognitive and behavioral abnormalities. A protein named *alpha-synuclein* (αS) was isolated from the electric organ of the Pacific electric ray in 1988 (3). Its relevance to dementia was not appreciated until a nonamyloid component (NAC) of amyloid plaques in Alzheimer's disease (AD) was discovered to be a fragment of the αS protein (also known as NACP) (3,4). αS was subsequently cloned and in 1997 was discovered to be a specific and common constituent of both cortical and subcortical Lewy bodies, as well as LNs (5,6).

Over the past decade, it has become clear that cortical LBs are present not only in dementia cases with motor and psychiatric symptoms, but also in most PD cases without dementia (7). Braak et al. (8), in a large autopsy series of predominantly PD cases, demonstrated a characteristic pattern of progressive cortical Lewy body involvement, a finding that implies that predictable pathologic staging may correlate with the clinical manifestations of PD (8). This chapter describes and correlates the neuropathologic and clinical features of the dementias that have diffuse cortical Lewy bodies. These dementias include both dementia with Lewy bodies (DLB) and idiopathic Parkinson's disease with dementia (PDD). DLB is now recognized as the second most common form of dementia. This chapter focuses on defining the pathology common to diseases with αS as a primary feature and the distinctions that separate them. Discussions of various clinical presentations of DLB and PDD follow, with clinicopathologic correlations.

LB PATHOLOGY IN THE SYNUCLEINOPATHIES

Lewy bodies are intracytoplasmic eosinophilic inclusions, which differ slightly in appearance in the brain stem and basal forebrain ("classical" or brain stem-type LB) from those in the cerebral neocortex. The brain stem or classical-type LBs typically are large (>15 micron diameter) and have an eosinophilic core surrounded by a less densely staining peripheral halo. These LBs are usually single and round. Ultrastructurally, brain-stem LBs have a dense osmiophilic core of granular and vesicular material and a concentric rim of radially or haphazardly arranged 8-nm to 10-nm diameter fibrils (9–12). These fibrils are composed of abnormally phosphorylated neurofilament proteins aggregated with ubiquitin and αS (13). The classical LB has been described in monoaminergic and cholinergic neurons (14–16).

Neocortical LBs, in contrast, are smaller and more difficult to discern on hematoxylin and eosin staining than those found in the brain stem. They are more homogeneous, with no distinct core, and have comparatively loosely arranged fibrils and granular material (17–21). Identification of neocortical LBs is greatly facilitated by immunohistochemical staining with ubiquitin and anti-αS antibodies (16). They are most often seen in the perikarya of nonpyramidal neurons in the deep cortical layers V and VI. The immunohistochemical profile of neocortical LBs appears similar to that of classical LBs (12,16,18). Cortical LBs have a predilection for the cingulate gyrus, insular and frontotemporal cortex, and amygdala, a distribution that correlates with mesolimbic dopaminergic projections (13,22,23). Extensive depletion of acetylcholine neurotransmission in neocortical areas occurs as a result of degeneration in the brain stem and basal forebrain cholinergic projection neurons (13). In addition to LBs, dystrophic neurons (LNs) are found in PD as well as Lewy body dementias (3). αS aggregation within dystrophic LNs is associated with regions rich in perikaryal LBs, particularly the CA2/3 region of the hippocampus. It is therefore likely that αS plays an important role in the loss of neuronal function (16). In addition, AD cases often have superimposed LB pathology. In fact, one series found that 57% of AD cases diagnosed by National Institute on Aging-Reagan Institute (NIA-RI) criterion had LBs or LNs on αS staining, predominantly in the amygdala (24), a finding that complicates the pathologic distinctions between these diseases.

LBs are derived from abnormally phosphorylated cytoskeletal elements, including medium and heavy neurofilaments and microtubules (11–13,18,25,26). Immunohistochemical evidence supports the concept that αS is the primary building block of the fibrillary component of LBs (16,27). Unlike the neurofibrillary tangles (NFTs) in AD, LBs do not stain with antibodies to microtubule-associated tau protein (11,12,28,29) but instead stain strongly to αS (3). The filamentous ultrastructural character of the LB and its immunohistochemical profile suggest that disturbed neurofilament metabolism or transportation is important in LB formation (30). αS is expressed in a number of neuronal and nonneuronal cell types such as cortical neurons, dopaminergic neurons, noradrenergic neurons, endothelial cells, and platelets. Its functions have been found to include the binding of fatty acids, the regulation of certain enzymes and transporters, the modulation of synaptic plasticity, and the production and regulation of neurotransmitter vesicles, including those for dopamine and acetylcholine (31,32).

In spite of the coexistence of cortical Lewy bodies and Alzheimer lesions in many brains (particularly cases of plaque-predominant AD), not many common biochemical features link these lesions. In some cases, beta-amyloid and senile plaques (SPs) are abundant, but with little Tau pathology and NFTs (16,33). Tau immunostaining, however, has been demonstrated at the periphery of LBs (34). Unlike LBs and LNs, NFTs do not contain αS. A few pathologic similarities between NFTs in AD and LBs are (a) ubiquitin is present in LBs and the NFTs in AD (21); (b) the multicatalytic proteinase or ingestin, a nonlysosomal ATP-dependent proteinase, has been immunohistochemically visualized in both LBs and loosely arranged globose NFTs (35); and (c) abnormal phosphorylation may play a role in cytoskeletal pathology in both conditions (36,37). Further differences between "classic" AD and Lewy body variant (LBV) have been reported as well. For example, whereas early AD typically has extensive degenerative changes in the CA1 area of the hippocampus (38), LBV sometimes shows relative sparing of this area with more neuritic degeneration in CA2/3 (39). Also, amyloid angiopathy is generally milder in cases of LBV than in pure AD (40). An interesting finding that may account for some of the memory impairment in LBV is temporal lobe vacuolation, common in the entorhinal cortex, amygdala, and superior temporal gyrus (41,42). Neurochemically, diffuse cortical LBs are associated with profound dopaminergic and acetylcholinergic changes (43). Striatal dopaminergic involvement is usually severe enough to cause extrapyramidal symptoms (EPS) in DLB, but these symptoms are less pronounced than those in PD. Compared to cases of pure AD, cases with isolated diffuse cortical LBs have less neocortical choline acetyltransferase (ChAT) activity but more functionally intact muscarinic receptors (44). Another commonality between AD and DLB is abnormal protein processing with pathologic structural conformations (e.g., Beta-amyloid peptide and αS) that foster neurodegeneration.

DEMENTIA WITH LEWY BODIES—WHAT'S IN A NAME?

A bewildering variety of appellations were initially applied to dementia cases with LBs; among these terms were "diffuse cortical Lewy body disease" (45), "diffuse Lewy body disease" (46), "senile dementia of the Lewy body type" (47), "Lewy body variant of Alzheimer's disease" (41), "diffuse Lewy body disease, common form, with plaques and/or tangles" (48), "Alzheimer's disease with Lewy bodies" (49), and "Parkinson's disease in Alzheimer's disease" (50). The clinical and pathological features reported under these various rubrics are generally similar but embody subtle differences. Since the establishment of consensus clinical criteria in 1996 (Table 11-1), DLB has become the predominant umbrella term to describe pathologic variations of two specific αS-laden dementias (51).

Newer insights into the pathologic characterizations of these disorders suggest that the distribution and severity of LBs at specific sites and the interaction with concomitant AD pathology may determine the precise symptoms and signs in individual patients. αS-rich subcortical LBs predominate in the mesencephon, particularly the substantia nigra pars compacta, of patients with PD (8). The presence of numerous cortical and subcortical LBs, SPs, and NFTs [meeting Consortium to Establish a Registry for Alzheimer Disease (CERAD) or NIA-RI criteria for AD (52)] defines a dementia subtype referred to as LBV, whereas the presence of abundant cortical LBs, without substantial numbers of NFTs or neuritic plaques, in patients with a dementia characterized by extrapyramidal signs and prominent neuropsychiatric features is now commonly referred to as "pure diffuse Lewy body disease" (pDLBD) (16). LBV appears to be far more common than pDLBD (43,53). The number of NFTs and neuritic plaques in LBV cases is often substantially less than in pure AD and closely resembles the changes seen in early stages of AD (54). In the past, there have been cases of AD described as "plaque-only" or "plaque predominant" (55).

TABLE 11-1. *Consensus criteria for the diagnosis of probable and possible DLB*

1) **Central Features**
   a. Progressive cognitive decline of sufficient magnitude to interfere with normal social and occupational function. Prominent or persistent memory impairment does not necessarily occur in the early stages but is evident with progression in most cases. Deficits on tests of attention and of frontal-subcortical skills and visuospatial abilities can be especially prominent.
2) **Core features (two core features essential for a diagnosis of probable, one for possible, DLB)**
   a. Fluctuating cognition with pronounced variations in attention and alertness
   b. Recurrent visual hallucinations that are typically well formed and detailed
   c. Spontaneous motor features of parkinsonism
3) **Feature supportive of the diagnosis**
   a. Repeated falls
   b. Syncope
   c. Transient loss of consciousness
   d. Neuroleptic sensitivity
   e. Systemized delusions
   f. Hallucinations in other modalities
4) **Features less likely to be present**
   a. History of stroke by neurologic exam or imaging
   b. Evidence on physical examination and investigation of any physical illness or other brain disorder sufficient to account for the clinical picture

[From McKeith et al. Consensus guidelines for the clinical and pathologic diagnosis of dementia with Lewy bodies (DLB): report of the consortium on DLB international workshop. *Neurology* 1996;47(5):1113–1124 (51), with permission.]

Hansen et al. (56) argue that most cases of "plaque-only" AD are in fact LBV (56). Some investigators have attributed cases with relatively sparse AD pathology to aging, implying that the LBs alone cause dementia in such cases (20). Supporting this possibility, good evidence exists that the degree of cortical LB concentration correlates well with the severity of dementia (57,58).

Given clear pathologic distinctions between the two diseases, a nosologic distinction has been made between LBV with and without pDLBD-prominent AD pathology. Although these entities are discrete pathologically, a clinical distinction between LBV and pDLBD is not easily made. Subsequently, the recent practice parameter for the diagnosis of dementia by the American Academy of Neurology uses the umbrella term DLB to describe both of these disorders as a group (59). Furthermore, DLB does not encompass PDD, in which the motor findings far precede dementia. There is no clear neuropathologic distinction between PDD and DLB, and clinical boundaries can be blurry (27). The ensuing discussion takes a combined descriptive clinocopathologic approach to clarify these classifications, using the terminology outlined above.

THE CLINICAL PRESENTATIONS OF PATIENTS WITH CORTICAL LEWY BODIES

A variety of clinical presentations is associated with LBs. These presentations include various combinations of dementia (often resembling dementia of the Alzheimer type), atypical parkinsonism (often lacking a resting tremor), and psychiatric features such as depression, hallucinations, and a fluctuating level of consciousness and cognition. The diseases most commonly associated with αS and dementia are LBV, pDLBD, and PD (with either mild subcortical dementia or more severe "global" dementia).

LBs IN PATIENTS WHO PRESENT WITH DEMENTIA

Clinical Characteristics

For those patients who present with dementia suggestive of AD and develop visual hallucinations and extrapyramidal signs, neuropathology is likely to show both AD and cortical Lewy bodies (LBV) and, less commonly, pDLBD. Regardless of nomenclature, dementia (20,41,60,61) and memory impairment (62) clearly are the major features of DLB. Also, a clinical distinction is increasingly recognized between AD and DLB, as described by the consensus guidelines (Table 11-1). Furthermore, methods of distinguishing between DLB and PDD are not well defined. An arbitrary "1-year rule" is often applied to separate PDD and DLB: onset of dementia within 1 year of parkinsonism qualifies as DLB, and more than 1 year of parkinsonism before dementia as PDD. This distinction is increasingly hard to justify from a neurobiologic point of view (27). Many authors have found relatively low diagnostic accuracy for DLB, with sensitivity ranging from 18% to 83% (27,53,63–66). Furthermore, when a higher degree of AD pathology is present in DLB cases, the occurrence of visual hallucinations and parkinsonism tends to be less common (67). Therefore, consensus criteria appear to be more sensitive and specific in pDLBD than in LBV (65). This disparity blurs clinical boundaries between AD and DLB, making clinical differentiation between these disorders difficult. Differences in methods, case selection, and referral practices may be responsible for the high variability in reported sensitivities and specificities [see McKeith et al, 2004 (27) for details]. Nonetheless, parkinsonism and neuropsychiatric symptoms have been the primary focus to distinguish DLB and AD clinically.

Most series report a mild (20,47) parkinsonian syndrome that lacks the entire classic triad of resting tremor, bradykinesia, and rigidity. A resting tremor is usually absent and has not been observed in more than 40 cases of LBV in the University of California, San Diego series, although a postural tremor was present in several (41,68). Merdes et al. (67), in a series of 98 pathologically proven DLB cases, found 55% to have spontaneous EPS (67). Burkhardt et al. (62) found rigidity to be more common than bradykinesia and tremor. Masked facies, along with bradykinesia and rigidity, appear most helpful in distinguishing LBV cases from pure

AD (68), and gait disorder was emphasized in another series (60). It is not yet clear whether patients with prominent diffuse Lewy bodies (either LBV or pDLBD) differ from typical patients with PD in their responsiveness to levodopa. A small number of diffuse Lewy body cases have been reported to have EPS unresponsive to levodopa (69,70), but other series have shown that most patients are levodopa responsive (57,61). In a pathologic series that did not restrict subjects to those who first presented with dementia, the proportion of patients who presented with parkinsonian signs followed by dementia was 14% (4 of 28 cases) in one series (43) and 40% (6 of 15 cases) in another (61). It has also been shown that a higher Braak stage of AD neurofibrillary pathology correlates to less frequent EPS (67). EPS, however, also commonly occurs in late-stage AD, and therefore the presence of EPS as the only core feature present (Table 11-1) should be interpreted with caution. Such cases can be classified as "possible DLB," but this group often includes many false positive cases (59).

In addition to the memory impairment central to the diagnosis of dementia, neuropsychological testing has shown that patients with LBV have impaired attention, verbal fluency, and visuospatial abilities (41). When matched for severity to subjects with pure AD using Blessed Information Memory Concentration (BIMC) scores, the LBV group performed more poorly on the Wechsler Adult Intelligence Scale-Revised (WAIS-R) Digit Span and Similarities subscales, letter fluency (not category fluency), the Wechsler Intelligence Scale for Children-Revised (WISC-R) Block Design, and the Copy-a-Cross Test. However, in most measures, the neuropsychological deficits of LBV did not differ from those of pure AD. This pattern of deficits, with disproportionate deficits on frontal (e.g., verbal fluency, attention) and visuospatial tasks, is also similar to that seen with PD dementia (71) and likely reflects the concomitant AD-like and PD-like pathology (72).

Distinctive psychiatric manifestations are common in LBV and pDLBD. A fluctuating course has been described, with frequent confusional states, visual hallucinations (27,47,73), agitation, and delusions (20,60). They often present early in the course of disease and persist. The hallucinations are similar to those reported in PDD, with vivid, colorful, three-dimensional, and generally mute images of animate objects (74). Kosaka (29) found psychosis or depression to be the initial symptom in 5 of 28 LBV cases (memory loss was the most common presentation and was the initial symptom in 16 of the 28 cases). Ferman et al. (75) found that the presence of three symptoms of neuropsychiatric fluctuation including daytime drowsiness, daytime sleep of 2 hours or more, staring episodes, or periods of disorganized speech were found in 63% of DLB patients (n = 70) (75). Merdes et al. (67) found that 42% of LBV subjects in one series had visual hallucinations during the course of their illness, and only 27% of subjects had both EPS and visual hallucinations. Those with low Braak Stages (stages 0–2) had a higher frequency of visual hallucinations (65%) than did subjects with higher Braak stages (33%) (67). Visual hallucinations appear to be associated with greater deficits in cortical acetylcholine (76) and may predict better response to cholinesterase inhibitors (77).

Improving Diagnostic Accuracy of DLB

Many efforts have been made to improve diagnostic accuracy by defining other clinical criteria and diagnostic techniques to identify unique features of DLB. These features include sleep disorders, electroencephalogram (EEG) evidence of neuropsychiatric fluctuations, autonomic failure, olfactory deficits, and neuroimaging findings. Rapid-eye-movement (REM) behavioral disorders (RBD) are often associated with synucleinopathies but not with tauopathies or amyloidopathies (78). Boeve et al., in a study of 14 neuropathologic cases, found that in the setting of dementia or parkinsonism, the presence of RBD often reflects an underlying synucleinopathy (78). REM sleep–wakefulness dissociation can explain several features of DLB and DLB fluctuations in level of consciousness as described above (75). In fact, several investigators reported neuropsychiatric fluctuations as a distinguishing feature in DLB (75,79). Ferman et al. (75) found fluctuations to be present about five times more frequently in DLB than in AD (75).

Because of these findings, attempts have been made to identify these fluctuations more accurately with EEGs. Abnormal EEGs with early background posterior slowing, fluctuations, and a frontally dominant burst pattern have been reported in patients with mild to moderate DLB (60,80–82). Walker et al. (83–85) showed substantially increased variability in EEG and attention in patients with DLB, compared to patients with AD (83,84). These same authors developed a "One Day Fluctuation Assessment Scale" that successfully identified fluctuations with a sensitivity and specificity that exceeded 80% (85). Autonomic dysfunctions, such as orthostatic hypotension and carotid hypersensitivity, are more common in DLB than in AD and may also help distinguish the two conditions (86). Another clinical feature that may help distinguish DLB from AD is the presence of anosmia. Prominent deficits of olfaction in PD have been well described (87), but only recently was anosmia shown to be more severe in autopsy-confirmed DLB than in pure AD (88). Olichney et al. (89) reported that the negative predictive value and specificity of anosmia were both good (92% and 78%). Sensitivity for DLB was fairly high (65%), but the positive predictive value was only 35% in an autopsy series of 108 dementia cases, most of whom (84%) had AD (89). Many features detectable by brain imaging may prove beneficial to support the diagnosis of DLB. These features include preservation (compared to AD) of hippocampal and medial temporal lobe volume on magnetic resonance imaging (90), and occipital hypoperfusion on single photon emission computed tomography (SPECT) (91). By using dopaminergic ligands with SPECT, dopamine transporter loss in the caudate and putamen can be detected in patients with DLB (92). A sensitivity of 83% and specificity of 100% has been reported when an abnormal scan is compared with autopsy findings (93).

Risk Factors and Prognosis for DLB

Risk factors for developing LBV or pDLBD are difficult to determine because of problems with nosology and with premortem identification of these patients. Advanced age and male sex are the strongest themes that emerge from the numerous case series (20,62). Patients with DLB who have severe AD pathology have poorer prognosis than those without AD changes (94). Patients with EPS that are unresponsive to levodopa may, in a sense, be at risk to have pDLBD or LBV. Interpreting studies of risk in DLB can be difficult, because many studies do not distinguish between LBV and pDLBD (95,96). There is some evidence of genetic associations between DLB and AD, which may imply overlapping risk factors. Apolipoprotein E epsilon 4 allele (APOE ε4) is known to reflect a non-Mendelian increased genetic risk in AD. It has also been demonstrated that the APOE ε4 allele is overrepresented in AD compared to healthy controls (97,98). APOE ε4 is associated with increased AD pathology in LBV (99). In contrast, APOE ε4 was not found to be overrepresented in pDLBD (97). Furthermore, pedigrees have been reported that feature LB pathology associated with AD, inherited in an autosomal dominant fashion. This pattern has been found in familial AD caused by β–amyloid precursor protein (APP) (100) and that caused by presenilin gene mutations (101,102). This genetic evidence supports the concept that αS and β-amyloid have convergent pathophysiologic pathways.

Olichney et al. showed that patients with LBV have faster mean rates of cognitive decline on the Mini Mental State Examination (MMSE) and shorter survival (by about 1.6 years) than patients with AD (103). Other studies have reported comparable survival in these groups (104), yet mean values from larger studies likely conceal disease heterogeneity: some cases of DLB clearly have a very rapid disease course (105,106). Ballard and colleagues (104) found that the presence of an APOE ε4 allele was the strongest predictor of accelerated cognitive decline in their DLB cohort (104).

Pathologic Correlates of DLB

With the discovery of αS as the common molecular building block for the lesions in several subtypes of dementias, nomenclature has evolved since Koska's description of dementias with diffuse cortical Lewy bodies in 1984. At that time, it was clear that the distribution and quantity of

LBs forms a spectrum. In 1984, on the basis of a study of 20 brains, Kosaka attempted to define three groups within this spectrum, denoted as Lewy body disease, groups A, B, and C (107). Group A was called "diffuse Lewy body disease" (DLBD) and was characterized by numerous and widespread neocortical LBs plus varying degrees of Alzheimer pathology. Group C denoted LBs restricted to the brain stem and diencephalon, equivalent to findings in idiopathic PD. Group B was intermediate between groups A and C, having some neocortical LBs, but fewer than in group A. Subsequently, several investigators found that all (18,108) or nearly all (96%) (109) brains of patients with PD have at least some neocortical LBs, thus making it difficult to distinguish between groups B and C. In 1990, Kosaka proposed a new classification of Lewy body disease (48) based on the density of neocortical LBs and on the presence or absence of concomitant AD pathology (senile plaques and NFTs). This initial schema divided Lewy body disease into "DLBD, pure form," with five or more neocortical LBs per 100 × field in the predilection sites but without AD pathology, and "DLBD, common form," with fewer than five neocortical LBs per 100 × field but with accompanying senile plaques and sometimes NFTs.

ChAT is commonly used as a marker for cholinergic activity. Similar to AD, dementias associated with LBs show decreased levels of cortical ChAT (43). In fact, several investigators have shown that ChAT levels in frontal, parietal, and temporal cortex are substantially lower in LBV subjects than in those with primary AD pathology (110,111). One study demonstrated that even though mean midfrontal cortex ChAT activity for LBV was less than half that for AD, hippocampal activity was not different between the two groups (43). This finding may explain why the deficits in memory for LBV and AD are difficult to distinguish. More recently, Tiraboschi et al. (111) reported that, unlike patients with AD, patients with LBV had decreased ChAT activity even in the earliest clinical stages of dementia. The degree of decreased activity across several cortical brain areas correlated with MMSE scores in a separate analysis of subjects with mild to moderate dementia (MMSE ≥10). These investigators also found that, unlike patients with LBV who had global cortical LB involvement, patients with AD had region-specific differences, with the superior temporal lobe declining earlier than the medial frontal and inferior parietal lobes (111). These examples of pathophysiologic differences between αS dementias and AD give strong evidence that LBs themselves, independent of AD pathology, contribute to clinical dementia.

With the advent of αS immunohistochemistry, detection of LBs and LNs has become more sensitive, making efforts toward defining characteristic patterns of distribution more plausible. Braak et al. (8) demonstrated a continuum of readily recognizable topographic patterns of LB pathology in subjects with idiopathic PD (8). There appeared to be a clear progression from pure subcortical involvement to diffuse cortical involvement. Stage 1 and 2 defined involvement virtually confined to the medulla oblongata, especially the dorsal motor nucleus of cranial nerves IX and X, and then primary olfactory areas (olfactory bulb and anterior olfactory nucleus). Stages 3 and 4 had involvement confined to the lower and upper brain stem, with no (stage 3) or very mild involvement (stage 4) of the anteromedial temporal mesocortex. Stages 5 and 6 showed additional severe involvement of neocortical structures. Although Braak et al. (8) make no claims of clinical correlation, and this was not a study of DLB, the later stages of cortical involvement included structures of key import to cognitive processing (i.e., structures such as amygdala, hippocampal formation, and anteromedial temporal mesocortex). This finding supports the idea that the density and location of αS pathology is of key importance in the clinical presentation and degree of dementia in DLB. Merdes et al. (67) demonstrated that, of demented subjects with LB pathology, those with a lesser degree of AD pathology (as measured by Braak staging) had a substantially higher frequency of visual hallucinations and EPS than subjects with high Braak stages (67). This finding suggests that the degree of AD pathology influences the clinical presentation of dementia, with more pDLBD cases having a more PD-like phenotype, and LBV cases more closely resembling AD. It also supports the notion that αS dementias are etiologically distinct from SP and NFT dementias. Improved understanding of these diseases has made a clinical and pathologic distinction between AD and DLB possible. However, distinguishing between cases of pDLBD and LBV, as defined neuropathologically, often remains a difficult clinical challenge, even for dementia specialists.

pDLBD as a Cause of Dementia

A few patients who present with dementia have pDLBD without substantial AD pathology at autopsy. A few well-described clinicopathologic reports exist. These rare patients are sometimes clinically indistinguishable from those with LBV. The initial clinical presentation of pDLBD usually includes parkinsonian movement abnormalities and, less commonly, dementia. For example, one series (73) described two diffuse Lewy body patients without SPs or NFTs, both of whom presented with fairly typical PD and developed dementia relatively late. The patients with pDLBD described by Kosaka (48) had clinical features different from those of patients with LBV. These patients were much younger (mean age of onset about 33 years) and predominantly presented with juvenile parkinsonism rather than dementia, although most became demented late in their illnesses. Hughes et al. (7), in their series of 100 PD cases, found four patients fulfilling quantitative criteria for pDLBD. Two of these patients presented with typical PD, then developed dementia late in their illnesses. The other two patients with DLBD had atypical presentations for PD, in that they had early confusion or dementia and were unresponsive to levodopa. These two patients, however, did not have pDLBD, in that SPs were present in both. Crystal et al. (60) reported a series of six demented patients with prominent psychiatric features as having DLBD. These patients all had SPs but were classified as having "DLBD alone" because neocortical NFTs were absent. In summary, although pDLBD seems capable of causing dementia, it is rarely seen in demented patients without preceding parkinsonism, in which case it is difficult to distinguish both clinically and pathologically from PDD.

DEMENTIA IN PATIENTS WHO PRESENT WITH PD

"Dementia" vs. Cognitive Impairment

Contrary to James Parkinson's original description, dementia is now recognized to occur fairly commonly in PD. The reported frequency of dementia has varied widely, from 8% (112) to 81% (113), owing largely to different populations, methods, and criteria for "dementia." Current criteria in the *Diagnostic Statistical Manual of Mental Disorders*, 4th Edition, Text Revision (DSM-IV-TR) for diagnosing dementia requires a "significant impairment in social or occupational functioning" because of impairments in multiple cognitive areas, generally consisting of memory impairment along with other cognitive deficits such as aphasia, apraxia, and agnosia, executive dysfunctioning, or both (114). The requirement of functional decline stemming from intellectual impairment is lacking from many earlier studies of dementia in PD (115). This is a particularly difficult assessment in a disease characterized by motor limitations that may also affect social and occupational function. If "fronto-subcortical" deficits alone are present in the absence of substantial memory deficits, then the DSM-IV-TR criteria may not be met, even if minor functional decline results. Although mild neurocognitive impairment is very common in PD [and has been demonstrated in up to 93% of patients with PD (116)], many are unlikely to satisfy DSM-IV-TR criteria for dementia. The nature of and degree to which these cognitive deficits often fit a "frontosubcortical" (117,118) pattern have been reviewed in detail by Brown and Marsden (119) and in Chapters 7 and 8 of this volume. Whether the cognitive impairment in PD is isolated to fronto-subcortical deficits or is more global or AD-like in presentation, no formal clinical diagnostic criteria have been proposed or validated for PDD (120).

Prevalence and Incidence of Dementia in PD

In 1984, Brown and Marsden (115) critically reviewed data from multiple prevalence studies. They discovered that varying diagnostic criteria for PD and dementia likely resulted in overestimation of the prevalence of dementia in PD. Before adjusting for the varying criteria used to diagnose dementia, the overall reported prevalence was 35% in 2,530 patients with PD. Retrospective application of diagnostic criteria from the *Diagnostic Statistical Manual of Mental Disorders*, 3rd Edition (DSM-III) estimated that only 20% to 24.5% of patients with PD were demented. Some of the difficulty in measuring the prevalence of dementia is illustrated by a series of studies carried out in New York. A review of clinic and hospital records of 339 patients with PD suggested that the prevalence of dementia was 10.5% (121), a percentage that was later revised upward to 15.9% when cases of incipient dementia were included (122). However, a population-based epidemiologic study (123) by the same investigators found that 41% (74 cases) of 179 patients identified as having PD actually met DSM-III criteria for dementia. The discrepant figures may be attributable to selection bias, varying mean ages, and the use of different diagnostic criteria among studies. To estimate the incidence of PDD, a clinic-based cohort was followed for a mean period of 4.75 years, during which time 65 new cases of dementia were identified, yielding an overall incidence of 69 cases per 1,000 person-years of observation (122). This incidence rate for dementia was more than five times that reported for age-matched control subjects and was greater than would be expected from most prevalence studies. This discrepancy is probably caused by a greater mortality rate for demented patients with PD, which may cause cases to be underestimated in prevalence surveys. More recent studies have also found significant increases in the prevalence of dementia in patients with PD compared to normal controls (124). Increased mortality attributable to dementia is well known to occur in AD (125) and other dementing illnesses (126) and has been shown to occur in a survival analysis of PD (127).

Risk Factors for Dementia in PD

Several risk factors for dementia in PD have been defined. The foremost of these is age, with many studies reporting a clear increase of dementia among elderly patients with PD (123, 128–132). For example, from their population-based study, Mayeaux et al. (123) estimated the prevalence of PD in people over 80 as 1,145 per 100,000. Of this group, they estimated that 787 subjects would be demented. This number corresponds to a dementia rate of more than 68% among patients with PD over 80, compared to 0% under 50 and 12% of those between 50 and 59 years old. These data clearly show age to be a strong risk factor for dementia in PD. Different age distributions likely account for much of the wide variation in prevalence reported across studies. Age of onset may be more important than duration of PD as a determinant of dementia. For example, onset of motor manifestations after age 70 (123), but not the overall duration of PD (133), has been found to be a significant predictor of dementia.

Certain types or profiles of extrapyramidal signs may also be associated with PDD. The severity of motor impairment has been shown to be a predictor of dementia (134). Zetusky et al. (135) described a higher risk of dementia and a poorer prognosis for patients with prominent postural instability and gait disorder (PIGD) and less motor or cognitive deterioration in those with a tremor-dominant pattern after several years of symptoms. Tremor at onset has been shown to be a less reliable predictor (136).

Analyses of nondemented patients with PD from the DATATOP study (137) compared two clusters of patients with EPS: those with PIGD, and those with predominant resting tremor (tremor-dominant). The PIGD group had more severe complaints of motor, functional, and occupational disability than did tremor-dominant patients with similar age and mental status scores. Several other studies have shown that both prominent rigidity and bradykinesia, but not tremor, are associated with poor cognitive function in PD (71,74,138). However, Mortimer and colleagues (139) found that among the classic triad of parkinsonian signs, only bradykinesia severity correlated with poor cognition. A factor analysis of the Unified Parkinson's Disease Research Scale (UPDRS) components found that the factor reflecting rigidity and slowed repetitive movement best correlated with impairment on neuropsychological tests (140). This factor and another factor reflecting gait, postural stability, and bradykinesia were more severely abnormal in the demented than the nondemented PD subgroups.

No clinical evidence exists to show that levodopa treatment promotes the development of PD dementia. Our increased appreciation of dementia in PD could be partly attributable to the introduction of levodopa therapy, which has prolonged the survival of patients with PD patients (141–143) and thereby increased the prevalence of dementia. The presence or absence of response to levodopa, *per se,* is extremely difficult to study prospectively as a risk factor for PD dementia. The available clinical information is confounded by selection bias, in which only responders are likely to be willing to continue on long-term levodopa. Rajput et al. (144) found that 94% of patients with pathologically confirmed PD had shown clinical benefit from levodopa, but that only 60% of patients with dual PD and AD pathology had improved on levodopa.

Shared Risk Factors for PD and AD

Other potential risk factors have been studied, particularly those associated with AD. In a pilot study of 71 patients with PD, a family history of dementia in a first-degree relative was five times more common (30% vs. 5.6%) in those with dementia than in nondemented patients (133). This study, along with a Dutch survey showing that patients with AD were about three times more likely to have a relative with PD than were control subjects (145), provides evidence of a shared risk between AD and PD. The overlap is likely attributable in part to the inclusion of DLB cases, which have pathologic evidence of both disease processes, in those studies. On the other hand, other risk factors for AD, such as head trauma, thyroid disease, Down's syndrome (133), female sex (123), hypertension, and diabetes mellitus (103), have not been found to be risk factors for dementia in PD. Although several studies have shown an inverse relationship between smoking and the development of PD, there is evidence of a positive association between smoking and PDD (103). Lastly, caffeine has been shown in some studies to be protective against PD, but no studies have demonstrated an effect on the incidence of PDD (146). PDD and AD are both age-associated conditions and may be linked by an as yet unidentified pathophysiologic processes. Alternatively, the linkage between AD and PDD could be an artifact of selection bias in clinical series: when the changes of PDD and AD are both present, clinical features of motor or cognitive dysfunction may become more readily apparent or severe.

Pathologic Correlates of Dementia in PD

Issues of central importance to this chapter are to what extent LBs alone account for dementia in PD and whether concomitant AD is necessary. Some studies suggest that AD pathology is necessary for severe dementia. Boller et al. (147), in a study of 36 patients with idiopathic PD, reported the presence of AD pathology in all 9 severely demented patients but also in 3 of 13 patients with normal mental status scores. Paulus and Jellinger (148) found that patients with PD who had moderate or severe dementia had more extensive AD lesions than those with mild or no dementia. Gaspar and Gray (149) confirmed more severe AD pathology in cases of more severe PDD, although no plaques or tangles were found in one severely demented case. Hakim and Mathieson (150) in 1979 found AD pathology in 33 of 34 autopsied PD cases. However, they found no neuropathologic difference between the demented and nondemented cases. Other studies (151–153) have failed to find an association between Alzheimer's lesions in the cortex and dementia in patients with PD. This apparent contradiction might be secondary to a threshold effect. Because some SPs accumulate during normal aging as well as in AD, the presence, SPs may not adequately identify dementia in this population. However, AD pathology appears to be present in most patients with PDD and is generally thought to be present in 10% to 60% of all patients with PD (154). A recent discovery of a family with autosomal dominant PD, early onset dementia, lack of AD pathology, and numerous cortical and subcortical LBs has revealed a novel mutation, E46K, in the αS gene. This discovery is the first proof that PDD is directly related to the mutation of αS (155).

Hughes and colleagues (7) reported a series of 100 pathologically confirmed PD cases. All patients had some detectable cortical Lewy bodies, most commonly in the anterior cingulate gyrus. Of the 71 patients with adequate clinical information, 31 (44%) were considered demented. Of the demented patients, pathologic examination revealed AD in 29%, DLBD [meeting Kosaka's quantitative criteria for DLBD (48)] in 10%, "plentiful" LBs (but insufficient for Kosaka's criteria) in another 16%, and vascular damage in 6%, but no definite features were found in 55% of patients. It is important to our understanding of the disease to explain this sizable proportion of PDD without a clear pathologic basis. Unfortunately, pathology in the nondemented patients was not adequately described, and subjects were not categorized according to severity of dementia. It remains unclear what number or special extent of cortical Lewy bodies is required to generally produce dementia, or whether limbic and subcortical LBs can be sufficient to cause PDD. Revisiting this issue with αS staining in large, well-characterized PD cohorts should prove illuminating in this regard.

Rinne et al. (156) suggested that demented patients with PD have more neuronal loss in the medial substantia nigra than nondemented patients with PD. This relationship held even when patients with plaques or tangles were removed from the analysis. In light of the association of rigidity and bradykinesia with dementia, cell loss in the medial substantia nigral may simply be a proxy for more severe motor manifestations (dementia is more likely in older patients with PD, who usually have more severe motor disability) or of more advanced-stage PD. Paulus and Jellinger (148) also found neuronal loss in the medial substantia nigra to be somewhat greater in demented patients with PD, but this loss was less strongly associated with dementia than was the degree of AD pathology. Some investigators have found neuronal loss in the nucleus basalis of Meynert (NBM) of patients with PD and have suggested this damage as a cause of PDD (149,157,158). However, many investigators have failed to find a relationship between NBM damage and dementia (159–161). Further evidence that cortical Lewy bodies are implicated as a primary underlying mechanism for dementia is shown by biochemical and pathologic differences between αS dementias and AD. Braak et al. (8) proposed a staging system for sporadic PD, based on Lewy body distribution. Although the presence of clinical dementia was not expressly reported in this series, the authors noted that concomitant AD-related pathology was within the expected range for the respective age groups (8).

MANAGEMENT

Much of the management of these patients should focus on symptomatic treatment. Nonpharmacologic measures are often useful. Target symptoms usually include neuropsychiatric and parkinsonian motor symptoms as well as the manifestations of cognitive impairment. Nonpharmocologic treatments include physical therapy, assistive devices, and assistance with activities of daily living, as well as frequent orientation cues.

In PDD, continuing to manage the underlying PD is primary. Some studies support the usefulness of cholinesterase inhibitors (e.g., Donepezil) in treating cognitive impairment in these patients, although the potential for worsening tremor exists (162,163). Newer-generation antipsychotics, if needed, should be used cautiously, because they often worsen parkinsonism and may be associated with a general deterioration in some patients with PD, as has been described in DLB.

Pharmacologic management of DLB should include trials of cholinesterase inhibitors and of dopaminergic therapy, started at separate times. Anti-parkinsonian medications should be titrated to the lowest effective therapeutic dose. The effectiveness of these medications has not been proven in DLB, and they are thought to be somewhat less effective in DLB than in idiopathic PD. This disparity may be attributable to additional intrinsic striatal pathology and dysfunction (164).

There is evidence that DLB patients benefit from cholinesterase inhibitors, which may be even more effective in DLB than in AD (33). In fact, fluctuating cognitive impairments, visual hallucinations, sleep disturbances, and anxiety are improved on cholinesterase inhibitors, and these drugs are considered first-line therapy (27). This efficacy has been demonstrated most clearly for Rivastigmine, in a large double-blinded, placebo-controlled trial that showed improvement in cognition and multiple psychiatric symptoms on 6–12 mg (165). However, little reason exists to think that other cholinesterase inhibitors are not equally effective, especially at higher doses.

Phenothiazides should be avoided in DLB, because D-2 receptor antagonists can provoke a severe neuroleptic sensitivity reaction in up to 50% of patients with DLB and may increase mortality (166). This hypersensitivity has been suggested as a clue to clinical diagnosis. Newer atypical antipsychotic medications are safer but should be used with caution, because hypersensitivity reactions have been noted with these agents as well (27). Again, use of D-2 antagonists carries a substantial risk of worsening parkinsonism.

It is also reasonable to treat DLB patients with vitamin E (1,000 IU, twice a day), because this dose reduced institutionalization and death in a large study of patients with AD (as did the MOAb-inhibitor selegeline, albeit with more side effects) (167). Other antioxidants are theoretically useful for both AD and PD, because oxidative damage from reactive oxygen species have been implicated in both. One recent study suggests that αS oligomerization is mediated by hydroxyl radicals produced through Cu, Zn-superoxide dismutase, and the hydrogen peroxide system (168). Also, memantine, a new glutamate antagonist approved for the treatment of moderate to severe AD, might show benefit in DLB, although no trials have been done. In the future, any disease-modifying therapies that prove effective for either AD or PD will be good candidates for improving the treatment of DLB patients.

"Incidental" Lewy Bodies

The prevalence of subcortical Lewy bodies in "normal" elderly populations has been reported to be about 5% to 10% for subjects older than 50 and appears to rise with increasing age (169). Challenging these figures is a report (170) in which elderly controls were rigorously defined to exclude neurologic or psychiatric symptoms. In the brains of 131 such control subjects, prevalence of LBs was very low, 2.3% overall, with a small age-associated increase (3.8%) for the subgroup between 70 and 100. Increasing neocortical SP concentration was associated with increasing age in these healthy controls, but none reached the diagnostic threshold for AD. A group of "quasicontrols," mostly patients who had been on a psychogeriatric ward, was also examined at autopsy and had an extremely high prevalence of LBs: 28%. Psychiatric symptoms in those patients who had LBs were scantily described but resembled those of senile dementia of the LB type, with episodic confusion, mild cognitive impairment, depression, and hallucinations reported. In addition, five patients had "mild EPS." This series was relatively small and based on nonstandardized clinical records of varying quality and detail. Nevertheless, this series suggests that neuropsychiatric symptoms may be the major correlate of "incidental" Lewy bodies and shows the need to further characterize the full spectrum of clinical manifestations of Lewy body disease in prospective series.

Other Disorders with Alpha-Synuclein Pathology

Alpha-synuclein pathology has been discovered in other disorders not commonly associated with dementia. αS has been implicated as a major component of tubulofilamentous inclusions found in oligodendrocytes [glial cytoplasmic inclusions (GCI)] and in neurons of patients with multiple systems atrophy (MSA), a Parkinson's-plus syndrome that includes Shy–Drager syndrome, striatonigral degeneration, and olivopontocerebellar atrophy (171). Neurodegeneration with brain iron accumulation, type I (Hallervorden–Spatz syndrome), is a rare neurodegenerative disorder in which αS-staining axonal swellings, LBs, and GCIs are easily detected. Axonal lesions seen after traumatic brain injury also consist of αS. This finding begs the question of whether αS is merely a marker of neuronal degeneration, or a true cause of it. For example, there are other neurodegenerative diseases in which αS staining is present but is not the primary pathologic constituent. Some cases of Pick's disease have αS in the dentate gyrus, and glial inclusions in amyotrophic lateral sclerosis (ALS) show αS immunoreactivity (171).

Dementias with Extrapyramidal Signs that are not Associated with DLBs

Some patients have clinical AD with EPS not attributable to diffuse Lewy bodies. A very common cause is AD with secondary parkinsonism caused by neuroleptic treatment. Therefore, prior treatment with neuroleptics must be diligently sought and ruled out before diagnosing diffuse Lewy body disease antemortem. In some patients with AD, severe substantia nigra degeneration is associated with NFTs in the nigra, and a few have substantia nigra neuron loss without inclusions. The differential diagnosis for dementia with EPS also includes "mixed" dementia caused by AD and cerebrovascular disease, vascular dementia, progressive supranuclear palsy, and, more rarely, Parkinson's-dementia complex of Guam, Wilson's disease, and atypical multiple sclerosis.

SUMMARY AND FUTURE QUESTIONS

Alpha-synuclein is found in LBs and LNs in cortical neurons, as well as in the classic subcortical and brain-stem sites that are associated with parkinsonism. Most patients have both cortical and subcortical LBs. Within the liberal confines of "Lewy body disease" are the commonly occurring combinations of diffuse Lewy bodies with AD pathology (LBV), which has received varying designations, pDLBD, and PD with or without dementia (PDD). DLB is the most commonly used term, now that consensus diagnostic criteria (51) have been developed and widely applied. DLB includes cases with either LBV or pDLBD pathology. LBV usually presents with dementia or neuropsychiatric symptoms (e.g. depression, visual hallucinations, fluctuating confusional states) rather than parkinsonism. Mild EPS are usually present, but their severity, responsiveness to levodopa, and rate of progression are still poorly defined. DLB, broadly defined, appears to be the second most common cause of cognitive impairment in the elderly, trailing only AD and exceeding the prevalence of vascular dementia. Some evidence supports a higher cortical LB load in patients with dementia than in those with predominantly motor syndromes. However, most demented patients with diffuse LBs also have AD lesions, and the relative degree of AD and LB pathologies affects the clinical presentation. Alpha-synuclein is the final pathologic denominator for two groups of patients: patients with PD who develop dementia, and demented patients who develop atypical parkinsonism.

In contrast, the rarer pDLBD cases seem to be within the PD spectrum, with greater motor than cognitive impairment early in the course. Patients with pDLBD appear to have a higher predilection for dementia than other patients with PD but less than those with LBV. Our ability to distinguish LBV from pDLBD or AD clinically has yet to be validated prospectively, although diagnostic accuracy is improving with better-defined clinical measures and supportive testing. Characterization of the clinical EPS and neuropsychiatric profiles in both forms of DLB needs further delineation. The concept of "incidental" or asymptomatic LBs has been questioned, because careful clinical review suggests that mild EPS or cognitive changes may be common in these patients. Advanced age is frequently associated with mild EPS and cognitive slowing, and perhaps some of those "normal" elderly people will prove to have not truly "incidental" LBs.

Many fundamental questions remain unanswered. What is the specific role and dysfunction of αS in these diseases? Does wild type αS cause disease? Does β-synuclein play a neuropathologic role? Are LBs causally related to subcortical and neocortical neuron loss, as might be implied by the presence of dystrophic Lewy neurites in some cases, or are they merely an epiphenomenon? What is the relationship between LB and concomitant AD pathologies, given the finding of NAC (αS fragment) as a common constituent, and the occasional colocalization of αS and Tau (at the periphery of LBs). Do AD and PD share common or interactive mechanisms of neurodegeneration? Which pathology, AD or LB, is primarily responsible for severity of dementia and its specific features? Are LBs sufficient to explain dementia in pure DLBD or idiopathic PDD when AD changes are minimal or absent? Does neuropathologic and epidemiologic evidence exist for an association of AD and PD in cases of LBV, and is LBV a unique disease rather than a "variant" of AD or PD? Dementia associated with LBs has now been identified as a common and important problem in elderly people. Answers to the above questions require further extensive investigation and must be found before we can have highly accurate diagnoses and more effective treatments.

ACKNOWLEDGMENTS

Supported by the Department of Veteran's Affairs and NIH grant NIH AG10483.

REFERENCES

1. Lewy F. Paralysis agitans. I. Pathologische anatomie. In: Lewandowsky M, ed. *Handbuch der neurologie*. Berlin, Germany: Springer, 1912:920–933.
2. Parkinson J. *An essay on the shaking palsy*. London: Whittingham and Rowland, 1817.
3. Dickson DW. α–Synucleinand the Lewy body disorders. *Curr Opin Neurol* 2001;14:423–432.
4. Ueda K, Fukushima H, Masliah E, et al. Molecular cloning of cDNA encoding an unrecognized component of amyloid in Alzheimer disease. *Proc Natl Acad Sci USA* 1993;90(23):11282–11286.
5. Polymeropoulus MH, Lavedan C, Leroy E, et al. Mutations in alpha synuclein gene identified in families with Parkinson's disease. *Science* 1997;276:2045–2047.
6. Galvin JE, Uryu K, Lee VM-Y, et al. Axon pathology in Parkinson's disease and Lewy body dementia hippocampus contain alpha, beta, and gamma synuclein. *Proc Natl Acad Sci USA* 1999;96:13450–13455.
7. Hughes A, Daniel S, Blankson S, et al. A clinicopathologic study of 100 cases of Parkinson's disease. *Arch Neurol* 1993;50:140–148.
8. Braak H, Del Tredici K, Rüb U, et al. Staging of brain pathology related to sporadic Parkinson's disease. *Neurobiol Aging* 2003;24:197–211.
9. Duffy P, Tennyson V. Phase and electron microscopic observations of Lewy bodies and melanin granules in the substantia nigra and locus coeruleus in Parkinson's disease. *J Neuropathol Exp Neurol* 1965;24:398–414.
10. Forno L. The Lewy body in Parkinson's disease. In: Yahr N, Bergmann K, eds. *Parkinson's disease. Advances in Neurology*, Vol. 45. New York: Raven Press, 1986:35–43.
11. Galloway P, Mulvihill P, Perry G. Filaments of Lewy bodies contain insoluble cytoskeletal elements. *Am J Pathol* 1992;140:809–822.
12. Hill W, Lee V-Y, Hurtig H, et al. Epitopes located in spatially separate domains of each neurofilament subunit are present in Parkinson's disease Lewy bodies. *J Comp Neurol* 1991;309:150–160.
13. McKeith I. Dementia with Lewy Bodies. *Br J Psychiatry* 2002;180:144–147.
14. Ohama E, Ikuta F. Parkinson's disease: distribution of Lewy bodies and monoamine neuron system. *Acta Neuropathol* 1976;34:311–319.
15. Zweig R, Jankel W, Hedreen J, et al. The pedunculopontine nucleus in Parkinson's disease. *Ann Neurol* 1989;26:41–46.
16. Galvin JE, Lee VM, Schmdt ML, et al. Pathobiology of the Lewy Body. *Adv Neurol* 1999;80:313–324.
17. Bergeron C, Pollanen M. Lewy bodies in Alzheimer disease. One or two diseases? *Alzheimer Dis Assoc Disord* 1989;3:197–204.
18. Schmidt M, Murray J, Lee V-Y, et al. Epitope map of neurofilament protein domains in cortical and peripheral nervous system Lewy bodies. *Am J Pathol* 1991;139:53–65.
19. Tiller-Borcich J, Forno L. Parkinson's disease and dementia with neuronal inclusions in the cerebral cortex: Lewy bodies or Pick bodies? *J Neuropathol Exp Neurol* 1988;47:526–535.
20. Dickson D, Crystal H, Mattiace L, et al. Diffuse Lewy body disease: light and electron microscopic immunocytochemistry of senile plaques. *Acta Neuropathol* 1989;78:572–584.
21. Kuzuhara S, Mori H, Izumiyama N, et al. Lewy bodies are ubiquitinated: a light and electron microscopic immunocytochemical study. *Acta Neuropathol* 1988;75:345–353.
22. De Keyser J, Herregodts P, Ebinger G. The mesoneocortical dopamine neuron system. *Neurology* 1990;40:1660–1662.
23. Eggertson D, Sima A. Dementia with cerebral Lewy bodies: a mesocortical dopaminergic defect? *Arch Neurol* 1986;43:524–527.
24. Hamilton RL. Lewy bodies in Alzheimer's disease: a neuropathological review of 145 cases using alpha-synuclein immunohistochemistry. *Brain Pathol*. 2000;10(3):378–384.

25. Pappolla M. Lewy bodies of Parkinson's disease: immune electron microscopic demonstration of neurofilament antigens in constituent filaments. *Arch Pathol Lab Med* 1986;110:1I60–1163.
26. Pollanen M, Bergeron C, Weyer L. Deposition of detergent-resistant neurofilaments into Lewy body fibrils. *Brain Res* 1993;603:121–124.
27. McKeith I, Reid W, et al. Dementia with Lewy bodies. *Lancet Neurol* 2004;3:19–28.
28. Galloway P, Grundke-Iqbal I, Iqbal K, et al. Lewy bodies contain epitopes both shared and distinct from Alzheimer neurofibrillary tangles. *J Neuropathol Exp Neurol* 1988;47:654–663.
29. Love S, Saitoh T, Quijada S, et al. Alz-50, ubiquitin, and tau immunoreactivity of neurofibrillary tangles, Pick bodies and Lewy bodies. *J Neuropathol Exp Neurol* 1988;47:393–405.
30. Pollanen M, Dickson D, Bergeron C. Pathology and biology of the Lewy body. *J Neuropathol Exp Neurol* 1993;52:183–191.
31. Dev KD, Hofele K, Barbieri S, et al. Part II: Alpha-Synuclein and its molecular pathophysiological role in neurodegenerative disease. *Neuropharmacology* 2003;45:14–44.
32. Kruger R, Schulz JB. The alpha-synuclein pathway to neurodegeneration. In: Tolosa E, Schulz B, McKeith IG et al., eds. *Neurodegenerative disorders associated with alpha-synuclein pathology.* Barcelona, Spain, Ars Medica, 2002:11–22.
33. Mosimann UP, McKeith IG. Dementia with Lewy bodies—diagnosis and treatment. *Swiss Med Wkly* 2003;133:131–142.
34. Ishizawa T, Mattila P, Davies P, et al. Colocalization of tau and alpha-synuclein epitopes in Lewy bodies. *J Neuropathol Exp Neurol* 2003;62(4):389–397.
35. Kwak S, Masaki T, Ishiuri S, et al. Multicatalytic proteinase is present in Lewy bodies and neurofibrillary tangles in diffuse Lewy body disease brains. *Neurosci Left* 1991;128:21–24.
36. Iwatsubo T, Nakano I, Fukunaga K, et al. Ca2+/calmodulin-dependent protein kinase II immunoreactivity in Lewy bodies. *Acta Neurol Pathol* 1991;82:159–163.
37. Lichtenberg-Kraag B, Mandelkow E, Biernat J, et al. Phosphorylation-dependent epitopes of neurofilament antibodies on tau protein and relationship with Alzheimer tau. *Proc Natl Acad Sci USA* 1992;89:5384–5388.
38. Hirano A, Zimmerman H. Alzheimer neurofibrillary changes: a topographic study. *Arch Neurol* 1962;7:227–247.
39. Dickson D, Ruan D, Crystal H, et al. Hippocampal degeneration differentiates diffuse Lewy body disease (DLBD) from Alzheimer's disease: light and electron microscopic immunocytochemistry of CA 2-3 neurites specific to DLBD. *Neurology* 1991;41:402–409.
40. Wu E, Lipton R, Dickson D. Amyloid angiopathy in diffuse Lewy body disease. *Neurology* 1992;42:2131–2135.
41. Hansen L, Salmon D, Galasko D, et al. The Lewy body variant of Alzheimer's disease: a clinical and pathological entity. *Neurology* 1990;40:1–8.
42. Hansen L, Masliah E, Terry R, et al. A neuropathological subset of Alzheimer's disease with concomitant Lewy body disease and spongiform change. *Acta Neuropathol* 1989;78:194–201.
43. Tiraboschi P, Hansen LA, Alford M, et al. Cholinergic dysfunction in diseases with Lewy bodies. *Neurology* 2000;54:407–411.
44. Piggott MA, Marshall EF, Thomas N, et al. Striatal dopaminergic markers in dementia with Lewy bodies, Alzheimer's and Parkinson's disease: rostrocaudal distribution. *Brain* 1999;122:1449–1468.
45. Gibb W, Ersi M, Lees A. Clinical and pathological features of diffuse cortical Lewy body disease (Lewy body dementia). *Brain* 1985;110:1131–1153.
46. Dickson D, Davies P, Mayeux R, et al. Diffuse Lewy body disease. *Acta Neuropathol* 1987;75:8–15.
47. Perry R, Irving D, Blessed G, et al. Senile dementia of Lewy body type. A clinical and neuropathologically distinct form of Lewy body dementia in the elderly. *J Neurol Sci* 1990;95:119–139.
48. Kosaka K. Diffuse Lewy body disease in Japan. *J Neurol* 1990;237(3):197–204.
49. Hansen L, Masliah E, Quijada-Fawcett S, et al. Entorhinal neurofibrillary tangles in Alzheimer disease with Lewy bodies. *Neurosci Left* 1991;129:269–272.
50. Ditter S, Mirra S. Neuropathologic and clinical features of Parkinson's disease in Alzheimer's disease patients. *Neurology* 1987;37:754–760.
51. McKeith IG, Galasko D, Kosaka K, et al. Consensus guidelines for the clinical and pathologic diagnosis of dementia with Lewy bodies (DLB): report of the consortium on DLB international workshop. *Neurology* 1996;47(5):1113–1124.
52. Khachaturian Z. Diagnosis of Alzheimer's disease. *Arch Neurol* 1985;42:1097–1105.
53. Hohl U, Tiraboschi P, Hansen L, et al. Diagnostic accuracy of dementia with Lewy bodies. *Arch Neurol* 2000;57:347–351.
54. Braak H, Braak E. Neuropathological staging of Alzheimer-related changes. *Acta Neuropathol* 1991;82:239–259.
55. Terry R, Hansen L, De Teresa R, et al. Senile dementia of the Alzheimer type without neocortical neurofibrillary tangles. *J Neuropathol Exp Neurol* 1987;46:262–268.
56. Hansen LA, Masliah E, Galasko D, et al. Plaque-only Alzheimer disease is usually the lewy body variant, and vice versa. *J Neuropathol Exp Neurol* 1993;52(6):648–654.
57. Aarsland D, Ballard C, McKeith I. et al. Comparison of extrapyramidal signs in dementia with Lewy bodies and Parkinson's disease. *J Neuropsychiatry Clin Neurosci* 2001;13(3):374–379.
58. Samuel W, Galasko D, Masliah E, et al. Neocortical Lewy body counts correlate with dementia in the Lewy body variant of Alzheimer's disease. *J Neuropathol Exp Neurol* 1996;55(1):44–52.
59. Doody RS, Stevens JC, Beck C, Dubinsky, et al. Practice parameter: management of dementia (an evidence-based review). Report of the Quality Standards Subcommittee of the American Academy of Neurology. *Neurology.* 2001;56(9):1154–1166.
60. Crystal H, Dickson D, Lizardi J, et al. Antemortem diagnosis of diffuse Lewy body disease. *Neurology* 1990;40:1523–1528.
61. Lennox G, Lowe J, Landon M, et al. Diffuse Lewy body disease: correlative neuropathology using antiubiquitin

immunocytochemistry. *J Neurol Neurosurg Psychiatry* 1989;52:1236–1247.
62. Burkhardt C, Filley C, Kleinschmidt-DeMasters B, et al. Diffuse Lewy body disease and progressive dementia. *Neurology* 1988;38:1520–1528.
63. Mega MS, Masterman DL, Benson DF, et al. Dementia with Lewy bodies: reliability and validity of clinical and pathologic criteria. *Neurology* 1996;47(6):1403–1409.
64. McKeith IG, Ballard CG, Perry RH, et al. Prospective validation of consensus criteria for the diagnosis of dementia with Lewy bodies. *Neurology* 2000;54(5):1050–1058.
65. Verghese J, Crystal HA, Dickson DW, et al. Validity of clinical criteria for the diagnosis of dementia with Lewy bodies. *Neurology* 1999;53(9):1974–1982.
66. Lopez OL, Becker JT, Kaufer DI, et al. Research evaluation and prospective diagnosis of dementia with Lewy bodies. *Arch Neurol* 2002;59(1):43–46.
67. Merdes AR, Hansen LA, Jeste DV, et al. Influence of Alzheimer pathology on clinical diagnostic accuracy in dementia with Lewy bodies. *Neurology* 2003;60(10):1586–1590.
68. Thai L, Galasko D, Katzman R, et al.. Clinical neurological findings predict Lewy bodies associated with AD at autopsy. *Neurology* 1993;43(4)(Suppl. 2):A336.
69. Mark M, Sage J, Dickson D, et al. Levodopa nonresponsive Lewy body parkinsonism: clinicopathologic study of two cases. *Neurology* 1992;42:1323–1327.
70. Sima A, Clark A, Sternberger N, et al. Lewy body dementia without Alzheimer changes. *Can J Neurol Sci* 1986;13:490–497.
71. Huber S, Paulson G, Shuttleworth E. Relationship of motor symptoms, intellectual impairment, and depression in Parkinson's disease. *J Neurol Neurosurg Psychiatry* 1988;51:855–858.
72. Connor DJ, Salmon DP, Sandy TJ, et al. Cognitive profiles of autopsy-confirmed Lewy body variant vs. pure Alzheimer disease. *Arch Neurol* 1998;55(7):994–1000 [published erratum appears in *Arch Neurol* 1998 Oct;55(10):1352].
73. Byrne E, Lennox G, Lowe J, et al. Diffuse Lewy body disease: clinical features in 15 cases. *J Neurol Neurosurg Psychiatry* 1989;52:709–717.
74. Lichter D, Corbett A, Fitzgibbon G, et al. Cognitive and motor dysfunction in Parkinson's disease. Clinical, performance, and computed tomographic correlations. *Arch Neurol* 1988;45:854–860.
75. Ferman TJ, Smith GE, Boeve BF, et al. DLB fluctuations: specific features that reliably differentiate DLB from AD and normal aging. *Neurology* 2004;62(2):181–187.
76. Perry EK, McKeith I, Thompson P, et al. Topography, extent, and clinical relevance of neurochemical deficits in dementia of Lewy body type, Parkinson's disease, and Alzheimer's disease. *Ann NY Acad Sci* 1991;640:197–202.
77. Wesnes K, McKeith I, Ferrara R, et al. Predicting response to Rivastigmine in dementia with Lewy bodies. *Eur Neuropsychopharmacol* 2002;2002:S373.
78. Boeve BF, Silber MH, Parisi JE, et al. Synucleinopathy pathology and REM sleep behavior disorder plus dementia or parkinsonism. *Neurology* 2003;61(1):40–45.
79. Ballard C, O'Brien J, Gray A, et al. Attention and fluctuating attention in patients with dementia with Lewy bodies and Alzheimer disease. *Arch Neurol* 2001;58(6):977–982.
80. Briel RC, McKeith IG, Barker WA, et al. EEG findings in dementia with Lewy bodies and Alzheimer's disease. *J Neurol Neurosurg Psychiatry* 1999;66(3):401–403.
81. Barber PA, Varma AR, Lloyd JJ, et al. The electroencephalogram in dementia with Lewy bodies. *Acta Neurol Scand* 2000;101(1):53–56.
82. Yamamoto T, Imai T. A case of diffuse Lewy body and Alzheimer's diseases with periodic synchronous discharges. *J Neuropathol Exp Neurol* 1988;47(5):536–548.
83. Walker MP, Ayre GA, Cummings JL, et al. Quantifying fluctuation in dementia with Lewy bodies, Alzheimer's disease, and vascular dementia. *Neurology* 2000;54(8):1616–1625.
84. Walker MP, Ayre GA, Perry EK, et al. Quantification and characterization of fluctuating cognition in dementia with Lewy bodies and Alzheimer's disease. *Dement Geriatr Cogn Disord* 2000;11(6):327–335.
85. Walker MP, Ayre GA, Cummings JL, et al. The clinician assessment of fluctuation and the one day fluctuation assessment scale. Two methods to assess fluctuating confusion in dementia. *Br J Psychiatry* 2000;177:252–256.
86. Ballard C, Shaw F, McKeith I, et al. High prevalence of neurovascular instability in neurodegenerative dementias. *Neurology* 1998;51(6):1760–1762.
87. Doty RL, Riklan M, Deems DA, et al. The olfactory and cognitive deficits of Parkinson's disease: evidence for independence. *Ann Neurol* 1989;25(2):166–171.
88. McShane RH, Nagy Z, Esiri MM. et al. Anosmia in dementia is associated with Lewy bodies rather than Alzheimer's pathology. *J Neurol Neurosurg Psychiatry* 2001;70(6):739–743.
89. Olichney JM, Murphy C, Hofstetter CR, et al. Anosmia is very common in Lewy body variant of Alzheimer's disease. *Neurology* 2002;58 (3):A486.
90. Barber R, Ballard C, McKeith IG, et al. MRI volumetric study of dementia with Lewy bodies: a comparison with AD and vascular dementia. *Neurology* 2000;54(6):1304–1309.
91. Lobotesis K, Fenwick JD, Phipps A, et al. Occipital hypoperfusion on SPECT in dementia with Lewy bodies but not AD. *Neurology* 2001;56(5):643–649.
92. Ransmayr G, Seppi K, Donnemiller E, et al. Striatal dopamine transporter function in dementia with Lewy bodies and Parkinson's disease. *Eur J Nucl Med*;28:1523–1528.
93. Walker Z, Costa DC, Walker RW, et al. Differentiation of dementia with Lewy bodies from Alzheimer's disease using a dopaminergic presynaptic ligand. *J Neurol Neurosurg Psychiatry* 2002;73(2):134–140.
94. Jellinger KA. Age-associated prevalence and risk factors of Lewy body pathology in a general population. *Acta Neuropathol (Berl)* 2003;106(4):383–384.
95. Cercy SP, Bylsma FW. Lewy bodies and progressive dementia: a critical review and mean-analysis. *J Int Neuropsychol Soc* 1997;3:179–194.
96. Walker Z, Allen RL, Shergill S, et al. Three year survival in patients with a clinical diagnosis of dementia with Lewy bodies. *Int Geriatr Psychiatry* 2000;15:267–273.
97. Galasko D, Saitoh T, Xia Y, et al. The apolipoprotein E allele epsilon 4 is overrepresented in patients with the Lewy body variant of Alzheimer's disease. *Neurology* 1994;44(10):1950–1951.

98. Katzman R, Galasko D, Saitoh T, et al. Genetic evidence that the Lewy body variant is indeed a phenotypic variant of Alzheimer's disease. *Brain Cogn* 1995; 28(3):259–265.
99. Olichney JM, Hansen LA, Galasko D, et al. The apolipoprotein E epsilon 4 allele is associated with increased neuritic plaques and cerebral amyloid angiopathy in Alzheimer's disease and Lewy body variant. *Neurology* 1996;47(1):190–196.
100. Rosenberg CK, Pericak-Vance MA, Saunders AM, et al. Lewy body and Alzheimer pathology in a family with the amyloid-beta precursor protein APP717 gene mutation. *Acta Neuropathol (Berl)* 2000;100(2):145–152.
101. Houlden H, Crook R, Dolan RJ, et al. A novel presenilin mutation (M233V) causing very early onset Alzheimer's disease with Lewy bodies. *Neurosci Lett* 2001;313(1-2):93–95.
102. Yokota O, Terada S, Ishizu H, et al. NACP/alpha-synuclein, NAC, and beta-amyloid pathology of familial Alzheimer's disease with the E184D presenilin-1 mutation: a clinicopathological study of two autopsy cases. *Acta Neuropathol (Berl)* 2002;104(6):637–648.
103. Levy G, Tang MX, Cote LJ, et al. Do risk factors for Alzheimer's disease predict dementia in Parkinson's disease? An exploratory study. *Mov Disord* 2002; 17(2):250–257.
104. Ballard C, O'Brien J, Morris CM, et al. The progression of cognitive impairment in dementia with Lewy bodies, vascular dementia and Alzheimer's disease. *Int J Geriatr Psychiatry* 2001;16(5):499–503.
105. Armstrong TP, Hansen LA, Salmon DP, et al. Rapidly progressive dementia in a patient with Lewy body variant of Alzheimer's disease. *Neurology* 1991;41: 1178–1180.
106. Lopez OL, Wisniewski S, Hamilton RL, et al. Predictors of progression in patients with AD and Lewy bodies. *Neurology* 2000;54:1774–1779.
107. Kosaka K, Yoshimura M, Ikeda K, et al. Diffuse type of Lewy body disease: progressive dementia with abundant cortical Lewy bodies and senile changes of varying degree. A new disease? *Clin Neuropathol* 1984;3:185–192.
108. Hughes A, Daniel S, Kilford L, et al. Accuracy of clinical diagnosis of idiopathic Parkinson's disease: a clinicopathological study of 100 cases. *J Neurol Neurosurg Psychiatry* 1992;55:181–184.
109. Perry E, McKeith I, Thompson P, et al. Topography, extent, and clinical relevance of neurochemical deficits in dementia of Lewy body type, Parkinson's disease, and Alzheimer's disease. *Ann NY Acad Sci* 1991; 640:197–202.
110. Langlais PJ, Thal L, Hansen L, et al. Neurotransmitters in basal ganglia and cortex of Alzheimer's disease with and without Lewy bodies. *Neurology* 1993;43(10): 1927–1934.
111. Tiraboschi P, Hansen LA, Alford M, et al. Early and widespread cholinergic losses differentiate dementia with Lewy bodies from Alzheimer disease. *Arch Gen Psychiatry* 2002;59(10):946–951.
112. Lees A. Parkinson's disease and dementia. *Lancet* 1985;1:43–44.
113. Martin W, Loewenson R, Resch J, et al. Parkinson's disease. A clinical analysis of 100 patients. *Neurology* 1973;23:783–790.
114. American Psychiatric Association. *Diagnostic and statistical manual of mental disorders*. 4th ed, text rev. Washington, DC: 2000.
115. Brown R, Marsden C. How common is dementia in Parkinson's disease? *Lancet* 1984;2:1262–1265.
116. Pirozzolo F, Hansch E, Mortimer J, et al. Dementia in Parkinson disease: a neuropsychological analysis. *Brain Cogn* 1982;1:71–83.
117. Albert M. Subcortical dementia. In: Katzman R, Terry R, Bick K, eds. *Aging*, Vol. 7. New York: Raven Press, 1978:173–180.
118. Albert M, Feldman R, Willis A. The 'subcortical dementia' of progressive supranuclear palsy. *J Neurol Neurosurg Psychiatry* 1974;37:121–130.
119. Brown R, Marsden C. 'Subcortical dementia': the neuropsychological evidence. *Neuroscience* 1988;25(2): 363–387.
120. Emre M. Dementia associated with Parkinson's disease. *Lancet Neurol* 2003;2:229–237.
121. Mayeux R, Stern Y, Rosenstein R, et al. An estimate of the prevalence of dementia in idiopathic Parkinson's disease. *Arch Neurol* 1988;45:260–262.
122. Mayeux R, Chen J, Mirabello E, et al. An estimate of the incidence of dementia in idiopathic Parkinson's disease. *Neurology* 1990;40:1573–1577.
123. Mayeux R, Denaro J, Hemenegildo N, et al. A population-based investigation of Parkinson's disease with and without dementia. *Arch Neurol* 1992;49:492–497.
124. Aarsland D, Andersen K, Larsen JP, et al. Prevalence and characteristics of dementia in Parkinson disease: an 8-year prospective study. *Arch Neurol* 2003;60(3): 387–392.
125. Aevarsson O, Svanborg A, Skoog, I. Seven-year survival rate after age 85 years: relation to Alzheimer disease and vascular dementia. *Arch Neurol* 1998;55: 1226–1232.
126. Katzman R. The prevalence and malignancy of Alzheimer disease: a major killer. *Arch Neurol* 1976; 33:217–218.
127. Levy G, Tang MX, Louis ED, et al. The association of incident dementia with mortality in PD. *Neurology* 2002;59(11):1708–1713.
128. Harada H, Nishikawa S, Takahaski K. Epidemiology of Parkinson's disease in a Japanese city. *Arch Neurol* 1983;40:151–154.
129. Kurland L. Epidemiology: incidence, geographic distribution and genetic considerations. In: Field W, ed. *Pathogenesis and treatment of parkinsonism*. Springfield, IL: Charles C Thomas Publisher, 1958:5–43.
130. Rajput A, Offord K, Beard C, et al. Epidemiology of parkinsonism: incidence, classification and mortality. *Ann Neurol* 1984;16:278–283.
131. Schoenberg B, Anderson D, Haerer A. Prevalence of Parkinson's disease in the biracial population of Copiah County, Mississippi. *Neurology* 1985;35:841–845.
132. Sutcliffe R. Parkinson's disease in the district of the Northampton Health Authority, United Kingdom: a study of prevalence and disability. *Acta Neurol Scand* 1985;72:363–379.
133. Marder K, Flood P, Cote L, et al. A pilot study of risk factors for dementia in Parkinson's disease. *Mov Disord* 1990;5:156–161.
134. Ebmeier K, Calder S, Crawford J, et al. Clinical features predicting dementia in idiopathic Parkinson's disease: a follow-up study. *Neurology* 1990;40:1222–1224.
135. Zetusky W, Jankovic J, Pirozzolo F. The heterogeneity of Parkinson's disease: clinical and prognostic implications. *Neurology* 1985;35:522–526.
136. Hershey L, Feldman B, Kim K, et al. Tremor at onset. *Arch Neurol* 1991;48:1049–1051.

137. Jankovic J, McDermott M, Carter J, et al. Variable expression of Parkinson's disease: a baseline analysis of the Datatop cohort. *Neurology* 1990;40:1529–1534.
138. Mayeux R, Stem Y. Intellectual dysfunction and dementia in Parkinson's disease. In: Mayeux R, Rosen W, eds. *Advances in neurology*, Vol. 38. New York: Raven Press, 1983:211–227.
139. Mortimer J, Pirozzolo F, Hansch E, et al. Relationship of motor symptoms to intellectual deficits in Parkinson's disease. *Neurology* 1982;32:133–137.
140. Richards M, Stem Y, Marder K, et al. Relationships between extrapyramidal signs and cognitive function in a community-dwelling cohort of patients with Parkinson's. *Ann Neurol* 1993;33:267–274.
141. Diamond S, Markham C, Hoehn M, et al. Multi-center study of Parkinson mortality with early versus late dopa treatment. *Ann Neurol* 1987;22:8–12.
142. Martilla R, Rinne U. Dementia in Parkinson's disease. *Acta Neurol Scand* 1976;54:431–441.
143. Kurtzke J, Murphy F. The changing patterns of death rates in parkinsonism. *Neurology* 1990;40:42–49.
144. Rajput A, Rozdilsky B, Rajput A, et al. Levodopa efficacy and pathological basis of Parkinson syndrome. *Clin Neuropharmacol* 1990;13:553–558.
145. Hofman A, Shulte W, Tarija T, et al. History of dementia and Parkinson's disease in 1st-degree relatives of patients with Alzheimer disease. *Neurology* 1989;39:1589–1592.
146. Ross GW, Abbott RD, Petrovitch H, et al. Association of coffee and caffeine intake with the risk of Parkinson disease. *JAMA* 2000;283(20):2674–2679.
147. Boller F, Mizutani T, Roessmann U. Parkinson disease, dementia, and Alzheimer's disease: clinicopathological correlations. *Ann Neurol* 1980;7:329–335.
148. Paulus W, Jellinger K. The neuropathologic basis of different clinical subgroups of Parkinson's disease. *J Neuropathol Exp Neurol* 1991;50(6):743–755.
149. Gaspar P, Gray F. Dementia in idiopathic Parkinson's disease. *Acta Neuropathol* 1984;64:43–52.
150. Hakim A, Mathieson G. Dementia and Parkinson disease: a neuropathologic study. *Neurology* 1979;29:1209–1214.
151. Heston L. Genetic studies of dementia: with emphasis on Parkinson's disease and Alzheimer neuropathology. In: Mortimer J Schuman L, eds. *Epidemiology of dementia*. New York: Oxford University Press, 1981.
152. Perry R, Tomlinson B, Candy J, et al. Cortical cholinergic deficit in mentally impaired parkinsonian patients. *Lancet* 1983;2:789–790.
153. Chui H, Mortimer J, Slager U, et al. Pathologic correlates of dementia in Parkinson's disease. *Arch Neurol* 1986;43:991–995.
154. Mahler M, Cummings J. Alzheimer disease and the dementia of Parkinson's disease: comparative investigations. *Alzheimer Dis Assoc Disord* 1990;4:133–149.
155. Zarranz JJ, Alegre J, Gomez-Esteban JC, et al. The new mutation, E46K, of alpha-synuclein causes parkinson and Lewy body dementia. *Ann Neurol* 2004;55(2):164–173.
156. Rinne J, Rummukainen J, Paljarvi L, et al. Dementia in Parkinson's disease is related to neuronal loss in the medial substantia nigra. *Ann Neurol* 1989;26:47–50.
157. Jellinger K. Pathology of parkinsonism. In: Fahn S, Marsden C, Jenner P et al., eds. *Recent developments in parkinsonism*. New York: Raven Press, 1986:33–66.
158. Whitehouse P, Hedreen J, White C, et al. Basal forebrain neurons in the dementia of Parkinson's disease. *Ann Neurol* 1983;13:243–248.
159. Candy J, Perry R, Perry E, et al. Pathological changes in the nucleus basalis of Meynert in Alzheimer's and Parkinson's disease. *J Neurol Sci* 1983;59:277–289.
160. Tagliavini F, Pilleri G, Bouras C, et al. The basal nucleus of Meynert in idiopathic Parkinson's disease. *Acta Neurol Scand* 1984;69:20–28.
161. Heilig C, Knopman D, Mastri A, Frey W. Dementia without Alzheimer pathology. *Neurology* 1985;35:762–765.
162. Leroi I, Brandt J, Reich SG, et al. Randomized placebo-controlled trial of donepezil in cognitive impairment in Parkinson's disease. *Int J Geriatr Psychiatry* 2004;19(1):1–8.
163. Aarsland D, Laake K, Larsen JP, et al. Donepezil for cognitive impairment in Parkinson's disease: a randomised controlled study. *J Neurol Neurosurg Psychiatry* 2002;72(6):708–712.
164. Duda JE, Giasson BI, Mabon ME, et al. Novel antibodies to synuclein show abundant striatal pathology in Lewy body diseases. *Ann Neurol* 2002;52(2):205–210.
165. McKeith I, Del Ser T, Spano P, et al. Efficacy of rivastigmine in dementia with Lewy bodies: a randomised, double-blind, placebo-controlled international study. *Lancet* 2000;356(9247):2031–2036.
166. McKeith I, Fairbairn A, Perry R, et al. Neuroleptic sensitivity in patients with senile dementia of Lewy body type. *Br Med J* 1992;305(6855):673–678.
167. Sano M, Ernesto C, Thomas RG, et al. A controlled trial of selegiline, alpha-tocopherol, or both as treatment for Alzheimer's disease. The Alzheimer's Disease Cooperative Study. *N Engl J Med* 1997;336(17):1216–1222.
168. Kang JH, Kim KS. Enhanced oligomerization of the alpha-synuclein mutant by the Cu, Zn-superoxide dismutase and hydrogen peroxide system. *Mol Cells* 2003;15(1):87–93.
169. Gibb W, Lees A. The relevance of the Lewy body to the pathogenesis of idiopathic Parkinson's disease. *J Neurol Neurosurg Psychiatry* 1988;51:745–752.
170. Perry R, Irving D, Tomlinson B. Lewy body prevalence in the aging brain: relationship to neuropsychiatric disorders, Alzheimer-type pathology and catecholaminergic nuclei. *J Neurol Sci* 1990;100:223–233.
171. Galvin JE, Lee VM, Trojanowski JQ. Synucleinopathies: clinical and pathological implications. *Arch Neurol* 2001;58(2):186–190.

12

Cognitive and Behavioral Changes in the Parkinson-Plus Syndromes

Sharon Cohen[1] and Morris Freedman[2]

[1]*Department of Medicine (Neurology) and Graduate Department of Speech Pathology, University of Toronto;* [2]*Department of Medicine (Neurology), Baycrest Centre for Geriatric Care, University of Toronto, Toronto, Canaada*

The parkinson-plus syndromes are akinetic-rigid disorders that are clinically and pathologically distinct from idiopathic Parkinson's disease (PD). Attention has recently been focused on characterizing the cognitive and behavioral abnormalities common to these syndromes, thereby further assisting in clinical diagnosis and enhancing our understanding of these conditions. Notwithstanding current debate regarding the relative merits of grouping versus separating out some of the parkinson-plus syndromes, this chapter addresses behavioral abnormalities reported for the following clinical entities: progressive supranuclear palsy, multiple-system atrophy (including olivopontocerebellar atrophy, striatonigral degeneration, and Shy–Drager syndrome), corticobasal degeneration, Machado–Joseph's disease, parkinsonism-dementia/amyotrophic lateral sclerosis (ALS), postencephalitic parkinsonism (PEP), Creutzfeldt–Jakob disease, and Gerstmann–Straussler–Scheinker disease. Other conditions in which parkinsonism may occur in association with cognitive and behavioral abnormalities are listed in Table 12-1.

PROGRESSIVE SUPRANUCLEAR PALSY (PSP)

Progressive supranuclear palsy (PSP) is a sporadic neurodegenerative disease that was first reported by Steele et al. in 1964 (1). Its characteristic clinical features include early gait disturbance with falls, axial rigidity with nuchal dystonia, cognitive and behavioral abnormalities, and supranuclear gaze abnormalities.

The nine patients described by Steele et al. (1) and Steele (2) developed personality changes and mild mental deterioration early in their clinical course. Most of the patients displayed mild to moderate cognitive impairment, whereas two developed severe dementia. Prominent features were irritability, indifference, lability of mood, and impairment of memory, calculation, abstract thinking, insight, attention, and comprehension. Steele (3) noted that the mental changes in PSP are rarely severe and are usually limited to altered personality and forgetfulness.

Albert et al. (4) studied 5 patients with PSP and reviewed 42 cases from the literature. The specific pattern of deficits led these authors to reintroduce the concept of *subcortical dementia*, a term coined earlier by von Stockert with reference to postencephalitic parkinsonism (5). Using PSP as a model, these authors described subcortical dementia as deficits in activation and timing characterized by bradyphrenia (slowness of thought processes), personality change (apathy or depression), forgetfulness rather than true memory impairment, and impaired manipulation of acquired knowledge (calculating and abstracting). Aphasia, apraxia, and agnosia, which are prominent in the "cortical dementias," were absent. They attributed subcortical dementia to a disruption of subcortical frontal connections

TABLE 12-1. Additional causes of parkinsonism and mental status alteration

Diagnosis	Cognitive abnormalities	Neuropsychiatric abnormalities[a]
Alzheimer's disease	+ + +	2
Pick's disease	+ + +	2p
Dementia with Lewy bodies	+ + +	2p
Normal pressure hydrocephalus[b]	+ + +	1
Binswanger's disease	+ + +	2
Multiinfarct state	+ +	2
Depression	+ +	always present
Dementia pugilistica	+ + +	2
Huntington's disease	+ + +	2p
Non-Guamanian amyotrophic lateral sclerosis	+	1
Pallidopontonigral degeneration	+ + +	1
Dentatorubropallido-\Lluysian atrophy	+ +	1
Familial parkinsonism with depression: hypoventilation	+ +	2p
Wilson's disease[b]	+ +	2p
Hallervorden–Spatz disease	+ + +	2
Basal ganglia calcification	+	1[c]
Manganese toxicity	+ +	2p

Others: Cerebral anoxia (including carbon monoxide poisoning), toxins (cyanide, disulfiram, valproate), central nervous system infections (sarcoid, toxoplasmosis, cryptococcosis, human immunodeficiency virus), subdural hematomas, obstructive hydrocephalus, brain tumors, multiple sclerosis, other rarer neurodegenerative and neurometabolic disorders

[a]Major changes in personality, mood, affect, or psychotic features resulting from the underlying disease.
[b]Untreated.
[c]May be prominent in some.
Cognitive abnormalities: + occasionally present; + + often present; + + + invariably present.
Major psychiatric abnormalities: 1, uncommon; 2, common; p, often prominent and early.

required for activating frontal lobe function. In 1985, Freedman and Albert (6) suggested that the terms *frontosubcortical* or *frontal system dementia* may be more appropriate. Notably, McHugh and Folstein (7) described a similar subcortical dementia syndrome in Huntington's disease.

Subsequent studies support the concept that frontal subcortical dementia characterizes the cognitive deficits in PSP (8–16). However, some evidence of cortical cognitive deficits has also been presented (17–23). A few investigators have found no evidence of substantial cognitive impairment in PSP (24–26).

Litvan (12) reported that the combination of severely slowed information processing and early, marked executive dysfunction was characteristic of dementia in PSP. Van der Hurk and Hodges (13) reported that episodic memory and recognition memory were relatively unharmed in patients with PSP compared to those with Alzheimer's disease. Pirtosek et al. (15) noted more prevalent deficits on selective attention tasks in PSP than in multiple-system atrophy (MSA), idiopathic Parkinson's disease (IPD), and corticobasal degeneration (CBD), using event-related potentials (ERP).

Maher et al. (8) found that 18 of 27 patients with PSP had intellectual impairment (9 mild and 9 marked), demonstrated by formal neuropsychological assessment, with particular difficulty performing frontal lobe tasks. Dubois et al. (9) found a frontal lobe profile of cognitive disturbance in patients with PSP, as evidenced by their performance on verbal fluency tasks, a revised version of the Wisconsin Card Sorting Test (WCST), and agraphic series, and during observation for imitation and utilization behavior. Impaired imitation and utilization behavior had previously been noted in PSP by Lhermitte (10), who postulated that the underlying mechanism was a loss of frontal lobe inhibition on parietal cortex.

Ghika et al. (23) described stimulus-oriented frontal behavioral signs in 17 patients with PSP. These signs included visual grasping, wherein gaze was attracted and involuntarily fixed to a mirror or TV set, compulsive utilization behaviors, such as picking up and replacing the telephone, echolalia, and echopraxia. Other stimulus-evoked behaviors included those of a patient who was unable to stand voluntarily, but who stood spontaneously when his lap belt was unbuckled or when a table in front of him was moved away.

Esmonde et al. (19) reported that selective language output deficits in PSP were compatible with the *dynamic aphasia* described in frontal lobe lesions, characterized by intact naming of pictures and verbal descriptions; intact word and sentence comprehension; impaired letter and category fluency; and impaired sentence completion.

Pillon et al. (11) compared severity of cognitive impairment in patients with PSP, Huntington's disease (HD), Parkinson's disease (PD), and Alzheimer's disease (AD) and looked for group-specific differences in the pattern of impairment after matching patients for overall degree of intellectual deterioration. Although it is unclear how selection bias was controlled, dementia was reported to be more severe in patients with PSP (n = 45) than in patients with PD (n = 164). In the earliest stages of cognitive impairment, the PSP group scored considerably lower on all frontal lobe tests (WCST, lexical fluency, and graphic series) than the groups with PD and AD. They also found more severe behavioral disorders in PSP than in the groups with PD or HD on tests of imitation, utilization behavior, and indifference. Patients with PSP had more difficulty performing mental control tasks (i.e, tests of attention) than did patients with PD matched for degree of dementia. Furthermore, patients with PSP performed more poorly on similarities testing than patients with HD or PD and achieved lower gestural and linguistic scores than did patients with AD or HD matched for mild degree of dementia. On the basis of their findings, the authors make a case for dividing subcortical dementia into the following subtypes: frontal lobe–like abnormalities in PSP, concentration and acquisition disorders in HD, and undifferentiated abnormalities in PD.

Robbins et al. (27) compared the performance of patients with PSP, PD, and MSA on tasks sensitive to frontal lobe function, including an attentional set-shifting test, a planning test (the Tower of London), and a test of spatial working memory. Although all groups were impaired on these tasks, patients with PSP demonstrated more severe disturbance than the other groups did on the attentional set-shifting test. On the planning task, patients with PSP demonstrated lengthened initial thinking time, unchanged subsequent thinking time, and impaired accuracy of problem solving. This pattern of impairment was similar to that seen in the PD group and dissimilar to that in the MSA group.

Litvan et al. (28) sought to clarify the extent and nature of memory impairment in PSP. Twelve patients with PSP and 12 age-matched healthy control subjects underwent a comprehensive battery of standardized tests to assess various aspects of verbal memory, including learning, information scanning, consolidation, and retrieval. Substantial impairment was found on several aspects of memory and included abnormally rapid forgetting, increased sensitivity to interference, and difficulty using strategic long-term memory search mechanisms. Recognition memory was less impaired than recall, in keeping with what has been reported for other subcortical dementias (5). Nevertheless, sufficient recognition and retrieval deficits were present to suggest that a loss of stored information also occurred, and that impairments were not merely the result of a disordered timing mechanism for recall, as postulated by Albert et al. (4).

Evidence for cortical involvement in cognitive dysfunction comes largely from case reports of PSP patients with aphasia and apraxia, deficits generally considered to represent cortical pathology. Mochizuki et al. (17) and Boeve et al. (18) report two separate cases of PSP presenting with primary progression aphasia (PPA). In both cases, language symptoms predated other PSP findings by years. In the case of PSP findings (18), apraxia of speech was also present.

Apraxia of eyelid opening in PSP has been reported by Ghika et al. (23). Ideomotor apraxia (IMA) has been assessed by Pharr et al. (21), using the Florida Apraxia Battery, and by Leiguarda et al. (22), using an alternative comprehensive apraxia battery. Pharr et al. (21) found evidence of IMA in patients with PSP and in patients with corticobasal degeneration in comparison to healthy control subjects. IMA was, however, less severe in patients with PSP than in patients with CBD, a difference that the authors found helpful in distinguishing these often confused syndromes. Leiguarda et al. (22) compared IMA in patients with PSP, IPD, and MSA and found more prevalent errors in the PSP group than in the IPD group, and no evidence of apraxia in the patients with MSA. PSP apractic errors were bilateral, mainly spatial, and present for transitive and intransitive limb items.

Mechanisms leading to cognitive impairment in PSP remain unknown. Pathologic findings include prominent neuronal loss, gliosis, and neurofibrillary tangles in several subcortical nuclei, with minimal changes in cerebral cortex (1,2). Cerebral atrophy, especially frontotemporal, has been noted (29). Bigio et al. (30) proposed that cortical tau burden is considerably greater in PSP patients with cognitive impairment than in those without cognitive impairment. Yamauchi et al. (31) implicated neurofibrillary degeneration in layer 3 of the association cortex and concluded that anterior corpus callosum atrophy is important in cognitive impairment and frontal subcortical hypometabolism associated with PSP.

Positron emission tomography (PET) scans demonstrate frontal lobe hypometabolism (32) and anterior cingulate gyrus hypometabolism (33). Single photon emission computerized tomography (SPECT) scans reveal frontal lobe hypoperfusion (29). Furthermore, magnetic resonance imaging (MRI) has been reported to be helpful in distinguishing PSP from CBD when comparing asymmetric frontoparietal atrophy and midline atrophy: frontoparietal asymmetry was documented in 0% of PSP patients compared to 87% of patients with CBD, whereas midline atrophy occurred in 89.3% of PSP patients compared to 6.3% of CBD patients (34). Dubinsky and Jankovic (35) found a higher incidence of cerebral ischemic lesions on imaging studies in patients with PSP compared to that found in controls. This finding raises the possibility that cognitive impairment in some patients with PSP may in part be caused by a multiple infarcts state. Notably, vascular dementia caused by lacunar disease typically conforms to a frontal system pattern of dementia (36).

Patients with PSP have markedly reduced dopamine in the caudate and putamen but normal levels of dopamine in the nucleus accumbens, frontal and temporal cortices, and hypothalamus, implying that mesocortical and mesolimbic dopamine systems are intact (37,38). Marked deficiency in choline acetyltransferase (ChAT) activity in the substantia innominata with only mild decreases in the frontal cortex has been reported by Ruberg et al. (38). Kish et al. (37) found normal ChAT activity in frontal and temporal cortex, hippocampus, and striatum in four of five patients, all four of whom were demented. Litvan et al. (28), finding no correlation between levels of cerebrospinal fluid dopamine and degree of memory impairment, reiterated the view of Ruberg et al. (38) that the cholinergic innominatocortical and septohippocampal systems are more likely than the dopaminergic deficiency to contribute to the memory difficulties in PSP. Litvan et al. (39) also demonstrated inconsistent improvement on memory tasks in patients with PSP who were given physostigmine. Furthermore, Kertzman et al. (40) demonstrated improved performance on visuospatial attentional tasks in a placebo-controlled study of seven patients with PSP and healthy controls, using physostigmine.

An alternative explanation for cognitive dysfunction in PSP was offered by Johnson et al. (26), who studied event-related potentials (ERPs) in patients with PSP. Delays occurred in both the early and late components of the ERP response, compatible with the pattern seen in subcortical dementia and distinct from the pattern in cortical dementia, in which only the late response is abnormal. However, the magnitude of delay and the increased number of response errors were more characteristic of results found with experimental reduction of stimulus discriminability.

Kimura et al. (24) examined seven patients with PSP and found impairment on tasks that relied heavily on visual and scanning ability, including various performance subtests of the Wechsler Adult Intelligence Scale (WAIS), such as the Digit Symbol subtest. They found no impairment of WAIS verbal IQ or of Wechsler Memory Scale (WMS) memory quotient, and concluded that intellectual decline and memory impairment were not distinguishing features of PSP. Fisk et al. (25) reached the same conclusion in a study of two additional patients with PSP. Although both studies employed standardized neuropsychological measures, they did not include tests sensitive to frontal system impairment.

The possibility cannot be excluded that the oculomotor abnormalities present in patients with PSP may account at least in part for findings such as those of Johnson et al. (26), Kimura et al. (24), and Fisk et al. (25). Furthermore, the validity of using formal neuropsychological tests that rely on visual stimuli in patients with considerable oculomotor dysfunction has not been adequately addressed.

Psychiatric and behavioral disturbances in PSP have been reviewed by Chiu (41) and Chiu and Li (42). Such disturbances were common in PSP and occasionally were presenting signs (41,42). Apathy can be particularly characteristic of PSP and is useful in distinguishing it from IPD (43) and CBD (44). Depression, when present in PSP, does not correlate with cognition, behavior, or motor deficits (14,44). Pseudobulbar affect (pathologic crying and laughing) was reported in one third of 19 patients with PSP, lending support to bifrontal pathway involvement (45).

Netzel and Sutor (46) reported electroconvulsive therapy (ECT) to be safe and effective for depression in one case of PSP, without affecting other neurologic symptoms. Fluoxetine has also been reported to be helpful for behavioral symptoms (aggression and restlessness) in PSP (42).

In 1996, Pareja et al. (47) reported the first case of prodromal symptoms of rapid eye movement (REM) sleep behavior disorder in PSP. Features consisted of speech inhibition during wakefulness and somniloquy with phasic muscle twitching during REM sleep.

Early personality change, with mild cognitive deficits that evolve into moderate dementia with prominent abnormalities on frontal system tasks, is most consistently reported for PSP. Psychiatric disturbance is common, and cortical cognitive symptoms may be present. Additional study will clarify the extent to which dementia in PSP differs from other dementias with subcortical (and cortical) pathology, the extent to which language disturbance and other cortical symptoms characterize PSP, and the extent to which biochemical deficiencies and other mechanisms contribute to the mental status changes.

MULTIPLE-SYSTEM ATROPHY (MSA)

The multiple-system atrophies (MSA) are a heterogeneous group of diseases whose pathology shows a combination of degenerative lesions in the pons, cerebellum, inferior olive, basal ganglia, and spinal cord. These atrophies have traditionally been divided into three main types: olivopontocerebellar atrophy, striatonigral degeneration, and Shy–Drager syndrome. Mental status abnormalities are generally held to be mild or absent in these disorders.

Olivopontocerebellar Atrophy (OPCA)

Olivopontocerebellar atrophy (OPCA) is a group of inherited and sporadic disorders associated with degeneration of the cerebellar cortex, inferior olives, and pons, and with frequent involvement of the basal ganglia and spinal cord. Progressive ataxia is accompanied by a number of additional neurologic features. Substantial clinical heterogeneity exists, even among individuals within the same family. Detailed cognitive studies, particularly in patients with the sporadic form of the disease, give conflicting results.

In classifying OPCA into five types, Konigsmark and Weiner (48) included dementia as a major feature of OPCA type V, an autosomal, dominantly inherited ataxia associated with dementia, ophthalmoplegia, and extrapyramidal signs, plus the distinguishing pathologic feature of neuronal loss in the cerebral cortex. Three families with this type of OPCA were described. In the first, one patient developed dementia after admission to a mental hospital at the age of 27 years, 12 years after the onset of ataxia. His condition deteriorated, and he died at age 30. Several other family members developed ataxia between the ages of 7 and 43; all of them eventually developed severe dementia. In the second family, mental deterioration characterized by disorientation and aphasia occurred in two of four affected individuals. In the third family, one individual developed paranoid ideation, visual hallucinations, and memory loss a few years after the onset of ataxia. A second family member was described as irritable, hallucinating, and with memory loss, eventually becoming completely disoriented. Hence, in most of these cases, dementia was severe and associated with memory loss, psychotic features, and aphasia.

Berciano (49) reviewed 54 cases of familial OPCA and 63 cases of sporadic OPCA and found dementia to be present in 57.4% of the familial OPCA group and 34.9% of the sporadic OPCA group, and a dominant feature in 22.2% and 11.1%, respectively. Dementia tended to occur in the mid-to-late stages of disease, although when it occurred early, it was often an outstanding feature leading to misdiagnosis.

Harding (50) presented the clinical features of 11 families with autosomal dominant cerebellar ataxia. Mental status abnormalities were the most commonly occurring feature after ophthalmoplegia. Marked euphoria, emotional lability, and severe dementia occurred. Dementia developed relatively early in the disease course.

Kish et al. (51) studied the neuropsychological profile of patients from a large pedigree with autosomal dominant OPCA (spinocerebellar ataxia type I) (52) who had previously been reported to be free of mental deterioration. The absence of obvious cognitive impairment in dominantly inherited OPCA was particularly surprising, because this disorder was associated with a cholinergic deficit as severe as that seen in Alzheimer's disease. The patients studied by Kish et al. obtained scores within the normal range on the Mini-Mental State Examination and tended not to be considered demented by family or those closely associated with them. They were independent in many aspects of day-to-day living, despite ataxia. Nevertheless, most patients showed changes in personality and mood, including emotional lability and impulsivity. Formal measures of depression (Hamilton and Beck Rating Scales) revealed that 7 of the 14 patients suffered from some degree of depression (3 moderate to severe), whereas only 1 control subject demonstrated depression.

Extensive formal neuropsychological testing revealed mild but definite cognitive abnormalities. Substantial differences in performance compared to that of normal controls were found for the Wechsler Adult Intelligence Scale-Revised (WAIS-R) verbal IQ, Hooper Visual Organization Test, WMS story recall, WCST (number of perseverative errors), and the Visual–Verbal Test. The more quantitatively severe deficits were evident on the latter three tests. The authors interpret the findings as being consistent with prominent frontal system dysfunction without evidence of aphasia, apraxia, or agnosia. On the basis of their neuropsychological findings and the comparable cholinergic deficit in OPCA and AD, they suggested that the cholinergic reduction in AD may account for only part of the cognitive deficits in AD.

In a separate study involving 12 patients from the same OPCA pedigree, El-Awar et al. (53) further characterized the nature of the frontal lobe dysfunction by using two tasks sensitive to different aspects of prefrontal pathology, delayed alternation (DA) and delayed response (DR). Whereas both tasks are sensitive to prefrontal cortex lesions involving dorsolateral and orbitofrontal pathology, DR is more sensitive to dorsolateral lesions. Furthermore, whereas both tasks measure spatial mnemonic factors, DA is also sensitive to perseveration. Perseveration on the DA task has been associated more with orbitofrontal than with dorsolateral lesions. The investigators found selective deficits on DA, but not on DR, in the OPCA subjects. They suggest that the deficits on DA could be attributable to a loss of cholinergic innervation to orbitofrontal cortex. Alternatively, they raise the possibility that damage to the integrity of cerebellofrontal connections may play a role. In addition, they could not exclude involvement of the temporal cortex, because deficits on DA, but not on DR, have been observed after bilateral temporal lobe lesions.

In a study of 12 patients with OPCA, Botez et al. (54) found frontal cognitive dysfunction similar to that reported by Kish et al. (51). In addition, they found considerable visuoconstructional deficits on block design tests and the Rey Complex Figure. Botez et al. (55,56) proposed that cerebellar impairment of a variety of etiologies interferes with visuospatial organization, planning and programming daily activities, and speed of information processing because of defective cerebelloparietal, cerebellofrontoparietal, and cerebellofrontal loops.

Hirono et al. (57) investigated 30 patients with "spinocerebellar degeneration." Their subjects consisted of a heterogeneous group (7 familial and 23 nonfamilial subjects) with insidious ataxia associated with cerebellar atrophy, with and without pontine atrophy. These subjects were compared with a control group, using a variety of cognitive tests. Their WAIS-R IQ scores showed considerable impairment, correlating with the severity of ataxia. Cognitive profiles were characteristic of those found in subcortical dementia. Specifically, the subjects were found to have anterograde memory deficits that are important for recall but not for recognition, reduced verbal fluency for both letters and categories without confrontation naming impairment, and a greater tendency toward depression than the control group, using the Zung Scale of Depression. Because no difference in cognitive performance was found between patients with pontine atrophy and those without, the authors concluded that cerebello–cerebral deactivation caused by cerebellar degeneration was the key underlying factor in cognitive impairment, and that brain stem projections did not contribute in any important way. Data was not presented separately for hereditary and nonhereditary patients.

The role of the cerebellum in cognition and frontal system cognitive tasks (58–63), and in parietal function, has been explored (60). Grafman et al. (58) found cognitive planning deficits on the Tower of Hanoi task in a heterogeneous group of 12 patients with cerebellar atrophy that included two patients with OPCA. Their findings were replicated by subgroup analysis for those patients having pure cerebellar cortical atrophy. Botez-Marquard and Botez (61) compared patients who had bilateral cerebellar disease, including OPCA, with patients who had unilateral cerebellar disease (mainly cerebellar stroke). Patients with bilateral disease demonstrated frontal executive dysfunction, slower information processing, decreased retrieval memory, decreased visuospatial organization, and decreased visuospatial working memory. Those patients with unilateral disease had transient deficits, which resolved within two to five months. Arroyo-Anllo and Botez-Marquard (60) compared OPCA patients with normal controls and found patients with OPCA to be deficient on frontal tasks (hand sequencing, verbal reasoning, and proverb interpretation) and deficient on measures that reflect parietal function (figure copy and immediate visual–spatial recall). Botez-Marquard et al. (62) found a correlation between degree of cerebellar atrophy, measured radiologically, and degree of cognitive impairment (attention, executive function, visuospatial function, memory). This correlation held true not only for neocerebellar atrophy but also for the vermis and fastigial nuclei, leading to the importance of neocerebellar–basal ganglia–associative cerebral cortex loops as well as fastigial–limbic loops.

Efforts toward molecular biologic definition of specific genetic disturbances in the progressive ataxias (52) may provide insight into the clinical heterogeneity that has been observed. At present, clinical variability in OPCA makes it difficult to come to any firm conclusions regarding the extent and nature of cognitive and behavioral changes. Nevertheless, disordered mood and intellectual function, both mild and late, as well as early and severe, have been documented in some inherited cases and to a lesser degree in sporadic cases. A frontal system pattern of cognitive impairment has been stressed. Mechanisms accounting for frontal system deficits may include damage to the cerebello–cerebral cortical pathways as well as a cholinergic deficit affecting the frontal cortex or caudate.

Striatonigral Degeneration (SND) and Shy–Drager Syndrome (SDS)

SND and SDS are sporadic neurodegenerative disorders characterized by bradykinesia, rigidity, minimal tremor, and poor response to dopaminergic therapy. SDS is additionally characterized by early and prominent autonomic nervous system dysfunction (64). Cognitive impairment has been reported in patients with SND. Some subjects with SND demonstrate sufficient autonomic dysfunction that conclusions about cognitive profiles cannot readily be drawn. The following discussion does not attempt to differentiate between SND and SDS.

In 1991, Sullivan et al. (65) reported a single case of SND with emphasis on neuropsychological aspects. Their patient was given a large number of neuropsychological tests and was found to have selective impairments on only a few tasks, without global dementia or mood disturbance. Many tests on which she performed normally included those that examine dorsolateral frontal lobe function (WCST and self-ordering tests), which often show impairment in patients with basal ganglia pathology.

Difficulties unrelated to motor impairment were demonstrated on the picture completion and picture arrangement subtests of the WAIS-R, sequencing for manual gestures, and memory span for serial arm movements. The authors interpreted these sequencing deficits as resulting from bilateral putaminal dysfunction that adversely affected frontal lobe activity. Letter fluency, but not semantic fluency, was also impaired; letter fluency is sensitive to inferior frontal lesions (66). Sullivan et al. (65) suggest that the putaminal portion of the ipsilateral frontal cortical–putaminal circuit may be the site of the abnormality that leads to impaired letter fluency. Alternatively, they suggest that connections between the insula and basal ganglia may be the critical lesion site. Finally, their patient did poorly on a distracter test of short-term memory (Brown–Peterson distracter task), showing particular difficulty after a short retention interval compared to her performance after longer intervals. This finding is similar to that found in tests of forgetfulness in PD and contrasts with normal forgetting or forgetting in other amnestic syndromes, in which longer intervals result in poorer retention.

Robbins et al. (67) compared the performance of 16 patients with MSA (SND, with or without autonomic disturbance) and of 16 control subjects on a variety of psychometric tests, with emphasis on three measures believed to be specific for frontal lobe dysfunction, which have been demonstrated to show quantitative and qualitative differences in performance between PD and AD patients. These three tests consisted of computerized adaptations of an attentional set-shifting paradigm, the Tower of London planning task, and a test of spatial working memory. Patients with MSA showed substantial deficits on all three of these tests, with a qualitative and quantitative pattern of performance that was more similar to that typical of patients with frontal lobe lesions than that of patients with PD. These deficits were found in the absence of substantial intellectual deterioration, perceptual difficulty, naming difficulty, or any consistent learning or memory abnormality. Furthermore, no correlation existed among extent of cognitive impairment, disease duration, and severity of motor deficits. The authors concluded that cognitive performance of patients with MSA follows a pattern of fronto-subcortical or frontostriatal impairment, but that given the differences in deficits between MSA and PD patients, subcortical dementia is likely not a unitary phenomenon. Similar conclusions were drawn in a subsequent study by Robbins et al. (27) in which the performance of patients with MSA on frontal lobe tasks was found to differ qualitatively from that of patients with PSP and PD.

De Volder et al. (68) performed PET scans on seven nondemented patients with probable SND. Marked glucose hypometabolism was found in the putamen and caudate and to a lesser extent in the prefrontal, premotor, and motor cortex. The degree of frontal lobe hypometabolism was less pronounced than that found in PSP, whereas the striatal hypometabolism was more severe. The authors suggest that frontal hypometabolism in SND results from subcortical–frontal deafferentation. Unfortunately, no measures of selective frontal cognitive deficits were reported.

Testa et al. (69) administered a battery of neuropsychological tests that emphasize visuospatial capabilities and memory to 19 patients with SND, 19 patients with PD, and 19 age- and education-matched normal control subjects. None of the subjects were demented by *Diagnostic and Statistical Manual of Mental Disorder, Version Three* (DSM-III) criteria. Patients with SND and PD showed similar cognitive dysfunction, performing especially poorly compared with control subjects on visuospatial organizational tests. These findings contrast with those of Sullivan et al. (65) and Robbins et al. (67), in which emphasis was placed on a frontal system pattern of cognitive abnormality with relative sparing of visuospatial function.

Sleep disorders have been described as common in MSA, affecting 70% of patients in one series reported by Ghorayeb et al. (70). These authors report sleep fragmentation in 52.5%, vocalizations in 60%, REM Sleep Behavior Disorder (RBD) in 47.5%, and nocturnal stridor in 19% of patients. Plazzi et al. (71) found that RBD occurred in patients with MSA (SDS type) but not in patients with pure autonomic failure. Boeve et al. (72) reviewed 3 studies dealing with RBD in neurodegenerative diseases with dementia or parkinsonism and concluded that RBD is characteristic of the synucleinopathies (MSA, PD, dementia with Lewy bodies), and of these, RBD is particularly associated with MSA.

Reports of mood disturbance in MSA give conflicting results. Goto et al. (73) report that depression may be the first symptom of MSA and may improve with anti-PD medication. Gill et al. (74), using the Beck Depression Inventory, reported depression as occurring in 88.7% of 15 patients with SDS. In 28.6%, depression was judged to be moderate to severe. Depression did not correlate with degree of physical disability on the Parkinson's Disease Disability Scale or Northwestern University Disability Scale for Parkinson's Disease. Others (75–77) report depression to be less common in MSA than in IPD. Fetoni et al. (75) described blunted affect as being more common in MSA (SND type) patients, whereas anxiety and depression were more common in IPD patients. The affective detachment of patients with MSA was reported not to improve with levodopa therapy.

MACHADO–JOSEPH'S DISEASE (MJD)

Machado–Joseph's disease (MJD) is an autosomal dominant degenerative disorder clinically similar to OPCA in motor findings but with a distinct pathologic profile. The age of onset is earlier, and progression is slower than for OPCA. Until recently, mental status has been thought to be normal. In a review by Rosenberg (78), all patients with this disease, regardless of phenotypes I-III, were said to be intellectually intact and lacking evidence of cognitive impairment or of cerebral cortex histologic abnormality. Nonetheless, more detailed neuropsychological and behavioral assessments have revealed cognitive deficits in at least some cohorts and have documented the presence of sleep disturbance as a common symptom in MJD.

In 1992, the National Institutes of Neurologic Disorders and Stroke sponsored an international workshop on MJD (79). An examination of phenotypic variability was conducted for approximately 900 patients. Sleep disturbances resembling RBD were described in almost 50% of 142 Portuguese patients. Nocturnal cries, nightmares, agitation, and disturbed REM sleep were reported, as seen on polygraphic sleep recordings. Sleep abnormalities were particularly common in type I patients and could develop early in the course of the disease. Subsequent cases of RBD in MJD patients have also been reported (80–82). Friedman (80) noted RBD in six out of seven patients with MJD. Recognizing that sleep disturbances similar to those described in the National Institute of Neurological Disorders and Stroke (NINDS) workshop are found in PD, the NINDS authors (79) suggested that the locus caeruleus may be the neuroanatomic substrate for the sleep disorder.

In addition to identifying sleep disturbance, the 1992 NINDS group reported cognitive impairment in a Brazilian cohort of Portuguese ancestry. Neuropsychological evaluation of 12 patients and 23 at-risk individuals demonstrated visuoperceptual dysfunction and constructional apraxia. Visual memory was impaired in the affected and at-risk groups. Some of the affected and at-risk patients showed a phenomenon referred to as the "fly eye" effect, consisting of multiplying of internal details.

Sequeiros and Coutinho (83) gave a detailed clinical description of 143 Portuguese patients with MJD but did not perform neuropsychological testing. Memory disturbance was found in only two patients, from different families. The rest were judged to be mentally intact because they were "completely alert, cooperative, and interested in surrounding events up to extreme situations of disability and inability to communicate."

Formal neurocognitive evaluation in MJD can reveal mild deficits in cognition and mood, compatible with a frontosubcortical pattern of impairment (84). Maruff et al. (85) found selective deficits in visual attention in six patients given a computerized cognitive battery (CANTAB). Deficits were independent of motor dysfunction and were felt to reflect frontosubcortical pathway disruption. Ishikawa et al. (86) report dementia with psychotic features in patients with longer-than-average numbers of MJD1 gene CAG repeats.

Formal neurocognitive assessment in MJD alerts us to the presence of mild but substantial dysfunction not previously recognized. How prevalent such cognitive and behavioral disturbance is in MJD requires additional study. Furthermore, comparison of MJD cognitive deficits with those in OPCA may provide insights regarding the role of the cerebellum in cognition.

CORTICOBASAL DEGENERATION (CBD)

Corticobasal degeneration (CBD) is a sporadic neurodegenerative disease characterized by insidious onset and gradually progressing asymmetric basal ganglionic and cerebrocortical dysfunction (87,88). Clinical features include asymmetric rigidity, akinesia, limb dystonia, postural instability, tremor, focal reflex myoclonus, and a variety of behavioral abnormalities, of which apraxia and alien limb phenomenon are the most striking. Characteristic pathology includes neuronal loss and gliosis in the substantia nigra, with achromatic neurons and degeneration of the cerebral cortex, especially in the frontoparietal regions (87). The question of whether CBD is a unique disease or a syndrome under the umbrella of Pick complex or frontotemporal lobar degeneration has been debated (89–92). Arguments rest largely on the relative importance assigned to clinical or pathologic features and are not likely to be resolved without future advances in molecular biology (89). Multiple clinical reports have strengthened our understanding of CBD (88,91,93,94). This chapter covers specific behavioral and cognitive abnormalities, well described in this disorder.

Apraxia

Ideomotor apraxia (IMA) is the inability to perform learned movements not explained by weakness, incoordination, sensory loss, incomprehension, or inattention to commands (95). Ideational apraxia (IA) is a disorder of planned action, which manifests itself through the faulty use of objects when a complex sequence of acts must be organized (96). In IA, the concept of the gesture is lacking (the patient does not know what to do), whereas in IMA, the implementation of the gesture in a precise motor program is disrupted (the patient knows what to do but not *how* to do it) (96). Both types of apraxia occur frequently in CBD (88,91,97). An example of IMA from the series reported by Riley et al. (88) includes a patient who was unable to perform any orofacial or limb movements except smiling to command. Examples of IA from the same series (88) include an individual who was unable to figure out how to put an electric plug into a socket, and how to push a vacuum cleaner, as well as a 61-year-old surgeon who developed difficulty gloving, tying knots, and manipulating instruments with his left hand. This latter patient actually stated that he had "forgotten how" to use the hand in performing these tasks.

IA and IMA occur early in CBD and are sometimes the presenting symptoms (88). The limbs are affected first, although a case of pathologically proven CBD has been described that presented with progressive loss of speech output and orofacial apraxia (98). As with other motor signs in CBD, limb apraxia may begin asymmetrically with the right upper extremity preferentially affected (88). Boeve et al. (99) report a tendency for unilateral upper extremity rigidity and apraxia to evolve together for a time before spreading to affect the ipsilateral lower limb or contralateral upper limb. In many cases of CBD, apraxia becomes severe, leading to extreme disability in which patients are totally unable to use their limbs voluntarily (88).

Apraxia has been reported in up to 71% of cases of CBD (88). This report included additional constructional apraxia, which is believed to represent a separate disturbance (100). Additional types of apraxia in CBD, distinct from IMA and IA, include apraxia of gaze, apraxia of the eyelids, apraxia of speech, and apraxia of gait. In traditional views of IMA, voluntary movements of the eyelids, eyes, and torso, which affect midline, axial, truncal, and locomotor activities, are thought to be spared (95).

Leiguarda et al. (101) demonstrated IMA in 7 of 10 patients in their series. Their decision to test the least affected limb to avoid confusion with other coexisting motor disturbances likely caused them to underestimate IMA prevalence, given the potential for asymmetry in CBD. Principal IMA error types reported were those of posture, orientation, sequencing, body part as object, and trajectory. None of the patients had buccofacial apraxia. IA, tested using sequential motor tasks and gesture discrimination, was present in only three subjects, two of whom had severe cognitive impairment, as measured by Mini-Mental State Examination scores, which suggested that these patients had advanced disease. This lower frequency and later development of IA in CBD contrasts with previous case descriptions. Furthermore, no patients in the series by Leiguarda et al. (101) had IA without IMA. Principal IA error types were perplexity, absent or unrecognizable responses, omissions, sequencing errors, and mislocations. The authors attempted to relate IMA to frontal lobe and specifically supplementary motor area dysfunction based on correlation with performance on the Picture Arrangement Task and the coexistence of alien limb phenomenon. In contrast, IA was believed to correlate with frontoparietal or diffuse cortical dysfunction.

Kertesz et al. (91) reported IMA and IA in 34 of 35 CBD patients. IMA was more common than IA and was often severe. IA was prominent in many and was found even in the absence of IMA.

Patients with CBD offer a unique opportunity to study IMA and IA, given their progressive courses and the relative absence of the usual confounding variables of substantial dementia and aphasia. Continued efforts to rigorously apply apraxia terminology, along with use of operational definitions and of formal apraxia test batteries with error analysis scoring, will shed greater light on mechanisms of motor planning.

Alien Limb Phenomenon (Alien Hand Sign)

Alien limb phenomenon is a limb that behaves in an uncooperative or foreign fashion, although ownership of the limb is not in question (102). Alien limb phenomenon has been reported in the left hand in the setting of corpus callosum section (102) and corpus callosum tumors (103) and in the right hand after left anterior cerebral artery territory infarction (104). In the latter cases, less complex involuntary movements were described, in which the affected hand rises toward the head or drifts upward purposelessly. Alien limb phenomenon has been attributed by some to lesions that affect the supplementary motor area (104,105) and is believed to represent faulty initiation, execution, and inhibition of preexisting, essentially intact, motor subroutines that are no longer coupled to external and internal inputs (105). In most cases, the degree of intermanual conflict initially present decreases with time.

Alien limb phenomenon is an unusual sign in neurology. Its presence, in the absence of a known callosal lesion, strongly suggests the diagnosis of CBD. Riley et al. (88) reported that alien limb phenomenon occurred in 50% of CBD patients studied. In these descriptions, alien limb phenomenon was a highly persistent sign, whereas Boeve et al. (99) characterized alien limb phenomenon in CBD as lasting a few months to a few years before progressive rigidity or dystonia supersedes. Kertesz et al. (91) reported alien limb phenomenon to be present in 27 of the 35 (77%) CBD patients studied.

Unilateral left limb apraxia and alien limb phenomenon are characteristic of the split-brain syndrome. Testing for other features of the split-brain syndrome (ipsilateral tactile anomia, ipsilateral hemi-alexia, ipsilateral agraphia) in patients with CBD would be of interest. The presence of these features would support the hypothesis that interhemispheric disconnection, rather than primary cortical lesions, accounts for some of the behavioral abnormalities in CBD.

Aphasia

Aphasia had been reported in 21% of patients with CBD (88). A variety of aphasic subtypes have been described in CBD, including "nominal" aphasia (106,107, Case 1), severe nonfluent aphasia (87, Case 1), and a case of pathologically proven CBD that presented with primary progressive aphasia in the form of transcortical motor aphasia (108). Detailed formal language assessments have recently suggested that language disturbances play a much more prominent role in CBD than previously recognized.

Kertesz et al. (91) reported language disturbance to be the most common cognitive symptom in CBD. Impaired naming and word fluency were described as common early features of the CBD language disturbance. PPA was described by these authors as a common corticosteroid-binding globulin (CBG)–related syndrome. Graham et al. (109) reviewed 10 cases of CBD and found phonologic impairment (verbal fluency, phoneme blending, and segmentation) to be prominent and typical even in nonaphasic patients. A few patients had deficits in semantic memory, naming, and reading, although these impairments were mild. Frattali et al. (110) reported 53% of patients (8 of 15) to have classifiable aphasic syndromes including Broca's, anomic, and transcortical motor aphasias. Aphasias were associated with MRI evidence of abnormalities in left frontal and left parietal cortical and subcortical white matter and in corpus callosum.

Although aphasia has been attributed to dominant hemisphere cortical pathology, subcortical lesions are well known to cause aphasic syndromes (111,112). Given the presence of both cortical and subcortical lesions in CBD, future study of language disturbance in CBD may serve to clarify the relative contributions of each of these lesion sites to the aphasic profiles seen.

Visuospatial and Constructional Deficits

Involvement of the right parietal cortex in CBD gives rise to visuospatial and constructional disturbances that are sometimes severe (107). A variety of visuospatial and constructional deficits have been reported in CBD, including impairment in copying shapes and figures (107,108), impairment on Block Design performance (107), and dressing apraxia (88).

Neglect

A few patients with CBD exhibit tactile and visual inattention (88, Case 2) or unilateral tactile extinction (87, Case 2). More detailed descriptions of neglect syndromes in CBD patients are not available. Given the extent to which right parietal cortex can be involved in this disease, a careful assessment for the spectrum of possible right hemisphere behavioral phenomena should prove rewarding.

Dementia

In addition to apraxia, aphasia, visuospatial and constructional deficits, alien hand sign, and neglect, impairment in personality, attention, calculation, recall, learning, abstract thinking, and left-right discrimination has been noted. The presence of multiple cognitive deficits constitutes dementia. However, early reports of CBD did not consider dementia to be a major feature (88,97).

Kertesz et al. (91) studied subjects longitudinally, using extensive neurocognitive testing, and found that 14 of 35 cases progressed to frontotemporal dementia, while 21 cases progressed to the syndrome of progressive aphasia. In 20 of the 35 cases, cognitive and behavioral symptoms developed before motor symptoms. In the remaining 15, motor features came first, followed by cognitive and behavioral change. Age of onset and disease duration were similar, regardless of whether the presenting symptoms were motor or cognitive and behavioral. However, those presenting with cognitive and behavioral change as a first symptom showed a male predominance of 14:6, whereas those presenting with motor symptoms had a female predominance of 10:5.

PARKINSONISM-DEMENTIA/ALS (P-D/ALS)

Parkinsonism-dementia/ALS is a particular syndrome of parkinsonism and dementia or amyotrophic lateral sclerosis (ALS), or both, which was recognized as endemic among the Chamorros of Guam and in the Kii Peninsula of Japan in the first half of this century. Its cause has been attributed variously to the neurotoxic effects of beta-*N*-methylamino-L-alanine (BMAA) contained in the cycad seed (113,114), defects in mineral metabolism (115), and the influenza A virus (116). Apart from a younger age of onset, the ALS component of the syndrome is clinically identical to ALS found elsewhere in the world. The P-D component is, however, distinct from idiopathic Parkinson's disease in that dementia is virtually always present, occurs earlier and to a more severe degree, and affects all aspects of mental functioning, leading to a vegetative state within a few years.

Elizan et al. (117) have described the clinical features of P-D. In one third of cases, dementia is the presenting or only feature. All of those who start with extrapyramidal features eventually develop dementia. Memory loss occurs early with most patients. One third develop early changes in personality and mood, including apathy, depression, irritability, restlessness, agitation, and antisocial or violent behavior. Most patients remain indifferent to their illness, even early in the disease, when insight is still relatively preserved. Sleep disturbances (hypersomnia or insomnia) occur throughout the disease course. As dementia progresses, acalculia, impaired comprehension, and concrete thinking are increasingly evident. Hallucinations have been reported in a few patients. Average age of onset of P-D is 54 years. Average disease duration is 4 years.

More recent descriptions of P-D/ALS come from Rogers-Johnson et al. (115) who examined Guamanian patients with onset of symptoms between 1950 and 1979. Other than an increased age of onset for ALS and P-D, a shorter duration of illness in ALS, and a longer duration in P-D, they found no major differences in physical or histopathologic findings compared to those in patients with onset before 1950. Of the 328 patients with P-D, dementia was documented in all but 5 patients who could not be tested. Early mental symptoms included laziness and forgetfulness. Excessive sleepiness occurred. Others developed sleep disturbance as the disease advanced. Dementia was relentlessly progressive, with obvious impairment of memory, calculation, comprehension, and personality.

Neuropathologic evidence supports the concept that Guamanian ALS and P-D are variants of the same disease (117). Five percent of patients with ALS develop clinical evidence of P-D within 6 years. At autopsy, a much higher percentage (at least 50%) of patients with ALS demonstrate pathologic features of P-D. Conversely, 38% of patients with P-D develop clinical ALS within 1.5 years, with additional cases showing ALS-related changes at autopsy.

The pathologic findings of the syndrome include motor neuron dropout as expected for ALS, plus cortical atrophy with neuronal loss, neurofibrillary tangles, granulovacuolar degeneration, and gliosis, which affect the frontal and temporal cortex as well as the hippocampus, hypothalamus, nucleus basalis, substantia nigra, globus pallidus, locus caeruleus, and thalamus. No Lewy bodies or senile plaques are seen (116).

In a study by Snow et al. (118) involving eight patients with Guamanian P-D, four with Guamanian ALS, and seven Guamanian apparently healthy control subjects, PET scanning demonstrated subclinical dopaminergic lesions in the ALS group and possibly in two of the controls. To classify patients at the outset, cognitive function was examined, and a mental state score (4 = normal, 20 = maximal severity) was derived, for each ALS and P-D subject. Scores in P-D distributed fairly evenly from 6 to 18. Two subjects with ALS had normal mental test scores. However, the remaining two had slightly elevated scores (5 and 7), suggesting that they may have entered the early clinical phase of P-D. Mental state scores were not included for the control subjects, an unfortunate omission, because PET scans demonstrated subclinical evidence of dopaminergic lesions in two of them.

Despite intensive neurologic surveillance in Guam, detailed investigations of cognitive function in P-D/ALS have not been conducted. Snow et al. (118) pointed out the difficulty of applying formal neuropsychological tests to non-English speaking individuals of a different cultural and educational background. Cummings and Benson (119) classified P-D among the subcortical dementias but acknowledged that the absence of aphasia, apraxia, and agnosia may be attributable to incomplete assessments.

The incidence of Guamanian P-D/ALS is declining, and the opportunity for formal neuropsychological evaluation of large numbers of individuals is therefore diminishing. Nonetheless, recognition has increased over the past 10 years that sporadic ALS itself is more than a motor disorder. Detailed neurocognitive assessment of sporadic ALS patients has revealed that mild frontal executive dysfunction may be common (120) and may progress to frontotemporal dementia (FTD) in some patients (121,122). Neary et al. (123) report that ALS patients presenting with bulbar palsy and amyotrophy are more susceptible than others to developing FTD. Furthermore, a non-Guamanian ALS-plus syndrome has been described (124), which involves ALS of usual age of onset followed by dementia, parkinsonism, or both, the latter unresponsive to levodopa. Spongiform changes in the superficial layers of the frontotemporal cortex have been reported in demented patients with ALS-plus (123,125–127). Further study of pathogenesis will be valuable to our understanding of the unifying disease mechanisms underlying destruction of motor and cognitive domains.

POSTENCEPHALITIC PARKINSONISM

Between 1915 and 1930, the world was struck by an epidemic of somnolent ophthalmoplegic encephalitis known as encephalitis lethargica. Although the etiologic agent was never fully established, the acute infection has been attributed by some to swine (Hswi1N1) influenza A virus and is estimated to have led to more than one million cases of severe neurologic disease (128). The nervous system was affected not only in the acute stage of the illness but also after recovery, giving rise to the syndrome of postencephalitic parkinsonism.

The acute illness began with a brief prodrome of fever, malaise, and pharyngitis, followed in short order by striking abnormalities in level of consciousness. The somnolence lasted days to months, with variable ability to arouse affected individuals. Less commonly, psychomotor excitation with extreme agitation, incoherent speech, and delusions were evident (129). Ophthalmoplegia, ptosis, and other cranial nerve abnormalities and focal signs, as well as parkinsonian rigidity, sometimes accompanied the acute illness. Among those who survived this stage, most patients went on to develop parkinsonism, mental status abnormalities, and other neurologic signs and symptoms weeks to years later. Young age of onset, tics, torticollis, pupillary dysfunction, ocular disturbances including oculogyric crises, and behavioral abnormalities distinguish the extrapyramidal syndrome from IPD (130).

In a 1924 follow-up of patients who had had encephalitis lethargica, Duncan (129) described mental sequelae ranging from minor to severe. Severe mental sequelae were more common in those with early onset of the postencephalitic syndrome following the acute illness and in those who contracted the acute disease at a young age. Forty percent of children under the age of 10 were reported to have developed severe mental sequelae. This rate declined to 20% for those over age 40. Furthermore, individuals with lethargy, somnolence, and coma were more likely to develop severe mental sequelae than were those with mania and delirium.

Minor mental sequelae were common but almost always mild. Both recent and remote memory were affected. Attentional difficulties were thought to be more disabling, in that they often led individuals to give up their jobs. Drowsiness, sometimes alternating with insomnia, was a common symptom and occurred more often in adults than in children. Sleep–wake cycles were often inverted. Personality change was common, with anxiety, irritability, and phobias. Severe behavioral abnormalities included schizophreniform states with delusions, hallucinations, catatonia, mania, hysteria, and obsessive–compulsive behavior. Attacks of compulsive thinking, counting, and speech were often associated with oculogyric crises (131). Many patients required institutionalization because of "insanity." Children under the age of 6 who experienced encephalitis lethargica occasionally developed mental retardation. Psychotic and neurotic behavior often appeared in phases of weeks to months, following which the individual might revert to a normal mental state or to a different abnormal mental state. Attacks of depression were also described.

In individuals who developed parkinsonism, mental sequelae were well correlated with the degree of motor impairment. In more severe cases, slowness of mental processing, catatonia, and dormant or unstable emotions predominated, while intellect, memory, and perception were relatively intact. Ziegler (132) found that patients tended to recover from behavioral sequelae, but only rarely recovered from parkinsonism. In 1965, Duvoisin and Yahr (133) assessed 31 long-term survivors and found behavioral disturbances in only 4. Whether this finding represents recovery over time, or merely a survival preference for those less severely afflicted, is unclear. Furthermore, the use of levodopa to treat parkinsonian symptoms revealed a striking propensity for patients with postencephalitic parkinsonism to develop or redevelop behavioral disturbance (as well as tics and other dyskinesias) (130,134), suggesting a latent, persisting abnormality.

Von Economo (135) attributed the abnormal levels of consciousness in the acute phase of the illness to inflammatory lesions in the upper midbrain. Hudson and Rice (116) reported pathologic findings in postencephalitic parkinsonism to consist of extensive inflammatory perivascular lymphocytic infiltration in acute and early postencephalitic cases, whereas late postencephalitic cases were characterized by extensive neuronal loss, gliosis, and neurofibrillary tangles with a predilection for the substantia nigra, locus caeruleus, midbrain including reticular formation, hippocampus, nucleus basalis, and to a lesser degree, frontotemporal cortex and hypothalamus. Because several of these sites are involved in behavior and cognitive function, lesions no doubt have relevance to the psychiatric and cognitive syndromes. The dramatic return to normality following weeks to months of severe psychiatric illness suggests that a reversible biochemical or physiologic component may also be present in addition to structural central nervous system changes. Ward (136) reviewed the literature on clinical–pathologic correlations in encephalitis lethargica and concluded that there was clear support for the concepts that (a) subcortical structures play an important role in complex behavior patterns and that (b) hysteria and obsessional neurosis have an organic etiology.

Although postencephalitic parkinsonism has essentially disappeared (137), it alerts us to the potential that other infectious agents might cause acute or delayed syndromes that combine extrapyramidal and behavioral features. Parkinsonism has been described in association with West Nile virus encephalitis (138) and Epstein–Barr encephalitis (139). Lance et al. (140) reported a young man who, following a minor illness, developed an akinetic-rigid syndrome with prominent rituals and stereotypies.

PRION-RELATED DISEASES

Prions are transmissible proteinaceous particles with little or no nucleic acid (141). They are responsible for spongiform dementing illnesses that can arise through genetic inheritance and infective transmission. Two of these diseases are discussed below.

CREUTZFELDT–JAKOB DISEASE (CJD)

Classic Creutzfeldt–Jakob disease (CJD) is a sporadic, rare disease. In 10% of patients, it is inherited in an autosomal dominant fashion. Rarely, CJD has been transmitted through contaminated corneal transplants, dural grafts, intracerebral electrodes, and human growth hormone preparations (142). A variant form of Creutzfeldt–Jakob Disease (vCJD), recognized since 1996, may share a common etiology or causative agent with bovine spongiform encephalopathy (143).

Brown et al. (144) reported 230 cases of neuropathologically verified CJD. Approximately one third of patients experienced a brief prodrome of malaise, impaired sleep, and altered eating pattern. Within weeks, this prodrome gave way to a rapidly progressive syndrome of mental deterioration associated with extrapyramidal, pyramidal, cerebellar, and visual changes. Lead pipe rigidity, myoclonus, and 1 Hz biphasic and phasic periodic electroencephalogram (EEG) complexes were seen in most of the patients. Few patients survived beyond 1 year.

Cognitive deficits in CJD conform to a profile of cortical dementia in which aphasia, agnosia, amnesia, apraxia, hallucinations, and delusions are prominent (145). In a rare report of detailed neuropsychological testing in a case of late CJD, Gass et al. (146) described patchy deficits with moderately severe impairment of verbal memory, word finding, and right-hand tactual performance, and relatively intact performance on other verbal, memory, and visuospatial tasks. In a small series, Snowden et al. (147) compared patients with sporadic and familial CJD and found the familial group to have a subcortical pattern of dementia. Common to both familial and sporadic CJD cases were episodic unresponsiveness, interference effects, and verbal and motor perseveration interpreted as evidence for a critical role of the thalamus in CJD dementia (148). Compared with familial and sporadic CJD, cases of CJD arising from cadaveric growth hormone tend to have predominant ataxia (149), with dementia being a milder and later feature (150).

The major difference in diagnosis for CJD is between rapidly progressive AD and thalamic dementia (145). AD is associated with myoclonus in more than 10% of cases (151), particularly when intellectual decline is rapid (152). Thalamic dementia runs a course of months to a few years and is associated with a variety of dyskinesias including myoclonus (153). A subcortical pattern of dementia and the absence of periodic EEG findings help differentiate thalamic dementia from CJD.

In contrast to CJD, vCJD affects young adults and is associated with sensory symptoms and pain (154). Presenting symptoms are typically psychiatric in nature, making the disease difficult to distinguish from primary psychiatric disorders of this age group for the first few months, until additional neurologic symptoms emerge (155). In reviewing the first 100 cases of vCJD in the United Kingdom, Spencer et al. (156) described early psychiatric features of dysphoria, anxiety, insomnia, and loss of interest. Similarly, Henry and Knight (154) reported depression as the dominant early symptom, with delusions and hallucinations also being common. Kapur et al. (148) provided one of the few reports of detailed neuropsychological testing in a case of vCJD. Early deficits were found in episodic memory, semantic memory retrieval, public knowledge, and executive tasks. Relative sparing was found in picture recognition memory, autobiographic memory, face perception, and complex copying. Postmortem pathologic findings included neuronal loss in the striatum, dorsal thalamus, cerebellum, and occipital cortex, prion protein (PrP) accumulation in the hippocampus, and widespread spongiform changes, including alterations in the entorhinal cortex and anterior thalamus.

Computed tomography (CT) and MRI of the brain in CJD are normal or reveal nonspecific atrophy (157,158). A "pulvinar sign" has been reported on MRI for vCJD (154). Pathologic examination in CJD reveals diffuse cerebral atrophy, neuronal loss, marked astrocytic proliferation in the cerebral cortex, and spongiform vacuolation in neuronal and astrocytic cytoplasm. Amyloid plaques containing PrP immunoreactivity are sometimes found in the cerebrum and cerebellum (159). In vCJD, the number of PrP-containing plaques is large, and the cerebellum displays confluent spongiform changes (160).

GERSTMANN–STRAUSSLER–SCHEINKER DISEASE (GSS)

Gerstmann–Straussler–Scheinker disease (GSS) was described clinically by Gerstmann in 1928 and further characterized by Gerstmann, Straussler, and Scheinker in 1936 in an Austrian family whose kindred now spans 9 generations and more than 220 members (161,162). The disease has been described in several other kindreds worldwide (163,164). GSS is an autosomal dominant illness related to point mutations in the PrP gene on chromosome 20 (165). Progressive ataxia is an early and universal feature, with dysarthria and oculomotor disturbances. Extrapyramidal signs, including rigidity and akinesia, become prominent as the disease evolves. Mental status changes, with progression to dementia, have been reported in most cases. The disease runs a course of 2 to 10 years.

In the large pedigree reported by Farlow et al. (164), all patients examined directly by the authors had dementia. Psychosis and severe depression were noted in several cases. Three subjects were reported in detail. In the first case, extreme confusion with fixed delusions, crying spells, impaired sleep, and poor appetite arose within a year and a half of onset of ataxia and dysarthria. Depressive features responded well to amitriptyline, without associated improvement in dementia. In the second case, early short-term memory impairment progressed to severe memory loss over a period of 3 years. Acalculia, impaired attention and concentration, perseveration, ideomotor and constructional apraxia, and finger agnosia were noted. Case 3 complained of forgetfulness within 3 years of onset of ataxia and dysarthria. This patient was agitated, had pressure of speech, and exhibited short-term memory impairment. He subsequently developed severe depression with vegetative signs, and still later, delusions, bizarre thought content, hallucinations, and mania. The psychiatric symptoms responded to lithium, but the dementia did not improve.

Unverzagt et al. (166) used a comprehensive neuropsychological test battery to compare 3 patients from a large Indiana kindred who had GSS and a mutation at codon 198 with healthy controls from the same kindred who did not have this mutation. Two of the three affected individuals demonstrated wide-ranging and severe deficits, which the authors felt reflected a global dementia. Intelligence, attention, memory, and executive abilities were among the domains affected. The third affected individual was earlier in his disease course and demonstrated more selective deficits, described by the authors as suggestive of early subcortical involvement.

Pathologic findings in patients with GSS consist of multicentric and unicentric PrP plaques, predominantly in the cerebral and cerebellar cortices (163) but also in subcortical structures such as hippocampus (167). Hyperphosphorylated tau, identical to that in Alzheimer's disease, has been identified around PrP plaques (167,168). Spongiform cortical changes may or may not be present (168). Degeneration of pyramidal and spinocerebellar tracts may be found (163).

Clinical subtypes of GSS associated with specific PrP gene mutations have been described (141,168,169). The most common GSS mutation is at codon 102 (P102L) (170) and is associated with the so-called ataxic form of GSS (141). A telencephalic form affecting codon 117 has also been described (141,171), as have two forms associated with neurofibrillary tangles (172). These two forms consist of clinical subtypes characterized by dementia (codon 217), and ataxia, parkinsonism, and dementia (codon 198). Additional mutations affecting codons 105, 145, 202, 212, 218 (168), codon 187 (173), and codon 131 (174) have been reported. The current thrust of research in GSS involves further molecular biological elucidation and clarification of the effect of different codon mutations on the variable clinical profiles seen in GSS.

ACKNOWLEDGMENTS

The authors gratefully acknowledge the secretarial support of Karen D'Sa in the preparation of this manuscript as well as the assistance of Vicki Giardino. Dr. Freedman was supported by the Saul A. Silverman Family Foundation, Toronto, Canada, as part of a Canada International Scientific Exchange Program (CISEPO) project.

REFERENCES

1. Steele JC, Richardson JC, Olszewski J. Progressive supranuclear palsy. *Arch Neurol* 1964;10:333–358.
2. Steele JC. Progressive supranuclear palsy. *Brain* 1972; 95:693–704.
3. Steele JC. Progressive supranuclear palsy. In: Vinken PJ, Bruyn GW, eds. *Handbook of clinical neurology, Part II.* Oxford: North Holland, 1975:217–229.
4. Albert ML, Feldman RG, Willis AL. The subcortical dementia of progressive supranuclear palsy. *J Neurol Neurosurg Psychiatry* 1974;37:121–130.
5. Cummings JL. Introduction. In: Cummings JL, ed. *Subcortical dementia.* New York: Oxford University Press, 1990:3–16.
6. Freedman M, Albert ML. Subcortical dementia. In: Vinken PJ, Bruyn GW, Klawans HL, eds. *Handbook of clinical neurology. Neurobehavioural disorders*, Vol 2(46). New York: Elsevier, 1985:311–316.
7. McHugh PR, Folstein MF. Psychiatric syndromes of Huntington's chorea: a clinical and phenomenologic study. In: Benson DF, Blumer D, eds. *Psychiatric aspects of neurologic disease.* New York: Grune & Stratton, 1975:267–286.
8. Maher ER, Smith EM, Lees AJ. Cognitive deficits in the Steele-Richardson-Olszewski syndrome (progressive supranuclear palsy). *J Neurol Neurosurg Psychiatry* 1985;48:1234–1239.
9. Dubois B, Pillon B, Legault F, et al. Slowing of cognitive processing in progressive supranuclear palsy. A comparison with Parkinson's disease. *Arch Neurol* 1988;45:1194–1199.
10. Lhermitte LL. Imitation and utilization behaviors. *Ann Neurol* 1986;19:326–334.
11. Pillon B, Dubois B, Ploska A, et al. Severity and specificity of cognitive impairment in Alzheimer's, Huntington's, and Parkinson's diseases and progressive supranuclear palsy. *Neurology* 1991;41:634–643.
12. Litvan I. Cognitive disturbances in progressive supranuclear palsy. *J Neural Transm Suppl* 1994;42:69–78.
13. Van der Hurk PR, Hodges JR. Episodic and semantic memory in Alzheimer's disease and progressive supranuclear palsy: a comparative study. *J Clin Exp Neuropsychol* 1995;17(3):451–471.
14. Esmond T, Giles E, Gibson M, et al. Neuropsychological performance, disease severity, and depression in progressive supranuclear palsy. *J Neurol* 1996;243(9):638–643.
15. Pirtosek Z, Jahanshahi M, Barrett G, et al. Attention and cognition in bradykinetic-rigid syndromes: an event-related potential study. *Ann Neurol* 2001;50(5): 567–573.
16. Soliveri P, Monza D, Paridi D, et al. Neuropsychological follow up in patients with Parkinson's disease, striatonigral degeneration-type multisystem atrophy, and progressive supranuclear palsy. *J Neurol Neurosurg Psychiatry* 2000;69(3):313–318.
17. Mochizuki A, Ueda Y, Komatsuzaki Y, et al. Progressive supranuclear palsy presenting with primary progressive

17. aphasia—clinicopathological report of an autopsy case. *Acta Neuropathol* 2003;105(6):610–614.
18. Boeve B, Dickson D, Duffy J, et al. Progressive nonfluent aphasia and subsequent aphasic dementia associated with atypical progressive supranuclear palsy pathology. *Eur Neurol* 2003;49(2):72–78.
19. Esmonde T, Giles E, Xuereb J, et al. Progressive supranuclear palsy presenting with dynamic aphasia. *J Neurol Neurosurg Psychiatry* 1996;60(4):403–410.
20. Pillon B, Gouider-Khouja N, Deweer B, et al. Neuropsychological pattern of striatonigral degeneration: comparison with Parkinson's disease and progressive supranuclear palsy. *J Neurol Neurosurg Psychiatry* 1995;58(2):174–179.
21. Pharr V, Uttl B, Stark M, et al. Comparison of apraxia in corticobasal degeneration and progressive supranuclear palsy. *Neurology* 2001;56(7):957–963.
22. Leiguarda RC, Pramstaller PP, Merello M, et al. Apraxia in Parkinson's disease, progressive supranuclear palsy, multiple system atrophy and neuroleptic-induced parkinsonism. *Brain* 1997;120(Pt 1):75–90.
23. Ghika J, Tennis M, Growdon J, et al. Environment-driven responses in progressive supranuclear palsy. *J Neurol Sci* 1995;130(1):104–111.
24. Kimura D, Barnett HJM, Burkhart G. The psychological test pattern in progressive supranuclear palsy. *Neuropsychologia* 1981;19:301–306.
25. Fisk JD, Goodale MZ, Burkhart G, et al. Progressive supranuclear palsy: the relationship between ocular motor dysfunction and psychological test performance. *Neurology* 1982;32:698–705.
26. Johnson R, Litvan I, Grafman J. PSP: altered sensory processing leads to degraded cognition. *Neurology* 1991;41:1257–1262.
27. Robbins TW, James M, Owen AM, et al. Cognitive deficits in progressive supranuclear palsy, Parkinson's disease, and multiple system atrophy in tests sensitive to frontal lobe dysfunction. *J Neurol Neurosurg Psychiatry* 1994;57:79–88.
28. Litvan I, Grafman J, Gomez C, et al. Memory impairment in patients with progressive supranuclear palsy. *Arch Neurol* 1989;46:765–767.
29. Lees AJ. Progressive supranuclear palsy (Steele-Richardson-Olszewski Syndrome). In: Cummings JL, ed. *Subcortical dementia*. New York: Oxford University Press, 1990:123–131.
30. Bigio EH, Brown DG, White CL III. Progressive supranuclear palsy with dementia: cortical pathology. *J Neuropathol Exp Neurol* 1999;58(4):359–364.
31. Yamauchi H, Fukuyama H, Nagahama Y, et al. Atrophy of the corpus callosum, cognitive impairment, and cortical hypometabolism in progressive supranuclear palsy. *Ann Neurol* 1997;41(5):606–614.
32. D'Antona R, Baron JC, Samson Y, et al. Subcortical dementia: frontal cortex hypometabolism detected by positron tomography in patients with progressive supranuclear palsy. *Brain* 1985;108:785–799.
33. Salmon E, Meulemans T, van der Linden M, et al. Anterior cingulate dysfunction in presenile dementia due to progressive supranuclear palsy. *Acta Neurol Belg* 1996;96(3):247–253.
34. Soliveri P, Monza D, Paridi D, et al. Cognitive and magnetic resonance imaging aspects of corticobasal degeneration and progressive supranuclear palsy. *Neurology* 1999;53(3):502–507.
35. Dubinsky RM, Jankovic J. Progressive supranuclear palsy and a multi-infarct state. *Neurology* 1987;37:570–576.
36. Ishii N, Nishihara Y, Imamura T. Why do frontal lobe symptoms predominate in vascular dementia with lacunes? *Neurology* 1986;36:340–345.
37. Kish SJ, Chang LJ, Mirchandani L, et al. Progressive supranuclear palsy: relationship between extrapyramidal disturbances, dementia, and brain neurotransmitter markers. *Ann Neurol* 1985;18:530–536.
38. Ruberg M, JavoY-Agid F, Hirsch E, et al. Dopaminergic and cholinergic lesions in progressive supranuclear palsy. *Ann Neurol* 1985;18:523–529.
39. Litvan I, Gomez C, Atack JR, et al. Physostigmine treatment of progressive supranuclear palsy. *Ann Neurol* 1989;26:404–407.
40. Kertzman C, Robinson DL, Litvan I. Effects of physostigmine on spatial attention in patients with PSP. *Arch Neurol* 1990;47:1346–1350.
41. Chiu HF. Psychiatric aspects of progressive supranuclear palsy. *Gen Hosp Psychiatry* 1995;17(2):135–143.
42. Chiu HF, Li SW. Progressive supranuclear palsy presenting with psychiatric features. *Br J Clin Pract* 1996;50(1):60–61.
43. Aarsland D, Litvan I, Larsen JP. Neuropsychiatric symptoms of patients with progressive supranuclear palsy in Parkinson's disease. *J Neuropsychiatry Clin Neurosci* 2001;13(1):42–49.
44. Litvan I, Cummings JL, Mega M. Neuropsychiatric features of corticobasal degeneration. *J Neurol Neurosurg Psychiatry* 1998;65(5):717–721.
45. Menza MA, Cocchiola J, Golbe LI. Psychiatric symptoms in progressive supranuclear palsy. *Psychosomatics* 1995;36(6):550–554.
46. Netzel PJ, Sutor B. Electroconvulsive therapy-responsive depression in a patient with progressive supranuclear palsy. *J ECT* 2001;17(1):68–70.
47. Pareja JA, Caminero AB, Masa JF, et al. A first case of progressive supranuclear palsy and pre-clinical REM sleep behavior disorder presenting as inhibition of speech during wakefulness and somniloquy with phasic muscle twitching during REM sleep. *Neurologia* 1996;11(8):304–306.
48. Konigsmark BW, Weiner LP. The olivopontocerebellar atrophies: a review. *Medicine* 1970;49:227–241.
49. Berciano J. Olivopontocerebellar atrophy. A review of 117 cases. *J Neurol Sci* 1982;53:253–272.
50. Harding AE. The clinical features and classification of the late onset autosomal dominant cerebellar ataxias—a study of 11 families, including descendents of "the Drew family of Walworth." *Brain* 1982;105:1–28.
51. Kish SJ, El-Awar M, Schut L, et al. Cognitive deficits in olivopontocerebellar atrophy: implications for the cholinergic hypothesis of Alzheimer's dementia. *Ann Neurol* 1988;24:200–206.
52. Orr HT, Chung M, Banfi S, et al. Expansion of an unstable trinucleotide CAG repeat in spinocerebellarataxia type 1. *Nat Genet* 1993;4:221–226.
53. El-Awar M, Kish S, Oscar-Berman M, et al. Selective delayed alternation deficits in dominantly inherited olivopontocerebellar atrophy. *Brain Cogn* 1991;16:121–129.
54. Botez MI, Leveille J, Botez T. Role of the cerebellum in cognitive thought: SPECT and neuropsychological findings. In: Matheson M, Newman H, eds. *Rehabilitation: the path back*. Richmond, Australia: Australian Society for the Study of Brain Impairment, 1989:179–195.
55. Botez MI, Botez T, Eli R, et al. Role of the cerebellum in complex human behavior. *Ital J Neurol Sci* 1989;10:291–300.

56. Botez MI, Gravel J, Attig E, et al. Reversible chronic cerebellar ataxia after phenytoin intoxication: possible role of cerebellum in cognitive thought. *Neurology* 1985; 35:1152–1157.
57. Hirono N, Yamadori A, Kameyama M, et al. Spinocerebellar degeneration (SCD): cognitive disturbances. *Acta Neurol Scand* 1991;84:226–230.
58. Grafman J, Litvan I, Massaquoi S, et al. Cognitive planning deficit in patients with cerebellar atrophy. *Neurology* 1992;42:1493–1496.
59. Moretti R, Torre P, Antonello RM, et al. Peculiar aspects of reading and writing performances in patients with olivopontocerebellar atrophy. *Percept Mot Skills* 2002;94(2):677–694.
60. Arroyo-Anllo EM, Botez-Marquard T. Neurobehavioral dimensions of olivopontocerebellar atrophy. *J Clin Exp Neuropsychol* 1998;20(1):52–59.
61. Botez-Marquard T, Botez MI. Olivopontocerebellar atrophy and Friedreich's ataxia: neuropsychological consequences of bilateral versus unilateral cerebellar lesions. *Int Rev Neurobiol* 1997;41:387–410.
62. Botez-Marquard T, Pedraza OL, Botez MI. Neuroradiological correlates of neuropsychological disorders in olivopontocerebellar atrophy (OPCA). *Eur J Neurol* 1996;3(2):89–97.
63. Botez-Marquard T, Routhier I. Reaction time and intelligence in patients with olivopontocerebellar atrophy. *Neuropsychiatry Neuropsychol Behav Neurol* 1995; 8(3):168–175.
64. Shy GM, Drager GA. A neurological syndrome associated with orthostatic hypotension. *Arch Neurol* 1960; 2:511–527.
65. Sullivan EV, De La Paz R, Zipursky RB, et al. Neuropsychological deficits accompanying striatonigral degeneration. *J Clin Exp Neuropsychiatry* 1991;13: 773–788.
66. Milner B. Some effects of frontal lobectomy in man. In: Warren JM, Akert K, eds. *Frontal granular cortex and behavior.* New York: McGraw-Hill, 1964:313–334.
67. Robbins TW, James M, Lange KW, et al. Cognitive performance in multiple system atrophy. *Brain* 1992; 115:271–291.
68. De Volder AG, Francart J, Laterre C, et al. Decreased glucose utilization in the striatum and frontal lobe in probable striatonigral degeneration. *Ann Neurol* 1989; 26:239–247.
69. Testa D, Fetoni V, Soliveri P, et al. Cognitive and motor performance in multiple system atrophy and Parkinson's disease compared. *Neuropsychologia* 1993;31:207–210.
70. Ghorayeb I, Yekhlef F, Chrysostome V, et al. Sleep disorders and their determinants in multiple system atrophy. *J Neurol Psychiatry* 2002;72(6):798–800.
71. Plazzi G, Cortelli P, Montagna P, et al. REM sleep behavior disorder differentiates pure autonomic failure from multiple system atrophy with parkinsonism. *J Neurol Neurosurg Psychiatry* 1998;64(5):683–685.
72. Boeve BF, Silber MH, Ferman TJ, et al. Association of REM sleep behavior disorder and neurodegenerative disease may reflect an underlying synucleinopathy. *Mov Disord* 2001;16(4):622–630.
73. Goto K, Ueki A, Shimode H, et al. Depression in multiple system atrophy: a case report. *Psychiatry Clin Neurosci* 2000;54(4):507–511.
74. Gill CE, Khurana RK, Hibler RJ. Occurrence of depressive symptoms in Shy-Drager syndrome. *Clin Auton Res* 1999;9(1):1–4.
75. Fetoni V, Soliveri P, Monza D, et al. Affective symptoms in multiple system atrophy and Parkinson's disease: response to levodopa therapy. *J Neurol Neurosurg Psychiatry* 1999;66(4):541–544.
76. Colosimo C, Albanese A, Hughes AJ, et al. Some specific clinical features differentiate multiple system atrophy (striatonigral variety) from Parkinson's disease. *Arch Neurol* 1995;52(3):294–298.
77. Pilo L, Ring H, Quinn N, et al. Depression in multiple system atrophy and in idiopathic Parkinson's disease: a pilot comparative study. *Biol Psychiatry* 199;39(9): 803–807.
78. Rosenberg R. Machado-Joseph disease: an autosomal dominant motor system degeneration. *Mov Disord* 1992; 7(3):193–203.
79. Spinella GM, Sheridan PH. Research initiatives on Machado-Joseph disease: National Institute of Neurological Disorders and Stroke Workshop summary. *Neurology* 1992;42:2048–2051.
80. Friedman JH. Presumed rapid eye movement behavior disorder in Machado-Joseph disease (spinocerebellar ataxia type 3). *Mov Disord* 2002;17(6):1350–1353.
81. Syed BH, Rye DB, Singh G. REM sleep behavior disorder and SCA-3 (Machado-Joseph disease). *Neurology* 2003;60(1):148.
82. Fukutake T, Shinotoh H, Nishino H, et al. Homozygous Machado-Joseph disease presenting as REM sleep behavior disorder and prominent psychiatric symptoms. *Eur J Neurol* 2002;9(1):97–100.
83. Sequeiros J, Coutinho P. Epidemiology and clinical aspects of Machado-Joseph disease. In: Harding AE, Deufel T, eds. *Advances in Neurology,* Vol 61. New York: Raven Press, 1993:139–153.
84. Zawacki TM, Grace J, Friedman JH, et al. Executive and emotional dysfunction in Machado-Joseph disease. *Mov Disord* 2002;17(5):1004–1010.
85. Maruff P, Tyler P, Burt T, et al. Cognitive deficits in Machado-Joseph disease. *Ann Neurol* 1996;40(3): 421–427.
86. Ishikawa A, Yamada M, Makino K, et al. Dementia and delirium in 4 patients with Machado-Joseph disease. *Arch Neurol* 2002;59(11):1804–1808.
87. Rebeiz JJ, Kolodny EH, Richardson EP. Corticodentatonigral degeneration with neuronal achromasia. *Arch Neurol* 1968;18:20–33.
88. Riley DE, Lang AE, Lewis A, et al. Cortical-basal ganglionic degeneration. *Neurology* 1990;40:1203–1212.
89. Neary D. Frontotemporal degeneration, Pick disease, and corticobasal degeneration. *Arch Neurol* 1997;54: 1425–1426.
90. Hachinski V. Frontotemporal degeneration, Pick disease, and corticobasal degeneration. *Arch Neurol* 1997;1429.
91. Kertesz A, Martinez-Lage P, Davidson BA, et al. The corticobasal degeneration syndrome overlaps progressive aphasia and frontotemporal dementia. *Neurology* 2000;55(1/2):1368–1375.
92. Mark MH. Lumping and splitting the parkinson plus syndromes: dementia with Lewy bodies, multiple system atrophy, progressive supranuclear palsy, and cortical-basal ganglionic degeneration. *Neurol Clin* 2001;19(3):1–19.
93. Rinne JO, Lee MS, Thompson PD, et al. Corticobasal degeneration: a clinical study of 36 cases. *Brain* 1994; 117:1183–1196.
94. Wenning GK, Litvan I, Jankovic J, et al. Natural history and survival of 14 patients with corticobasal

degeneration confirmed at postmortem examination. *J Neurol Neurosurg Psychiatry* 1998;64:184–189.
95. Geschwind N. The apraxias: neural mechanisms of disorders of learned movement. *Am Sci* 1975;63:188–195.
96. De Renzi E. Apraxia. In: Boller F, Grafman J, eds. *Handbook of neuropsychology*, Vol. 2. Amsterdam: Elsevier, 1989:245–263.
97. Watts RL, Williams RS, Growdon JD, et al. Corticobasal ganglionic degeneration. *Neurology* 1986; 35(Suppl. 1):178.
98. Lang AE. Cortical basal ganglionic degeneration presenting with "progressive loss of speech output and orofacial dyspraxia." *J Neurol Neurosurg Psychiatry* 1992;55:11101.
99. Boeve BF, Lang AE, Litvan I. Corticobasal degeneration and its relationship to progressive supranuclear palsy and frontotemporal dementia. *Ann Neurol* 2003; 54(Suppl. 5):S15–S19.
100. Poeck K. Clues to the nature of disruptions to limb praxis. In: Roy EA, ed. *Neuropsychological studies of apraxia and related disorders.* Amsterdam: Elsevier, 1985:99–109.
101. Leiguarda R, Lees AJ, Merello M, et al. The nature of apraxia in corticobasal degeneration. *J Neurol Neurosurg Psychiatry* 1994;57:455–459.
102. Bogen JE. Split-brain syndrome. In: Frederiks JAM, ed. *Handbook of clinical neurology*, Vol. 1(45), *Clinical neuropsychology.* Amsterdam: Elsevier, 1985:99–106.
103. Brion S. Jedynak CPo Troubles du transfert interhemispherique (callosal disconnection). *Rev Neurol (Paris)* 1972;126:257–266.
104. McNabb AW, Carroll WM, Mastaglia FL. "Alien hand" and loss of bimanual coordination after dominant anterior cerebral artery territory infarction. *J Neurol Neurosurg Psychiatry* 1988;51:218–222.
105. Goldberg G, Mayer NH, Toglia JU. Medical frontal cortex infarction and the alien hand sign. *Arch Neurol* 1981;38:683–686.
106. Scully RE, Mark EJ, McNeely BU. Case records of the Massachusetts General Hospital. *N Engl J Med* 1985; 313:739–748.
107. Gibb WRG, Luthert PJ, Marsden CD. Corticobasal degeneration. *Brain* 1989;112:1171–1192.
108. Lippa CF, Cohen R, Smith TW, et al. Primary progressive aphasia with focal neuronal achromasia. *Neurology* 1991;41:882–886.
109. Graham NL, Bak T, Patterson K, et al. Language function and dysfunction in corticobasal degeneration. *Neurology* 2003;61(4):493–499.
110. Frattali CM, Grafman J, Patronas N, et al. Language disturbances in corticobasal degeneration. *Neurology* 2000;54(4):990–992.
111. Naeser MA, Alexander MP, Helm-Estabrooks N, et al. Aphasia with predominantly subcortical lesion sites. *Arch Neurol* 1982;39:2–14.
112. Damasio AR, Damasio H, Rizzo M, et al. Aphasia with nonhemorrhagic lesions in the basal ganglia and internal capsule. *Arch Neurol* 1982;39:15–20.
113. Spencer PS, Nunn PB, Hugon J, et al. Guam amyotrophic lateral sclerosis-parkinsonism-dementia linked to a plant excitant neurotoxin. *Science* 1987;237:517–522.
114. Cox PA, Sacks OW. Cycad neurotoxins, consumption of flying foxes, and ALS-PDC disease in Guam. *Neurology* 2002;58:956–959.
115. Rogers-Johnson P, Garruto R, Yanagihara R, et al. Amyotrophic lateral sclerosis and parkinsonism dementia on Guam: a thirty-year evaluation of clinical and neuropathological trends. *Neurology* 1986;36:7–13.
116. Hudson AJ, Rice GPA. Similarities of Guamanian ALS/PD to post-encephalitic parkinsonism/ALS: possible viral cause. *Can J Neurol Sci* 1990;17:427–433.
117. Elizan TS, Hirano A, Abrams BM, et al. Amyotrophic lateral sclerosis and parkinsonism-dementia complex of Guam. *Arch Neurol* 1966;14:356–368.
118. Snow BJ, Peppard RF, Guttman M. et al. Positron emission tomographic scanning demonstrates a presynaptic dopaminergic lesion in lytico-bodig. *Arch Neurol* 1990;47:870–874.
119. Cummings JL, Benson DF, eds. *Dementia: a clinical approach*, 2nd ed. Boston, MA: Butterworth-Heinemann, 1992:139.
120. Caselli RJ, Smith BE, Osborne D. Primary lateral sclerosis; a neuropsychological study. *Neurology* 1995; 45(11):2005–2009.
121. Mantovan MC, Baggio L, Dalla Barba G, et al. Memory deficits and retrieval processes in ALS. *Eur J Neurol* 2003;10(3):221–227.
122. Lomen-Hoerth C, Murphy J, Langmore S, et al. Are amyotrophic lateral sclerosis patients cognitively normal? *Neurology* 2003;60(7):1094–1097.
123. Neary D, Snowden JS, Mann DM. Cognitive change in motor neuron disease/amyotrophic lateral sclerosis (MND/ALS). *J Neurol Sci* 2000;180(1-2):15–20.
124. Zoccolella S, Palagano G, Fraddosio A, et al. ALS-Plus: 5 cases of concomitant amyotrophic lateral sclerosis and parkinsonism. *Neurol Sci* 2002;23 (Suppl. 2):S123–S124.
125. Wilson CM, Grace GM, Munoz DG, et al. Cognitive impairment in sporadic ALS: a pathologic continuum underlying a multisystem disorder. *Neurology* 2001; 57(4):651–657.
126. Tomik B, Adamek D, Lechwacka A, et al. ALS-Plus syndrome. A clinical and neuropathological case study. *Pol J Pathol* 2000; 51(4):191–196.
127. de Brito-Marques PR, de Mello RV. Amyotrophic lateral sclerosis with dementia. Case report. *Arq Neuropsiquiatr* 1999;57(2A):277–283.
128. Ravenholt RT, Foege WH. 1918 Influenza, encephalitis lethargica, parkinsonism. *Lancet* 1982;2:860–864.
129. Duncan AG. The sequelae of encephalitis lethargica. *Brain* 1924;47:76–95.
130. Weiner WJ, Lang AE, eds. *Movement disorders—a comprehensive survey.* New York: Futura, 1989:52.
131. Devinsky O. Neuroanatomy of Gilles de la Tourette's syndrome. *Arch Neurol* 1983;40:508–514.
132. Ziegler LH. Follow-up studies on persons who have had epidemic encephalitis. *JAMA* 1928;91:138–141.
133. Duvoisin RC, Yahr MD. Encephalitis and parkinsonism. *Arch Neurol* 1965;12:227–239.
134. Sacks OW. Acquired Tourettism in adult life. In: Friedhoff AJ, Chase TN, eds. *Gilles de la Tourette syndrome.* New York: Raven Press, 1982:89–92.
135. Von Econono C. *Encephalitis lethargica: its sequelae and treatment.* London: Oxford University Press, 1931.
136. Ward CD. Neuropsychiatric interpretations of postencephalitic movement disorders. *Mov Disord* 2003;18(6): 623–630.
137. Riley M, Esiri MM. A contemporary case of encephalitis lethargica. *Clin Neuropathol* 2001;20(1):2–7.
138. Robinson RL, Shahida S, Madan N, et al. Transient parkinsonism in West Nile virus encephalitis. *Am J Med* 2003;115(3):252–253.

139. Hsieh JC, Lue KH, Lee YL. Parkinson-like syndrome as the major presenting symptom of Epstein-Barr virus encephalitis. *Arch Dis Child* 2002;87(4):358.
140. Lance JW, Hickie I, Wakefield D, et al. An akinetic-rigid syndrome, depression, an stereotypies in a young man. *Mov Disord* 1998;13(5):835–844.
141. Hsiao K, Cass C, Schellenberg GD, et al. A prion protein variant in a family with the telencephalic form of Gerstmann-Straussler-Scheinker syndrome. *Neurology* 1991;41:681–684.
142. Berger JR, David NJ. Creutzfeldt-Jakob disease in a physician: a review of the disorder in health care workers. *Neurology* 1993;43:205–206.
143. Weihl CC, Roos RP. Creutzfeldt-Jakob disease, new variant Creutzfeldt-Jakob disease, and bovine spongiform encephalopathy. *Neurol Clin* 1999;17(4):835–859.
144. Brown P, Cathala F, Castaigne P, et al. Creutzfeldt-Jakob disease: clinical analysis of a consecutive series of 230 neuropathologically verified cases. *Ann Neurol* 1986;20:597–602.
145. Cummings JL, Benson FD, eds. *Dementia: A clinical approach*, 2nd ed. Boston, MA: Butterworth-Heinemann, 1992:189–198.
146. Gass CS, Luis CA, Meyers TL, et al. Familial Creutzfeldt-Jakob disease. A neuropsychological case study. *Arch Clin Neuropsychol* 2000;15(2):165–175.
147. Snowden JS, Mann DM, Neary D. Distinct neuropsychological characteristics in Creutzfeldt-Jakob disease. *J Neurol Neurosurg Psychiatry* 2002;73(6):686–694.
148. Kapur N, Ironside J, Abbott P, et al. A neuropsychological-neuropathological case study of variant Creutzfeldt-Jakob disease. *Neurocase* 2001;7(3):261–267.
149. Brown P, Preece M, Brandel JP, et al. Iatrogenic Creutzfeldt-Jakob disease at the millennium. *Neurology* 2000;55(8):1075–1081.
150. Cordery RJ, Hall M, Cipolotti L, et al. Early cognitive decline in Creutzfeldt-Jakob disease associated with human growth hormone treatment. *J Neurol Neurosurg Psychiatry* 2003;74(10):1412–1416.
151. Hauser WA, Morris ML, Heston LL, et al. Seizures and myoclonus in patients with Alzheimer's disease. *Neurology* 1986;36:1226–1230.
152. Mayeux R, Stem Y, Spanton S. Heterogeneity in dementia of the Alzheimer type: evidence of subgroups. *Neurology* 1985;35:453–461.
153. McDaniel KD. Thalamic degeneration. In: Cummings LJ, ed. *Subcortical dementia*. New York: Oxford University Press, 1990:132–144.
154. Henry C, Knight R. Clinical features of variant Creutzfeldt-Jakob disease. *Rev Med Virol* 2002;12(3):143–150.
155. Will RG, Stewart G, Zeidler M, et al. Psychiatric features of new variant Creutzfeldt-Jakob disease. *Psychiatr Bull* 1999;23(5):264–267.
156. Spencer MD, Knight RS, Will RG. First hundred cases of variant Creutzfeldt-Jakob disease: retrospective case note review of early psychiatric and neurological features. *Br Med J* 2002;324(7352):1479–1482.
157. Galvez S, Cartier L. Computed tomographic findings in 15 cases of Creutzfeldt-Jakob disease with histologic verification. *J Neurol Neurosurg Psychiatry* 1984;47:1244–1246.
158. Kovanen J, Erkinjuntti T, Iivanainen M, et al. Cerebral MR and CT imaging in Creutzfeldt-Jakob disease. *J Comput Assist Tomogr* 1985;9:125–128.
159. Roberts GW, Lofthouse R, Allsop D, et al. CNS amyloid proteins in neurodegenerative diseases. *Neurology* 1988;38:1534–1540.
160. Narang HK. A critical review of atypical cerebellum-type Creutzfeldt-Jakob disease: its relationship to "new variant" CJD and bovine spongiform encephalopathy. *Exp Biol Med* 2001;226(7):629–639.
161. Masters DL, Gajdusek DC, Gibbs CJ. Creutzfeldt-Jakob disease virus isolations from the Gerstmann-Straussler syndrome. *Brain* 1981;104:559–588.
162. Hainfellner JA, Brantner-Inthaler S, Cervenakova L, et al. The original Gerstmann-Straussler-Scheinker family of Austria: divergent clinicopathological phenotypes but constant PrP genotype. *Brain Pathol* 1995;5(3):201–211.
163. Kuzuhara S, Kanazawa I, Sasaki H, et al. Gerstmann-Straussler-Scheinker's disease. *Ann Neurol* 1983;14:216–225.
164. Farlow MR, Yee RD, Dlouhy SR, et al. Gerstmann-Straussler-Scheinker disease. I. Extending the clinical spectrum. *Neurology* 1989;39:1446–1452.
165. Collins S, McLean CA, Masters CL. Gerstmann-Straussler-Scheinker syndrome, fatal familial insomnia, and kuru: a review of these less common human transmissible spongiform encephalopathies. *J Clin Neurosci* 2001;8(5):387–397.
166. Unverzagt FW, Farlow MR, Norton J, et al. Neuropsychological function in patients with Gerstmann-Straussler disease from the Indiana kindred (F198S). *J Int Neuropsychol Soc* 1997;3(2):169–178.
167. Ishizawa K, Komori T, Shimazu T, et al. Hyperphosphorylated tau deposition parallels prion protein burden in a case of Gerstmann-Straussler-Scheinker syndrome P102L mutation complicated with dementia. *Acta Neuropathol* 2002;104(4):342–350.
168. Mohr M, Tranchant C, Steinmetz G, et al. Gerstmann-Straussler-Scheinker disease and the French-Alsatian A117V variant. *Clin Exp Pathol* 1999;47(3-4):161–175.
169. Boellaard JW, Brown P, Tateishi J. Gerstmann-Straussler-Scheinker disease—the dilemma of molecular and clinical correlations. *Clin Neuropathol* 1999;18(6):271–285.
170. Young K, Clark HB, Piccardo P, et al. Gerstmann-Straussler-Scheinker disease with the PRNP P102L mutation and valine at codon 129. *Brain Res Mol Brain Res* 1997;44(1):147–150.
171. Heldt N, Boellaard JW, Brown P, et al. *Clin Neuropathol* 1998;17(4):229–234.
172. Hsiao K, Dlouhy SR, Farlow MR, et al. Mutant prion proteins in Gerstmann-Straussler-Scheinker disease with neurofibrillary tangles. *Nat Genet* 1992;1(1):68–71.
173. Cervenakova L, Buetefisch C, Lee HS, et al. Novel PRNP sequence variant associated with familial encephalopathy. *Am J Med Genet* 1999;88(6):653–656.
174. Panegyres PK, Toufexis K, Kakulas BA, et al. A new PRNP mutation (G131V) associated with Gerstmann-Straussler-Scheinker disease. *Arch Neurol* 2001;58(11):1899–1902.

13
Behavioral Changes in Frontotemporal Dementia with Parkinsonism

Catherine E. Pace-Savitsky, Julene K. Johnson, and Bruce L. Miller

University of California, San Francisco, San Francisco, California

This chapter focuses on frontotemporal lobar degeneration (FTLD), a spectrum of heterogeneous disorders that affect the anterior frontal and temporal lobes. Patients with FTLD are clinically classified on the basis of cortical clinical syndromes associated with behavioral and language abnormalities, but many patients exhibit extrapyramidal or motor neuron syndromes early in the course of the illness. FTLD, first described by Pick in 1892, is now recognized as a leading cause of dementia, particularly in the presenium (1). As understanding of FTLD has improved, the diagnosis and treatment of this spectrum of disorders has also improved. However, 101 years after Pick's initial description of this spectrum of disorders, a study in 1993 noted that 18 out of 21 patients with autopsy-confirmed FTLD had been misdiagnosed with Alzheimer's disease (AD) (2). Also, the behavioral disturbances characteristic of FTLD often result in it being misdiagnosed as psychiatric disorders such as depression, schizophrenia, and obsessive–compulsive disorder, personality disorder, or both. Additionally, despite the new diagnostic criteria for FTLD, there has been ongoing controversy amongst clinicians about the classification of the disorder (3), which has contributed to confusion about prevalence, prognosis, education, and treatment of FTLD.

In 1998, Neary et al. published a consensus on clinical diagnostic criteria, which divided FTLD into three prototypic neurobehavioral syndromes (1). The most common syndrome is frontotemporal dementia (FTD), the core characteristics of which include early decline in social and personal conduct, emotional blunting, and loss of insight. The second syndrome is a disorder of expressive language, termed progressive nonfluent aphasia (PA). Like FTD, PA has an insidious onset with gradual progression and exhibits nonfluent spontaneous speech with agrammatism, phonemic paraphasias, anomia, or some combination of these features. The third syndrome, semantic dementia (SD), which is also a progressive language disorder, is characterized by severe comprehension and naming deficits, loss of word meaning, or perceptual impairments, including prosopagnosia, associative agnosia, or both.

Most cases of FTLD are sporadic, though our knowledge of the genetic basis of this disease is progressing. Wilhelmsen et al. were the first to link FTLD to chromosome 17. These authors coined the term "dementia–disinhibition–parkinsonism–amy trophy syndrome" to describe a family with presenile dementia associated with frontal lobe features and prominent motor deficits, including parkinsonism, amyotrophic lateral sclerosis (ALS), or both (4). Later, this family and other patients with presenile dementia were shown to have mutations in the exon and intron regions of the tau gene. This discovery strongly linked FTLD to tau and led to the rethinking of the clinical features and neuropathology of FTLD and other tau-related disorders, including progressive supranuclear palsy (PSP) and corticobasal degeneration (CBD) (3). Most of the first families with tau mutations had prominent parkinsonian features (5). In some familial cases, clinical features compatible with

PSP and CBD were evident. Similarly, some patients with familial or sporadic forms of FTLD exhibited PSP or CBD neuropathology. Also, longitudinal clinical studies of FTLD suggested that many patients who did not have parkinsonian features went on to develop PSP or CBD disorders, whereas similar studies of PSP and CBD showed prominent cognitive and behavioral deficits reminiscent of FTLD. The overlap between FTLD, PSP, and CBD has led some authors to lump the three disorders under the term "the Pick-Complex" (3). Many others continue to separate these syndromes. No differences have been determined between the behavioral features of chromosome-linked FTDP-17 and those of the sporadic form of FTLD (6).

FTLD with parkinsonism is both clinically and pathologically heterogeneous. The neuropathology is characterized by neuronal loss, gliosis, and tau-positive accumulations in both neurons and glia. The filamentous tau inclusions are the hallmark of patients who have FTDP-17. Neuropathologic changes are found predominantly in the frontal and temporal cortices and are also common in limbic and midbrain structures, such as the caudate, amygdala, substantia nigra, globus pallidus, and pons (7,8). Degeneration of the basal ganglia and substantia nigra is likely related to the clinical symptoms of parkinsonism (9).

The distribution and type of neuropathology in FTLD with parkinsonism can overlap with that of other tauopathies, such as CBD and PSP (5). There is also heterogeneity within and between families with the same mutation. For example, Bird et al. (10) described two families with the same chromosome 17 mutation that had different patterns of pathology: one patient had neurofibrillary tangle pathology that was similar to that of PSP, whereas another patient had pathology similar to that of Pick's disease. The differences in location and type of neuropathology most likely reflect underlying selective vulnerability and is not yet well understood.

FRONTOTEMPORAL DEMENTIA

In contrast to AD, FTD is considered to be an early-onset dementia, with mean onset between 53 and 56 years. Duration of the disease is reported to be approximately 8 years from onset (1). Although FTD was previously believed to be a disease affecting both sexes equally (11,12), more recent studies suggest that it is more common in men than in women (13). Our own clinical experience has also suggested a male predominance, and 67% of our patients with clinically diagnosed FTD are men.

Behavioral Features

As in many degenerative brain disorders, the asymmetric degeneration in FTD contributes to a wide array of clinical and neuropsychological presentations. In the research criteria for FTD, the disorder is defined as a behavioral syndrome, although neuropsychological deficits and motor syndromes are common. Most imaging studies of FTD cohorts have found bilateral atrophy or hypoperfusion of the cingulate, dorsolateral, and orbitofrontal cortex and the insula, with greater right-sided than left-sided involvement (14). Although maintaining appropriate social behavior is a complex process with many contributing factors, the right frontal and temporal lobes have been shown to vigorously affect emotional processing, global attention, self-awareness, and regulation of one's sense of self (15). As described later, the progressive aphasia syndromes associated with FTLD are more likely to involve the left hemisphere of the cerebral cortex.

The Neary criteria for FTD include four core features: decline in social conduct, decline in personal conduct, emotional blunting, and loss of insight. Patients with FTD exhibit slow, insidious changes in personality, with increasing social withdrawal and passivity. Using personality scales, Rankin et al. have shown that patients with FTD become progressively more submissive and passive as the disease progresses (16). Antisocial behaviors emerge in most patients, and theft, infidelity, and indecent exposure characterize the early stages of the illness. Rudeness, loss of social etiquette, and inappropriate behaviors in public settings are common. Loss of insight is among the core criteria for FTD, and many patients are distinctly unaware of their behavioral deficits.

Loss of empathy is common, and family members report that patients show a puzzling lack of interest in the well-being of their family. Emotional blunting is extremely common, and patients exhibit profound apathy, spending hours in front of the television or shuffling paper at work. Patients with FTD often fail to respond with appropriate emotions to loss of employment, financial crises, or health problems of their friends and relatives. Some of the loss of empathy is explained by apathy, whereas other aspects may arise from the patient's inability to identify emotions in others (17,18).

These patients commonly have poor insight into what is socially acceptable behavior, even in the case of those patients whose premorbid social etiquette had been exceptional. Patients with FTD can exhibit a profound loss of personal boundaries—they can be withdrawn and disengaged at home but can be overly friendly with strangers. For example, one patient was thrown out of several shopping centers for offering women back massages while standing in check-out lines, and another patient approached strangers and discussed intimate details of his strained marital situation. Not only is the patient's sense of social etiquette disturbed, but insight into the needs of others becomes impaired as well. One patient gave his wife an empty shoe box for Christmas one year, thinking the box was something that she needed and could truly use, whereas the year before he had given her diamond earrings. Another patient left her grandchild unattended in a high chair at the shopping mall food court while she went in search of her other family members, who were shopping at the other end of the mall. Despite the grave nature of some of these behaviors, patients typically are able to offer explanations for their actions, which seem completely normal and justified to them. These justifications can be profoundly upsetting to caregivers, who are unable to reason with the patient or help the patient understand the consequences of their actions.

Compulsions and overeating are common with all variants of FTLD but are particularly common in patients with FTD. Compulsive behaviors include counting or hoarding items (especially food), drinking beverages in a specific order or at a specific time, picking up coins, and counting rituals. Patients who develop one compulsion often go on to develop others and can become rigid and inflexible, especially if they are untreated. One patient's compulsions began 5 to 6 years before other notable FTD-like symptoms developed. He began collecting cans, going out of his way to obtain them even when it was extremely inconvenient. Counting and sorting the cans occupied many hours of his time, and soon this compulsion extended to coin collecting and eating sweets. He began walking 6 miles each day, passing by phone booths looking for coins that people might have dropped or left behind, checking trash receptacles for cans, and passing by bakeries and candy shops looking for sweets (19).

Other frequently reported behavioral changes include alterations in eating habits and food preferences. The most common change is toward a preference for sweets and, notably, patients tend to eat more rapidly, often "shoveling" food or failing to use utensils properly. Carbohydrate craving and changes in diet are seen in up to two-thirds of patients (20). Less commonly seen are "food fads" in which patients refuse to eat anything but one or two particular foods. For example, one patient would eat only lobster, avocado, and bacon, whereas another preferred eating only condiments—particularly ketchup.

In the mid-to-late stages of FTD, patients exhibit poor personal hygiene. Caregivers consistently report that patients with FTD exhibit decreased interest in their personal appearance and that they often do not bathe or change their clothes for many days unless forced to do so. In a smaller percentage of patients, dress style or color preferences change. For example, one patient developed a new passion for purple and would wear only purple clothes, day or night, regardless of the occasion. The patient was known for being an impeccable dresser before her illness, but now she would mix and match prints and intermix shades of purple that, to those around her, were seen as rather unbecoming.

Cognitive Features

Loss of executive function is very common in FTD, and problems with future planning and logical thinking have profound effects on the patients and their families. Many patients have lost their jobs, financial savings, and social relationships by the time they are diagnosed. On neuropsychological testing, patients with FTD exhibit difficulty with frontal lobe functions such as word generation (phonemic fluency), alternating sequences, abstraction, and inhibition. Disorganized approaches to cognitive testing affect performance. The Mini-Mental State Examination (MMSE) does not identify these deficits, and many patients can be profoundly impaired, despite normal MMSE results. Patients with FTD are not typically amnesic, though poor memory may be a complaint of patients, caregivers, or both. Poor memory can be attributed to an increase in distractibility that leads to poor encoding of information and weakened learning strategies.

Motor Symptoms

Although most patients have FTD with cognitive and behavioral dysfunction, motor symptoms also commonly develop early in the illness. Studies on the parkinsonian features of FTD are still limited, but the general consensus is that the parkinsonism found in FTLD differs from that found in idiopathic parkinsonism. Tremor is less common, and patients tend to show axial rigidity and eye movement abnormalities. Indeed, in some patients the distinction between FTD and PSP is difficult because of the overlap of the two syndromes. Some other patients develop CBD-like syndromes with alien hand, dystonia, and focal paralysis, although CBD is more common in the PA subgroup (2). A strong link also exists between FTD and ALS. Approximately 15% of patients in an FTD cohort also met the research criteria for ALS. Similarly, considerably few ALS patients show frontal-executive features compatible with FTD (21).

Neuroanatomy

An example of a magnetic resonance imaging (MRI) from a patient diagnosed with FTD is shown in Figure 13.1. It illustrates degeneration most prominently in the left frontal region of the brain. FTD can affect both the right and left frontal and temporal lobes in varying degrees, and support for localization is derived from functional imaging. Degeneration in the dorsolateral prefrontal cortex is associated with impaired judgment, perseveration, difficulty with set shifting, poor planning, impaired abstraction,

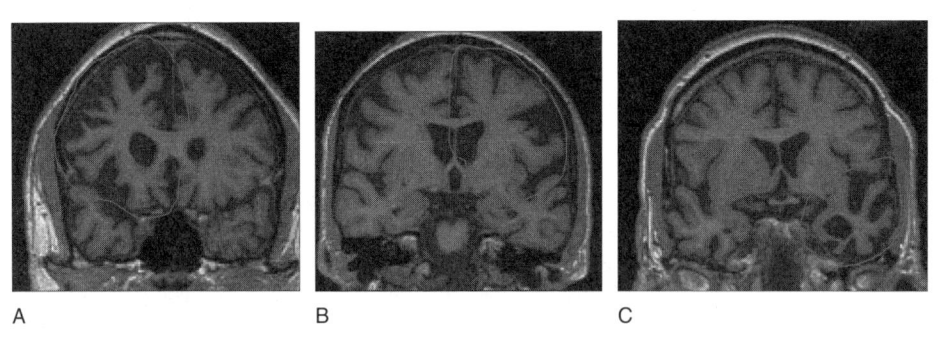

FIG. 13-1. Coronal sections from T1-weighted magnetic resonance images showing differences among the atrophy patterns of patients with frontotemporal dementia (FTD), progressive nonfluent aphasia (PA), and semantic dementia (SD). A is the image of a patient in later stages of FTD. Note that there is considerably greater right frontal atrophy than left frontal atrophy. Patient first presented with decreased personal hygiene, increased irritability, and new compulsions, such as watching television for hours while simultaneously taping other shows with two VCRs so as not to miss anything. B is an image of a patient diagnosed with nonfluent progressive aphasia. Note that there is considerably greater left frontal atrophy than right frontal atrophy. This patient's first symptom was an occasional stuttering of speech and slowly progressed to word-finding difficulty and halting speech. C is an image of a patient diagnosed with SD. Note considerable left temporal atrophy. This patient presented with speech and language dysfunction and slowly developed behavioral symptoms that included entering the homes of neighbors unannounced and limiting his food choices to only chicken, broccoli, and carrots.

and reduced verbal output. Loss of function in orbito-frontal cortex leads to disinhibition, impulsivity, euphoria, and socially inappropriate behavior. Injury to anterior cingulate cortex is linked to apathy and reduced motivation (20).

Case History

Patient 1, a 54-year-old male college graduate with a strong family history of FTD with parkinsonism, was referred for an evaluation with complaints of changing personality and disturbances in organizational skills. Cognitive loss and disinhibition were first noticed approximately 7 years earlier, when the family was preparing to repaint their kitchen; he required family members to explain to him, several times, how to use the paint brush. Gradually, he developed trouble multitasking, planning, and following through on tasks. This impairment began to affect his performance as a store manager, and employees began noticing that he was frequently over-ordering inventory. When the stress of store management became too great, he began looking for nonmanagerial positions such as park ranger and farm laborer, which he felt would "be high paying enough to allow his family to move" to a more upscale community. During the same time, personality changes appeared. He became more socially withdrawn, rarely speaking unless spoken to, and began distancing himself from his wife. At one point, his wife was hospitalized, and he seemed to show very little interest in her well-being or recovery. Other family members also noticed increasing apathy, including a loss of interest in his young grandchildren, upon whom he had previously lavished his attention.

About 5 years after the first signs of personality change began, rigidity about his daily schedule became increasingly problematic. It began with a desire to have his meals served at specific times each day. Changes in the schedule caused him to become irritable and agitated, though he never became violent. Soon he insisted on watching a television show that came on each day at 5:00 PM. He would not turn on the television until the clock read precisely 5:00 PM. He would also walk up and down the stairs at exactly 11:50 AM each day.

It was at about this time that the patient's sister died at the age of 57 from FTD with parkinsonism and motor neuron disease (MND). Her autopsy demonstrated FTD pathology. A further detailed family history revealed that his mother had died at the age of 59 from what was believed to be dementia with parkinsonism, though this diagnosis was never confirmed by autopsy. His father had died at 62 years from a stroke, and it was unclear whether any of the father's family members had had dementia. In Patient 1's generation, there were 7 children, of which he was the youngest. The two eldest children, a daughter and a son, had died in their late 50s to early 60s from dementia with parkinsonism. The third child (the second daughter) began developing symptoms of cognitive disturbance and ALS in her late 30s and died of a head injury at the age of 37. The next child, a son, died at age 50 from pancreatic cancer and was believed to have not been affected by dementia, and one surviving sister, the fifth child, self-reports to have no related symptoms, although cognitive and neurological evaluations have indicated that early stages of a dementialike syndrome may be developing. One woman from the third generation had also developed symptoms of dementia in her early 40s and has since died. (See Fig. 13-2.)

Subsequently, Patient 1 developed symptoms of environmental dependence along with stereotypic behaviors. If objects were placed in front of him, he would invariably play with them. On an airplane flight, he watched the flight attendant demonstrate how to pull the oxygen mask down from the ceiling. He mimicked this behavior and continued demonstrating it throughout the duration of the flight. The family also noticed a new propensity for fidgeting with his hand and playing with his wedding ring.

Apathy became increasingly prominent, as did changes in his food preferences. He would no longer help out around the house or do other chores as he previously had done. He was content watching television all day, except at the exact time when he expected his meals. He developed a preference for sweets, which was a change from his premorbid state. For example, when a large bag of candy was purchased for Halloween, all of the Snickers were found missing from the bowl.

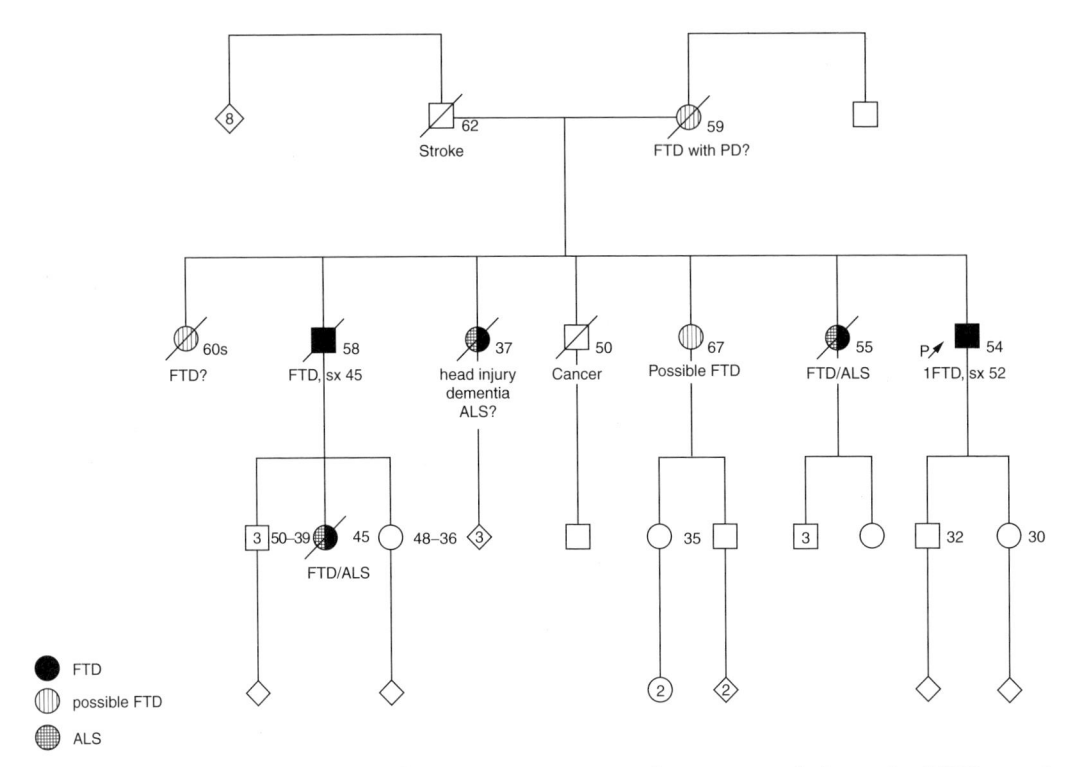

FIG. 13-2. Pedigree of Patient 1. Solid figures represent frontotemporal dementia (FTD); mesh figures represent amyotropic lateral sclerosis (ALS); vertical striped figures represent possible FTD.

The family later found one of his drawers filled with empty wrappers. He could barely wait for a meal to be finished before he got up from the table to get sweets from the kitchen.

Neuropsychological testing demonstrated considerable impairment of executive functioning, including areas such as working memory, set shifting, response inhibition, generation of verbal and nonverbal information, stimulus boundedness, perseveration, and lack of abstract reasoning. His deficits in the area of visuospatial functioning were inconsistent, though many of his difficulties may have been attributable to poor organization of visuospatial material. Memory, language, and comprehension were intact. He had no deficits in praxis, and he could calculate. He evinced no symptoms when screened for depression.

Neurological examination revealed a number of physical findings consistent with dysfunction in frontal lobe–basal ganglia circuit. Initiation of saccades was slow, and smooth pursuit was saccadic. Finger taps were slowed and tone was increased in the left greater than right upper extremity. Gait testing revealed decreased arm swing on the left side. In light of the family history of ALS, nerve conduction studies and a swallowing study were performed; results were normal. MRI showed evidence of bilateral frontal lobe and striatal atrophy. There were no ischemic white matter changes.

This case illustrates the behavioral and executive abnormalities that are the hallmark of this disease, especially in the early to middle stages. In these familial cases, the syndrome is remarkably transferred through generations. However, because this disease was not well characterized and was poorly understood in past years, it is difficult to be certain of possible cases in earlier generations—many of which were dismissed as psychiatric illness or atypical forms of AD.

PROGRESSIVE NONFLUENT APHASIA

Individuals with PA develop a nonfluent aphasia with prominent word-finding difficulties and altered speech output that includes agrammatism, phonemic paraphasias, anomia, or some combination of these features (1). Language and speech deficits precede the development of dementia or behavioral abnormalities by many years. Some patients develop characteristic Broca's aphasia, some show profound abnormalities in speech production, whereas verbal apraxia is the presenting syndrome in other patients. Imaging shows left-sided atrophy, as seen in Figure 13-1.

Most patients with PA describe a frustration with "losing" their words. Speech is effortful and eventually becomes void of content. Object naming becomes severely impaired, though it is common for patients to have partial knowledge of the word, such as the first letter, and will make attempts to use a word that come close to the correct one. For example, a picture of an apple is presented to the patient and he says, "atter . . . no . . . attle . . . no . . . apper . . ." (1). Low frequency words are more difficult for these patients to retrieve, but unlike patients with SD (discussed later), the patient remembers the meaning of the word. For example, when a patient is presented with a picture of a harmonica, although he is unable to say the word "harmonica," he is able to mime how a harmonica is used and is able to describe some of its attributes, such as "it makes music" or "you play with your mouth."

Articulation is effortful, and single word repetition is often impaired in PA, leading to decreased verbal output and social withdrawal. Polysyllabic words become increasingly difficult to repeat, as are long word sequences.

Formal neuropsychological testing typically demonstrates deficits in expressive language, oral apraxia, and some executive tasks, with preservation of visuospatial skills and visual memory. Language impairment can compromise performance on verbal memory tasks and tasks that require verbal expression.

Changes in Behavior

The behavioral changes typically seen in the frontal variants of FTD are not usually present in the early stages of PA. Social withdrawal, depression, and apathy are the most common behavioral symptoms, whereas insight and social awareness remain relatively preserved. Initially, the disease is localized unilaterally to the left frontal, left frontoparietal, or left frontotemporal regions, but as the disease spreads to the right side of the brain, more FTD-like symptoms develop, such as irritability, loss of insight, and rigidity (20). Eventually patients with PA develop FTD syndromes. Not all patients who begin with a progressive aphasia syndrome have FTLD pathology, and a left angular gyrus–predominant AD can present as PA.

A strong overlap exists between CBD, PSP, and PA, and many patients who initially have focal left frontal lobe aphasia syndromes go on to develop focal motor syndromes suggestive of CBD or PSP. Similarly, some of these patients show CBD or PSP pathology at postmortem.

SEMANTIC DEMENTIA

SD represents a temporal variant of FTD (tvFTD) and is characterized as a progressive loss of semantic knowledge, that is, knowledge about words, objects, facts, and their meaning (22). As the disease progresses, the patient's speech becomes "empty" and is characterized by frequent, vague references to people, places, and things. Speech is fluent, except for occasional word-finding pauses. However, it lacks content, and phrases such as "that thing" and "that place" are used in substitution for precise nominal terms. The most distinct characteristic is the patient's loss of word meaning, often asking, "What's a ___?" in common conversation. For example, when one patient's wife asked him what he preferred for dinner—pasta or salmon, he replied, "What's pasta?"

Idiosyncratic word usage commonly develops. Patients adopt words or phrases that are repeated over and over, typically at the beginning or end of sentences. For example, one patient would say, "There again" nearly every time he started a sentence, despite that fact that the particular phrase added no value or had no relevance to the idea he was trying to convey. Press of speech is also common, where the patient speaks without interruption—talking louder than the others when an attempt is made to enter the conversation.

Often, patients with considerable right temporal lobe involvement develop prosopagnosia, or difficulty recognizing familiar faces. This symptom can extend into other sensory modalities, such as associating names with voices or even identifying familiar animal sounds. Patients often complain of difficulty identifying familiar voices over the telephone and become very distressed in social situations when it becomes apparent that they are unable to identify the faces of even very close friends and associates.

Cognitive testing reveals profound anomia to confrontation naming. The anomia leads to comprehension deficits, even when speech remains fluent. General knowledge becomes severely impaired. Depending upon the severity of the right temporal lobe injury, facial recognition and emotion recognition are impaired (14). Skills spared in this population include preserved working memory, repetition, ability to read aloud and write orthographically regular words, visuospatial skills, and day-to-day memory.

As with patients with FTD, patients with SD are often described as lacking sympathy or empathy. Yet, unlike FTD, this deficit is replaced with coldness rather than apathy. Irritability and mental rigidity become increasingly problematic, and food fads, hyperorality, and eccentric clothing choices are often reported (18).

Parsimony, an abnormal preoccupation with money or financial economy, is commonly reported. Patients may hoard or constantly count their money, make attempts to avoid spending, and force family members to engage in similar behavior (such as restricting water and electricity usage) in order to save money (1).

As with the other variants of FTLD, motor manifestations are seen, including parkinsonism and motor neuron changes. However, it is our impression that motor manifestations are less common with SD than with FTD and PA.

OTHER FTLD-SPECTRUM DISORDERS LINKED TO TAU GENE

The link between FTLD and the tau gene, expressed as "tauopathy," warrants a brief description of PSP and CBD because they can often present with very similar symptoms and can be difficult to distinguish while making a differential diagnosis. Table 13-1 offers a brief

TABLE 13-1. *Characteristics of FTLD and related disorders*

Disease	Behavioral symptoms	Cognitive symptoms	Motor symptoms	Neuroimaging
Frontotemporal dementia	Early disinhibition, loss of empathy and insight, emotional blunting, apathy, mental rigidity, and perseveration	Impairment of executive function: set shifting, abstraction and reasoning, response generation, and organization and planning	Cogwheel rigidity and hypokinesia (late stages)	Focal (can be asymmetric) temporal or frontal atrophy or hypometabolism
Semantic dementia	Indifference to the needs of others, narrowed spectrum of interests, and preoccupation with money or finances	Press of speech, semantic impairment, idiosyncratic word usage, and preserved phonology and syntax	Primitive reflexes are absent or late, akinesia, tremor, and rigidity	Anterior temporal abnormalities, can be symmetrical or asymmetrical
Progressive nonfluent aphasia	Early preservation of social skills and late-stage changes in behavior	Anomia, phonemic paraphasias, agrammatism, and impaired repetition	Contralateral primitive reflexes (late stages), akinesia, tremor, and rigidity	Asymmetrical deterioration in dominant hemisphere
Corticobasal degeneration	Some disinhibition, personality changes, irritability	Progressive aphasia, progressive visuospatial deficits	Alien hand syndrome, asymmetric manual apraxia, ocular apraxia, falls, myoclonus, rigidity	Frontal or parietal atrophy or hypometabolism, may be asymmetric
Progressive supranuclear palsy	Apathy and depression	Frontal dysexecutive syndrome, forgetfulness, and slowed thinking	Early falls, rigidity, and slow saccades (vertical greater than horizontal)	Frontal and subcortical hypometabolism and atrophy

description and comparison of each disorder within this spectrum.

PSP is considered to be a movement disorder with pathology particularly localized to the brain stem and basal ganglia (although cortical involvement is increasingly recognized). Core features of PSP include vertical supranuclear gaze palsy with intact reflex eye movements but impaired voluntary ocular pursuits and saccades, axial rigidity, postural instability (which often leads to falls), and increased tone (which results in an upright neck and body posture). However, most patients with PSP also exhibit cognitive and behavioral syndromes that have considerable parallels with FTLD. Apathy, depression, and chronic fatigue are common in many patients before other features of the illness begin. Similarly, frontal or executive disorders are also present in many patients, and impaired judgment may be an early feature of PSP.

CBD, also known as corticobasal ganglionic degeneration (CBGD), was first described as a motor disorder with sparing of cognitive function (23), but more recently, CBD has been better understood to cause motor abnormalities with "generalized intellectual impairment" (24), and it is now recognized that cognitive dysfunction may actually be a common presenting manifestation of the disease. As the name suggests, patients typically have symptoms indicating dysfunction in the cerebral cortex and basal ganglia, with symptoms usually being worse on one side of the body. Core features include limb apraxia, cortical sensory loss, myoclonus, aphasia, bradykinesia, rigidity, dystonia and, less frequently, alien limb. Patients who have pronounced left-sided involvement can present with language dysfunction, which could easily be misdiagnosed as AD. Neuropsychologically, patients who have CBD show impaired attention and executive dysfunction similar to that in patients who have FTD, yet they have higher scores on memory testing than patients who have AD (25). Depression is extremely common in CBD.

FINAL DISCUSSION

FTLD is a family of non-AD dementias whose behavioral disturbances are a central component of diagnosis. Because the diseases can originate in the left or right temporal lobes or in the frontal lobe, symptoms are quite variable and make diagnosis challenging (26). The most important tool in making a diagnosis of FTLD is a detailed clinical history focusing on cognitive and behavioral features. Neuroimaging is also mandatory.

Many patients with FTLD exhibit atypical parkinsonian features at presentation, or go on to develop them. Similarly, many patients who have CBD or PSP have clinical features that suggest FTLD. Sporadic and genetic cases (caused by tau mutations) are clinically difficult to distinguish. Fewer than 10% of familial cases exhibit tau mutations. A better understanding of the biologic factors that influence FTLD, CBD, and PSP will help clarify issues related to nomenclature.

The medical therapies for FTLD are directed at symptoms. In the future, molecule-based therapies are likely to emerge, offering hope for patients suffering from these devastating illnesses.

ACKNOWLEDGMENTS

Supported by the McBean Foundation, the National Institute on Aging (NIA) grant AG10129, NIA grant P50-AG05142, NIA grant AG16570, Alzheimer's Disease Research Centers, and the State of California, Alzheimer's Disease Research Center of California (ARCC) grant 01-154-20 and M01 RR00079 General Clinical Research Center.

REFERENCES

1. Neary D, Snowden JS, Gustafson L, et al. Frontotemporal lobar degeneration: a consensus on clinical diagnostic criteria. *Neurology* 1998;51:1546–1554.
2. Mendez MF, Selwood A, Mastri AR, et al. Pick's disease versus Alzheimer's disease: a comparison of clinical characteristics. *Neurology* 1993;43:289–292.
3. Kertesz A. Frontotemporal dementia, Pick disease, and corticobasal degeneration. One entity or 3? *Arch Neurol* 1997;54:1427–1429.
4. Wilhelmsen KC, Lynch T, Pavlou E, et al. Localization of disinhibition-dementia-parkinsonism-atrophy complex to 17q21-22. *Am J Hum Genet* 1994;55:1159–1165.
5. Reed LA, Schmidt ML, Wszolek ZK, et al. The neuropathology of a chromosome 17-linked autosomal dominant parkinsonism and dementia ("pallido-ponto-nigral degeneration"). *J Neuropathol Exp Neurol* 1998; 57(6):588–601.
6. van Swieten JC, Heutink P. Frontotemporal dementia with Parkinsonism-17. *Gene Rev*, http://www.geneclinics.org/profiles/ftdp-17/details.html, 2000.
7. Hulette CM, Pericak-Vance MA, Roses AD, et al. Neuropathological features of frontotemporal dementia and

parkinsonism linked to chromosome 17q-22 (FTDP-17). *J Neuropathol Exp Neurol* 1999;58(8):859–866.
8. Foster NL, Wilhelmsen K, Sima AAF, et al. Frontotemporal dementia and parkinsonism linked to chromosome 17: a consensus conference. *Ann Neurol* 1997; 41:706–715.
9. Sima AAF, Defendini R, Keohane C, et al. The neuropathology of chromosome 17-linked dementia. *Ann Neurol* 1996;39:734–743.
10. Bird TD, Nochlin D, Parvoneh P, et al. A clinical pathological comparison of three families with frontotemporal dementia and identical mutations in the tau gene (P301L). *Brain* 1999;122:741–756.
11. Gustafson L. The clinical picture of frontal lobe degeneration of the non-Alzheimer type. *Dementia* 1993; 4:143–148.
12. Stevens M, Van Duijn CM, Kamphorst W, et al. Familial aggregation in frontotemporal dementia. *Neurology* 1998;50:1541–1545.
13. Ratnavalli E, Brayne C, et al. The prevalence of frontotemporal dementia. *Neurology* 2002;58:1615–1621.
14. Rosen HJ, Perry RJ, Murphy J, et al. Emotion comprehension in the temporal variant of frontotemporal dementia. *Brain* 2002;125(Pt 10):2286–2295.
15. Mychack P, Kramer JH, Boone KB, et al. The influence of right frontotemporal dysfunction on social behavior in frontotemporal dementia. *Neurology* 2001;56: S11–S15.
16. Rankin K, Kramer JH, Mychack P, et al. Double dissociation of social functioning in frontotemporal dementia. *Neurology* 2003;60:266–271.
17. Rosen HJ, Perry RJ, Murphy J, et al. Emotion comprehension in the temporal variant of frontotemporal dementia. *Brain* 2002;125(Pt 10):2286–2295.
18. Edwards-Lee T, Miller B, et al. The temporal variant of frontotemporal dementia. *Brain* 1997;120:1027–1040.
19. Swartz JR, Miller BL, Lesser IM, et al. Behavioral phenomenology in Alzheimer's disease, frontotemporal dementia and late-life depression: a retrospective analysis. *J Geriatr Psychiatry Neurol* 1997;10:67–74.
20. Levy ML, Miller BL, Cummings JL. Frontal and frontotemporal dementia. In: Growdon JH, Rossor MN, eds. *The dementias*. Boston, MA: Butterworth-Heinemann, 1998:45–65.
21. Lomen-Hoerth C, Murphy J, Langmore S, et al. Are amyotrophic lateral sclerosis patients cognitively normal? *Neurology* 2003;60:1094–1097.
22. Snowden JS, Neary D, Mann DMA. Semantic dementia. In: Snowden JS, Neary D, Mann DMA, eds. *Frontotemporal lobar degeneration*. New York: Churchill Livingstone, 1996:91–114.
23. Rebeiz JJ, Kolodny EH, Richardson EPJR. Corticodentatonigral degeneration with neuronal achromasia. *Arch Neurol* 1968;18:20–33.
24. Gibb WR, Luthert PJ, Marsden CD. Corticobasal degeneration. *Brain* 1989;112:1171–1192.
25. Pillon B, Blin J, Vidailhet M, et al. The neuropsychological pattern of corticobasal degeneration: comparison with progressive supranuclear palsy and Alzheimer's disease. *Neurology* 1995;45:1477–1483.
26. Rosen HS, Lengenfelder J, Miller BL. Frontotemporal dementia. *Neurol Clin* 2000;18:979–992.

14

Behavioral Symptoms Associated with Huntington's Disease

Karen E. Anderson[1] and Frederick J. Marshall[2]

[1]*Department of Neurology, Movement Disorders Division, University of Maryland, School of Medicine, Baltimore, Maryland;* [2]*Department of Neurology, University of Rochester School of Medicine and Dentistry, Rochester, New York*

Huntington's disease (HD) is an autosomal dominant, progressive neurodegenerative disorder characterized by chorea and dystonia. Cognitive impairment and psychiatric symptoms occur in almost all patients. These behavioral changes are often more troubling than the movement disorder and can greatly augment caregiver burden. This chapter examines the neurologic and cognitive symptoms in HD and focuses on the psychiatric conditions. Clinical studies are used to guide treatment recommendations. However, because behavioral changes in HD have received little attention, the authors share their clinical experience.

CLINICAL FEATURES

Prevalence of HD is estimated at approximately 5 to 10 per 100,000, with approximately 30,000 affected individuals in the United States. The disorder is seen less commonly among those of non-European ancestry (1,2). Onset is in the 4th or 5th decade of life, but may occur from childhood through the 8th decade (3,4).

Neurologic abnormalities include involuntary movements (chorea and dystonia) and gait disorders, impairment of saccades and smooth pursuit, dysarthria, and impaired swallowing. These symptoms progress over 10 to 15 years, leading in most cases to severe disability. Chorea, the rapid and involuntary dancelike movement that is the hallmark of the disease, typically worsens in the middle stages of the illness and then decreases as the patient becomes more debilitated.

Dystonia, bradykinesia, and rigidity worsen as the disease progresses. Patients with juvenile onset HD often have parkinsonism as the predominant neurologic feature, sometimes accompanied by seizures and myoclonus. The absence of chorea in these cases makes the diagnosis challenging if no available family history is available. Deterioration of function is more rapid in juvenile onset cases than in others. Patients with onset later in life have a slowly progressive course. Older patients are sometimes misdiagnosed as having a parkinsonian syndrome, and their symptoms occasionally respond to levodopa (5).

GENETICS AND DISEASE MECHANISM

HD is caused by an abnormal expansion of trinucleotide repeats coding for glutamine at the N-terminus of the *huntingtin* protein. The increase occurs in sequences of cytosine, adenine, and guanine (CAG) in exon 1 of the HD gene, which is located on chromosome 4. The gene is expressed throughout the body (6). The normal function of *huntingtin* is unknown. Excitotoxic effects of glutamatergic transmission, mitochondrial dysfunction, and dysregulation of CREB-binding protein-mediated gene expression have all been suggested as disease mechanisms in HD (7–9). The HD gene is transmitted as an autosomal dominant trait, so that each child of an affected individual has a 50% chance of inheriting the gene. Healthy individuals have between 9 and 26 CAG repeats, with most having approximately 18 repeats on each allele. Those individuals who develop clinically apparent symptoms of HD have a higher number of repeats, usually greater than 39. CAG repeat number is inversely correlated with the age of disease onset. Predicting the exact age of disease onset in any individual patient based on CAG repeat length is impossible. Those individuals who have an HD gene with 36 to 39 repeats may or may not develop the symptoms of HD, but if they do, they have a later disease onset. They are, however, at risk of transmitting the disorder to their children, because the CAG repeats expand in each successive generation. No individual with 35 or fewer CAG repeats has been reported to develop HD symptoms, but those with 27 to 35 repeats may pass a clinically important mutation on to their children through repeated CAG expansion in successive generations. Genetic counseling at a certified testing program is recommended by the Huntington's Disease Society of America (HDSA) for presymptomatic at-risk individuals seeking to be tested for the HD gene (see Chapter 16, this volume). The HDSA advises against testing for the HD gene in minors. Adverse outcomes, including precipitation of major psychiatric illness and suicidality, have occurred following genetic testing for HD (10,11).

NEUROPATHOLOGIC SUBSTRATES OF BEHAVIOR

A decline in the number of medium spiny striatal neurons is the main pathological change in HD. Caudate changes predominate, but cell death also occurs in the globus pallidus. As the disease advances, widespread atrophy occurs (12,13). Because the first neuropathology in HD occurs in the associative areas of the striatum, cognitive and psychiatric symptoms may develop earlier than motor symptoms in the course of the illness (14,15).

Attempts have been made to parse out the behavioral effects of changes in various circuitry thought to be damaged by HD pathology. Cummings (16) has described three distinct frontal–subcortical circuits that may modulate behavior. Paulsen et al. (17) have expanded this description and applied it to specific psychiatric symptoms in HD. They described three circuits, the dorsolateral–subcortical circuit, the orbitofrontal circuit, and the medial prefrontal circuit. The dorsolateral–subcortical circuit projects from the dorsal, anterior, and lateral prefrontal cortex through the dorsolateral head of the caudate and into the ventral anterior and medial dorsal thalamic nuclei. This circuit is involved in regulating working memory and also has the ability to modulate behavior on the basis of environmental cues, an ability called "set shifting." These are basic executive functions, and dysregulation of these functions may have a negative effect on behavior. For example, if a patient with HD cannot adjust to a new circumstance and becomes frustrated, irritability may ensue. The orbitofrontal circuit projects from the anterior and lateral orbitofrontal cortex through the ventromedial caudate nucleus to the ventral anterior and medial dorsal thalamic nuclei. Dysfunction in this circuit has been linked to the development of affective and of obsessive and compulsive symptoms. Finally, the medial prefrontal circuit projects from the paralimbic cortical regions through the nucleus accumbens to the medial dorsal nucleus of the thalamus and is involved in regulating response inhibition. Damage to this circuit produces apathy, which generally increases with duration of disease in HD (18–20).

BRAIN IMAGING FINDINGS

Basal ganglia atrophy correlates positively with CAG repeat length in structural and volumetric magnetic resonance imaging (MRI) studies (21–23). Both generalized atrophy and focal frontal lobe changes occur (24). Decrease in caudate volume over time has also been observed in presymptomatic at-risk individuals (25). More recent work suggests that cortical thinning and volume reductions in other regions are present even in early stages of HD, which may explain some of the heterogeneity seen in behavioral symptoms (26,27).

Functional studies have demonstrated caudate and putaminal hypometabolism, along with some frontal metabolic reductions that correlate with decline in function (28–31). Positron emission tomography (PET) studies of dopamine function have found striatal and cortical receptor abnormalities, some of which relate to behavior

(32,33). Abnormal response to passive sensory stimulation in both the cortex and the striatum have been seen in PET studies of HD, and this abnormality could contribute to motor abnormalities (34). Only two imaging studies have related changes in brain function to psychiatric symptoms in HD. Mayberg et al. (35) used PET to compare patients with early-onset HD, with and without depression, to a group of healthy volunteers. Brain metabolism was found to be reduced in the basal ganglia and cingulate in both groups of patients with HD, compared with metabolism in controls. The patients with HD who had depressed mood had lower orbital frontal–inferior prefrontal cortex metabolism than those who did not have mood changes. Another group found decreased anterior-posterior brain metabolic ratios in patients with HD and psychotic symptoms, suggesting that hypofrontality contributes to the development of psychotic symptoms in HD (36).

COGNITIVE SYMPTOMS

Visuospatial performance deficits may be some of the earliest cognitive changes seen in HD (37–39). Memory deficits in HD include slowed rates of learning and impaired recall (40,41); however, free recall improves with cuing (42–44). Retention is relatively normal in HD compared to that in Alzheimer's disease (AD) (42,43). Executive dysfunction is also reported consistently in studies of patients with HD (37,45–48). Procedural memory is impaired, as is seen in tests of skill and motor learning (49) (see Chapter 15, this volume).

PSYCHIATRIC SYMPTOMS

There is no predictable time for onset of psychiatric symptoms in HD; they may occur prior to neurological impairment (50). Overall prevalence of psychiatric symptoms in HD has been reported to be anywhere from 30% to more than 70%. A study of 52 consecutive outpatients, using careful evaluation with standard measures and information from caregivers, found that 98% of patients with HD in this group had at least one psychiatric symptom, demonstrating that as evaluation continues and more information is gathered, most patients are likely to demonstrate some behavioral disturbances (17). Virtually all psychiatric symptoms described in the general population may be seen in persons with HD, although some appear to be more particular to the illness than others.

Unlike the somewhat predictable progression of motor and cognitive symptoms, no generalized time course has been demonstrated for psychiatric disease; the severity of these symptoms varies throughout the course of illness in individual patients (51). Depression is generally concurrent with, or follows onset of, motor symptoms, and apathy may increase as the illness progresses (17,20). Presence of psychiatric disorders has not been shown to relate to CAG repeat length, and time of onset of psychiatric symptoms is not correlated with CAG repeat number (52–56). Psychiatric symptoms add greatly to caregivers' burdens and patients' distress and are often one of the main considerations in deciding to institutionalize a patient (57). Psychiatric symptoms have been cited as the most disturbing aspect of HD by family members (58). Because psychiatric symptoms are often amenable to treatment with standard psychopharmacologic agents, providing relief from these symptoms can greatly affect quality of life for both patients and caregivers. Table 14-1, at the end of the next section, provides information to help guide treatment of behavioral symptoms in patients with HD.

IRRITABILITY AND AGGRESSION

Over 50% of patients with HD will exhibit irritability at some point during the illness, making it one of the most common and problematic behavioral symptoms (19,59,60). Early work by Rosenbaum (61) reported irritability in almost 90% of 46 patients with HD who were admitted for psychiatric treatment. Folstein (3) found that, of 186 patients, 30% met *Diagnostic and Statistical Manual of Mental Disorders* (DSM) (62) criteria for intermittent explosive disorder, and 6% met criteria for antisocial personality disorder. A study of 960 patients with HD found that more than 60% of patients with HD or their caregivers reported aggressive behavior by the patient when questioned at their first visit to an HD clinic (63). A retrospective study found that more than

60% of patients with HD or their caregivers reported agressive behavior by the patient when questioned (64). Although a clear time course is not apparent for development of irritability, it may manifest itself before the onset of motor symptoms. Berrios et al. (65) compared asymptomatic, gene-positive individuals to gene-negative controls from families at risk for HD. All evaluation was carried out before genetic testing results were known. The investigators observed that irritability measures were significantly elevated in the gene-positive group, suggesting that irritability can appear quite early in the course of the illness. The biologic underpinnings of irritability in HD are unclear, but dysfunction of the circuit linking the orbitofrontal cortex to the basal ganglia and thalamus may contribute, specifically if the ventrobasal striatal area is affected (16). Early PET work supported this theory (36).

TABLE 14-1. *Pharmacotherapy for psychiatric symptoms in Huntington's disease (HD)*

Class of agent	Indications	Example/Typical dosing range	Comments
SSRIs	Depression, irritability, aggression, anxiety, obsessive–compulsive disorder	Escitalopram 10–20 mg qd Fluoxetine 20–40 mg qd Sertraline 50–200 mg qd Paroxetine 20–40 mg qd	Higher doses may be needed for anxiety disorders (e.g., 60–80 mg fluoxetine qd)
Atypical neuroleptics	Irritability, aggression, psychosis	Quetiapine 50–200 mg qd Olanzapine 5–20 mg qd Ziprasidone 20–80 mg b.i.d.	Should start first with an SSRI for cases of mild to moderate irritability and aggression. In select patients, quetiapine dosing may increase; upper dosing range, 600–800 mg qd. Weight gain, a common side effect of olanzapine, may be beneficial in HD.
Standard neuroleptics	Suppression of chorea in select cases, extreme agitation requiring rapid sedation	Haloperidol 2–10 mg qd	May worsen gait disorders and swallowing problems; may cause akathisia and tardive dyskinesia. Should try haloperidol for agitation only if atypical neuroleptics fail.
Mood stabilizers	Treatment of mania, irritability	Divalproex 500–1000 mg b.i.d. Lamotrigine 100 mg b.i.d.	Should try mood stabilizers for irritability only after trial of antidepressants, atypical neuroleptics, or both. With divalproex, must follow blood levels, check liver function tests periodically. Advise patients about possibility of severe rash, including Stevens–Johnson syndrome, with lamotrigine.
Benzodiazepines	Suppression of movements so that patients can fall asleep, extreme agitation, anxiety	Clonazepam 0.5–1 mg qhs	May cause paradoxical disinhibition. May worsen apathy.
Tricyclic antidepressants	Depression, obsessive–compulsive disorder, insomnia	Nortriptyline 50–150 mg qd Amitriptyline 25–100 mg qd Clomipramine 50–150 mg qd Trazodone 50–200 mg qhs	Check blood levels of NTP for therapeutic range. Potential for anticholinergic side-effects. All are sedating; trazodone is most helpful for sleep but has minimal antidepressant effect.
Other antidepressants	Depression; may be helpful for apathy in a few cases	Bupropion XL 150–300 mg qd	May cause anxiety, especially when treatment is initiated.

qd, each day; qhs, each pm; b.i.d., twice a day; NTP, Nortriptyline; SSRIs, Selective Serotonin Reuptake Inhibitors.

Aggression, when it occurs in HD, usually accompanies irritability. Burns et al. (59) reported that 59% of patients with HD were aggressive when assessed with a standardized scale. Dewhurst et al. (66,67) found that violence was the main reason for hospitalization in 25% of 102 psychiatric inpatients with HD. In another study of 46 psychiatric inpatients with HD, more than 10% had attempted to commit homicide, and 65% assaulted someone during hospitalization (61). Aggression in HD occurred with similar frequency in men and women in a nursing home study (68). Of these patients, 26% were mildly aggressive, and 11% were moderately aggressive, but aggression seldom resulted in serious injury to the patients or to others. In a broader clinician-based survey, frequent and severe physical aggression occurred among only 10% of patients (69). Discrepancy in estimates of the burden of aggression in HD may be attributable to selection bias, with institutionalized patients showing higher rates of aggression than others because aggression prompts institutionalization.

Behavioral techniques, such as adhering to a schedule to minimize unexpected events, may help to decrease aggression (70). Because irritability is often directed toward individuals known to the patients, especially caregivers, educating caregivers in how to identify and avoid situations that trigger irritability, and how to minimize its effects if it does occur, is extremely important. If the irritability escalates into physical aggression, caregivers should be encouraged to contact emergency medical services for assistance. Patients should be carefully evaluated to rule out medical illness, delirium, medication toxicity, or physical discomfort, especially those patients who have not been disruptive previously, or those who may have impaired ability to communicate (71). Underlying psychiatric illness should also be considered. Akathisia may occur, with concomitant restlessness and irritability, in patients who are being treated with neuroleptics or tetrabenazine to suppress chorea. Irritability and aggression respond to pharmacotherapy in many cases, sometimes in combination with behavioral interventions. Table 14-1 provides an overview of medications used to treat these symptoms. Starting in the lower end of the dosing range for medications is important when treating any patient with HD. Exceptions may occur in patients who are particularly aggressive; these patients may require high dosages of medication to control behavioral problems.

PERSONALITY ALTERATIONS

Development of personality alterations that are not specific to one psychiatric diagnosis have been reported for many years by those who study HD (50,66). Personality changes are probably one of the most common, and least studied, of all behavioral abnormalities in HD. Reports indicate that personality changes occur in 10% to 41% of patients with HD (60,66,72–75). Aside from aggression and irritability, these changes have not been examined in depth; areas that have received less study include impulsivity, emotional lability, and lack of empathy for others. Criminal behavior also occurs in conjunction with personality change in some patients; generally, these acts are misdemeanors, such as indecent exposure, drunkenness, and disturbing the peace, although more serious crimes, such as assault and shooting, were reported in a survey of nearly 500 patients with HD in South Africa (2,60).

Personality changes have been described in gene-positive, asymptomatic individuals. Anger and hostility have been reported to be elevated among family members most at risk to develop HD, and irritability has been shown to be increased in asymptomatic, gene-positive individuals (65,76). Several groups concluded that personality changes are among the earliest signs of HD, often occurring before onset of motor and cognitive changes (66,73,74,77,78). A recent study comparing asymptomatic carriers to individuals from families at risk for HD who were gene negative found that both groups had elevated scores on tests for personality disorders, suggesting a role for environment (65). Kirkwood et al. (79) also found increasing irritability and cynical hostility in presymptomatic gene carriers before onset of motor symptoms. Few data are available on treating personality changes in HD. If irritability is part of the personality change in an individual patient, antidepressants, especially selective serotonin reuptake inhibitor (SSRIs), or low doses of atypical neuroleptics may be helpful.

APATHY

Apathy is an extremely common and treatment-resistant symptom of HD. In a retrospective study of reports to a specific health board, apathy was found in more than 50% of patients with HD (80). In a more recent study using standard psychiatric assessments and information from caregivers, 50% of the patients were also found to have apathy (17). Apathy has been shown to increase as the illness progresses (18,20). Unlike other behavioral features in HD, apathy correlates positively with progression of cognitive and motor impairment, perhaps attributable to derangement in the striatofrontal projections underlying executive function (81). Apathy is often difficult to differentiate from depression, especially as the disease progresses and communication diminishes because of dysarthria or impaired cognition. Apathy is often more distressing to caregivers than to patients. Few treatments are effective for apathy, although structuring daily activities may be useful, as with irritability and aggression. Presenting patients with limited choices to simplify decision making may also help. Some apathetic patients participate in activities if guided but do not initiate participation (18). Educating family members to promote reasonable expectations for patient behavior is often the most meaningful intervention. Table 14-1 outlines pharmacologic treatments for apathy; these agents generally provide minimal benefit.

AFFECTIVE DISORDERS

Changes in mood are quite common in HD. A review by Slaughter et al. (82) found 16 English language studies on depression in HD. Overall prevalence of depression in HD was 30%, and prevalence of dysthymia was 5.6%. Depression is reported to occur either with or following onset of motor abnormalities, arguing against purely reactive mood changes (17,65,76,83). Earlier studies, before genetic testing became available, suggested mood changes often occurred before onset of motor symptoms, but these studies were retrospective assessments of subjects who were already showing neurologic symptoms (66). Mayberg et al. (35) did not find a positive correlation between depression and duration of illness or activities of daily living in HD, arguing against purely reactive depression. Brain imaging data from the same study suggest depressed mood could arise from disruption of frontal–striatal circuitry. A study of cerebrospinal fluid (CSF) found that, unlike neurologically intact patients with depressed mood, patients with HD who had depressive disorders (major depression or dysthymia) did not differ from patients without depression in CSF concentrations of 5-hydroxyindole acetic acid (5-HIAA) or corticotrophin-releasing factor (CRF) (84). However, a positive correlation was seen between severity of depression and CRF concentration. These findings suggest that the neurochemical basis of depression in HD may differ from that seen in other major depressive disorders.

Suicide rates in HD are increased fourfold compared with rates in the general population (85). Completed suicide rates from 3% to 7% have been reported, with more than a quarter of patients exhibiting suicidal behavior at some point in the illness; suicide risk is particularly increased among those HD patients who live to be in their 50s or 60s (86,87). This overall increase in suicidality in HD may be partly attributable to the high rate of impulsivity seen in these patients (88). Risk factors for suicidal behavior in patients with HD are similar to those in the general population, and include depression, living alone, childlessness, and being unmarried (89). Thus, patients with HD who express suicidal ideation should be evaluated immediately. Suicide may occur early in the illness (86,90). Suicidal ideation may occur in conjunction with genetic testing in at-risk persons (10). The prevalence of mania and hypomania are increased in HD. From the limited data available, mania appears to occur in approximately 5% of patients; if hypomania is included, 10% of patients are affected with these symptoms (3).

Treatment of mood disorders in HD is particularly important, given the high rate of suicide seen in the disorder. Although depressed mood is by far the predominant mood disorder in HD, identifying and treating mania and hypomania is important, given that both of these conditions may increase impulsivity and could lead to self harm. Many patients will improve greatly with standard doses of antidepressants (Table 14-1). If irritability or psychosis accompanies depression, the addition of a small dose of an atypical neuroleptic can be helpful.

ANXIETY DISORDERS

Little is known about anxiety disorders in HD. Older studies report anxiety as a frequent prodromal symptom (66). Occurrence of obsessive and compulsive symptoms are common in patients with HD. Such symptoms have been reported in 20% to 50% of patients with HD, depending on the measure used for assessment (17,63,91). De Marchi et al. reported a family at risk for HD with a high prevalence of obsessive–compulsive disorder (OCD). OCD and obsessive gambling have been reported in an HD pedigree (92). The possible relationship of obsessive and compulsive symptoms to frontal–striatal changes in HD is supported by PET studies in primary OCD. This work showed orbitofrontal or caudate hypermetabolism, or both, in patients with OCD, which decreased in response to treatment (93). Obsessions and compulsions are also seen with increased frequency in other illnesses affecting basal ganglia, including Tourette's syndrome, basal ganglia lesions, and Sydenham's chorea (94–96). Anxiety disorders usually respond to standard treatments (Table 14-1). As in the general population, when antidepressants are used, especially selective serotonin reuptake inhibitors (SSRIs), higher doses may be needed to achieve maximal control of these symptoms. No studies have been conducted of behavior therapy, such as systematic desensitization or cognitive behavioral therapy, for anxiety disorders in HD.

HALLUCINATIONS, PARANOIA, AND PSYCHOSIS

Psychotic symptoms are seen in 3% to 12% of patients (97); the rates of psychosis and actual schizophrenia reported in older studies of patients in psychiatric hospitals may have been misleading, and newer work suggests that the prevalence of psychosis is probably closer to 3% (98). Isolated delusions have also been reported (50).

Psychosis is thought to be more prevalent in patients with early onset of disease than in others (17). Delusions of persecution are probably the most common psychotic symptoms. Most patients with HD and psychosis do not meet diagnostic criteria for schizophrenia (65). The symptoms may result from effects of dopaminergic hyperactivity, interacting with subcortical limbic pathology. Tsuang et al. suggest that patients with HD and psychosis may have a familial predisposition to develop psychosis, because of multiple genetic factors that may influence development of a particular phenotype in the HD gene (99). Functional imaging studies have shown reduced anterior-posterior metabolic ratios in patients with HD and psychosis, suggesting hypofrontality, which is also reported in schizophrenia (36).

Psychosis and paranoia in patients with HD respond to standard treatment (Table 14-1). Starting with an atypical neuroleptic is preferable because of the favorable side effect profile of this drug class. Neuroleptics are best given at bedtime to avoid worsening daytime sedation and confusion. If daytime agitation is an issue, morning dosing or divided dosing may be indicated.

OTHER BEHAVIORAL ABNORMALITIES

Impaired insight is seen in many patients with HD. Snowden at al. (100) found that patients with HD were poor at reporting their involuntary movements. This deficit did not relate to degree of motor or cognitive impairment. Patients with HD have a tendency to draw erroneous inferences in social interactions (101).

Many HD patients suffer from disrupted sleep. Patients may have difficulty falling asleep because their movements disturb them. Poor overall quality of sleep is seen in studies of sleep changes in HD, and sleep quality worsens as the disease progresses (102–104).

Both increases and decreases in sexual desire are reported in HD. Hypersexuality was reported in 12% of men and 7% of women in an early study (67). Members of families at risk for HD who ultimately develop HD have more children than those who do not (3). However, impotence is also increased (3). Paraphilias including exhibitionism, voyeurism, pedophilia, and sexual aggression were noted in very early work on HD (105). Promiscuous behavior and sexual abuse of children are seen, and infidelity commonly occurs early in the illness (61,105).

Anecdotally, patients with HD are thought to be at high risk for substance abuse. However, little work has been done in this area. King (106) studied 42 consecutive patients at an HD clinic. Prevalence of current or past alcohol abuse was 24% for men, 5.9% for women, and 16.7% overall, rates that were similar to those in the local community. When alcohol abuse occurred in persons at risk for HD, it was often concurrent with depressive symptoms. Berrios et al. (65) did not find a substantial difference in the incidence of alcohol abuse when comparing asymptomatic gene carriers to those from families at risk for HD who were gene negative.

THE FAMILIAL ENVIRONMENT

Patients with HD often come from chaotic families, because of the destabilizing effects of a dominantly inherited condition with such profound effects on behavior and function. This environment contributes to development of psychopathology (65,107–109). Conduct disorder has been reported to be increased among children of patients with HD who did not develop HD (107,108). However, other work has found no increased risk of psychiatric disorders in unaffected relatives of HD patients (98).

RELATIONSHIP OF PSYCHIATRIC SYMPTOMS TO COGNITIVE CHANGES

Impaired executive function probably contributes to psychiatric morbidity in HD and results in decreased flexibility in changing behavior to suit an evolving environment. Dysfunction of striatofrontal pathways is implicated in the development of many psychiatric symptoms in HD, including impulsivity, apathy, depression, and obsessive–compulsive behavior [see (16) for a discussion of this circuitry and its relationship to psychiatric symptoms]. However, little evidence exists of a relationship between the degree of cognitive decline and psychiatric symptoms. Psychiatric symptoms regularly occur before onset of cognitive changes. Using a global rating of psychiatric symptomatology, Caine and Shoulson (18) found no relationship between severity of cognitive impairment and psychopathology. Degree of psychopathology did correlate with disability in this study. Paulsen et al. (17) also did not find a relationship between psychiatric symptoms and dementia. In another study of 11 patients, rank order scores on the Minnesota Multiphasic Personality Disorder Inventory correlated with a measure of cognitive decline (110). In their study of HD patients in nursing homes, Shiwach and Patel found that aggression correlated with the degree of functional impairment (68). Work comparing patients with progressive supranuclear palsy, a hypokinetic disorder, to those with HD, which causes hyperkinesis in most patients, suggests that, early in basal ganglia disorders, psychiatric symptoms are independent of both cognitive and motor abnormalities (111).

RELATIONSHIP OF PSYCHIATRIC SYMPTOMS TO MOTOR SYMPTOMS

Thompson et al. suggest that apathy may correlate with progression of cognitive and motor symptoms (81). Other symptoms that have received extensive study in HD, such as depression and irritability, have not been reliably shown to correlate with progression of motor and functional impairment (51,56,111). Early work by Dewhurst et al. (66) found that anxiety-depressive disorder was the most common psychiatric disorder in HD patients with rigidity as a prominent motor symptom. No recent study has been conducted on behavioral symptoms in the rigid form of the illness.

RELATIONSHIP OF PSYCHIATRIC SYMPTOMS TO ONE ANOTHER

Little attention has been given to the study of whether certain psychiatric symptoms are related. No relationship was found between irritability, aggression, and apathy in the study by Burns et al. (59). Another study found no correlation between presence of depression and apathy or irritability (35).

TREATMENT

Currently, no treatment is proven to prevent the onset of HD symptoms or slow disease progression. However, treating psychiatric symptoms is extremely important and can greatly improve quality of life in these patients and reduce the burden on their caregivers. Specific recommendations on treatment of psychiatric symptoms are outlined in Table 14-1. Prior reviews have summarized the limited research on treatment of behavioral symptoms in HD (112,113), and Anderson and Marder (114) outlined suggestions for a stepwise approach to evaluating and treating various problematic behaviors. Treatment recommendations may also be found in publications from the Huntington's Disease Society of America (115).

Other measures to improve quality of life and maintain function in HD patients include physical therapy, speech, and swallowing assessment and therapy, and dietary interventions include increasing calorie intake to maintain weight, modifying diet to prevent choking, and paying attention to food presentation to enhance appetite. As in all neurodegenerative illness, maintaining physical function and independence at the highest possible level may greatly affect overall quality of life and mental outlook.

SUMMARY

In addition to the abnormal movements most commonly associated with HD, cognitive impairment and psychiatric symptoms occur in almost all patients. These behavioral symptoms contribute to morbidity and augment what is often an overwhelming caregiver burden. Behavioral interventions may be useful in managing some HD patients with behavioral symptoms, especially irritability and apathy. Patients should be evaluated for underlying medical illness that might contribute to psychiatric symptoms, especially if onset of behavioral change is rapid. According to clinical observation, HD patients with psychiatric symptoms respond to standard pharmacotherapy. Controlled studies are needed to determine the true efficacy of these agents for use in treating people with HD.

REFERENCES

1. Folstein SE, Chase GA, Wahl WE, et al. Huntington's disease in Maryland: clinical aspects of racial variation. *Am J Hum Genet* 1987;41:168–179.
2. Hayden MR, MacGregor JM, Beighton PH. The prevalence of Huntington's chorea in South Africa. *S Afr Med J* 1980;58(5):193–196.
3. Folstein SE. *Huntington disease: a disorder of families (ed1).* Baltimore, MD: The Johns Hopkins Press, 1989.
4. Gilstad J, Reich SG. Chorea in an octogenarian. *Neurologist* 2003;9(3):165–166.
5. Reuter I, Hu MTM, Andrew TC, et al. Late onset levodopa responsive Huntington's disease with minimal chorea masquerading as Parkinson plus syndrome. *J Neurol Neurosurg Psychiatry* 2000;68:238–241.
6. Strong TV, Tagle DA, Valdes JM, et al. Widespread expression of the human and rat Huntington's disease gene in brain and nonneural tissues. *Nat Genet* 1993;5:259–265.
7. Difiglia M. Excitotoxic injury of the neostriatum is a model for Huntington's disease. *Trends Neurosci* 1990;13:286–289.
8. Beal MF. Does impairment of energy metabolism result in excitotoxic neuronal death in neurodegenerative illnesses? *Ann Neurol* 1992;31:119–130.
9. Nucifora FC, Sasaki M, Peters MF Jr, et al. Interference by huntingtin and atrophin-1 with cbp-mediated transcription leading to cellular toxicity. *Science* 2001;291(5512):2423–2428.
10. Almqvist EW, Bloch M, Brinkman R, et al. A worldwide assessment of the frequency of suicide, suicide attempts or psychiatric hospitalization after predictive testing for Huntington disease. *Am J Hum Genet* 1999;64:1293–1304.
11. Decruyenaere M, Evers-Kiebooms G, Cloostermans T, et al. Psychological distress in the 5-year period after predictive testing for Huntington's disease. *Eur J Hum Genet* 2003;11(1):30–38.
12. Vonsattel JM, Myers RH, Stevens TJ, et al. Neuropathological classification of Huntington's disease. *J Neuropathol Exp Neurol* 1985;44:559–577.
13. Rosas HD, Feigin AS, and Hersch SM. Using advances in neuroimaging to detect, understand, and monitor disease progression in Huntington's disease. *NeuroRx*, Apr 2004;1:263–272.
14. Vonsattel JP, Difiglia M. Huntington's disease. *J Neuropathol Exp Neurol* 1998;57:369–384.
15. Middleton FA, Strick PL. Basal ganglia and cerebellar loops: motor and cognitive circuits. *Brain Res Rev* 2000;31:236–250.
16. Cummings JL. Fronto-subcortical circuits and human behavior. *Arch Neurol* 1993;50:873–880.
17. Paulsen JS, Ready RE, Hamilton JM, et al. Neuropsychiatric aspects of Huntington's disease. *J Neurol Neurosurg Psychiatry* 2001;71(3):310–314.
18. Caine ED, Shoulson I. Psychiatric syndromes in Huntington's disease. *Am J Psychiatry* 1983;140(6):728–733.
19. Paulsen JS, Stout JC, Delapena J, et al. Frontal behavioral syndromes in cortical and subcortical dementia. *Assessment* 1996;3:327–337.
20. Levy ML, Cummings JL, Fairbanks LA, et al. Apathy is not depression. *J Neuropsychiatry Clin Neurosci* 1998;10(3):314–319.
21. Harris GJ, Pearlson GD, Peyser CE, et al. Putamen volume reduction on magnetic resonance imaging

exceeds caudate changes in mild Huntington's disease. *Ann Neurol* 1992;31(1):69–75.
22. Aylward EH, Li Q, Stine OC, et al. Longitudinal change in basal ganglia volume in patients with Huntington's disease. *Neurology* 1997;48(2):394–399.
23. Rosas HD, Goodman J, Chen YI, et al. Striatal volume loss in HD as measured by MRI and the influence of CAG repeat. *Neurology* 2001;57(6):1025–1028.
24. Aylward EH, Anderson NB, Bylsma FW, et al. Frontal lobe volume in patients with Huntington's disease. *Neurology* 1998;50(1):252–258.
25. Aylward EH, Codori AM, Rosenblatt A, et al. Rate of caudate atrophy in presymptomatic and symptomatic stages of Huntington's disease. *Mov Disord* 2000; 15(3):552–560.
26. Rosas HD, Liu AK, Hersch S, et al. Regional and progressive thinning of the cortical ribbon in Huntington's disease. *Neurology* 2002;58(5):695–701.
27. Rosas HD, Koroshetz WJ, Chen YI, et al. Evidence for more widespread cerebral pathology in early HD: an MRI-based morphometric analysis. *Neurology*. 2003; 60(10):1615–1620.
28. Kuhl DE, Phelps ME, Markham CH, et al. Cerebral metabolism and atrophy in Huntington's disease determined by 18FDG and computed tomographic scan. *Ann Neurol* 1982;12(5):425–434.
29. Berent S, Giordani B, Lehtinen S, et al. Positron emission tomographic scan investigations of Huntington's disease: cerebral metabolic correlates of cognitive function. *Ann Neurol* 1988;23(6):541–546.
30. Young AB, Penney JB, Starosta-Rubinstein S, et al. PET scan investigations of Huntington's disease: cerebral metabolic correlates of neurological features and functional decline. *Ann Neurol* 1986;20(3):296–303.
31. Bartenstein P, Weindl A, Spiegel S, et al. Central motor processing in Huntington's disease. A PET study. *Brain* 1997;120(Pt 9):1553–1567.
32. Pavese N, Andrews TC, Brooks DJ, et al. Progressive striatal and cortical dopamine receptor dysfunction in Huntington's disease: a PET study. *Brain* 2003;126 (Pt 5):1127–1135.
33. Backman L, Robins-Wahlin TB, Lundin A, et al. Cognitive deficits in Huntington's disease are predicted by dopaminergic PET markers and brain volumes. *Brain* 1997;120(Pt 12):2207–2217.
34. Boecker H, Ceballos-Baumann A, Bartenstein P, et al. Sensory processing in Parkinson's and Huntington's disease: investigations with 3D H(2)(15)O-PET. *Brain* 1999;122(Pt 9):1651–1665.
35. Mayberg HS, Starkstein SE, Peyser CE, et al. Paralimbic frontal lobe hypometabolism in depression associated with Huntington's disease. *Neurology* 1992;42(9): 1791–1797.
36. Kuwert T, Lange TW, Langen KJ, et al. Cerebral glucose consumption measured by PET in patients with and without psychiatric symptoms of Huntington's disease. *Psychiatry Res* 1989;29:361–362.
37. Josiassen RC, Curry LM, Mancall EL. Development of neuropsychological deficits in Huntington's disease. *Arch Neurol* 1983;40:791–796.
38. Hodges JR, Salmon DP, Butters N. Differential impairment of semantic and episodic memory in Alzheimer's and Huntington's diseases: a controlled prospective study. *J Neurol Neurosurg Psychiatry* 1990; 53:1089–1095.
39. Pillon B, Dubois B, Lhermitte F, et al. Heterogeneity of cognitive impairment in progressive supranuclear palsy, Parkinson's disease, and Alzheimer's disease. *Neurology* 1986;36:1179–1185.
40. Weingartner H, Caine ED, Ebert MH, et al. Imagery, encoding, and retrieval of information from memory: some specific encoding-retrieval changes in Huntington's disease. *J Abnorm Psychol* 1979;88:52–58.
41. Butters N. The clinical aspects of memory disorders: contributions from experimental studies of amnesia and dementia. *J Clin Neuropsychol* 1984;6:17–36.
42. Massman PJ, Delis DC, Butters N, et al. Are all subcortical dementias alike? Verbal learning and memory in Parkinson's and Huntington's disease patients. *J Clin Exp Neuropsychol* 1990;12:729–744.
43. Butters N, Salmon DP, Cullum CM, et al. Differentiation of amnesic and demented patients with the Wechsler memory scale-revised. *Clin Neuropsychol* 1988;2:133–148.
44. Pillon B, Deweer B, Michon A, et al. Are explicit memory disorders of progressive supranuclear palsy related to damage to striatofrontal circuits? Comparison with Alzheimer's, Parkinson's, and Huntington's diseases. *Neurology* 1994;44:1264–1270.
45. Lange KW, Paul GM, Robbins TW, et al. L-DOPA and frontal cognitive function in Parkinson's disease. *Adv Neurol* 1993;60:475–478.
46. Brandt J. Cognitive impairments in Huntington's disease: insights into the neuropsychology of the striatum. In: Corkin S, Grafman J, Boller F, eds. *Handbook of neuropsychology*, Vol. 5. Amsterdam: Elsevier, 1991.
47. Lange KW, Sahakian BJ, Quinn NP, et al. Comparison of executive and visuospatial memory function in Huntington's disease and dementia of Alzheimer type matched for degree of dementia. *J Neurol Neurosurg Psychiatry* 1995;58:598–606.
48. Pillon B, Dubois B, Ploska A, et al. Severity and specificity of cognitive impairment in Alzheimer's, Huntington's and Parkinson's diseases and progressive supranuclear palsy. *Neurology* 1991;41:634–643.
49. Knopman D, Nissen MJ. Procedural learning is impaired in Huntington's disease: evidence from the serial reaction time task. *Neuropsychologia* 1991;29:245–254.
50. Morris M. Psychiatric aspects of Huntington's disease. In: Haper PS, cd. *Huntington's disease*. Philadelphia, PA: WB Saunders, 1991:81–126.
51. Huntington Study Group. Unified Huntington's disease rating scale: reliability and consistency. *Mov Disord* 1996;11:136–142.
52. Weigel-Weber M, Schmid W, et al. Psychiatric symptoms and CAG expansion in Huntington's disease. *Am J Med Genet* 1996;67:53–57.
53. Andrew SE, Goldberg YP, Kremer B, et al. The relationship between trinucleotide (CAG) repeat length and clinical features of Huntington's disease. *Nat Genet* 1993;4(4):398–403.
54. MacMillan JC, Snell RG, Tyler A, et al. Molecular analysis and clinical correlations of the Huntington's disease mutation. *Lancet* 1993;342(8877):954–958.
55. Berrios GE, Wagle AC, Markova IS, et al. Psychiatric symptoms and CAG repeats in neurologically asymptomatic Huntington's disease gene carriers. *Psychiatry Res* 2001;102(3):217–225.
56. Zappacosta B, Monza D, Meoni C, et al. Psychiatric symptoms do not correlate with cognitive decline,

motor symptoms, or CAG repeat length in Huntington's disease. *Arch Neurol* 1996;53:493–497.
57. Wheelock VL, Tempkin T, Marder K et al., Huntington Study Group. Predictors of nursing home placement in Huntington disease. *Neurology.* 2003;60(6): 998–1001.
58. Stern R, Eldridge R. Attitudes of patients and their relatives to Huntington's disease. *J Med Genet* 1975; 12(3):217–223.
59. Burns A, Folstein S, Brandt J, et al. Clinical assessment of irritability, aggression, and apathy in Huntington disease and Alzheimer disease. *J Nerv Ment Dis* 1990; 178:20–26.
60. Bolt JMW. Huntington's disease in the west of Scotland. *Br J Psychiatry* 1970;116:259–270.
61. Rosenbaum D. Psychosis with Huntington's chorea. *Psychiatr Q* 1941;15:93–99.
62. *Diagnostic and statistical manual*. APA Press.
63. Marder K, Zhao H, Myers RH et al., Huntington Study Group Rate of functional decline in Huntington's disease. *Neurology* 2000;54(2):452–458.
64. Nance MA, Sanders G. Characteristics of individuals with Huntington disease in long-term care. *Mov Disord* 1996;11(5):542–548.
65. Berrios GE, Wagle AC, Markova IS, et al. Psychiatric symptoms in neurologically asymptomatic Huntington's disease gene carriers: a comparison with gene negative at risk subjects. *Acta Psychiatr Scand* 2002; 105(3):224–230.
66. Dewhurst K, Oliver J, Trick KLK, et al. Neuropsychiatric aspects of Huntington's disease. *Confin Neurol* 1969;31:258–268.
67. Dewhurst K, Oliver JE, McKnight AL. Socio-psychiatric consequences of Huntington's disease. *Br J Psychiatry* 1970;116:255–258.
68. Shiwach RS, Patel V. Aggressive behavior in Huntington's disease: a cross-sectional study in a nursing home population. *Behav Neurol* 1993;6:43–47.
69. Marshall FJ, Taylor S, Huntington Study Group. Aggression and irritability in Huntington's disease: a survey of treatment patterns. *Neurology*1997;48(Suppl.3):A49.
70. Moskowitz CB, Marder K. Palliative care for people with late-stage Huntington's disease. *Neurol Clin* 2001; 19(4):849–865.
71. Ranen NG, Peyser CE, Folstein SE. A physician's guide to the management of Huntington's disease. *Pharmacologic and nonpharmacologic interventions*. New York: Huntington's Disease Society of America, 1993.
72. Brothers CRD. Huntington's chorea in Victoria and Tasmania. *J Neurol Sci* 1964;1:405–450.
73. Heathfield KW. Huntington's chorea. Investigation into the prevalence of this disease in the area covered by the North East Metropolitan Regional Hospital Board. *Brain* 1967;90(1):203–232.
74. Mattsson B. Huntington's chorea in Sweden. *Acta Psychiatr Scand Suppl* 1974;255:221–235.
75. Saugstad L, Odegard O. Huntington's chorea in Norway. *Psychol Med* 1986;16(1):39–48.
76. Baxter LR, Mazziotta JC, Pahl JJ, et al. Psychiatric, genetic, and positron emission tomographic evaluation of persons at risk for Huntington's disease. *Arch Gen Psychiatry* 1992;49:148–152.
77. Brothers CRD, Meadows AW. An investigation of Huntington's chorea in Victoria. *J Ment Sci* 1955;101: 548–563.

78. Lishman AW. Senile dementias, presenile dementias, and pseudodementias. In: Lishman AW, ed. *Organic psychiatry: the psychological consequences of cerebral disorder*. Oxford: Blackwell Science, 1998:468–469.
79. Kirkwood SC, Siemers E, Viken R, et al. Longitudinal personality changes among presymptomatic Huntington disease gene carriers. *Neuropsychiatry Neuropsychol Behav Neurol* 2002;15(3):192–197.
80. Pflanz S, Besson JAO, Ebmeier KP, et al. The clinical manifestation of mental disorder in Huntington's disease: a retrospective case record study of disease progression. *Acta Psychiatr Scand* 1991;83:53–60.
81. Thompson JC, Snowden JS, Craufurd D, et al. Behavior in Huntington's disease: dissociating cognition-based and mood-based changes. *J Neuropsychiatry Clin Neurosci* 2002;14(1):37–43.
82. Slaughter JR, Martens MP, Slaughter KA. Depression and Huntington's disease: prevalence, clinical manifestations, etiology, and treatment. *CNS Spectrums* 2001; 6:306–326.
83. Shiwach RS, Norbury CG. A controlled psychiatric study of individuals at risk for Huntington's disease. *Br J Psychiatry* 1994;165(4):500–505.
84. Kurlan R, Caine E, Rubin A, et al. Cerebrospinal fluid correlates of depression in Huntington's disease. *Arch Neurol* 1988;45(8):881–883.
85. Di Maio L, Squitieri F, Napolitano G, et al. Suicide risk in Huntington's disease. *J Med Genet* 1993;30: 293–295.
86. Schoenfeld M, Myers RH, Cupples LA, et al. Increased rate of suicide among patients with Huntington's disease. *J Neurol Neurosurg Psychiatry* 1984;47: 1283–1287.
87. Farrer LA. Suicide and attempted suicide in Huntington disease: implications for preclinical testing of persons at risk. *Am J Med Genet* 1986;24(2):305–311.
88. Leonard DP, Kidson MA, Brown JG, et al. A double blind trial of lithium carbonate and haloperidol in Huntington's chorea. *Aust N Z J Psychiatry*. 1975;9(2): 115–118.
89. Lipe H, Schultz A, Bird TD. Risk factors for suicide in Huntington's disease: a retrospective case controlled study. *Am J Med Genet* 1993;48(4):231–233.
90. Turner TH. Huntington's chorea without dementia; a problem case. *Br J Psychiatry* 1985;146:548–550.
91. Anderson KE, Marder KS. An overview of psychiatric symptoms in Huntington's disease. *Curr Psychiatry Rep* 2001;3:379–388.
92. De Marchi N, Morris M, Mennella R, et al. Association of obsessive–compulsive disorder and pathological gambling with Huntington's disease in an Italian pedigree: possible association with Huntington's disease mutation. *Acta Psychiatr Scand* 1998;97(1):62–65.
93. Benkelfat C, Nordahl TE, Semple WE, et al. Local cerebral glucose metabolic rates in obsessive–compulsive disorder. Patients treated with clomipramine. *Arch Gen Psychiatry* 1990;47(9):840–848.
94. Cath DC, Spinhoven P, van Woerkom TC, et al. Gilles de la Tourette's syndrome with and without obsessive–compulsive disorder compared with obsessive–compulsive disorder without tics: which symptoms discriminate? *J Nerv Ment Dis* 2001;189(4):219–228.
95. Laplane D, Levasseur M, Pillon B, et al. Obsessive–compulsive and other behavioral changes with bilateral basal ganglia lesions. A neuropsychological, magnetic

resonance imaging and positron tomography study. *Brain* 1989;112(Pt 3):699–725.
96. Swedo SE, Leonard HL, Garvey M, et al. Pediatric autoimmune neuropsychiatric disorders associated with streptococcal infections: clinical description of the first 50 cases. *Am J Psychiatry* 1998;155(2):264–271.
97. Mendez MF. Huntington's disease: update and review of neuropsychiatric aspects. *Int J Psychiatry Med* 1994; 24:189–208.
98. Jensen P, Sorenson SA, Fenger K, et al. A study of psychiatric morbidity in patients with Huntington's disease, their relatives, and controls: admissions to psychiatric hospitals in Denmark from 1969–1991. *Br J Psychiatry* 1993;163:790–797.
99. Tsuang D, Almqvist EW, Lipe H, et al. Familial aggregation of psychotic symptoms in Huntington's disease. *Am J Psychiatry* 2000;157(12):1955–1959.
100. Snowden JS, Craufurd D, Griffiths HL, et al. Awareness of involuntary movements in Huntington disease. *Arch Neurol* 1998;55(6):801–805.
101. Snowden JS, Gibbons ZC, Blackshaw A, et al. Social cognition in frontotemporal dementia and Huntington's disease. *Neuropsychologia* 2003;41(6):688–701.
102. Silvestri R, Raffaele M, De Domenico P, et al. Sleep features in Tourette's syndrome, neuroacanthocytosis and Huntington's chorea. *Neurophysiol Clin* 1995; 25(2):66–77.
103. Wiegand M, Moller AA, Lauer CJ, et al. Nocturnal sleep in Huntington's disease. *J Neurol* 1991;238(4):203–208.
104. Hansotia P, Wall R, Berendes J. Sleep disturbances and severity of Huntington's disease. *Neurology* 1985; 35(11):1672–1674.
105. Lion EG, Kahn E. Experiential aspects of Huntington's chorea. *Am J Psychiatry* 1938;95:717–727.
106. King M. Alcohol abuse in Huntington's disease. *Psychol Med* 1985;15(4):815–819.
107. Folstein SE, Franz ML, Jensen BA, et al. Conduct disorder and affective disorder among the offspring of patients with Huntington's disease. *Psychol Med* 1983;13:45–52.
108. Folstein SE, Abbott MH, Chase GA, et al. The association of affective disorder with Huntington's disease in a case series and in families. *Psychol Med* 1983;13: 537–542.
119. Berrios GE, Markova IS, Gimbert R. The role of psychiatry in genetic prediction programmes for Huntington's disease. *Psychiatr Bull* 1995;19:203–206.
110. Boll TJ, Heaton R, Reitan RM. Neuropsychological and emotional correlates of Huntington's disease. *J Nerv Ment Dis* 1974;158:61–68.
111. Litvan I, Paulsen JS, Mega MS, et al. Neuropsychiatric assessment of patients with hyperkinetic and hypokinetic movement disorders. *Arch Neurol* 1998;55(10): 1313–1319.
112. Anderson KE, Louis ED, Stern Y, et al. Cognitive correlates of obsessive and compulsive symptoms in Huntington's disease. *Am J Psychiatry* 2001;158(5):799–801.
113. Leroi I, Michalon M. Treatment of the psychiatric manifestations of Huntington's disease: a review of the literature. *Can J Psychiatry* 1998;43:933–940.
114. Anderson KE, Marder KM. Huntington's disease. In: Johnson RT, Griffin JW, McArthur JC, eds. *Current therapy in neurologic disease*, 6th ed. St. Louis, London, Philadelphia, Toronto: Mosby, 2002:282–287.
115. Rosenblatt A, Ranen NG, Nance MA, et al. *A physician's guide to the management of Huntington's disease*. New York: Huntington's Disease Society of America, 1999.

15
Cognitive Changes in Huntington's Disease

Jane S. Paulsen and Rachel A. Conybeare

University of Iowa, Department of Psychiatry and Neurology, Iowa City, Iowa

Huntington's disease (HD) is a genetically transmitted neurodegenerative disease of the basal ganglia characterized by a triad of clinical symptoms including choreoathetosis, cognitive decline, and psychiatric features. The typical symptoms of HD are presented in Table 15-1. Pathogenically, patients with HD present with marked neuronal loss in the striatum, with considerable loss of medium-sized spiny neurons. The prevalence of HD varies across studies but, generally, is thought to be 5 to 10 cases per 100,000 population, which is about one tenth of the prevalence of Parkinson's disease (PD) (1). Since 1993, a genetic test has been available that can accurately detect the presence of the mutation [i.e., 37 or more cytosine–adenine–guanine (CAG) repeats on the IT 15 gene on chromosome 4]. This mutation, transmitted through autosomal dominant inheritance, is an example of genetic "anticipation"; later generations tend to manifest the disease at a younger age, particularly in the case of paternal inheritance.

The diagnosis of symptomatic HD is based upon a neurologic evaluation along with a family history of the disease and the presence of unequivocal movement disorder. Early signs of HD may include involuntary movements, changes in saccadic eye movements, inability to suppress reflexive glances to novel visual stimuli, motor impersistence, impaired rapid alternating movements, balance problems, and akathisia (2). Patients with HD may attempt to mask early chorea, the rapid and involuntary dance-like movement that is the hallmark of the disease, with purposeful movements (e.g., crossing their legs and arms), but as the disease progresses, the choreic movements become noticeable. Some patients do not recognize these movements (see the section Other Behavioral Abnormalities in Chapter 14), a phenomenon known as *anosagnosia*, but family members notice them and often report that the patient with HD is fidgety and is unable to sit still or concentrate on a task for an extended period. Regardless of whether the patient recognizes the choreic movements the movements are more disturbing in many cases to family members than to the patient.

The clinical characteristics of HD are assessed using the Unified Huntington's Disease Rating Scale (UHDRS) (3). The UHDRS assesses four characteristics of HD: motor function, cognition, behavior, and functional abilities. This rating scale has been used since 1994, and data have been collected prospectively from more than 8,000 patients with symptomatic HD and from 1,000 individuals at risk for HD. Although the UHDRS enables generalizations about the symptoms and presentation of HD, HD can present very differently across individuals. Some patients exhibit only a set of characteristic symptoms predominantly. Some families with HD have shown consistency between generations in the type of symptoms and degree of severity, whereas in other families HD presents with marked differences between generations. The clinician working with patients who have HD must understand that each patient will have a different form of the disease, and that patient needs thus will differ.

After the onset of HD in patients, cognitive deficits may not develop uniformly. According to Snowden et al. (4), as HD progresses from preclinical to early stages, the patient exhibits a gradual decline in the performance of psychomotor tasks, but the memory function of these patients decreases rapidly soon after clinical onset of HD. The insidious nature of the disease adds to the difficulty of distinguishing

TABLE 15-1. *Features of Huntington's disease*

Cognitive Features
  Decreased selective and sustained attention
  Decreased performance IQ with verbal performance discrepancy
  Decreased verbal fluency and verbal output
  Faulty memory retrieval strategies; better recognition, cuing, and priming
  Equivalent remote memory deficits, i.e., absent temporal gradient
  Deficient memory requiring effortful processing
  Decreased procedural learning
  Abnormal egocentric spatial orientation and visuomotor integration
  Executive deficits: planning, organizing, sequencing, abstraction, and judgment

Psychiatric Features
  Irritability, aggression, and alterations in personality
  Depression, anxiety, apathy, and increased risk of suicide
  Decreased initiation, spontaneity, and engagement
  Obsessive thinking and compulsive behavior
  Hallucinations, delusions, paranoia, and psychosis
  Impaired insight

Motor Features
  Involuntary movements
  Change in saccadic eye movements
  Inability to suppress reflexive glances
  Tongue motor impersistence
  Impaired rapid alternating movements
  Balance problems and akathisia

---

cognitive symptoms from everyday cognitive shortcomings that people exhibit when they are stressed, tired, and overworked (e.g., forgetfulness, clumsiness, and inability to concentrate). Such cognitive shortcomings evoke anxiety in patients even when they are presymptomatic, which underscores the importance of learning more about the cognitive changes associated with HD. This chapter describes the different areas of cognitive function that are impaired in HD and discusses one way to understand these cognitive changes.

"DEMENTIA" IN HUNTINGTON'S DISEASE

Before 1700, dementia was defined as "being out of one's mind" (5). In addition to the word dementia, terms such as amentia, imbecility, morosis, foolishness, stupidity, simplicity, idiocy, dotage, and senility were used to indicate cognitive and behavioral decline (5). As the understanding of the brain and its effect on cognition and behavior has steadily increased, the definition of "dementia" has also evolved. In the 1970s, the word dementia was distinguished from "senility." Put simply, dementia can be defined as "a syndrome of acquired intellectual impairment produced by brain dysfunction" (6). More specific diagnostic criteria are set forth in the Diagnostic and Statistical Manual of Mental Disorders, 4th edition (DSM-IV) definition, "dementia must include memory impairment and an additional cognitive impairment (aphasia, apraxia, agnosia or problems with executive functioning). The deficits in cognitive abilities must develop gradually and represent a distinct decline from past abilities as well as cause a significant impairment in social or occupational functioning" (7).

HD has historically been cited as the best model of "subcortical" dementia (8) [in contrast to the prototypical "cortical" dementia, Alzheimer's disease (AD)]. The use of the terms cortical and subcortical dementia and the differences between these terms are not widely agreed upon, but the large amount of literature on these types of dementia makes addressing them important. Dementia of the "subcortical" type presents with an inability to activate cognitive processes, including slowed psychomotor speed, difficulty with recall, and impaired ability to solve complex problems. This type of dementia typically lacks features of "cortical" dementias such as the primary language, memory, and visual-spatial deficits (9,10). Features that typically distinguish cortical and subcortical dementias are outlined in Table 15-2.

TABLE 15-2. *Features distinguishing subcortical from cortical dementia*

Feature	Subcortical dementia Huntington's disease (HD)	Cortical dementia (Alzheimer's disease)
Mental status		
Language	No aphasia	Aphasia
Learning	Disorganized and slow, but can learn	Rapid forgetting and defective storage of information
Memory	Forgetful	Amnesia
Speed of processing	Slow, but relatively accurate	Slow, often inaccurate
Motor systems		
Speech	Dysarthric, but accurate	Normal clarity and rate, but often inaccurate
Motor speed	Slow	Normal
Anatomy		
Cortex	Largely spared	Involved
Basal ganglia	Involved	Largely spared

[From Morris M. Dementia and cognitive changes in Huntington's disease. In: Weiner WJ, Lang AE, eds. *Behavioral neurology of movement disorders*, Vol. 65. New York: Raven Press, 1995:187–200, with permission.]

The general syndrome of dementia was last defined in the DSM-IV in 1994, and this definition was found to have several limitations (6). First, certain dementias may have preserved memory but multiple intellectual impairments, as is evident in frontal–temporal dementia. Second, stating that dementia substantially impairs social or occupational function can possibly be an arbitrary judgement of a diagnosis of dementia. Lastly, defining dementia on the basis of only two areas of cognitive impairment makes it difficult to distinguish dementia from a lesion that might affect conterminous brain areas. Mendez and Cummings (6) provide a definition of dementia without these limitations.

> "Dementia" means a loss of mental functions. It is an acquired, persistent impairment in multiple areas of intellectual function, not caused by delirium. Operationally, three or more of the following nine spheres of mental activity are compromised: memory, language, perception (especially visuospatial), praxis, calculations, conceptual or semantic knowledge, executive function, personality or social behaviour, and emotional awareness or expression. The compromise in mental functions is documented by mental status assessment, either by bedside mental status evaluation, clinical rating scales, or neuropsychological testing. (Page 4)

Because the definition of "dementia" is constantly evolving, research on the prevalence of dementia in patients with HD is minimal, and reports are varied. Past studies report the prevalence of dementia at rates ranging from 15% (11) to 95% (12). One study reports that patients with HD complain of dementia in approximately 10% of cases, and that 90% of patients with HD will develop dementia over the course of the illness (10). The variations in prevalence are likely attributable to inconsistencies in diagnostic criteria and definitions and to differences in patient populations and study paradigms.

In light of the broad spectrum of definitions of dementia and inconsistency in measuring the prevalence of dementia in HD, the literature should move away from using the term "dementia" in conjunction with HD. Dementia is a broad term, which carries with it a major stigma. A diagnosis of dementia does little to inform the treatment of a patient with HD because the diagnosis can be based on various definitions or can simply be the clinician's judgment. Until a widely accepted definition of dementia is agreed upon, and studies confirm that dementia is prevalent to a considerable degree in HD, it seems reasonable to focus on the specific symptoms of HD (i.e., motor, cognitive, and psychiatric) as they are presented in the literature, rather than rely on the meaning of a term that is widely disputed.

The cognitive symptoms in a patient with HD that are described by the term "dementia" might

TABLE 15-3. *Clinical criteria for amnestic mild cognitive impairment*

1. Memory complaint, preferably corroborated by an informant
2. Impaired memory function for age and education
3. Preserved general cognitive function
4. Intact activities of daily living
5. Not demented

[From Petersen RC, Doody R, Kurz A, et al. Current concepts in mild cognitive impairment. *Arch Neurol* 2001;58(12):1985–1992, with permission.]

be better summarized using the criteria for mild cognitive impairment (MCI). Criteria for MCI are presented in Table 15-3. The criteria here are specific for the amnesic form of MCI, most often referred to in relation to Alzheimer's disease, but can be used in reference to HD as well. Subtle memory impairment is common in patients with HD and is often one of the initial symptoms (10). Notably, the definition of MCI includes subtle memory impairment, but generally, patients exhibit intact cognitive function and ability to perform activities of daily living. Most patients who report mild memory impairments in the early stages of HD perform well in jobs and social activities. The deficits these patients are experiencing would not be captured in the DSM-IV definition of dementia, which requires a comorbid disturbance of social and occupational functioning. In sum, the definition for MCI is more sensitive to the memory symptoms of HD than the definition for dementia and seems appropriate for describing the beginning cognitive changes associated with HD.

THE COGNITIVE DISORDER

Zakzanis (13) performed an effect size analysis incorporating meta-analytic principles to review neuropsychological findings in HD. The analysis included 760 patients with HD and 943 healthy controls. The results indicated that patients with HD were most deficient in areas of delayed recall and memory acquisition. Other substantial deficiencies were in the areas of cognitive flexibility and abstraction, manual dexterity, attention and concentration, performance skill, and verbal skill. Although Zakzanis provided a rank-order list of specific neuropsychological tests in order of HD sensitivity to aid in the interpretation of the quantitative results, she also reported that executive dyscontrol may be an overriding deficit that contributes to poor performance on numerous specific tests. An additional confounding factor in testing performance is the presence of neurologically based unawareness or anosognosia. Often, a patient appearing stubborn or uncooperative, or a patient not performing at the level of which he or she is capable, is experiencing anosognosia, apathy, depression, or some combination of these states (see Chapter 14). Anosognosia has been shown to be much more common in HD than in healthy controls (14), and apathy and depression are present in 50% and 30% of patients with HD, respectively, (see Chapter 14). In contrast, some patients with HD are aware of their initial cognitive decline and become very frustrated and depressed because of things they are no longer able to do. Together, these factors may cause patients to withdraw from neuropsychological testing before the assessment is complete, to fail to perform at the level which they are capable, or to refuse testing altogether.

Despite the difficulties involved in the test, neuropsychological assessment can dramatically improve the understanding of HD in patients. Cognitive functions are among the most robust predictors of functional capacity (15). For instance, Rothlind and Brandt (16) examined motor and cognitive measures as predictors of independence in activities of daily living and reported that cognitive measures were more highly correlated with functioning than were other clinical measures of disease, including motor symptoms. Although the presence of unequivocal motor symptoms is the current criterion for diagnosing HD, research indicates that psychiatric and cognitive changes often present as symptoms of HD several years before motor symptoms do (14,15). Table 15-4 lists the primary cognitive deficits found in patients with HD, along with the neuropsychological tests that showed the highest percent discrimination between patients with HD and healthy controls (13). Notably, tests of memory do not reveal primary memory impairment, but rather, a retrieval deficit. The area of attention and concentration shows a general cognitive slowing but not a

TABLE 15-4. *Primary cognitive deficits in Huntington's disease (HD) and most effective neuropsychological test*

Cognitive deficit	Neuropsychological test(s)	Percent discrimination between HD patients and controls
Delayed recall	WMS—R visual reproduction	95
	WMS—R logical memory	95
	CVLT—long delay free recall	91
	CVLT—long delay cued recall	89
Memory acquisition	CVLT—list a total recall	93
Cognitive	WCST	82
Flexibility	Tower of London	79
Manual dexterity	Purdue Pegboard (right hand)	95
	Finger tapping test (right hand)	82
Attention and concentration	Trails A	80
	Trails B	78
	Stroop Color Reading	90
	Stroop Color Word	82
	Stroop Interference	79
Performance skill	WAIS-R Digit-Symbol	82
	WAIS-R Block Design	71
	Rey-O Figure	56
Verbal skill	WAIS-R Verbal IQ	71

WMS, Wechsler Memory Scale; CVLT, California Verbal Learning Test.

major deficit of selective attention or concentration. Although performance IQ tests are sensitive to HD, a primary visuospatial task, the Rey-O Figure, appears to discriminate only 56% of patients with HD from healthy controls. The most sensitive tasks require timed performances.

EXECUTIVE FUNCTIONS

Among the most prominent cognitive impairments in HD are the so-called "executive functions." These fundamental abilities control performance in many cognitive areas, including reasoning, planning, judgment, decision making, attention, learning, memory, flexibility, and timing.

Patients with HD demonstrate impairment on the Wisconsin Card Sorting Test (17) and the Stroop Color Word Test (18), and on clinical rating scales of executive dyscontrol (19,20). They also show impairment on the Tower of London test, a measure of the planning component of executive functioning (21). In fact, brief tests of executive function have been suggested as sensitive tools for differential diagnosis: the Serial Sevens item on the Mini-Mental Status Exam (22), the Initiation and Perseveration subtest of the Dementia Rating Scale (23), and an abbreviated battery of frontal lobe tests have been demonstrated to be distinctly sensitive to patients with HD (16,24,25).

Some recent research has evaluated the performance of patients with HD in clinically relevant, face-valid tests of judgment and decision making. Stout et al. (26) used a simulated gambling task to quantify decision-making deficits in patients with HD. The gambling task involved repeatedly choosing from four decks of cards, two with good consequences and two with poor outcomes. Patients with HD made fewer advantageous selections than age- and education-matched healthy controls or patients with Parkinson's disease (PD) matched for cognitive impairment severity (see Fig. 15-1). The number of advantageous selections made by the patients with HD was not associated with overall severity of the disease, but it was correlated significantly with brief measures of conceptualization and memory. Several patients with HD indicated that one or more of the card decks were "bad" but continued to make selections from the decks that they identified as "bad." Patients with focal ventromedial frontal lobe damage demonstrated similar responses to the gambling task (27), indicating that dysfunction at the level of the caudate can result in behavioral disturbances similar to the disturbances seen in patients with primary cortical damage.

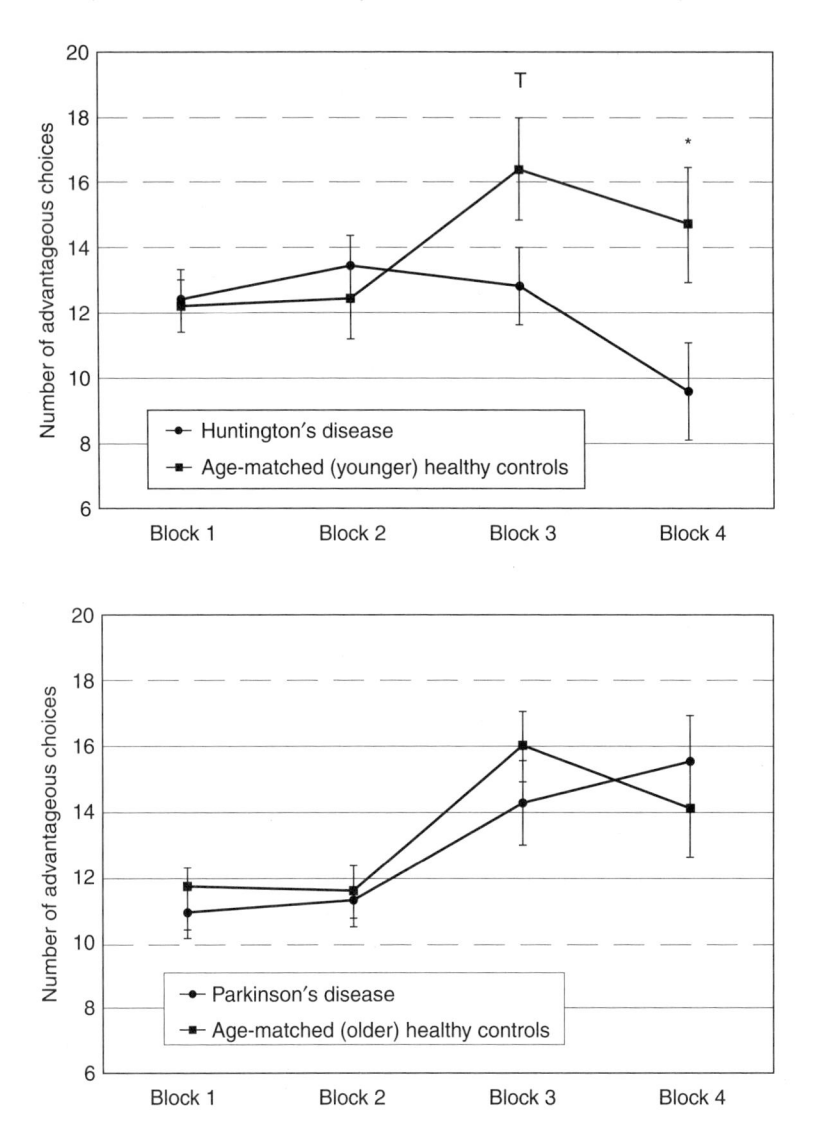

FIG. 15-1. Gambling task outcomes for Huntington's disease (HD), Parkinson's disease (PD), and healthy controls. [From Stout J, Rodawalt W, Siemers E, et al. Risky decision making in Huntington's disease. *J Int Neuropsychol Soc* 2001;7(1):92–101, with permission.]

The striatum has also been identified as contributing to the behavioral, social, or psychiatric disturbances seen in patients with HD. A study found that when patients with frontotemporal dementia (FTD) and HD were given tests of theory of mind to explore their ability to interpret social situations and describe mental states, the patients with FTD were severely impaired, whereas patients with HD exhibited milder impairment while interpreting cartoons and stories and had normal preference judgments (28). However, qualitatively, patients with FTD tended to construct concrete, literal interpretations of cartoons and stories, whereas patients with HD were more likely to misconstrue situations. The authors concluded that the breakdown of social skills in patients with FTD and those with HD may have different underlying bases, and that the frontal neocortex and striatum may contribute to social behavior in distinctly different ways.

Another study used an experimental version of Twenty Questions, the well-known parlor game (29). Patients with HD were instructed to ask as few yes–no questions as possible to determine which item in an array, consisting of line drawings of common living and nonliving things, was the preselected target. Patients with HD asked fewer (e.g., "Is it living/nonliving?" or "Is it in the top half of the page?"), less relevant (e.g., "Is it yellow?") and more restrictive, which eliminated only one item, constraint-seeking questions (e.g., "Does it buzz and sting you?"), than age- and education-matched healthy controls.

Decision-making tasks may be impaired because of cognitive decrements in learning, attention, inhibition, or appreciation for future consequences. The findings of the Gambling and Twenty Questions tests can also be interpreted as further evidence that patients with HD are less able than healthy controls to benefit from feedback and have difficulty varying output on the basis of previous response (30). Despite evidence that they had explicit knowledge that could be used to perform the tasks, patients with HD were unable to update existing "programs" on the basis of new experience or to alter their responses. Numerous wide-ranging consequences of these types of executive deficits are self-evident.

Patients with HD and those with PD have subcortical damage within the frontal–subcortical circuits; however, specific areas of damage may explain why HD but not PD is associated with poor responses in the simulated gambling task (31). In patients with HD, loss of the medium spiny neurons occurs more in the caudate nucleus than in the putamen. Behavior changes similar to those exhibited by patients with damage to the ventromedial frontal lobe or to other areas of prefrontal cortex may occur in HD, because caudate efferents ultimately affect the prefrontal cortex, which is important in cognitive and personality functions. In contrast, loss of neurons in the substantia nigra pars compacta in PD primarily affects the putamenal efferents, which project more strongly to the premotor regions of the frontal cortex (32) and are involved more in response selection for executing movement than in cognitive and personality functions.

ATTENTION AND WORKING MEMORY

Early neuropsychological studies using the Wechsler Adult Intelligence Scales (33) consistently reported that patients with HD performed most poorly on the subtests that require attention and working memory (e.g., Arithmetic, Digit Span, and Digit Symbol) (34–36). More recent studies on patients with HD have emphasized dysfunction in unique aspects of attention, including resource allocation, response flexibility, and vigilance (37–39). For instance, Lawrence et al. (40) reported that patients with HD are able to maintain attention for a previously learned response set but have difficulty shifting attention to a new set. The difficulty of patients with HD in task switching may also be due to inadequate inhibition of responding before the task is switched (41). Sprengelmeyer et al. (39) reported that patients with HD are able to maintain alertness when the task involves an external cue but fail when internal self-generated vigilance is required. The authors emphasized the potential effect of this impairment on a number of other "higher-order" cognitive deficits described in patients with HD.

Recent studies on working memory have also demonstrated that patients with HD tend to perseverate on previously correct responses and demonstrate difficulty maintaining attention on updated information in immediate memory (38). Tests of attention and working memory, such as the Brief Test of Attention, have been so well established as being sensitive to HD that these types of tests are incorporated into longitudinal research programs and clinical trials for studying HD (42).

LEARNING AND MEMORY

Hahn-Barma et al. (43) administered a comprehensive neuropsychological battery of tests to 91 asymptomatic at-risk individuals. CAG repeat lengths were measured to separate individuals with the HD mutation from those with normal expansion sizes. Performances on learning and memory tests divided the individuals with the gene mutation into two groups, those who had cognitive deficits and those who did not, without overlap. The performance of individuals without cognitive deficits was similar to that of healthy normal controls on all tests. The individuals with cognitive deficits differed from the other groups on several tests, and performances were significantly associated with CAG repeat length. These data suggest that impairments of learning and memory may be early manifestations of disease in patients with the HD mutation who do not yet have motor abnormalities.

Deficits in learning and memory are the most frequently reported cognitive complaints from patients with HD and their family members. Patients with HD exhibit verbal learning deficits even in the earliest stages of the illness (44). Most studies have described memory impairment in patients with HD as a primary encoding and retrieval deficit, because recognition memory is often relatively preserved (45,46). That is, most studies show that patients with HD consistently have problems learning new information and also experience difficulty when asked to use free recall to remember what they have learned; in contrast, their performance is close to that of normal controls when a less effortful memory strategy is used, such as offering choices of, or recognition of, various learned items. Although the preservation of recognition memory has been demonstrated in several studies of patients with HD, some investigators have questioned the consistency of this finding across tests (47) and through middle and last stages of the disease (48,49), with one study indicating that deficits in recognition memory are apparent in asymptomatic gene carriers (50).

Patients with HD manifest relatively intact retention over a delay period, indicating no abnormal forgetting or rapid loss of information (46,51). When tested on memory for information acquired long ago, they demonstrate no temporal gradient in performance, indicating that memory performance is equivalent, though mildly impaired, for all periods of their lives (52).

Research in HD patients has made substantial contributions to our understanding of memory over the past few decades (53). Briefly, observations that skill learning is intact in patients with medial–temporal and diencephalic damage but is deficient in patients with HD led to an explosion of research investigating the existence of multiple, independent memory systems in the brain. It is well documented that skill learning depends on the integrity of the basal ganglia. Recently, however, Gabrieli et al. (54) documented dissociable skill-learning performances in patients with HD, suggesting the existence of separable neural circuits for skill learning. They propose that a striatal memory system may be essential for sequence or open-loop skill learning but not for skills that involve closed-loop learning of novel visual-response mappings. Moreover, impairments in "open-loop" skill learning may be attributable to limitations in working memory. For instance, Goldman-Rakic (55) suggested that a fundamental feature of working memory is that it guides behavior on the basis of internal, symbolic models rather than external, perceptual feedback. Consistent with this interpretation, Paulsen et al. (30) reported that skill learning was impaired only when external immediate feedback was no longer available. Similarly, Willingham et al. (56) showed that patients with HD exhibited intact skill learning when visual feedback was available but showed defective skill learning when their performance relied on sequence learning without feedback. These findings are consistent with those from animal studies of the basal ganglia, which suggest that the striatum can "chunk," or combine, the representations of motor and cognitive action sequences so they can be implemented as units. The models put forth by Gabrieli et al. (54) and Willingham et al. (56) offer a concise explanation for the learning and memory impairment profile found in patients with HD.

In summary, the memory impairment in patients with HD is characterized by a mild encoding deficit (likely caused by impaired organization of the information to be learned and by ineffective working memory) and moderately impaired retrieval in the context of relatively intact memory storage when measured with a less effortful strategy (i.e., recognition). Frontostriatal disruption secondary to HD possibly diminishes learning and memory performance when internally guided, open-loop thoughts or skills are required. Other learning and memory skills that are less dependent on internal working memory capacity may be relatively intact.

PRIMARY SENSORY PROCESSING

Several studies using the University of Pennsylvania Smell Identification Test (UPSIT) have shown olfaction impairments in patients with HD (57). In the most comprehensive research to date, Nordin et al. (58) assessed absolute detection, intensity discrimination, quality discrimination, short-term recognition memory, and lexical-based and picture-based identification for odor in patients with HD, using taste and vision as comparison modalities. Results suggested that although odor-recognition memory is not affected in patients with HD, absolute detection, intensity discrimination, quality discrimination, and identification were considerably impaired. Poor detection sensitivity explained the poor performance on several other olfactory tasks in which odor identification was the function most impaired. Moberg and Doty (59) evaluated olfactory functions in people at risk for HD. Findings were not significant, and the authors argue that olfaction cannot serve as an indicator of genetic vulnerability in persons at risk for HD. Recent research suggests that neuropsychological impairments become evident in patients at risk for HD when they are close to disease onset (versus far from onset). Thus, some studies of at-risk patients have likely included a preponderance of participants far from onset, resulting in false-negative findings. The utility of olfactory assessment for identifying people close to onset of HD remains an empiric question.

SPATIAL–PERCEPTUAL SKILL

Deficits in the ability to copy simple geometric designs, to copy block designs, and to put together puzzles are evident in patients with HD. Although some of these impairments likely reflect motor abnormalities, performance on motor-free untimed perceptual tasks is also impaired (60). A consistent and primary spatial impairment has been identified in the perception of personal, or egocentric, space (61). Mohr et al. (62) recently examined whether visuospatial deficits in basal ganglia disease are a nonspecific function of dementia severity or whether they reflect disease-specific impairments. Findings suggested that general visuospatial processing capacity is impaired as a nonspecific dementia effect in patients with HD and those with PD, whereas only patients with HD show specific impairment in person-centered spatial judgment. For instance, patients with HD (but not PD) experience difficulty with map reading, directional sense, and varying their motor responses following alterations in space. Patients with HD typically misjudge distances and the relation between their body and walls, curbs, and other potential obstacles.

The theory of differential visuospatial memory impairment based on the stage of disease was studied by assessing memory for hand positions (egocentric memory) and memory for spatial locations (allocentric memory) in patients with HD and in normal controls (63). Patients with HD were impaired, compared to normal controls. Correlation analyses indicated that the performances of patients with HD on the two tasks were not associated with each other, and that performance on the Hand Position Memory task was associated with global cognitive status and disease severity. These results are consistent with the notion that patients with HD present with a deficit in a variety of visual stimuli and suggest that the caudate nucleus plays a role in both types of visual memory. If neurodegeneration in HD proceeds from the tail of the caudate (interconnected with the inferotemporal cortex) to the head (interconnected with the frontal cortex), allocentric spatial memory may be impaired early in the disease, and egocentric spatial memory may be impaired later. The fact that only performance on the Hand Position Memory task (egocentric memory) was correlated with disease severity supports a differential visuospatial impairment based on stage of disease.

Although the underlying basis for the visual perceptual impairments in patients with HD is not fully understood, disruptions in corticostriatal circuitry may make it difficult to update spatial relations on the basis of feedback. Cortico–cortico connections to the parietal cortex may also be compromised, secondary to disruption of the prefrontal cortex.

LANGUAGE

One of the most prominent features of HD is the motor speech impairment, or dysarthria, that is characteristic of the illness. Early speech changes may include insufficient breath support, varying prosody, increased response latencies, and mild misarticulations. As HD progresses, phrase length becomes reduced, and pauses in speech output lengthen (64). Patients with HD exhibit impaired letter and category fluency early in the disease (45,65), although the integrity of word associations remains relatively intact, with little evidence of intrusion or perseveration errors (66,67). Patients with HD may be at risk for productive syntax impairments, which are most likely a product of motor speech as well as underlying cognitive impairment of executive processes (68). Syntax errors are typically evident only with complex sentences. Although some patients with late-stage HD report mild deterioration in semantic knowledge structure, several other studies have shown that errors in confrontation naming are more likely caused by visual–perceptual deficits (69) and slow retrieval (70).

In longitudinal studies of verbal fluency, patients with HD exhibit reduced capacity to use correct words over time and increased instances of word repetitions (71). These deficits can be understood in terms of the two underlying components of verbal fluency tasks: clustering (the ability to generate successive words within a subcategory) and switching (the ability to shift from one subcategory to another). Patients with HD display decreased switching ability over time, whereas clustering ability remains stable. The impaired switching ability is consistent with the progressive reduction in cognitive flexibility attributed to disruption of frontal subcortical circuits in patients with HD; letter fluency tests have been shown to be especially sensitive to such disruption (71,72).

Speech output becomes severely impaired as HD progresses, typically resulting in a profound communication deficit. Assistive devices for language expression are recommended for patients in the early stages of HD to ensure that preferences are understood and needs are met in later stages when traditional communication is no longer possible. Computer devices are useful for a brief period, after which motor dyscontrol limits use of a keyboard or joystick. Infrared detectors are often prone to error because it also detects involuntary movements of patients. Alphabet boards and pictures that summarize frequently requested needs are adaptive and can be used throughout the illness. Simple computer response keys and large YES–NO cards are critical for patients in the late stages of HD.

Although motor output of speech is the primary impairment in patients with HD, several more subtle language impairments are associated with the disease. The patient's ability to comprehend conversation is limited by its length and complexity. Poor executive control impairs the patient's ability to sequence and organize the information that is communicated. In addition, there is some evidence that patients with HD cannot benefit from affective and propositional prosody (73). Murray and Stout (74) observed that patients with HD and those with PD adequately perceived main information on a discourse comprehension test but had problems processing detailed or implied information. These comprehension deficits correlated with performances on tests of selective and sustained attention abilities, verbal memory, and with dementia severity. Accordingly, speech-language pathology services should not only address motor problems but should also evaluate potential communication difficulties, offering compensatory strategies to maximize and maintain patients' communication functioning. For instance, patients could be taught to capitalize on their discourse strengths, and caregivers could be taught to use direct statements rather than rely on the patients' ability to infer important information.

TIME PERCEPTION AND PRODUCTION

Recent findings have suggested that people with basal ganglia dysfunction, and specifically patients with HD, have difficulty in estimating and using time (75). These findings are corroborated clinically; people often complain that their once-punctual spouses have become frequently late and often misestimate how long activities will take. The clinical relevance of these findings to patients' daily activities, such as driving, is unknown, but research is underway to better characterize these observations.

ADVANCES IN HUNTINGTON'S DISEASE RESEARCH

Cognitive Changes

Despite some mixed findings (76–78), the overall evidence is strong that cognitive and behavioral changes can be detected before diagnosis in individuals at risk for HD (2,4,43,79–84). The available studies on patients with HD have varied considerably in terms of study samples and specific cognitive measures used, however, limiting comparison across studies. Thus, the magnitude and time course of early changes in patients with HD are still unclear. Despite these limitations, some recent studies have suggested that inhibitory control mechanisms (i.e., set shifting and fluency) and speed of processing (e.g., Digit Symbol) are among the first impairments in individuals at risk for HD.

Collaborative research by the Huntington Study Group (HSG) has shed light on the cognitive profile of presymptomatic HD. There are 155 individuals in the HSG database who have not been gene tested, who showed no HD symptoms on first testing, and who have had at least one follow-up evaluation at an average of 21 months after the first testing. Thirty-four of these individuals have been diagnosed with HD at subsequent visits. Initial values and rates of change in cognitive variables among the 121 individuals who did not exhibit symptoms of HD (nonconverters) and the 34 patients who demonstrated HD at follow-up visit(s) (converters) are given in Table 15-5. Rates of change and their standard deviations were estimated from a mixed-model analysis. Findings suggest that clear differences exist in cognitive performance change rates between individuals at risk for HD who were close to onset of the disease and those far from onset of the disease (or without CAG expansion). In individuals at risk for HD who were close to the onset of disease, neuropsychological performances declined at a much more rapid rate than in those individuals who were far from the onset of HD, and effect sizes of the group differences were robust with every cognitive measure, ranging from 0.8 to 1.9.

PREDICT-HD

Predict-HD is a longitudinal study, conducted by the HSG, designed to examine neurobiologic and neurobehavioral markers of HD in 600 genetically tested, presymptomatic individuals (NINDS 40068, Paulsen JS, Principal Investigator). The measures used in the study include a comprehensive neuropsychological battery composed of tests that are well established in the literature and tests designed specifically for the presymptomatic cohort. Other measures include an magnetic resonance imaging (MRI) scan, blood tests, and psychiatric surveys. This study is the first designed to use all these measures to research this large a sample of gene-tested individuals who are presymptomatic for HD. The results of the Predict-HD study will help determine the earliest signs of HD and when these signs begin, the most accurate tests for detecting the onset of HD, and the factors that influence the age at which a person carrying the HD gene develops the illness.

TABLE 15-5. *Baseline performance and estimated change rate in presymptomatic Huntington's disease (HD)*

Cognitive measure	Nonconverters (n = 121) Initial value (SD)	Change rate (SD)	Converters (n = 34) Initial value (SD)	Change rate (SD)
Verbal Fluency	32.3 (12.1)	1.7 (2.4)	33.9 (13.2)	−0.5 (1.2)
Symbol Digit	48.8 (11.4)	0.1 (2.2)	40.4 (13.6)	−1.8 (1.6)
Stroop	70.8 (14.2)	0.6 (3.0)	62.9 (15.9)	−2.0 (2.5)
Stroop Reading	85.6 (16.2)	0.7 (3.3)	78.7 (17.1)	−2.1 (3.5)
Stroop Interference	40.9 (11.7)	0.5 (2.8)	37.3 (13.8)	−2.2 (0.4)

[From Paulsen JS, Zhao H, Stout JC, et al. Clinical markers of early disease in persons near onset of Huntington's disease. *Neurology* 2001;57:658–662, with permission.]

Preliminary data reported from the Predict-HD study shows an association between estimated years before onset of HD in patients and cognitive decline (85). The recognition of fear during both static and dynamic tasks has been associated with years to onset of HD (86). Computerized tests of finger tapping and self-paced tapping exhibited variability between patients with HD that was associated with estimated years to onset of disease (87). Lack of initiation is frequently cited as a behavioral and cognitive symptom in patients with HD. A subtest of the Predict-HD study supported this observation, finding that initiation times on tasks assessing response time were more related than movement times to estimated age of onset (88). A three-disk and four-disk Tower of London task provided evidence that estimated years to onset of HD is correlated with trial completion time and average time per move on the four-disk task. These findings suggest that individuals who are closer to onset of HD may be performing differently from others in the timing of decisions, supporting the finding that initiation is lacking. Overall, data from 123 patients who were examined at their baseline visit for the Predict-HD study show evidence of associations between estimated years to onset of HD and poorer performance on several cognitive task-assessing domains including choice reaction time, finger tapping, facial recognition of emotions, smell identification, and decision making (85).

Neuroimaging

Neuroimaging has made a large contribution to understanding the cognitive changes associated with HD. Structural and functional neuroimaging studies indicate clear basal ganglia abnormalities in patients with HD (see Figs. 15-2 and 15-3).

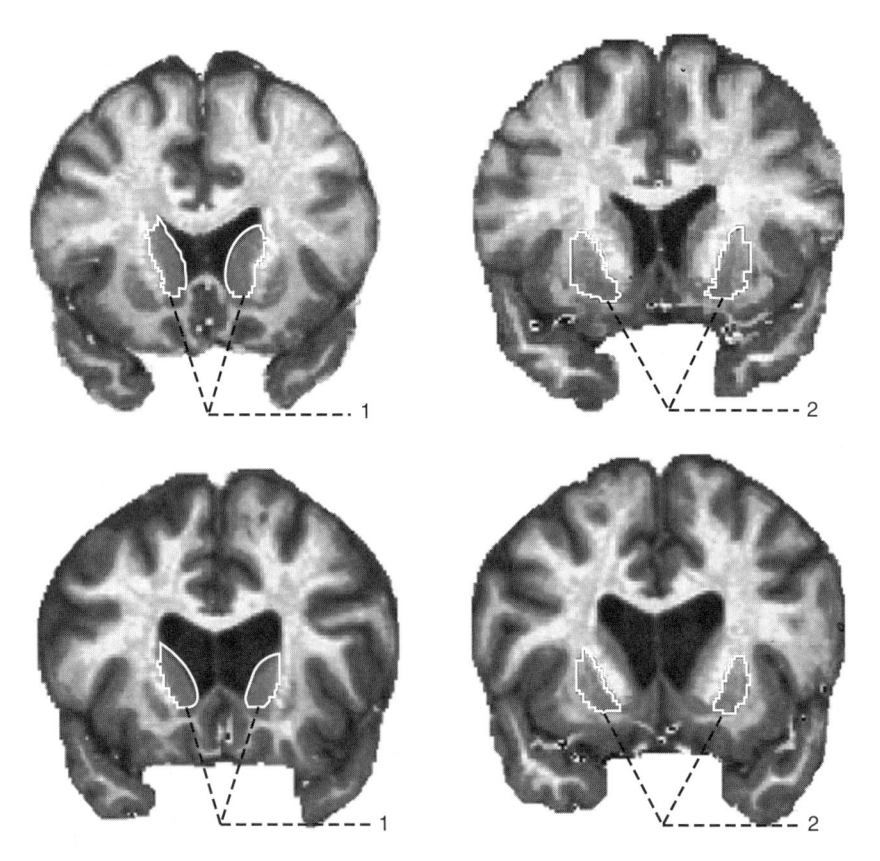

FIG. 15-2. Magnetic resonance image of healthy control **(top)** and patient with Huntington's disease (HD) **(bottom)**. 1 and 2 represent areas traced for volumetric analysis; 1 traces the caudate and 2 traces the putamen. From Jane S. Paulsen, University of Iowa. Printed with permission.

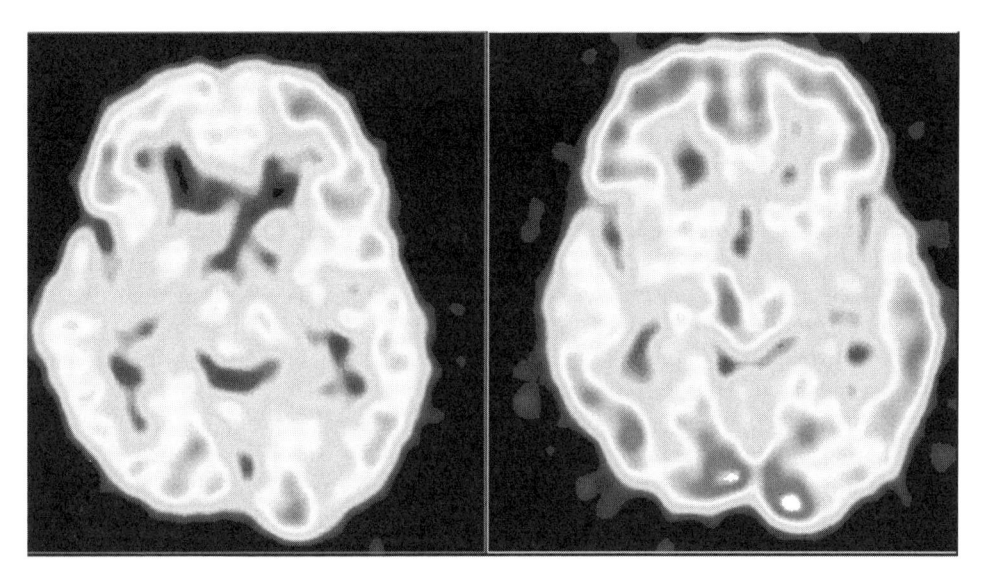

FIG. 15-3. Positron emission tomography using F-deoxy-D-glucose (FDG): patients with HD **(left)** and healthy controls **(right)**. (From Mark Guttman, Centre for Addiction and Mental Health, with permission.)

MRI (Fig. 15-2) reveals volume reduction in subcortical structures, including the caudate and putamen (89–97). Positron emission tomography (PET) (Fig. 15-3) shows reduced glucose metabolism (94,98–102) and dopamine receptor–binding deficiencies in the caudate and putamen (103–106) before the development of clinical symptoms in patients with HD. A few studies found no significant differences between controls and presymptomatic individuals in glucose metabolism or dopamine receptor binding (107,108). Recent studies using indices of quantitative volumetric MRI and PET raclopride binding potential, however, suggest that striatal dysfunction is evident within a decade before onset of HD symptoms and that function declines further as subjects approach the onset of HD (97,109). Kirkwood et al. (110) conducted a study measuring motor function and reaction time among presymptomatic HD gene carriers and noted a tendency toward greater physiologic abnormalities as neurologic symptoms increased in patients. The authors also suggested that some essentially static motor function and reaction time abnormalities may be present from birth in people who later develop HD, although gene carriers may still show normal neuronal functioning for a long period of life (108).

A number of reports have demonstrated significant associations between imaging indices and clinical correlates of the disease, including illness duration (98,111), functional capacity (112), motor symptoms (113), cognitive impairment (114), and CAG repeat length (115). Progressive basal ganglia atrophy, demonstrated by quantitative neuroimaging with serial MRI, suggests that progression is more rapid in patients with an early age of HD onset and a long CAG repeat length (115). Abnormalities in the basal ganglia are associated negatively with the estimated number of years to onset of HD and positively associated with CAG length in presymptomatic CAG-expanded individuals (93, 108). Data from the Predict-HD Study (85) has found that striatal volumes in presymptomatic people are associated with declining performances on traditional and computerized tests of cognition. Lawrence et al. (116) found a significant relation between striatal dopamine receptor binding (visualized by PET) and cognitive performances in 17 presymptomatic gene carriers with a median of 8 years until estimated onset of HD. Striatal dopamine receptor levels and cognitive performance declined as subjects approached their estimated ages of onset.

Using functional MRI, Paulsen et al. (117) demonstrated that presymptomatic individuals more than 12 years from estimated onset of motor symptoms showed a decrease in caudate activity and a compensatory increase in supplementary motor area and anterior cingulate activities during a time discrimination task. The functional changes exhibited in patients with HD preceded changes in cognitive task performance and structural brain changes. This pattern of brain activation may represent an early neurobiologic marker of HD. Presymptomatic patients estimated to be less than 12 years from HD onset showed abnormalities in brain activation, task performance, and volumetric measurements. Functional imaging findings also demonstrated that the patients estimated to be close to onset of HD displayed considerably less activation in subcortical regions than controls did, whereas the participants estimated to be 12 years or more from onset of HD demonstrated an intermediate level of activation. Images of the functional scans completed in this study are presented in Figure 15-4. Unlike structural imaging, which detects only changes in the caudate in patients who are close to onset of HD, the results of this study suggest that functional neuroimaging may provide a useful means of detecting the evolution of changes in neural function during the earliest stages of HD.

In summary, both cognitive changes and neuroimaging analyses reveal that subtle changes in the function and structure of the brain begin years before the onset of the movement disorder in HD. Large-scale efforts are underway to further delineate the earliest cognitive and brain structure changes in patients with HD in the prodromal phase. Drug development has pushed beyond the goal of providing palliative interventions to the goal of delaying onset or slowing disease progression. Detecting cognitive decline and understanding the morphological changes to the striatum in patients with HD are therefore essential to determining when to initiate clinical trials to delay motor onset.

ACKNOWLEDGMENTS

This project was supported by National Institutes of Health Grant N540068 and the Howard Hughes Medical Institute and the Roy Carver Medical Trust.

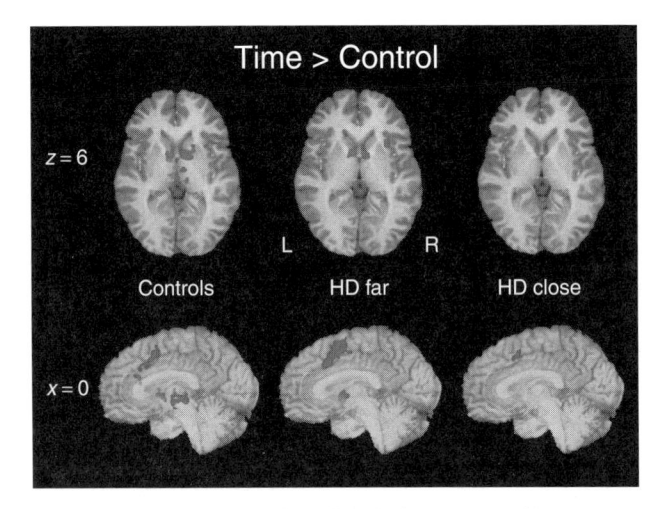

FIG. 15-4. Volume of activation (microliters) in the thalamus, caudate, or putamen **(top)** and the supplementary motor area or cingulate **(bottom)**. The three groups are controls, 12 years or more from onset of motor symptoms (*far*) in patients with HD, and 12 years or less from onset of motor symptoms (*close*) of HD. (From Paulsen JS, Zimbelman JL, Hinton, SC, et al. An fMRI biomarker of early neuronal dysfunction in presymptomatic Huntington's disease. *Am J Neuroradiol*, 2004 Nov/Dec;25:1715–1721, with permission.)

REFERENCES

1. Qilibash N, ed. *Evidence-based dementia practice*. Malden, MA: Blackwell Science, 2002.
2. Siemers E, Foroud T, Bill DJ, et al. Motor changes in presymptomatic Huntington disease gene carriers. *Arch Neurol* 1996;53:487–492.
3. Group HS. Unified Huntington's disease rating scale: reliability and consistency. *Mov Disord* 1996;11:136–142.
4. Snowden JS, Craufurd D, Thompson J, et al. Psychomotor, executive, and memory function in preclinical Huntington's disease. *J Clin Exp Neuropsychol* 2002;24:133–145.
5. Berrios GE. Historical aspects of psychoses: 19th century issues. *Br Med Bull* 1987;43:484–498.
6. Mendez MF, Cummings JL. *Dementia: a clinical approach*. Philadelphia, PA: Butterworth-Heinemann, 2003.
7. Diagnostic and Statistical Manual of Mental Disorders: Fourth edition DSM-IV. Washington, DC: American Psychiatric Association, 1994.
8. Folstein SE, Brandt J, Folstein MF. Subcortical dementia. In: Cummings J, ed. *Huntington's disease*. London: Oxford University Press, 1990:87–107.
9. Spar JE, La Rue A. *Concise guide to geriatric psychiatry*. Los Angeles, CA: American Psychiatric Press Concise Guides, 1990.
10. Gontkovsky ST. Huntington's disease: a neuropsychological overview. *J Cogn Rehab* 1998;16:6–9.
11. Oliver JE. Huntington's chorea in Northamptonshire. *Br J Psychiatry* 1970;116:241–253.
12. Heathfield KW. Huntington's chorea. Investigation into the prevalence of this disease in the area covered by the North East Metropolitan Regional Hospital Board. *Brain* 1967;90:203–232.
13. Zakzanis KK. The subcortical dementia of Huntington's disease. *J Clin Exp Neuropsychol* 1998;20:565–578.
14. Snowden JS, Craufurd D, Griffiths HL, et al. Awareness of involuntary movements in Huntington's disease. *Arch Neurol* 1998;55:801–805.
15. Holtzer R, Wegesin DJ, Albert SM, et al. The rate of cognitive decline and risk of reaching clinical milestones in Alzheimer disease. *Arch Neurol* 2003;60:1137–1142.
16. Rothlind JC, Brandt J. A brief assessment of frontal and subcortical functions in dementia. *J Neuropsychiatry Clin Neurosci* 1993;5:73–77.
17. Savage CR. Neuropsychology of subcortical dementias. *Psychiatr Clin North Am* 1997;20:911–931.
18. Paulsen JS, Como P, Rey G, et al. The clinical utility of the Stroop test in a multicenter study of Huntington's disease. *J Int Neuropsychol Soc* 1996;2:35.
19. Paulsen JS, Stout JC, Delapena J, et al. Frontal behavioral syndromes in cortical and subcortical dementia. *Assessment* 1996;3:327–337.
20. Paulsen JS, Mega MS, Cummings JL. The spectrum of behavioral changes in Huntington's disease. *J Neurospychiatry* 1997;9:655–656.
21. Watkins LH, Rogers RD, Lawrence AD, et al. Impaired planning but intact decision making in early Huntington's disease: implications for specific fronto-striatal pathology. *Neuropsychologia* 2000;38:1112–1125.
22. Folstein MF, Folstein SE, McHugh PR. Mini-Mental State: a practical method for grading the cognitive state of patients for the clinician. *J Pschiatr Res* 1975;12:189–198.
23. Mattis S. Mental status examination for organic mental syndrome in the elderly patient. In: Bellak L, Karasu TB, eds. *Geriatric psychiatry*. New York: Grune & Stratton, 1976:77–122.
24. Brandt J, Folstein SE, Folstein MF. Differential cognitive impairment in Alzheimer's disease and Huntington's disease. *Ann Neurol* 1988;23:555–561.
25. Paulsen JS, Butters N, Sadek JR, et al. Distinct cognitive profiles of cortical and subcortical dementia in advanced illness. *Neurology* 1995;45:951–956.
26. Stout JC, Rodawalt WC, Siemers ER. Risky decision making in Huntington's disease. *J Int Neuropsychol Soc* 2001;7:92–101.
27. Bechara A, Damasio H, Tranel D, et al. Insensitivity to future consequences following damage to human prefrontal cortex. *Cognition* 1994;50:7–15.
28. Snowden JS, Gibbons ZC, Blackshaw A, et al. Social cognition in frontotemporal dementia and Huntington's disease. *Neuropsychologia* 2003;41:688–701.
29. Stout JC, Paulsen JS, Tawfik-Reedy Z, et al. The nature of problem-solving deficits in patients with early Huntington's disease. *J Int Neuropsychol Soc* 1996;2:35.
30. Paulsen JS, Butters N, Salmon DP, et al. Prism adaptation in Alzheimer's and Huntington's disease. *Neuropsychology* 1993;7:73–81.
31. Alexander GE, Crutcher MD. Functional architecture of basal ganglia circuits: neural substrates of parallel processing. *Trends Neurosci* 1990;13:266–271.
32. Alexander GE. Anatomy of the basal ganglia and related motor structures. In: Watts RL, Koller WC, eds. *Movement disorders: neurological principles and practice*. New York: McGraw-Hill, 1997.
33. Wechsler D. *Wechsler adult intelligence scale*, 3rd ed. San Antonio, TX: The Psychological Corporation, 1997.
34. Boll TJ, Heaton R, Reitan R. Neuropsychological and emotional correlates of Huntington's disease. *J Ment Nerv Disord* 1974;158:61–69.
35. Josiassen RC, Curry LM, Mancall EL. Development of neuropsychological deficits in Huntington's disease. *Arch Neurol* 1983;40:791–796.
36. Strauss ME, Brandt J. An attempt at presymptomatic identification of Huntington's disease with the WAIS. *J Clin Exp Neuropsychol* 1986;8:210–228.
37. Hanes KR, Andrewes DG, Pantelis C. Cognitive flexibility and complex integration in Parkinson's disease, Huntington's disease, and schizophrenia. *J Int Neuropsychol Soc* 1995;1:545–553.
38. Lange KW, Sahakian BJ, Quinn NP, et al. Comparison of executive and visuospatial memory function in Huntington's disease and dementia of Alzheimer type matched for degree of dementia. *J Neurol Neurosurg Psychiatry* 1995;58:598–606.
39. Sprengelmeyer R, Lange H, Homberg V. The pattern of attentional deficits in Huntington's disease. *Brain* 1995;118:145–152.
40. Lawrence AD, Sahakian BJ, Hodges JR, et al. Executive and mnemonic functions in early Huntington's disease. *Brain* 1996;119:1633–1645.
41. Aron AR, Watkins L, Sahakian BJ, et al. Task-set switching deficits in early stage Huntington's disease: implications for basal ganglia function. *J Cogn Neurosci* 2003;15:629–642.
42. The Huntington Study Group. Safety and tolerability of the free-radical scavenger OPC-14117 in Huntington's disease. *Neurology* 1998;50:1366–1373.
43. Hahn-Barma V, Deweer B, Durr A, et al. Are cognitive changes the first symptoms of Huntington's disease? A study of gene carriers. *J Neurol Neurosurg Psychiatry* 1998;64:172–177.

44. Hamilton JM. Cognitive, motor, and behavioral correlates of functional decline in Huntington's disease. *Clinical Psychology*. San Diego, CA: University of California, 1998:58.
45. Butters N, Wolfe J, Granholm E, et al. An assessment of verbal recall, recognition, and fluency abilities in patients with Huntington's disease. *Cortex* 1986;22:11–32.
46. Delis DC, Massman PJ, Butters N, et al. Profiles of demented and amnesic patients on the California verbal learning test: implications for the assessment of memory disorders. *Psychol Assess: J Consult Clin Psychol* 1991;3:19–26.
47. Brandt J, Corwin J, Krafft L. Is verbal recognition memory really different in Huntington's and Alzheimer's disease? *J Clin Exp Neuropsychol* 1992;14:773–784.
48. Kramer JH, Delis DC, Blusewicz MJ, et al. Verbal memory errors in Alzheimer's and Huntington's dementias. *Dev Neuropsychol* 1988;4:1–15.
49. Lang CJG, Majer M, Balan P. Recall and recognition in Huntington's disease. *Arch Clin Neuropsychology* 2000;15:361–371.
50. Berrios GE, Wagle AC, Markova IS, et al. Psychiatric symptoms in neurologically asymptomatic Huntington's disease gene carriers: a comparison with gene negative at risk subjects. *Acta Psychiatr Scand* 2002;105:224–230.
51. Massman PJ, Delis DC, Butters N, et al. Are all subcortical dementias alike? Verbal learning and memory in Parkinson's and Huntington's disease patients. *J Clin Exp Neuropsychol* 1990;12:729–744.
52. Butters N, Albert MS. Processes underlying failures to recall remote events. In: Cermak LS, ed. *Human, memory, and amnesia*. Hillsdale, NJ: Erlbaum, 1982:257–274.
53. Gabrieli JD. Cognitive neuroscience of human memory. *Annu Rev Psychol* 1998;49:87–115.
54. Gabrieli JD, Stebbins GT, Singh J, et al. Intact mirror-tracing and impaired rotary-pursuit skill learning in patients with Huntington's disease: evidence for dissociable memory systems in skill learning. *Neuropsychology* 1997;11:272–281.
55. Goldman-Rakic PS. In: Plum F, Mountcastle V, eds. *Handbook of physiology*, Vol. 5. Bethesda, MD: American Physiological Society, 1987:373–417.
56. Willingham DB, Koroshetz WJ, Peterson EW. Motor skills have diverse neural bases: spared and impaired skill acquisition in Huntington's disease. *Neuropsychology* 1996;10:315–321.
57. Doty RL. Olfactory dysfunction in neurodegenerative disorders. In: Getchell TV, Doty RL, Bartoshuk LM et al., eds. *Smell and taste in health and disease*. New York: Raven Press, 1991:735–751.
58. Nordin S, Paulsen JS, Murphy C. Sensory- and memory-mediated olfactory dysfunction in Huntington's disease. *J Int Neuropsychol Soc* 1995;1:271–280.
59. Moberg PJ, Doty RL. Olfactory function in Huntington's disease patients and at-risk offspring. *Int J Neurosci* 1997;89:133–139.
60. Mohr E, Brouwers P, Claus JJ, et al. Visuospatial cognition in Huntington's disease. *Mov Disord* 1991;6:127–132.
61. Potegal M. A note on spatial motor deficits in patients with Huntington's disease: a test of a hypothesis. *Neuropsychologia* 1971;9:233–235.
62. Mohr E, Claus JJ, Brouwers P. Basal ganglia disease and visuospatial cognition: are these disease-specific impairments? *Behav Neurol* 1997;10:67–75.
63. Davis JD, Filoteo JV, Kesner RP, et al. Recognition memory for hand positions and spatial locations in patients with Huntington's disease: differential visuospatial memory impairment? *Cortex* 2003;39:239–253.
64. Podoll K, Caspary P, Lange HW, et al. Language functions in Huntington's disease. *Brain* 1988;111:1475–1503.
65. Randolph C, Braun AR, Goldberg TE, et al. Semantic fluency in Alzheimer's, Parkinson's, Huntington's disease: dissociation of storage and retrieval failures. *Neuropsychology* 1993;7:82–88.
66. Butters N, Granholm E, Salmon DP, et al. Episodic and semantic memory: a comparison of amnesic and demented patients. *J Clin Exp Neuropsychol* 1987;9:479–497.
67. Randolph C. Implicit, explicit, and semantic memory functions in Alzheimer's disease and Huntington's disease. *J Clin Exp Neuropsychol* 1991;13:479–494.
68. Murray LL, Lenz LP. Productive syntax abilities in Huntington's and Parkinson's diseases. *Brain Cogn* 2001;46:213–219.
69. Hodges JR, Salmon DP, Butters N. The nature of the naming deficit in Alzheimer's and Huntington's disease. *Brain* 1991;114:1547–1558.
70. Rohrer D, Salmon DP, Wixted JT, et al. The disparate effects of Alzheimer's disease and Huntington's disease on semantic memory. *Neuropsychology* 1999;13:381–388.
71. Ho AK, Sahakian BJ, Robbins TW, et al. Verbal fluency in Huntington's disease: a longitudinal analysis of phonemic and semantic clustering and switching. *Neuropsychologia* 2002;40:1277–1284.
72. Rich JB, Troyer AK, Bylsma FW, et al. Longitudinal analysis of phonemic clustering and switching during word-list generation in Huntington's disease. *Neuropsychology* 1999;13:525–531.
73. Speedie LJ, Brake N, Folstein SE, et al. Comprehension of prosody in Huntington's disease. *J Neurol Neurosurg Psychiatry* 1990;53:607–610.
74. Murray LL and Stout JC. Discourse comprehension in Huntington's and Parkinson's diseases. *American Journal of Speech-Language Pathology* 1999;8:137–148.
75. Meck WH. Neuropharmacology of timing and time perception. *Brain Res Cogn Brain Res* 1996;3:227–242.
76. de Boo GM, Tibben AA, Hermans JA, et al. Memory and learning are not impaired in presymptomatic individuals with an increased risk of Huntington's disease. *J Clin Exp Neuropsychol* 1999;21:831–836.
77. Strauss ME, Brandt J. Are there neuropsychologic manifestations of the gene for Huntington's disease in asymptomatic, at-risk individuals? *Arch Neurol* 1990;47:905–908.
78. Giordani B, Berent S, Boivin MJ, et al. Longitudinal neuropsychological and genetic linkage analysis of persons at risk for Huntington's disease. *Arch Neurol* 1995;52:59–64.
79. Lyle OE, Gottesman II. Premorbid psychometric indicators of the gene for Huntington's disease. *J Consult Clin Psychol* 1977;45:1011–1022.
80. Jason GW, Pajurkova EM, Suchowersky O, et al. Presymptomatic neuropsychological impairment in Huntington's disease. *Arch Neurol* 1988;45:769–773.
81. Diamond R, White RF, Myers RH, et al. Evidence of presymptomatic cognitive decline in Huntington's disease. *J Clin Exp Neuropsychol* 1992;14:961–975.
82. Foroud T, Siemers E, Kleindorfer D, et al. Cognitive scores in carriers of Huntington's disease gene compared to noncarriers. *Ann Neurol* 1995;37:657–664.

83. Campodonico JR, Codori AM, Brandt J. Neuropsychological stability over two years in asymptomatic carriers of the Huntington's disease mutation. *J Neurol Neurosurg Psychiatry* 1996;61:621–624.
84. Kirkwood SC, Siemers E, Stout JC, et al. Longitudinal cognitive and motor changes among presymptomatic Huntington disease gene carriers. *Arch Neurol* 1999;56:563–568.
85. Johnson SA, Stout JC, Paulsen JS, et al. PREDICT-HD: A cognitive neuroscience approach to the study of cognition in presymptomatic Huntington's disease (HD). 32nd Annual meeting of the International Neuropsychological Association, Baltimore, MD, 2004:123.
86. Johnson SA, Stout JC, Langbehn D, et al. Recognition of static and dynamic facial expression in the Predict-HD cohort at baseline. 32nd Annual meeting of the International Neuropsychological Society, Baltimore, MD, 2004:71.
87. Nehl C, Paulsen JS, Johnson SA, et al. Predict-HD. Early changes in psychomotor speed in presymptomatic Huntington's disease. 32nd Annual meeting of the International Neuropsychological Society, Baltimore, MD, 2004:71.
88. Hoth KF, Stout JC, Johnson SA, et al. Simple and choice reaction time is associated with estimated nearness to symptom onset in presymptomatic Huntington's disease (HD). 32nd Annual meeting of the International Neuropsychological Society, Baltimore, MD, 2004:71.
89. Fennema-Notestine C, Archibald SL, Jacobson MW, et al. Cerebellar atrophy and cerebral white matter loss in Huntington's disease. *Neurology* 2003 *(submitted)*.
90. Starkstein SE, Brandt J, Bylsma FW, et al. Neuropsychological correlates of brain atrophy in Huntington's disease: a magnetic resonance study. *Neuroradiology* 1992;34:487–489.
91. Harris GJ, Pearlson GD, Peyser CE, et al. Putamen volume reduction on magnetic resonance imaging exceeds caudate changes in mild Huntington's disease. *Ann Neurol* 1992;31:69–75.
92. Rosas HD, Goodman J, Chen YI, et al. Striatal volume loss in HD as measured by MRI and the influence of CAG repeat. *Neurology* 2001;57:1025–1028.
93. Aylward EH, Codori A, Barta P, et al. Basal ganglia volume and proximity to onset in presymptomatic Huntington's disease. *Arch Neurol* 1996;53:1293–1296.
94. Grafton ST, Mazziotta JC, Pahl JJ, et al. Serial changes of cerebral glucose metabolism and caudate size in persons at risk for Huntington's disease. *Arch Neurol* 1992;49:1161–1167.
95. Thieben MJ, Duggins AJ, Good CD, et al. The distribution of structural neuropathology in pre-clinical Huntington's disease. *Brain* 2002;125:1815–1828.
96. Gomez-Tortosa E, MacDonald ME, Friend JC, et al. Quantitative neuropathological changes in presymptomatic Huntington's disease. *Ann Neurol* 2001;49:29–34.
97. Aylward EH, Codori AM, Rosenblatt A, et al. Rate of caudate atrophy in presymptomatic and symptomatic stages of Huntington's disease. *Mov Disord* 2000;15:552–560.
98. Mazziotta JC, Wapenski J, Phelps ME, et al. Cerebral glucose utilization and blood flow in Huntington's disease: symptomatic and at-risk subjects. *J Cereb Blood Flow Metab* 1985;5:S25–S26.
99. Mazziotta JC, Phelps ME, Pahl JJ, et al. Reduced cerebral glucose metabolism in asymptomatic subjects at risk for Huntington's disease. *N Engl J Med* 1987;316:357–362.
100. Feigin A, Fukuda M, Dahawan V, et al. Metabolic correlates of levodopa response in Parkinson's disease. *Neurology* 2001;57:2083–2088.
101. Young AB, Penney JB, Starosta-Rubenstein S, et al. PET scan investigations of Huntington's disease: cerebral metabolic correlates of neurological features and functional decline. *Ann Neurol* 1986;20:296–303.
102. Reynolds NC Jr, Hellman RS, Tikofsky RS, et al. Single photon emission computerized tomography (SPECT) in detecting neurodegeneration in Huntington's disease. *Nucl Med Commun* 2002;23:13–18.
103. Sedvall G, Karlsson P, Lundin A, et al. Dopamine D1 receptor number—a sensitive PET marker for early brain degeneration in Huntington's disease. *Eur Arch Psychiatry Clin Neurosci* 1994;243:249–255.
104. Ginovart N, Farde L, Halldin C, et al. Effect of reserpine-induced depletion of synaptic dopamine on [11C]raclopride binding to D2-dopamine receptors in the monkey brain. *Synapse* 1997;25:321–325.
105. Weeks RA. Striatal D1 and D2 dopamine receptor loss in asymptomatic mutation carriers of Huntington's disease. *Ann Neurol* 1996;40:49–54.
106. Pavese N, Andrews TC, Brooks DJ, et al. Progressive striatal and cortical dopamine receptor dysfunction in Huntington's disease: a PET study. *Brain* 2003;126:1127–1135.
107. Andrews TC, Weeks RA, Turjanski N, et al. Huntington's disease progression. PET and clinical observations. *Brain* 1999;122(Pt 12):2353–2363.
108. Antonini A, Leenders KL, Spiegel R, et al. Striatal glucose metabolism and dopamine D2 receptor binding in asymptomatic gene carriers and patients with Huntington's disease. *Brain* 1996;119:2085–2095.
109. Lawrence AD, Hodges JR, Rosser AE, et al. Evidence for specific cognitive deficits in preclinical Huntington's disease. *Brain* 1998;121:1329–1341.
110. Kirkwood SC, Siemers E, Bond C, et al. Confirmation of subtle motor changes among presymptomatic carriers of the Huntington disease gene. *Arch Neurol* 2000;57:1040–1044.
111. Lang C. Is direct CT caudatometry superior to indirect parameters in confirming Huntington's disease? *Neuroradiology* 1985;27:161–163.
112. Young AB, Shoulson I, Penney JB, et al. Huntington's disease in Venezuela: neurological features and functional decline. *Neurology* 1986;36:244–249.
113. Kuwert T, Lange HW, Langen KJ, et al. Cortical and subcortical glucose consumption measured by PET in patients with Huntington's disease. *Brain* 1990;113:1405–1423.
114. Hasselbalch SG, Oberg G, Sorensen SA, et al. Reduced regional cerebral blood flow in Huntington's disease studied by SPECT. *J Neurol Neurosurg Psychiatry* 1992;55:1018–1023.
115. Aylward EH, Li Q, Stine OC, et al. Longitudinal change in basal ganglia volume in patients with Huntington's disease. *Neurology* 1997;48:394–399.
116. Lawrence AD, Weeks RA, Brooks DJ, et al. The relationship between striatal dopamine receptor binding and cognitive performance in Huntington's disease. *Brain* 1998;121:1343–1355.
117. Paulsen JS, Zimbelman, JL, Hinton SC, et al. An fMRI biomarker of early neuronal dysfunction in presymptomatic Huntington's disease. *Am J Neuroradiol* 2004 Nov/Dec;25:1715–1721.

16
Psychosocial Effects of Predictive Testing for Huntington's Disease

Michael R. Hayden and Yvonne Bombard

Department of Medical Genetics, Centre for Molecular Medicine and Therapeutics, Children's and Women's Health Centre of British Columbia, University of British Columbia, Vancouver, Canada

Huntington's disease (HD) is an autosomal dominant, inherited neuropsychiatric disorder that usually presents in adult life with mood and personality changes, clumsiness, and chorea. This disease is progressive, with cognitive decline and worsening movement disorder, ending in death approximately 15 to 20 years from onset (1,2). The discovery in 1983 of the first DNA marker linked to HD, and later identification of additional highly polymorphic DNA markers, facilitated the development of predictive testing programs for persons at risk for HD (3,4).

Major concerns have been raised in the past about whether it was ethical to offer a predictive test without treatment being available to prevent or interrupt the progress of the disease (5,6). Concerns have also been raised that disclosing the results of predictive tests might precipitate depression, breakdown of family relationships, or suicide attempts (7,8). Important concerns have also been expressed that predictive testing would result in worsening the quality of life for families at risk for this disorder. After substantial debate and consultation between scientists, families, and the lay groups that represent patients with HD worldwide, the first predictive test was offered in 1986 (9).

The discovery of a novel gene containing a trinucleotide repeat that is expanded on HD chromosomes (10) facilitated highly accurate predictive testing, using direct analysis for the cytosine-adenine-guanine (CAG) repeat in persons at risk for HD. This test enables individuals to know with near-complete certainty that they have, or have not, inherited the HD gene. The direct test also allowed reassessment for those individuals who had previously participated in the less specific predictive testing program. In particular, this test was useful for people whose previous testing using linked markers was uninformative and for those who did not have any blood samples from crucial family relatives.

The clinical manifestations associated with HD are caused by a CAG trinucleotide expansion in the HD gene. Persons affected with HD have a CAG repeat length greater than 36. Anyone with a CAG repeat length greater than 36 is considered to be at increased risk for developing HD in his or her lifetime, should he or she live long enough. Some individuals with repeat lengths between 36 and 41 may never develop symptoms of HD in their lifetimes, however, even if they live to an advanced age. CAG repeat lengths between 27 and 35 are called *intermediate alleles*. Individuals with intermediate alleles are not at risk of developing symptoms of HD but may be at risk of having a child with an allele in the HD range. The risk of CAG expansion in intermediate alleles has only been observed in cases when the parent transmitting the allele is male (11).

For patients at risk for HD, participating in predictive testing permits individuals to learn whether they have inherited a CAG expansion. However, for those who have, the question shifts from "will I get HD?" to "when will I get HD?" A substantial inverse relationship exists between CAG repeat lengths and age at onset of HD. A larger CAG expansion is associated with an earlier age of onset, given a person's current age and clinical presentation (Fig. 16-1). For example,

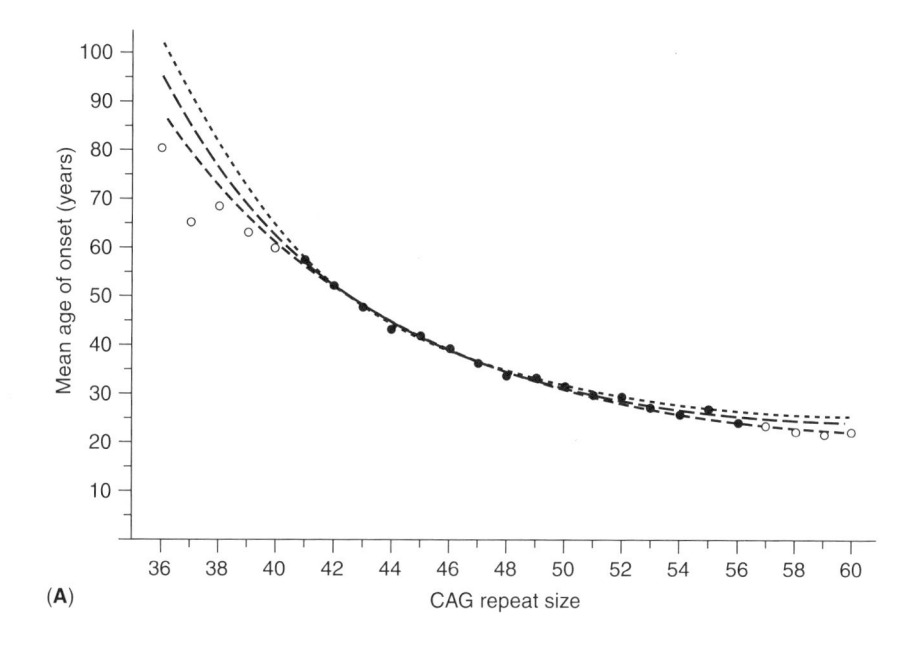

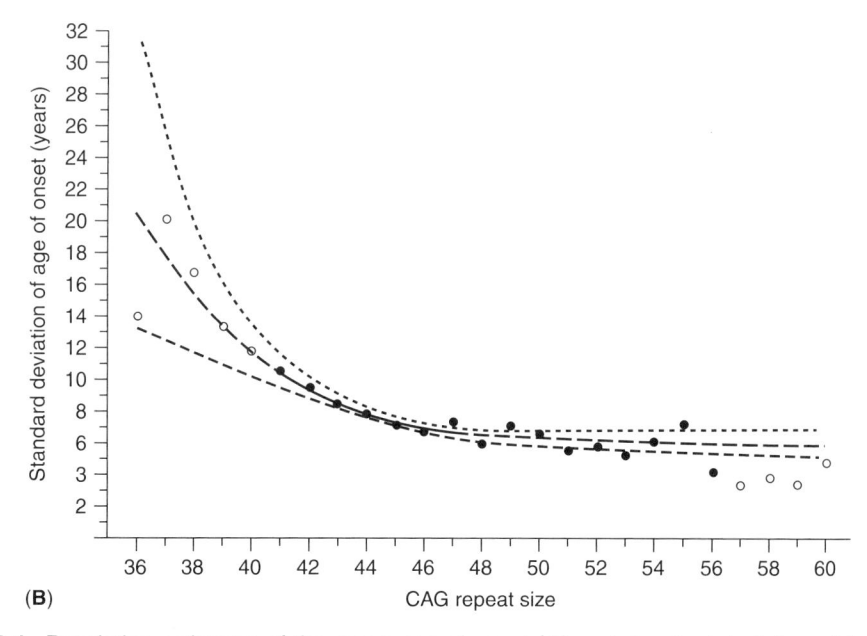

FIG. 16-1. Population estimates of the mean age of onset **(A)** and standard deviation of the age of onset **(B)** for CAG repeat lengths 36–60. The ● symbols and solid line indicate the range of data that was used to fit the exponential curves. The ○ symbols and long dashed lines indicate CAG lengths for which the model's predictions were extrapolated. Lines with small dashes indicate 95% confidence intervals; lines with larger spaces between dashes indicate the region where the model's predictions were extrapolated. (From Langbehn DR, Brinkman RR, Falush D, et al. *Clin Genet* 2004;65:267–277, with permission.)

current parametric survival models predict that a 40-year-old individual with 42 CAG repeats has a 80% chance of disease onset by the age of 60, while a 40-year-old individual with 45 CAG repeats is almost certain to be affected by that age (with 95% confidence intervals from 78–82 and 98–99, respectively) (12). However, caution must be exercised when predicting age of onset for a particular CAG repeat length, because the precision of the predictions is relatively low, with wide confidence limits. Furthermore, CAG length is only one of numerous determinants of HD onset. Additional genetic and environmental factors, such as genetic polymorphisms and sibship, contribute to variations in HD onset.

In this chapter, the psychosocial effects of HD on persons at risk for this disorder, and on their families, are outlined. The impact of genetic testing is described, particularly in the 5% to 10% of people who enter predictive testing programs already manifesting signs and symptoms of this disease. By carefully assessing these individuals and their psychological responses to this information, suitable approaches have been developed to provide the diagnosis of HD to affected persons; genetic testing is also relevant for providing predictive information to people at risk from other incurable or serious disorders.

PSYCHOLOGICAL CONSEQUENCES OF PREDICTIVE TESTING FOR HD

Short-term Psychological Responses to Predictive Testing of Those Receiving a Decreased-Risk Result

Most people who participate in a predictive testing program for HD will receive a result that indicates decreased risk. Approximately 55% of persons at risk who have received a predictive testing have received a decreased-risk result (13), primarily because people who present to predictive testing programs do so at a relatively old mean age [39 years in our series and 37 years worldwide (13, 14)], which means that most of these people have already passed through a substantial period of their lives without manifesting signs and symptoms. The mean age at presentation for predictive testing has selected for persons who are more likely not to have inherited the HD gene. Before predictive testing programs were implemented, predictive testing was expected to promise the clearest benefits to those found not to have inherited the HD gene (15–17). Although psychological function inmost people who receive a decreased-risk result has improved; a considerable proportion (10%) of people have also needed additional support because of difficulty coping with their decreased-risk results (18). These individuals may be particularly vulnerable to adverse psychological effects if the test result contradicts the individual's conscious or unconscious expectations about the outcome.

Short-term Psychological Responses to Predictive Testing among Those Receiving an Increased-Risk Result

Candidates who have received results indicating increased risk are considered to be at high risk for emotional difficulties. Our clinical experience with these individuals suggests that many of them undergo a difficult period of adjustment, and some experience a prolonged period of considerable emotional distress (19). During the early follow-up period of up to 1 year, a few candidates have expressed regret in taking the test. However, most have reiterated their commitment to the process and stated that it had been helpful and that given the choice, they would do it again. The highest level of stress occurred immediately after receiving test results. Within the first year, however, this period is followed in most instances by adjustment, and stress and features of depression return to baseline levels (19).

Numerous factors contribute to stress in adjusting to this information. The person's past patterns of communication and modes of dealing with major stress have emerged as crucial variables. A history of psychiatric disorder is also a risk factor for unsuccessful adjustment to results of predictive testing. A history of substantial and prolonged adverse psychological response to other difficult or threatening situations, such as the death of a loved one or a change in employment status, increases the likelihood of an adverse response to predictive testing (19).

Individuals who have increased-risk results seem particularly worried by normal episodes of clumsiness or mild depressive symptoms and, in some instances, have sought repeated neurologic assessments. Neurologists and other physicians faced with clinical examination of these individuals need to be particularly mindful that the increased-risk result merely provides an indication of genetic risk for disease, whereas the diagnosis of HD or onset of illness is clinical and depends on the presentation of signs and symptoms characteristic of this illness. The distinction between the risk presented by inheriting a gene, demonstrated by DNA analysis, and the criteria for clinical diagnosis must be kept clearly in mind. A most damaging scenario for these individuals would be a premature diagnosis of HD, which can affect the individuals, their families, and their employment (19).

Long-term Psychological Responses to Predictive Testing for HD

Long-term follow-up in the largest known cohort, which examined psychological consequences of receiving the results of predictive testing, demonstrated that psychological distress was reduced significantly from baseline and that this reduction was sustained throughout a 5-year follow-up period, both for groups with increased and decreased-risk results (20). An overall improvement in general severity index (GSI) scores during the follow-up periods (up to 2 years, $p < 0.001$; at 5 years, $p = 0.002$, Fig. 16-2) was detected in both risk groups.

These results, as evaluated by the GSI (one of the primary measures of psychological status)

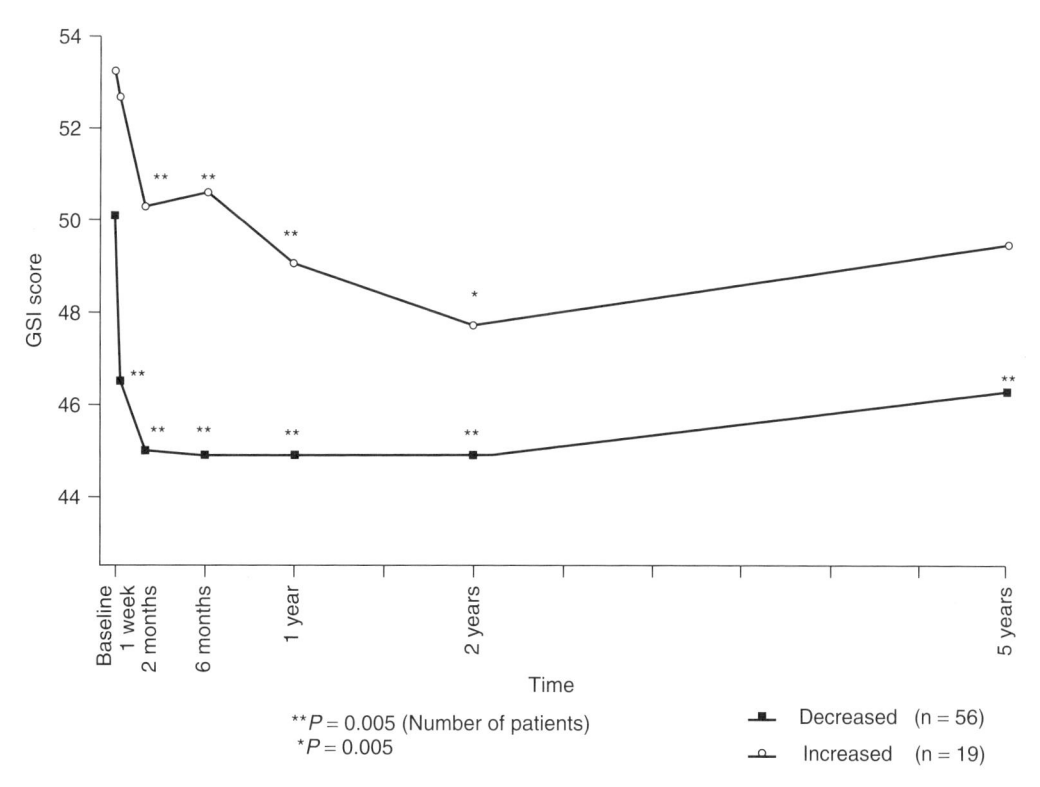

FIG. 16-2. Repeated measures analysis on the GSI scores for all individuals who completed the questionnaires at all visits (n = 75). The *P* values for the paired t-tests for the total cohort (n = 202) at each assessment are also included. Lower scores indicate less psychological distress. There was no significant difference in scores over the 5 years follow-up between the two results groups (repeated measures analysis). The GSI scores improved significantly compared to baseline for both results groups until 2 years and were sustained through 5 years for the decreased risk group. (From Almqvist EW, Brinkman R, Wiggins S, et al. *Clin Genet* 2003; 64:300–309, with permission.)

suggest that, in general, psychological health improves for people who undergo predictive testing. Other investigators also found few negative psychological consequences of predictive testing for HD (21–23). Knowing the results of the predictive test, even if it indicates an increased risk, reduces uncertainty and provides an opportunity for appropriate planning. Furthermore, detailed pretest counseling has clearly excluded many individuals who might have suffered an adverse event, particularly those who were taking the test to satisfy a request from others, such as an employer or a spouse, and those who were uncertain as to whether they truly wanted to participate. Many have also reasoned that people coming forward for predictive testing are a self-selected group, better equipped than others to handle "bad" news (24,25). Other hypotheses suggest that pretest expectations of receiving an increased-risk result may help to mobilize coping mechanisms such as denial (6,26). Often a person's social context shapes the way a test result is perceived. The perception of a test result as positive or negative may be contingent upon a person's family dynamics, because often test results affect the family system as a whole (15,27). A final explanation of these psychological consequences is that receiving predictive test results, although undoubtedly an emotional experience, eventually becomes understood as one of many other experiences that affect an individual's life over time.

Adverse Events Following Predictive Testing for HD

The threat to quality of life among those who received an increased-risk result was seriously considered when developing test protocols. Serious concern was expressed that an increased-risk result could precipitate catastrophic reactions (16–18).

Some individuals have had considerable difficulty incorporating the results of predictive testing into their lives. The prevalence of clinically defined adverse events—namely, clinical depression, psychiatric hospitalization, attempted suicide, a marked increase in alcohol consumption, planned suicide, and breakdown of a serious relationship, with negative consequences—found in our longitudinal psychological assessments was 6.9% (14 of 202 individuals) (20). The adverse event most commonly diagnosed was clinical depression requiring antidepressants (6 of 202 participants, 3.0%). Other adverse events, such as attempted suicide (1.5%); breakdown of a serious relationship with negative consequences for the participants (1%); and psychiatric hospitalization, sustained or increased use of alcohol during the follow-up period, or development of a suicide plan (0.5% for each category), were less common. However, the proportion of individuals in the increased-risk group who had a clinically important adverse event (7 of 68, 10.3%) was twice as great as that in the decreased-risk group (7 of 134, 5.2%; $p = 0.24$).

An estimate of the worldwide prevalence of catastrophic events (CE)—namely, suicide, suicide attempt, and psychiatric hospitalization—after predictive testing for HD was 0.97% (44 of 4,527, $p = 0.3$) (14). Worldwide, more female participants experienced a CE than male participants [70.4% (31/44) of women, vs. 29.5% (13/44) of men, $p = 0.18$] (14). Most of the participants [37/44 (84.1%)] who experienced a CE had received an increased-risk result. Approximately 2% of all persons with an increased-risk result experienced a CE, a significantly higher percentage than in the group with decreased-risk results ($p < 0.0001$). Notably, a few individuals (7/2,601, approximately 0.3%) who received a decreased-risk result also experienced a CE. In fact, individuals in the decreased-risk group experienced the most severe events (4 suicide attempts and 4 psychiatric hospitalizations). Notably, 50% of those who received an increased-risk result were already symptomatic at the time of the catastrophic event (14). These findings highlight features that may predict and possibly prevent an adverse event.

Predictors of Adverse Events Following Predictive Testing for HD

Assessment of baseline parameters among individuals who experienced an adverse outcome following a predictive test result identified factors associated with an increased prevalence of such outcomes. Several variables in the worldwide assessment of CE clearly discriminated between participants who experienced an adverse event and those who did not. Individuals who have received an increased-risk result and begin manifesting signs and symptoms are a particularly vulnerable group. Of persons who experienced a CE, 54% were symptomatic at the time of the event (14). In fact, four of five persons who committed suicide had signs of HD, a finding that highlights the particular vulnerability of some individuals during the period immediately after a diagnosis of HD. Indeed, 11 of 21 persons (52.4%) who attempted suicide and 8 of 18 (44.4%) who were hospitalized for psychiatric disorders also had symptoms of HD (14). In addition to clinical status, a psychiatric history within 5 years before testing is associated with increased risk of CE. After the predictive testing program, 38.5% of persons who experienced a CE had a psychiatric history as compared to a predictive testing comparison group (p less than 0.0005). Unemployment status is an additional factor associated with an increased prevalence of CE after predictive testing; more than 50% of those worldwide who experienced a CE, as well as all those who committed suicide, had been unemployed (14). Further, predictor models identified elevated baseline scores for depression and psychological distress, low scores on measures of general well being [Beck Depression Inventory (BDI), GSI, and General Well Being Scale (GWB), respectively] and an increased-risk result as further predictive of depressive symptoms following testing (20). Clearly, evaluating the individuals' psychological profile at baseline can identify those individuals who are especially vulnerable and may require additional support. However, the predictors identified in these models represent a small part of the reality of the testing process.

Timing of Adverse Events Following Predictive Testing for HD

The mean incidence of CE identified in a worldwide assessment was 0.44% per year (range, 0.35%–0.65% per year) (14). Most individuals who experienced a CE did so within a year of receiving increased-risk results. By contrast, after the first year, most of the CE occurred in persons who received a decreased-risk result [Fig. 16-3; (14,20)]. These findings point to predictive test results as the precipitating factor for a CE among those identified at increased risk. However, the longer the time that elapses after results, the more likely it is that factors other than, or in addition to, the test results contributed to the adverse outcomes.

Psychological Effects of Predictive Testing for HD

The prevalence of clinically defined adverse events suggests that some individuals will have considerable difficulty incorporating predictive test results into their lives. This difficulty is exemplified, in particular, by a case report of an individual who attempted suicide after receiving a decreased-risk result, who had not otherwise displayed any indication of previous or current psychological distress (20). For many, including the professional or lay public, an adverse outcome to a decreased risk may be unexpected. Our experience suggests that some participants with a decreased-risk result (10%) may be particularly vulnerable to adverse effects, especially if the test result contradicts the individual's consciously or unconsciously expected outcome (20). Many individuals at risk for HD have made important, and in some instances, irreversible decisions based on the belief that they were likely to develop HD in the future. These include financial decisions, as well as decisions with regard to child rearing and marriage, such as a vasectomy or tubal ligation. A decreased-risk result may substantially alter these expectations but may leave individuals with the difficulty of trying to reverse what, in many instances, are irreversible actions. In some instances, siblings may participate in predictive testing, but the response of other siblings cannot be predicted from that of one particular sibling. When one sibling receives a decreased-risk result, survivor guilt may be present, particularly if another sibling is already showing signs and symptoms of this illness. However, survivor guilt does not appear to be a major cause of distress or depression among participants with decreased risk of HD.

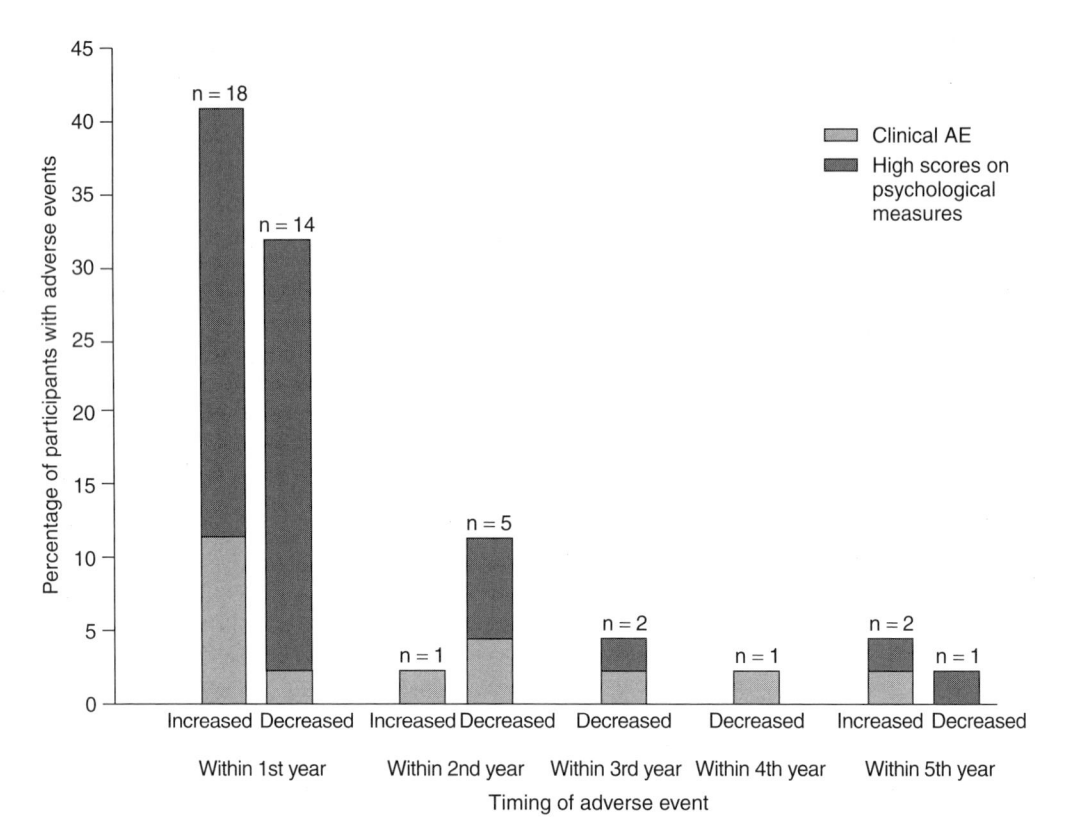

FIG. 16-3. Timing of adverse events. The number of participants with clinical adverse events (subset of AEs defined as high scores on the psychological measures is identified in bar graph) for the individuals in the increased and decreased risk groups are shown relative to when the event occurred. Most adverse events occurred in the first year of follow-up ($p = 0.00005$). (From Almqvist EW, Brinkman R, Wiggins S, et al. *Clin Genet* 2003; 64:300–309, with permission.)

In some situations, predictive testing results may contradict a firmly held belief of preselection, the expectation of the candidate or a relative that a particular person will develop HD (28). In some instances, this expectation can impose considerable stress on a family that may have already acted as if one child was destined to develop HD, whereas another child was not. Inability to accept the outcome of testing that contradicts preselection may be a major impediment to successful coping in a family with this result. This change is particularly difficult to assimilate when it is unexpected or contrary to perceived plans and dreams.

Another major cause of psychological disturbance in persons at risk is related to unrealistic expectations of a decreased-risk result. For many, being at risk has created an all-pervading fear that has permeated different aspects of their lives, such as career plans and decisions about marriage and procreation. The expectations raised by a decreased-risk result include freedom from fear and anxiety and a new hope for a disease-free future. However, receiving a decreased-risk result does not confer any new powers or abilities. Old habits and behaviors remain, and making changes is as difficult as it was previously. Moreover, the possibility of developing HD in the future can no longer be used as a psychological crutch for different decisions or behaviors. In general, the most critical time for persons receiving a decreased-risk result occurs some time distant from the time that they receive results, usually between 1 and 4 years (20) (Fig. 16-3). This finding contrasts with that for individuals who receive an increased-risk result, in whom the critical time for adverse events is generally within the first 12 months of receiving the result (14,20).

The protocol of precounseling and assessment enables the clinician to determine the psychosocial status of each person participating in the test and makes it easier to develop a rapport and to identify those persons who might require further assessment and possible additional psychological treatment before proceeding in the program. Establishing open communication allows the clinician to explore the person's motivation for taking the test and allows those who are uncertain to withdraw from predictive testing.

Another factor in the pretest counseling phase that might affect the outcome or the ability to provide appropriate care is to discuss individuals' attitudes about sharing information with others. Improving communication is likely to enhance the candidate's chances of coping successfully with predictive testing. Some candidates talk freely and openly about HD with their colleagues and family, whereas others are more circumspect and choose not to communicate this information with others. Reasons for this reticence include not wanting the pity of others, not wanting friends and family to relate differently, being unable to bear the thought of others watching for symptoms, not feeling close enough to others, and wanting to protect others from the distress and the possible anguish that predictive testing may cause (19).

Assessing the candidate's social support network includes evaluating his or her willingness to reach out for support. In general, open communication should be encouraged, because it tends to facilitate intimacy, support, and understanding. However, the risks of open communication must also be discussed, because it may leave the person vulnerable to rejection, to discriminating policies by employers, and to additional emotional distress (29).

The individuals we have studied have been followed for a period of only 1 to 5 years; clearly, longitudinal evaluation will provide much needed information about the long-term effect of living at increased risk for HD, particularly as these persons get close to the expected age of disease onset.

PSYCHOLOGICAL EFFECTS FOR THOSE FOUND TO BE AFFECTED WITH HD DURING A PREDICTIVE TESTING PROGRAM

Approximately 5% to 10% of persons who participate in the predictive testing program have been found to have signs and symptoms of HD. In some instances, these persons have not consciously acknowledged the presence of early signs and symptoms. We have been able to observe some of the characteristic ways in which individuals adapt to living at risk for HD, undergoing further adaptive and sometimes maladaptive responses as the disease becomes manifest (30).

As a result of this longitudinal assessment, different stages of response to HD have been recognized in persons at risk. In the earliest phase (warning stage), individuals become aware of the threat of disease, usually as their at-risk status is appreciated. Some individuals respond by seeking information about the disease. Usually, following this initial phase of concern, the person's realization that the threat, although profound, is not imminent allows the person to integrate the information into his or her life. When signs and symptoms develop, including mild involuntary movements, subtle cognitive changes, or personality changes such as increased irritability and depression, some individuals become aware that the disease is present (the incipient stage). Reaching this awareness is a profound event, and often the response is one of shock, an increase in fear and anxiety, and a massive mobilization and entrenchment of psychological defense mechanisms. During this early phase of the illness, symptoms are mild, and the effect on function is usually minimal; thus, individuals are initially successful in using denial, rationalization, and repression as defenses. At this stage, projection or displacement is also observed, as when an individual casts blame on other people or situations to explain changes. In some instances, depression may be present, and many such individuals are highly sensitive and resistant to anyone confronting them on the subject of HD. Although these responses may seem maladaptive on the surface, they represent important emotional work, being done to come to terms with the onset of illness. Over a period of months or years, the reality is slowly assimilated, and the groundwork is laid for conscious acceptance of a diagnosis of HD (30).

The breakthrough stage occurs when the symptoms of HD become more pronounced and intrude on daily activities. The presence of the disease can no longer be denied, and function in many areas may be compromised. Business decisions may be less judicious than formerly, and family and social relationships may become strained. Knowledge of the symptoms reduces fear and anxiety, enabling individuals to lower defensive postures. Individuals then must confront a degree of conscious fear and anxiety about their own future, the genetic effect on their children, and the general long-term implications of this disease. However, this breakthrough enables the patient to openly discuss and deal with the disease and its implications (30). Following this phase and usually after professional contact is made, the formal diagnosis marks a crucial transition for the affected person. After diagnosis, the adjustment stage represents the challenge of living with this debilitating degenerative illness. Adjustment occurs in the short and long term and includes internal psychological adjustments as well as adjustments to external realities.

Because of the progressive nature of the disease, the process of adjustment is repeated after each loss, a process that places repeated strain on the individual. The psychological effect of the diagnosis affects especially the patient's definition of self in relation to time. A fundamental reassessment of priorities and attitudes occurs; the effect on family relationships, employment, financial status, and insurance all have to be considered in light of the functional changes and expected rate of illness progression.

In the small number of persons whose psychological readiness lags behind symptoms, prematurely presenting the diagnosis may cause great psychological distress. Individuals enter predictive testing programs because they wish to know whether they have inherited the gene, but some do not wish to know that they currently have signs and symptoms. These individuals may truly be unaware of onset, which can be subtle and insidious and, in some cases, not marked by a movement disorder. In other instances, family members or even an employer may have coerced the individual to see an attending physician. Clearly, an important part of the treatment of such patients is a sensitive assessment of the patient's psychological readiness to hear the diagnosis of HD. When such an assessment is not done, disastrous consequences may ensue (29,30).

In one instance, a patient who clearly was only just coming to terms with her risk status and had not appreciated her signs and symptoms of HD, receiving the diagnosis of HD precipitated an acute depression, resulting in a serious suicide attempt and an extended period of psychiatric hospitalization (31). This woman had been hospitalized for psychiatric disorder 15 years previously, but at the time of diagnosis she was in a stable marriage and had children and a career. The diagnosis of HD was delivered before she had psychologically reached the breakthrough phase. She was emotionally unprepared to receive the diagnosis, and this lack of readiness precipitated her depression. Major adverse psychological responses have been seen in other persons who have received the diagnosis of HD. In two instances, patients made serious suicide attempts, and two other patients became psychotic within 3 months of being diagnosed. In each of these instances, these individuals had a history of clinically important psychiatric illness at some time in the past. In retrospect, at the time of diagnosis none of these patients were firmly placed in the breakthrough phase of their response to signs and symptoms of illness (30).

The situation in which a person is psychologically unprepared to learn of their clinical status is more likely to occur for people in predictive testing programs. In some instances, individuals may present earlier than usual and may be truly unaware of very early signs and symptoms of HD. Our approach derives from the principle of patient autonomy and supports the patient's right to determine the amount of information (whether to be fully informed and when the information should be given). Some patients who are clearly affected with early signs of HD do not immediately wish to know the results of a physical examination. In many instances, these patients will choose at a later phase, sometimes within a year or two, to hear the results of neurologic assessment. However, on very rare occasions, presenting the diagnosis might be important, even when the patient is not firmly in the breakthrough phase. For example, an individual's psychological state might lag behind the development of symptoms to the extent that the effects of the disease cause harm to the patient, threaten the well-being or integrity of his or her family, or cause serious problems at work. If the disease in its early phase also manifests as a serious psychiatric illness, a clear diagnosis of HD may enable the family to deal appropriately with the patient and understand him or her within the context of a psychiatric diagnosis secondary to HD (30).

The family, at the same time, will be faced with the genetic implications of the diagnosis of HD for each of its family members. In most instances, however, it is appropriate to give primacy to patients' autonomy, to enable them to voluntarily request the diagnosis and to make decisions about disseminating the information to other persons, such as a relative or an employer. Only in rare situations would the public interest override such concerns, such as in the case of a commercial airline pilot or bus driver.

The model of stages of response, based on our predictive testing experience, present a useful psychological map of patient response to the threat of being diagnosed with other severe incurable illnesses. The question of how and when to give the diagnosis of HD to these persons may also have relevance for other conditions, especially genetic conditions with adult onset for which there is no treatment, such as familial Alzheimer's disease or other genetic causes of late-onset neurologic illnesses. Providing adequate support before delivering a diagnosis might also help to decrease or avoid CE following the diagnosis of HD.

PSYCHOLOGICAL EFFECTS OF PRENATAL TESTING FOR HUNTINGTON'S DISEASE

In general, demand for prenatal testing has been low, ranging between 2% and 3% worldwide (32–35). In Canada, only approximately 18% of such eligible and pregnant individuals chose to have prenatal testing, which is below the expected demand based on previous studies conducted before these programs were developed (15–17,34). The most commonly cited reason for not choosing prenatal testing was the belief that a cure would be found in time to benefit the children (34). In addition, the prospect of terminating a fetus at increased risk for a late-onset illness also has prevented numerous persons from choosing this option, which has created many stressful dilemmas for persons at risk.

The options available for prenatal testing depend on whether the at-risk parent has undergone predictive testing. A parent who has received an increased-risk result may request prenatal testing to directly test the fetal DNA. For those persons who do not wish to undergo testing but wish to test their fetus, an exclusion test may be performed. Exclusion testing is performed by linkage analysis, which compares the chromosomes obtained from the blood samples of several family members to those of the fetus. In this way, the risk that the fetus is carrying the gene for HD can be estimated without revealing the parent's risk. For the at-risk parent, prenatal testing becomes a complex decision that balances the parent's predictive information with that of the at-risk fetus.

Parents who do not accept termination of pregnancy as an option, but who wish to have a prenatal test to ensure that they do not have offspring at risk for this illness, must balance the complexities and difficulties associated with the birth of a child at known high risk for HD against the possibility of obtaining information that their continuing pregnancy might be at low risk. The situation becomes more complicated for exclusion testing in which the child's risk may be close to 50% and similar to that of the at-risk parent. In this situation, the onset of symptoms in the parent would be equivalent to a definitive predictive test on the child, because each of them would have inherited the same chromosome 4. When the implications of prenatal testing for HD are explained to parents who do not consider the termination of pregnancy an option, they usually decide not to pursue this approach.

The small number of participants in our study who participated in prenatal testing have coped reasonably well, although participation has been quite stressful (34). Some couples who participated in the test had felt the stress related to the technology, with the technological imperative being to repeat the test once they had used it for one pregnancy; having used the test in the first pregnancy, they can justify that initial use of prenatal testing only if they continue to use the same technology in future pregnancies. For this reason, some couples have repeated prenatal tests. In-depth, careful counseling is necessary to free couples from feeling that they must make the same choice they made in previous pregnancies. The psychological suffering that might result from the successive loss of repeated pregnancies has to be balanced against the possible relief of hearing that the current pregnancy is at low risk for having inherited the gene for HD.

In a substantial number of persons in the cohort previously studied, the inaccuracy of the test was deemed an important factor in dissuading them from using prenatal diagnosis, because doing so might result in termination of a potentially healthy child. The discovery of a mutation in HD that allows definitive testing has not resulted in increases in the request for prenatal testing (13). In fact, the improvement in the test's accuracy has likely been offset by optimism about a potential treatment, which is the predominant reason for not considering prenatal testing. Cloning the gene for HD has led some to assume that effective therapy will not remain in the distant future. This hope that this possibility will be realized is likely to reduce still further the demand for prenatal testing, because terminating a pregnancy for a potentially curable adult-onset illness is likely to be even less acceptable. As further research developments occur, patients will likely become more hopeful that effective therapy is imminent, and prenatal testing for HD and other late-onset genetic disorders is unlikely to be a frequently chosen option.

PARTICIPATION RATE IN PREDICTIVE TESTING FOR HD

The participation rate in predictive testing for HD has been below the demand anticipated on the basis of previous studies conducted before these programs were developed. The participation rate worldwide ranges between 3% and 24% (13) (Table 16-1). A number of explanations for this discrepancy have been given. The cost of testing may be an impediment for those seeking predictive testing in countries where a universal health care system does not cover the testing costs. The acceptability of predictive testing for a late-onset illness is also likely to depend on the burden of this disease in families (35). For a severe illness for which there is no treatment, such as HD, familial Alzheimer's disease, prion diseases, and hereditary motor sensory neuropathy, prediction of future risk for the disease is unlikely to be accepted by most at-risk persons. However, as new approaches to or hopes for therapy that is likely to delay the onset of illness or affect the prognosis become available, testing for these adult onset disorders will become more acceptable. Another impediment to predictive testing for HD concerns genetic discrimination. Fear of discriminatory practices in the areas of insurance or employment may prevent persons from using predictive testing, especially in light of the current legislative climate and the general lack of understanding about genetic test results.

TABLE 16-1. *Predictive testing uptake in Canada: comparison with other countries*

Country	Testing uptake (%)	Reported prevalence of HD
Canada	18	8.4/100,000
United Kingdom	18	7.5/100,000
The Netherlands	24	6.5/100,000
France	5	5/100,000
Worldwide study	5	4/100,000
Germany, Austria, Switzerland	<3–4	1/100,000

HD, Huntington's disease.
(From Creighton S, Almqvist EW, MacGregor D et al. *Clin Genet* 2003; 63:462–475, with permission.)

GENETIC DISCRIMINATION

Genetic discrimination is different treatment of individuals or their family members based on genotype rather than phenotype (36). The consequences of genetic discrimination, both for the individual concerned and society as a whole, are widespread. Discrimination on the basis of genetic status has the potential to create substantial social, health, and economic burdens for society by reducing opportunities for genetically at-risk individuals in a range of contexts (e.g., insurance and employment) (29). For some, the potential for genetic discrimination may hinder potentially helpful engagement with preventative genetic medicine or eventual prophylactic treatment. For example, many women at increased risk for breast cancer do not undergo genetic testing, for fear of its social implications for themselves and their families (37).

These fears have precipitated new strategies and dilemmas for predictive testing for HD, one of which is the request for anonymous predictive testing. Several individuals have sought predictive testing under the auspices of anonymity for fear of genetic discrimination against themselves and their families (38). However, anonymous testing raises salient issues. Although social discrimination based on a genetic status is ethically questionable, clinicians cooperate in excluding insurance companies from risk information, even though a public policy response would be preferable. Furthermore, the quality of patient care, such as appropriate counseling and follow-up, is compromised when results are provided anonymously (38).

NEGATIVE FAMILY HISTORIES OF HD ARE FREQUENT

Introducing the direct mutation test also permits identifying a previously unrecognizable symptomatic HD population, including patients with atypical manifestations or those without a family history. In fact, 25% of persons presenting for diagnostic testing in Canada lack a family history of HD (13,39). Several explanations may apply when patients with an expanded trinucleotide repeat of the HD gene lack a family history of the disease, including a new mutation, prior misdiagnosis within the family, nonpenetrance, or nonpaternity. Further investigations into the mutational flow of disease alleles uncovered a new mutation rate for HD of at least 10% in each generation (40). The occurrence of new mutations has subsequently required new counseling protocols concerning new mutations and intermediate alleles—larger forms of an allele that are not clinically important for the individual being tested but may be associated with the disease if the allele expands upon transmission to an offspring. Moreover, the direct mutation analysis has ascertained late-onset cases—elderly people with signs and symptoms of HD—who were previously not thought to have HD by virtue of the late onset. This form of testing has transformed the direct mutation test into a clinically important diagnostic tool.

HD PREDICTIVE TESTING AS A MODEL FOR TESTING FOR OTHER LATE ONSET ILLNESSES

HD represents one of the first diseases where the ability to identify genetic risk has now moved from the use of closely linked genetic markers to a direct approach and assessment of the mutation. The predictive test for HD represents the first test for any adult onset genetic disease. Fundamental principles that have emerged from presymptomatic testing for HD have already been incorporated into testing for other diseases, such as breast cancer, polycystic kidney disease, Alzheimer's disease, and AIDS (41). These principles include the importance of pre- and posttest counseling, the priority of individuals at 25% *a priori* risk, assessment of symptomatic individuals, and counseling of persons from families who represent new mutations (42). Clinical protocol consists of several sessions that deal with the risks and benefits of testing, psychosocial assessment of the person's available support systems, the confidentiality of the test process, and the potential for genetic discrimination, particularly in the areas of insurance and employment.

Today, predictive testing for HD is accepted worldwide, and its practice is based on guidelines that have been approved by patients, families, lay organizations, governments, and health-insurance providers (43,44). These guidelines delineate recommendations ranging from the use of predictive testing to appropriate laboratory and counseling protocols. The guidelines also outline essential information that is to be provided to all testing candidates, such as general information on HD, the testing procedures, and the consequences of testing (44). The predictive testing guidelines for HD represent a standard for similar testing in other disorders, both genetic and nongenetic, in which a blood test may reveal a future risk.

ACKNOWLEDGMENTS

We gratefully acknowledge the support of the Michael Smith Foundation for Health Research for YB. MRH is a principal investigator of the National Institute of Neurological Disorders and Stroke (NINDS)-funded study Neurobiological *Predict*ors of *H*untington *d*isease, known as PREDICT-HD. MRH holds a Canada Research Chair in Human Genetics.

REFERENCES

1. Hayden MR. *Huntington's chorea*. New York: Springer Verlag, 1981.
2. Harper PS. *Huntington's disease*. London: WB Saunders, 1991.
3. Gussella JF, Wexler NS, Conneally PM, et al. A polymorphic DNA marker genetically linked to Huntington's disease. *Nature* 1983;308:234–238.
4. Wassmuth J, Hewitt J, Smith B, et al. A highly polymorphic DNA locus very tightly linked to the Huntington gene. *Nature* 1988;332:734–736.
5. Crauford DIO, Harris R. Ethics of predictive testing for Huntington's chorea: the need for more information. *Br Med J* 1986;293:249–251.
6. Kessler S, Bloch M. Social system responses to Huntington disease. *Fam Proc* 1989;28:59–67.
7. Farrer CA. Suicide and attempted suicide in Huntington disease: implications for preclinical testing of persons at risk. *Am J Med Genet* 1986;24:305–311.
8. Perry TL. Some ethical problems in Huntington chorea. *CMAJ* 1981;125:1098–1100.
9. Hayden MR. Predictive testing for Huntington's disease: the calm after the storm. *Lancet* 2000;356:1944–1945.
10. The Huntington Disease Collaborative Group. A novel gene containing a trinucleotide repeat that is expanded and unstable on Huntington's disease chromosomes. *Cell* 1993;72:971–983.
11. Goldberg YP, Kremer B, Andrew SE, et al. Molecular analysis of new mutations for Huntington's disease: intermediate alleles and sex of origin effects. *Nat Genet* 1993;5:174–179.
12. Langbehn DR, Brinkman RR, Falush D, et al. A new model for prediction of the age of onset and penetrance for Huntington's disease based on CAG length. *Clin Genet* 2004;65:267–277.
13. Creighton S, Almqvist EW, MacGregor D, et al. Predictive, prenatal and diagnostic genetic testing for Huntington's disease: the experience in Canada from 1987–2000. *Clin Genet* 2003;63:462–475.
14. Almqvist EW, Bloch M, Brinkman R, et al. A worldwide assessment of the frequency of suicide, suicide attempts or psychiatric hospitalizations following predictive testing for Huntington disease. *Am J Hum Genet* 1999;64:1293–1304.
15. Meissen GJ, Berchek RL. Intended use of predictive testing by those at risk for Huntington disease. *Am J Med Genet* 1987;26:283–293.
16. Mastromauro C, Myers RH, Berkman B. Attitudes towards presymptomatic testing in Huntington disease. *Am J Med Genet* 1987;26:271–282.
17. Kessler S, Field T, Worth L, et al. Attitudes of persons at risk for Huntington disease toward predictive testing. *Am J Med Genet* 1987;26:259–270.
18. Huggins M, Bloch M, Wiggins S, et al. Predictive testing for Huntington disease in Canada: adverse effects and unexpected results in those receiving a decreased risk. *Am J Med Genet* 1992;42:508–515.
19. Bloch M, Adam S, Wiggins S, et al. Predictive testing for Huntington disease in Canada: the experience of those receiving an increased risk. *Am J Med Genet* 1992;42:499–507.
20. Almqvist EW, Brinkman R, Wiggins S, et al. Psychological consequences and predictors of adverse events for five years after testing for Huntington disease. *Clin Genet* 2003;64:300–309.
21. Bundey S. Few psychological consequences of presymptomatic testing for Huntington disease. *Lancet* 1997;4:4.
22. Broadstock M, Michie S, Marteau T. Psychological consequences of predictive genetic testing: a systematic review. *Eur J Hum Genet* 2000;10:731–738.
23. Meiser B, Dunn S. Psychological effect of genetic testing for Huntington's disease: an update of the literature. *J Neurol Neurosurg Psychiatry* 2000;174:336–340.
24. Bloch M, Fahy M, Fox S, et al. Predictive testing for Huntington's disease: II. Demographic lifestyle patterns, attitudes and psychosocial assessments of first 51 test candidates. *Am J Med Genet* 1989;32:217–224.
25. Codori AM, Hanson R, Brandt J. Self-selection in predictive testing for Huntington's disease. *Am J Med Genet* 1994;54:167–173.
26. Marteau TM, Croyle RT. The new genetics. Psychological responses to genetic testing. *Br Med J* 1998;316:693–696.
27. Williams JK, Schutte DL, Holkup PA, et al. Psychosocial impact of predictive testing for Huntington disease on support persons. *Am J Med Genet* 2000;96:353–359.
28. Kessler S. Psychiatric implications of presymptomatic testing for Huntington's disease. *Am J Orthopsychiatry* 1987;57:212–219.
29. Creighton S, Bombard Y, Hayden MR. Predictive testing for Huntington disease: the crystal ball is not crystal clear. *Lancet Neurol* 2004;3:249–252.
30. Bloch M, Adam S, Fuller A, et al. Diagnosis of Huntington disease: a model for the stages of psychological response based on experience of a predictive testing program. *Am J Med Genet* 1993;47:368–374.
31. Lam RW, Bloch M, Jones BD, et al. Psychiatric morbidity associated with early clinical diagnosis of Huntington disease in a predictive testing program. *J Clin Psychiatry* 1988;49:444–447.
32. Tyler A, Quarrell OW, Lazarou LP, et al. Exclusion testing in pregnancy for Huntington's disease. *J Med Genet* 1990;27:488–495.
33. Maat-Kievit A, Vegter-van der Vlis M, Zoeteweij M, et al. Paradox of a better test for Huntington's disease. *J Neurol Neurosurg Psychiatry* 2000;69:579–583.

34. Adam S, Wiggins S, Whyte P, et al. Five year study of prenatal testing for Huntington's disease: demand, attitudes, and psychological assessment. *J Med Genet* 1993;30:549–556.
35. Babul R, Wiggins S, Adam S, et al. Attitudes toward predictive testing after the cloning of the Huntington's disease gene: relevance for other adult onset disorders. *JAMA* 1993;270:2321–2325.
36. Billings PR, Kohn MA, de Cuevas M, et al. Discrimination as a consequence of genetic testing. *Am J Hum Genet* 1992;50:476–482.
37. Armstrong K, Weber B, Fitzgerald G, et al. Life insurance and breast cancer risk assessment: adverse selection, genetic testing decisions, and discrimination. *Am J Med Genet* 2003;120A:359–364.
38. Burgess MM, Adam S, Bloch M, et al. The dilemmas of anonymous predictive testing for Huntington disease: privacy versus optimal care. *Am J Med Genet* 1997;71: 197–201.
39. Almquist EW, Elterman DS, MacLeod PM, et al. High incidence rate and absent family histories in one quarter of patients newly diagnosed with Huntington disease in British Columbia. *Clin Genet* 2001;60:198–205.
40. Falush D, Almqvist E, Brinkman R, et al. Measurement of mutational flow implies a high new mutation rate for Huntington disease and substantial underascertainment of late onset cases. *Am J Hum Genet* 2001;68:373–385.
41. Hayden MR. Predictive testing for Huntington's disease: a universal model? [Comment] *Lancet Neurol* 2003;2: 141–142.
42. Benjamin CM, Adam S, Wiggins S, et al. Proceed with care: direct predictive testing for Huntington disease. *Am J Hum Genet* 1994;55:606–617.
43. Copley TT, Wiggins S, Dufrasne S, et al. Are we all of one mind? Clinicians' and patients' opinions regarding the development of a service protocol for predictive testing for Huntington disease. Canadian collaborative study for predictive testing for Huntington disease. *Am J Med Genet* 1995;58:59–69.
44. Went LJ, International Huntington Association (IHA) and the World Federation of Neurology (WFN) Research Group on Huntington's Chorea. Guidelines for the molecular genetics predictive test in Huntington's disease. *Neurology* 1994;44:1533–1536.

17

Public Health Significance of Tic Disorders in Children and Adolescents

Lawrence Scahill, Denis G. Sukhodolsky,
Susan K. Williams, and James F. Leckman

*Child Study Center, Yale University School of Medicine,
New Haven, Connecticut*

Tourette's syndrome (TS) is a neuropsychiatric disorder of childhood onset characterized by motor and vocal tics. The tics of TS range from mild to severe, and conditions such as Chronic Motor or Chronic Vocal Disorder are presumed to be etiologically related variants (1). Following onset in childhood, TS follows a fluctuating course, with periods of exacerbation and periods when the tics are milder (2). Independent of tic severity in childhood, most patients with TS show a decline in tics during middle to late adolescence (3). Despite the decline in tics after puberty, however, in clinical samples disability often endures into adulthood. In addition to tics, children and adolescents with clinically ascertained tic disorders often have problems with obsessive–compulsive symptoms, inattention, impulsiveness, and hyperactivity, as well as problems with disruptive behavior, low frustration tolerance, and anxiety regulation (4–6). Whether these co-occurring characteristics are also present in community-ascertained samples is less clear. The etiology of TS is unknown, but both genetic and environmental factors appear to play a role (1). Results from family studies strongly suggest that TS is vertically transmitted in families (7). In an affected sib-pair study, specific regions on chromosome 4 and chromosome 8 appeared to be associated—though both findings fell short of the usual statistical significance level (8). Taken together, these data suggest that TS may be a heterogeneous disorder in which the pathophysiology is shared but has multiple causes (9).

Epidemiology is concerned with the prevalence, distribution, and determinants of disease in the population. The results of epidemiologic inquiry in neuropsychiatric disorders such as TS can inform public policy by describing the prevalence of the disorder in the general population. In addition, by examining the entire spectrum of the disorder in a community sample systematically, epidemiologic surveys can help delineate people that have the disorder from those who do not. This delineation may be especially useful for a disorder such as TS, which appears to reside on a continuum, from mild and inconsequential tics to more severe forms involving frequent and multiple tics that interfere with everyday living. Examining the full TS spectrum in a community sample may also help detect gaps in mental health services. Finally, by identifying the factors that increase the risk of developing a disorder such as TS, epidemiologic studies may identify secondary prevention strategies to reduce the likelihood of developing the disorder. The purpose of this chapter is to document the public health impact of tics and TS in children. We begin with a review of recent epidemiologic studies in TS to establish the scope of the problem. We also examine data from informative community surveys and large clinical series to elucidate the types of neuropsychiatric disabilities that may be associated with tics and TS.

COMMUNITY STUDIES: SCOPE OF THE PROBLEM

Tics are common in school-age children, affecting 4% to 24% in this population (10–13). The highest estimate of 24% comes from the study by Snider et al. (13). In this study, trained raters observed 553 children in a suburban elementary school during an 8-month period. The children ranged from 5 to 12 years of age, and each child was observed on multiple occasions. During the study period, 18% of the children (n = 101) were rated as having an isolated or transient tic on at least one observation. A much smaller number of children (n = 34 or 6% of the sample) were rated as having persistent tics. In a similar age group, Lapouse and Monk (11) assessed the prevalence of tics in 482 randomly selected children between 6 and 12 years of age. On the basis of parent interviews, the investigators identified 12.2% of the children (n = 59) with at least one tic but only 0.4% (n = 19) with multiple tics. The difference in the prevalence of single isolated tics and more prominent tics across these two studies is probably attributable to the different methods employed: direct observation and parent reports. Despite the difference in the prevalence of tics across these two studies, the dramatic decrease in prevalence between a single tic and multiple or persistent tics is evident in both studies.

The estimated prevalence of TS also varies, from 5 to 300 per 10,000 [(14,15); also see (16) for a review]. From a public health perspective, this level of imprecision in estimating prevalence is unsatisfactory. Fortunately, the consensus emerging from several recent studies narrows the estimate to a range of 10 to 100 per 10,000. Table 17-1 shows the prevalence estimates for all published studies since 1990. The differences across these studies and earlier estimates arise from several factors. First, earlier estimates were based on clinically ascertained cases, an approach that failed to count cases that had not come to clinical attention, such as mild cases or those with poor access to treatment. More recent studies have tried to correct this systematic undercount by ascertaining community samples. This strategy has resulted in higher estimates of prevalence. Second, rather than simply relying on patient registries and checklists to identify cases, several recent studies have used detailed parent interviews and, in some instances, direct observation of the child to confirm the presence of tics. This approach has provided support for the notion that TS does indeed reside on a continuum from mild tics to more severe forms. Third, given that tics often subside in the later teenage years, the age of the children surveyed could also influence the detection of tic disorders—even when direct observation is employed. For example, Apter et al. (17) systematically evaluated 28,000 16- and 17-year-old inductees in the Israeli Defense Force and estimated a prevalence of 5 cases per 10,000. By contrast, in a community sample that included over 4,000 children between the ages of 7 and 15 years, Khalifa and von Knorring (18) observed an overall prevalence of 60 per 10,000. Within this sample, the prevalence of TS among the 7- to 9-year-olds was three times greater than that observed in the 13- to 15-year-olds, suggesting a clear age effect for case identification.

Fourth, the definition of tic disorders, including TS, changed with the introduction of *The Diagnostic and Statistical Manual of Mental Disorders*, 3rd edition (DSM-III) (27). Thus, even relatively large community surveys done before 1980 found much lower prevalences of TS. For example, Rutter et al. (12) evaluated a sample of 3,000 children that included all 10- to 12-year-olds from the Isle of Wight. In this sample, 4.4% of the children were identified as having tics, but no cases of TS were identified. It seems likely that, if this study had used current definitions of tic disorders, some children would have met diagnostic criteria for a tic disorder. Using DSM-III-R criteria, Costello et al. (21) reported a prevalence of 4.2% for all tic disorders combined (Transient Tic Disorder, Chronic Tic Disorder, and TS) in a similar age group of children in the Great Smoky Mountains project. The similarity of these estimates across the two studies is striking and implies differences in classification rather than true differences in prevalence between these two samples.

TABLE 17-1. *Prevalence studies in tics and tic disorders in pediatric samples published since 1990*

Author/Year	N	Source of sample	Age	Informant	Diagnostic criteria	No. of cases of TS	Prevalence
Comings et al., 1990 (19)	3,034	Three selected schools	5–14	Teacher, trained observer	DSM-III-R	23 of TS	63/10,000 TS
Apter et al., 1993 (17)	28,037	Military inductees	16–17	Subject, trained observer	DSM-III-R	12 of TS	5/10,000 TS
Landgren et al., 1996 (20)	589	Community	6–7	Parent and examination	DSM-III-R	2 of TS	34/10,000 TS
Costello et al., 1996 (21)	4,500	Community (random)	9–13	Parent	DSM-III-R	Not reported	10/10,000 TS 420/10,000 all tic disorders
Verhulst et al., 1997 (22)	780	Community (random)	13–18	Parent + child	DSM-III-R	Not reported	10/10,000 TS 400/10,000 all tic disorders
Mason et al., 1998 (15)	167	Community single school	13–14	Parent, child, trained observer	DSM-III-R	5 of TS	299/10,000 TS
Kadesjo and Gillberg, 2000 (23)	435	Birth cohort	10–11	Parent and examination	DSM-IV	5 of TS	115/10,000 TS
Peterson et al., 2001 (24)	776	Community (random)	9–20	Parent, subject	DSM-III	2 of TS	26/10,000 TS
Kurlan et al., 2001 (25)	1,596	Community	8–17	Parent, teacher, trained observer	DSM-IV	Not reported	150/10,000 TS[a] 80/10,000 TS[b]
Hornsey et al., 2001 (26)	918	Community mainstream classes	13–14	Parent, child, trained observer, clinician	DSM-III-R	7 of TS	76/10,000 TS
Khalifa and von Knorring, 2003 (18)	4,479	Community all available in a township	6–16	Parent, teacher, examination	DSM-IV	25 of TS	60/10,000 TS 660/10,000 all tic disorders

[a]In Special Education classes.
[b]In Regular Education classes.

A closer look at the surveys in Table 17-1 indicates that the highest estimates of prevalence come from studies that use direct observation (for example, 15,19,25). Still, the trustworthiness of the findings of these studies is under threat. The study by Mason et al. (15) based their estimate on a sample of 167 children from a single school. Kurlan et al. (25) set out to ascertain a large randomly selected sample through public school rosters. Unfortunately, only 11% of the randomly selected sample agreed to participate, and it may well be that those with tics were more likely to participate. Nonetheless, the findings from community-based samples suggest that tic disorders are relatively common in school-age children and often undetected. An important remaining consideration is whether the presence of tics—even mild tics—places a child at higher risk for other problems with behavior, learning, or both.

ASSOCIATED PROBLEMS

The common occurrence of inattention, impulsiveness, and overactivity (i.e., core symptoms of Attention-Deficit Hyperactivity Disorder, ADHD), other disruptive behavior problems, and obsessive–compulsive symptoms in children with TS is well documented (5,6,28). The extent to which these clinical characteristics are etiologically related to TS or to the comorbid features that prompt referral for treatment is unclear. Caine et al. (29) estimated the prevalence of TS on the basis of patient registries and a public information campaign to identify previously undetected cases of TS in the Rochester, New York region. Nearly 50% of the children identified from patient registries had comorbid ADHD. By contrast, nearly all of the previously unidentified cases were free of comorbid conditions—suggesting that comorbidity is indeed associated with help seeking. Similarly, Kadesjo and Gillberg (23) identified 5 cases from a community sample of 435 eleven-year-old children. Of these, four had learning problems, and two had symptoms consistent with ADHD. By contrast, a cohort of 58 children from the same region had been previously diagnosed with TS. In this group of clinically ascertained children with TS, nearly two thirds also had ADHD and one third had disruptive behavior problems. Given the possibility that parents of children with a tic disorder and co-occurring behavioral problems are more likely to seek treatment than parents of children with a tic disorder alone, it is inappropriate to draw conclusions about the etiologic relationship between these additional behaviors and TS found in clinical samples. On the other hand, clinical samples may provide access to large numbers of TS patients with and without comorbid conditions. By dividing large clinical samples into more homogeneous subgroups (e.g., TS only, compared to TS plus ADHD), it may be possible to compare the level of disability across subgroups. Thus, to examine the functional impairment associated with tics and TS with and without other behavioral problems, clinical and community samples can be complementary.

Associated Problems in Community Samples

The association between the tics and other behavioral problems has been observed in several epidemiologic samples over the past three decades. The first of these samples was from the Isle of Wight study (12). Although no cases of TS were identified (presumably because of the diagnostic conventions at the time), the presence of tics was highly associated with disruptive behavior and anxiety. The more recent study by Mason et al. (15) observed that four of five children with previously unidentified TS had disruptive behavior problems. Snider et al. (13) noted no significant difference in the rate of parent- and teacher-rated disruptive behavior problems between the group of children with an isolated or transitory tic (approximately 23%) and the sample as a whole (approximately 25%). In the group of children with persistent tics, however, the rate of disruptive behavior was nearly twice as high, at 41%.

Gadow et al. (10) ascertained a sample of 3,006 children between the ages of 3 and 18 from three communities across the eastern half of the United States. One hundred and sixty-one teachers in selected schools voluntarily completed rating scales on 10 to 15 students from their classroom rosters. The teachers were asked to rate consecutive children, starting with first name on the class list. The DSM-IV-based instrument asked teachers to score symptom observation on a 0 to 3 scale, in which 0 = never; 1 = sometimes; 2 = often; 3 = very often. In the subsample of 1,520 children between the ages of 6 and 12 years, 7.8% of children (n = 118) were rated by teachers as having tics (a score of at least 1 on either of the tic questions). To be classified as indicating ADHD, item scores had to be 2 or greater on the number of symptoms specified in DSM-IV (30). One hundred and seventy-seven children (11.6%) were rated as having probable ADHD; only 65 (4.3%) were rated as having both tics and ADHD. This sample of 65 children with tics and ADHD was just more than 50% (65/118) of the entire sample of school-age children with tics. Expressed as an odds ratio, these data indicate that children with tics were 8.5 times more likely to have ADHD than children without tics. Given that ADHD usually has an earlier age of onset than tics, it would not be appropriate to claim that tics are a risk factor for ADHD. Nonetheless, these observations suggest that tics and ADHD are associated in community samples.

The study by Peterson et al. (24) provides longitudinal data on the association between tics and other psychiatric problems in a community sample of children followed over a 17-year period. At Time 1, the study evaluated 976 randomly selected children between the ages of 1 and 10 years and followed them forward to the ages 17 to 28 years. Subsequent evaluations were conducted 8, 10, and 17 years later. (N.B. The prevalence data presented in Table 17-1 were derived from the Time 2 survey, when this sample ranged in age from 9 to 20 years.) At Time 2, these investigators did not observe an association between tics and ADHD, but the presence of ADHD at Time 2 did predict the emergence of tics at Time 3.

Other community-based studies have shown an association with tic disorders and learning disability (23) and the use of special education services (25). Clearly, the presence of TS can interfere with educational progress, resulting in the need for special education services at a higher than expected rate in the population. Children with TS and ADHD are presumably more likely than others to have learning problems, but learning difficulties in TS can occur in the absence of ADHD (31). In addition to the higher than expected rate of children with TS in special education environments (25,29,31), Baron-Cohen et al. (32) found a rate of 4.3% of TS in a sample of nearly 450 children with pervasive developmental disorders from special schools in London.

A two-stage community study in Connecticut evaluated the prevalence of mental health disorders and mental health service needs for children from the ages of 6 to 12 (33–35). In the first stage, parents and teachers provided data for 910 children. On the basis of standard cut-off scores for the Child Behavior Checklist (CBCL) (36) or the stated impression by parent or teacher that the child needed mental health services, 460 children screened positive, and 450 children screened negative. The investigators attempted to recruit all children screened positive and a 20% randomly selected sample of those screened negative. A total of 449 children actually participated in the second stage, which included 359 children screened positive and 90 screened negative (roughly 78% from each screening group).

The second stage included a parent-on-child Diagnostic Interview Schedule for Children (DISC). On the DISC, the parents of 58 children answered "yes" to screening questions about tics. The interview included more detailed questions about the onset, duration, type, and frequency of tics as well as a written description of the reported abnormal movements or vocalizations. Using all available information, two independent clinicians assessed tic disorders according to DSM-III-R criteria. Diagnostic disagreements were resolved by consensus (37). Following the case-by-case review, 32 subjects were identified as having a possible (n = 11) or definite (n = 21) tic disorder. Of the 21 children with a definite tic disorder, 3 children met criteria for TS; 11 for either Chronic Motor or Chronic Vocal Tic Disorder; and 7 for Transient Tic Disorder. These data suggest a prevalence of 3 per 1,000 for TS, 8 per 1,000 for Chronic Motor Tic Disorder, 4 per 1,000 for Chronic Vocal Tic Disorder, and 8 per 1,000 for Transient Tic Disorder (34).

The sample of 21 children with a definite tic disorder was divided into two groups, those with a tic disorder only (n = 13) and those with a tic disorder plus ADHD (n = 8). These groups were compared by parent and teacher ratings to a group of children with ADHD (no tics) and a control group with no psychiatric illnesses, randomly selected from the same community sample. A clear pattern emerges from these ratings. On both the Conners' Parent and Teacher Questionnaires, children with tic disorders accompanied by ADHD were indistinguishable from the group with ADHD without tics. By contrast, the group of children with tic disorders only was intermediate on all measures between the group with ADHD and the control group (37). The only exceptions to this pattern were parent and teacher ratings on the Learning Problems scale. On this scale, both parents and teachers rated children with tic disorders with or without ADHD as having considerably greater problems with learning than controls without psychiatric illness. These data suggest that children with only a tic disorder may not show disruptive behavior, but may have learning difficulties that are evident to both parents and teachers.

Associated Problems in Clinical Samples

The association of TS with other psychiatric diagnoses, disruptive behavior, and functional impairment has been observed in numerous clinical series during the past three decades [see (38) for review]. Since this review, investigators from several centers have presented data on well-characterized, clinically ascertained samples (4–6,28,39). Because these investigators used systematic assessment methods and contrast groups (e.g., unaffected controls and children with ADHD without tics), these reports provide valuable insight concerning the effects of tic severity and comorbid conditions on functional status in children with TS derived from clinical samples (see Table 17-2).

Carter et al. (39) evaluated 72 eight- to fourteen-year-old children, including 16 with TS only, 33 with TS and ADHD, and 23 normal controls (NC). The TS only group did not differ from normal controls, whereas the group with TS and ADHD scored significantly higher on the CBCL subscales of aggression and delinquent behavior. Social and adaptive deficits were evident only in a group of children with TS and comorbid ADHD as measured by the Vineland and the CBCL. The group with TS but without ADHD did not differ significantly from the controls in the measures of disruptive behavior or adaptive functioning. The authors concluded that social and adaptive impairments in children with TS and ADHD are similar to those in children with ADHD alone.

Coffey et al. (4) evaluated 190 consecutive cases of children and adolescents with TS (mean age 10.6) from a clinical setting and reported that more than 95% of children had one or more comorbid diagnoses. The three most common co-occurring conditions were ADHD (77%), oppositional defiant disorder (ODD) (61%), and major depressive disorder (52%). In a sample of 97 cases of children with well-characterized TS from a regional referral center, Spencer et al. (6) observed rates of 81% for ADHD, 65% for ODD, and 22% for obsessive–compulsive disorder (OCD). The presence of ADHD with TS was strongly associated with ODD, but the prevalence of OCD across the groups with TS with or without ADHD did not differ. Children with TS and ADHD were more likely to be placed in special education. Compared to unaffected controls, however, both those with TS and ADHD and those with TS and no ADHD showed significantly greater overall impairment, as measured by the Global Assessment of Functioning (30). These data suggest that, although TS with ADHD results in greater disability than TS without ADHD, the presence of TS can be associated with functional impairment—even in the absence of ADHD.

Sukhodolsky et al. (5) examined the association of disruptive behavior with social, family, and adaptive functioning in 94 children (mean age, 11 years) with TS. The sample included 42 children with TS but not ADHD and 52 children

TABLE 17-2. *Selected reports of clinically ascertained children with TS with and without ADHD*

Author/Year	No. of TS	Mean age	Contrast groups	Informants	Measures	Primary findings
Carter et al., 2000 (39)	49	10.9	ADHD NC	Parents Children Teachers	K-SADS, CBCL Vineland FES	Social and behavioral dysfunction is ADHD specific
Coffey et al., 2000 (4)	190	10.6	None	Parents	K-SADS GAF	High rates of comorbidity: ADHD—77% ODD—61% Depression—52%
Spencer et al., 2001 (6)	97	10.9	ADHD Psychiatric controls NC	Parents	K-SADS GAF	Severity of ADHD symptoms in TS + ADHD associated with higher rate of mood disorder and lower GAF
Sukhodolsky et al., 2003 (5)	94	10.9	ADHD NC	Parents Children Teachers	K-SADS, CBCL Vineland FES	TS only more impaired than NC in socialization and daily living skills; TS + ADHD are impaired in all domains of family and adaptive functioning

ADHD, Attention-Deficit Hyperactivity Disorder; ODD, Oppositional Defiant Disorder; NC, normal controls; K-SADS, Schedule for Affective Disorders and Schizophrenia for School-Age Children; GAF, Global Assessment of Functioning Scale; CBCL, Child Behavior Checklist; Vineland, Vineland Adaptive Behavior Scales; FES, Family Environment Scale.

with TS and ADHD. These TS groups were compared to age-matched children with ADHD (no tics) and unaffected controls on various parent and teacher measures. Children with TS uncomplicated by ADHD did not differ from unaffected controls on the parent and teacher ratings of disruptive behavior. By contrast, children with TS and ADHD scored significantly higher than unaffected controls and similarly to children with ADHD alone on measures of disruptive behavior. Children with TS and ADHD also demonstrated significantly lower scores in adaptive functioning on the Vineland Adaptive Behavior Scales, compared to those with TS but not ADHD and unaffected controls. Nonetheless, children with TS uncomplicated by ADHD were significantly more impaired than unaffected controls on measures of social competence and daily living skills.

Increasingly, parents and clinicians have expressed concern about explosive behavior in children and adolescents with TS. Explosive behavior, which has been dubbed "rage attacks" in the TS community, is a chief complaint for many families. These episodic outbursts are described as dramatic expressions of anger and frustration marked by yelling, property destruction, and threats of harm or self-injury—though patients are typically not aggressive. Parents often report that the outbursts have a rapid onset in response to minor provocation and may last minutes to hours. Budman et al. reported explosive behavior in more than 50% of 68 clinically referred children with TS (40). The inherent limitation of studying this behavior in TS is the problem of ascertainment—children with explosive behavior are more likely to come to clinical attention. Thus, it is not clear that the findings in the clinical samples are generalizable. In addition, it is unclear whether the problems of low frustration tolerance and explosive behavior are part of TS, a secondary problem related to the burden of chronic disease, or a separate problem related to comorbid conditions, such as a mood disorder or anxiety disorder. Clearly, anger, aggression, and explosive behavior are common in other psychiatric disorders and not unique to TS (41). Thus, the underlying cause and treatment of explosive behavior need not be unique to TS.

A full discussion of the treatment for TS, including these cooccurring problems, is beyond the scope of this chapter [for reviews, see (42) and (43)]. Despite the common occurrence of complaints regarding disruptive and explosive behavior in TS, few treatment studies have been conducted in children and adolescents with tic disorders. Reasonable candidates for intervention might be parent-management training for younger children and anger-control training for adolescents (44,45). Indeed, studies to evaluate these interventions in children with TS are currently underway.

SUMMARY

In conclusion, data from community surveys suggest that tic disorders, including TS, exist on a spectrum from transient to persistent, multiple motor, and vocal tics that interfere with activities of daily living. The presence of isolated and transitory tics is common and appears to be of minimal consequence. On the other hand, persistent tics, even mild tics, appear to be associated with ADHD, disruptive behavior, and learning problems (though not necessarily formal learning disability). The presence of ADHD with tics increases the likelihood of disruptive behavior and learning problems, but learning problems can be observed in community samples of children with tic disorders, even in the absence of ADHD. To date, few studies have clearly defined the nature of the learning problems in children with tic disorders. Nonetheless, the data do suggest that having chronic tics is associated with impairment independent of ADHD. Community samples and recent investigations in clinical samples confirm that the presence of ADHD predicts greater disability than that associated with tic disorders alone.

ACKNOWLEDGMENTS

This work was supported in part by the following federal grants: Program Project MH-49351 (Dr. Leckman); RUPP-PI U10 MH66764; R03MH67845; R15NR007637; M01RR06022 (Dr. Scahill).

The authors acknowledge the advice and collaboration of Drs. Robert A. King, M.D., George Anderson, Ph.D., Diane Findley, Ph.D., Paul J.

Lombroso, M.D., and Mary Schwab-Stone, M.D. Thanks also to Erin Kustan for assistance in preparing this manuscript.

REFERENCES

1. Leckman JF. Tourette's syndrome. *Lancet* 2002;360: 1577–1586.
2. Lin H, Yeh CB, Peterson BS, et al. Assessment of symptom exacerbations in a longitudinal study of children with Tourette syndrome or obsessive–compulsive disorder. *J Am Acad Child Adolesc Psychiatry* 2002;41: 1070–1077.
3. Leckman JF, Zhang H, Vitale A, et al. Course of tic severity in Tourette syndrome: the first two decades. *Pediatrics* 1998;102:14–19.
4. Coffey BJ, Geller D, Biederman J, et al. Anxiety disorders and tic severity in juveniles with Tourette's disorder. *J Am Acad Child Adolesc Psychiatry* 2000;39:562–568.
5. Sukhodolsky DG, Scahill L, Zhang H, et al. Disruptive behavior in children with Tourette's syndrome: association of ADHD comorbidity, tic severity, and functional impairment. *J Am Acad Child Adolesc Psychiatry* 2003; 42:98–105.
6. Spencer T, Biederman J, Coffey BJ, et al. Tourette disorder and ADHD. *Adv Neurol* 2001;85:57–77.
7. Pauls DL, Tourette Syndrome Association International Consortium on Genetics. Update on the genetics of Tourette syndrome. *Adv Neurol* 2001;85:281–293.
8. Tourette Syndrome Association International Consortium for Genetics. A complete genome screen in sib pairs affected by Gilles de la Tourette syndrome. *Am J Hum Genet* 1999;65:1428–1436.
9. Palumbo D, Maughan A, Kurlan R. Hypothesis III—Tourette syndrome is only one of several causes of a developmental basal ganglia syndrome. *Arch Neurol* 1997;54:475–483.
10. Gadow KD, Nolan EE, Sprafkin J, et al. Tic and psychiatric comorbidity and adolescents. *Dev Med Child Neurol* 2002;44:330–338.
11. Lapouse R, Monk MA. Behavior deviations in a representative sample of children: variation by sex, age, race, social class and family size. *Am J Orthopsychiatry* 1964;34:436–446.
12. Rutter M, Tizard J, Whitmore K. *Education, health, and behavior*. London: Longman, 1970.
13. Snider LA, Seligman LD, Ketchen BR, et al. Tics and problem behaviors in school children: prevalence, characterization, and associations. *Pediatrics* 2002;110: 331–336.
14. Burd L, Kerbeshian J, Wikenheiser M, et al. Prevalence of Gilles de la Tourette's syndrome in North Dakota children. *J Am Acad Child Adolesc Psychiatry* 1986;25:552–553.
15. Mason A, Banerjee S, Eapen V, et al. The prevalence of Tourette syndrome in a mainstream school. *Dev Med Child Neurol* 1998;40:292–296.
16. Scahill L, Tanner C, Dure L. The epidemiology of tics and Tourette syndrome in children and adolescents. *Adv Neurol* 2001;85:261–271.
17. Apter A, Pauls DL, Bleich A, et al. An epidemiological study of Gilles de la Tourette's syndrome in Israel. *Arch Gen Psychiatry* 1993;50:734–738.
18. Khalifa N, von Knorring AL. Prevalence of tic disorders and Tourette syndrome in a Swedish school population. *Dev Med Child Neurol* 2003;45:315–319.
19. Comings DE, Himes JA, Comings BG. An epidemiological study of Tourette's syndrome in a single school district. *J Clin Psychiatry* 1990;51:463–469.
20. Landgren M, Petterson R, Kjellman B, et al. ADHD, DAMP, and other neurodevelopmental/psychiatric disorders in 6-year-old children: epidemiology and comorbidity. *Dev Med Child Neurol* 1996;38:891–906.
21. Costello EJ, Angold A, Burns BJ, et al. The Great Smoky Mountains study of youth: goals, design, methods, and the prevalence of DSM-III-R disorders. *Arch Gen Psychiatry* 1996;53:1129–1136.
22. Verhulst FC, van der Ende J, Ferdinand RF, et al. The prevalence of DSM-III-R diagnoses in a national sample of Dutch adolescents. *Arch Gen Psychiatry* 1997; 54:329–336.
23. Kadesjo B, Gillberg C. Tourette's disorder: epidemiology and comorbidity in primary school children. *J Am Acad Child Adolesc Psychiatry* 2000;39:548–555.
24. Peterson BS, Pine DS, Cohen P, et al. Prospective, longitudinal study of tic, obsessive–compulsive, and attention-deficit hyperactivity disorders in an epidemiological sample. *J Am Acad Child Adolesc Psychiatry* 2001;40: 685–695.
25. Kurlan R, McDermott MP, Deeley C, et al. Prevalence of tics in school children and association with placement in special education. *Neurology* 2001;57:1383–1388.
26. Hornsey H, Banerjee S, Zeitlin H, et al. The prevalence of Tourette syndrome in 13–14-year-olds in mainstream schools. *J Child Psychol Psychiat* 2001;42: 1033–1039.
27. American Psychiatric Association. *Diagnostic and statistical manual*, 3rd ed. Washington, DC: American Psychiatric Association, 1980.
28. Coffey BJ, Biederman J, Geller DA, et al. Distinguishing illness severity from tic severity in children and adolescents with Tourette's disorder. *J Am Acad Child Adolesc Psychiatry* 2000;39:556–561.
29. Caine ED, McBride MC, Chiverton P, et al. Tourette's syndrome in Monroe county. *Neurology* 1988;38: 472–475.
30. American Psychiatric Association. *Diagnostic and statistical manual*, 4th ed. Washington, DC: American Psychiatric Association, 1994.
31. Eapen V, Robertson MM, Zeitlin H, et al. Gilles de la Tourette's syndrome in a special education schools: a United Kingdom study. *J Neurol* 1997;244:378–382.
32. Baron-Cohen S, Scahill VL, Izaguirre J, et al. The prevalence of Gilles de la Tourette syndrome in children and adolescents with autism: a large scale study. *Psychol Med* 1999;29:1151–1159.
33. Scahill L, Schwab-Stone M, Merikangas K, et al. Psychosocial and clinical correlates of ADHD in a community sample of young school-age children. *J Am Acad Child Adolesc Psychiatry* 1999;38:976–983.
34. Schwab-Stone M, Fallon T, Briggs M, et al. Reliability of diagnostic reporting for children aged 6-11 years: a test-retest study of the diagnostic interview schedule for children—revised. *Am J Psychiatry* 1994;151:1048–1054.
35. Zahner GE, Jacobs JH, Freeman DH, et al. Rural and urban child psychopathology in a northeastern U.S. state: 1986–1989. *J Am Acad Child Adolesc Psychiatry* 1993;32:378–387.

36. Achenbach TM. *Manual for the child behavior checklist.* Burlington, VT: University of Vermont Press, 1983.
37. Scahill L, Williams SK, Schwab-Stone M, et al. Learning and behavioral problems in a community sample of children with tic disorders. *Adv Neurol* (in press).
38. Walkup JT, Scahill L, Riddle MA. Disruptive behavior, hyperactivity, and learning disorders in children with Tourette's syndrome. *Adv Neurol* 1995;65:259–272.
39. Carter AS, O'Donnell D, Schultz RT, et al. Social and emotional adjustment in children affected with Gilles de la Tourette's syndrome: associations with ADHD and functioning. *J Child Psychol Psychiatry* 2000;41:215–223.
40. Budman C, Bruun R, Park K, et al. Explosive outbursts in children with Tourette's disorder. *J Am Acad Child Adolesc Psychiatry* 2000;39:1270–126.
41. Connor DF. *Aggression and antisocial behavior in children and adolescents: research and treatment.* New York: Guilford, 2002.
42. Riddle MA, Carlson J. Clinical psychopharmacology for Tourette Syndrome and associated disorders. *Adv Neurol* 2001;85:343–354.
43. Piacentini J, Chang S. Behavioral treatments for Tourette Syndrome and tic disorders: state of the art. *Adv Neurol* 2001;85:319–332.
44. Kazdin AE. Problem-solving skills training and parent management training for conduct disorder. In: Kazdin AE, ed. *Evidence-based psychotherapies for children and adolescents.* New York: Guilford Press, 2003:241–262.
45. Sukhodolsky DG, Kassinove H, Gorman B. Cognitive behavioral therapy for anger in children and adolescents: a meta-analysis. *Aggress Violent Behav* 2004;9:247–269.

18

Obsessive–Compulsive Disorder in Tourette's Syndrome

Peter G. Como,[1] Jennifer LaMarsh,[2] and Katherine A. O'Brien[3]

[1]*Departments of Neurology, Psychiatry, and Brain and Cognitive Science, University of Rochester Medical Center, Rochester, New York;*
[2]*Psychology and Social Sciences, University of Rochester, Rochester, New York;*
[3]*Brain and Cognitive Science, University of Rochester, Rochester, New York*

The relationship between Tourette's syndrome (TS) and obsessive–compulsive disorder (OCD) dates back to the original description of TS by Itard (1), who reported the case of the Marquise de Dampierre, who developed symptoms of TS at age seven. Many years later, the French neurologist Charcot examined the same patient; his observations were published in 1885 by his student, Georges Gilles de la Tourette (2), in a paper that described nine cases of the syndrome that would later bear his name. In his account of the case of the Marquise, Tourette described obsessive thoughts that tormented her, in addition to the motor and vocal tics that were observed (3). Charcot, however, was the first neurologist to characterize obsessive–compulsive behavior as involuntary "impulsive" ideas, such as doubting, checking, touching, and repetitive counting, as part of the tic disorder (4) that would later become known as Tourette's syndrome. A rather convincing case has been made that the 18th-century English lexicographer and critic, Dr. Samuel Johnson, also had TS and OCD (5). Dr. Johnson reportedly felt compelled to measure his footsteps, to perform complex gestures when he crossed a threshold, and to touch objects repetitively. Robertson and Reinstein (6) translated the early writings of Gilles de la Tourette, Guinon, and Grasset, which described many psychiatric features in patients with tic disorders, with particular emphasis on OCD, including checking rituals, counting compulsions, compulsive touching, a need for explanations of commonplace facts, and a need for order and routine. In the modern era, studies have been conducted to determine whether obsessive–compulsive behaviors (OCB) seen in patients with comorbid TS are similar to or different from those seen in patients who have a primary psychiatric diagnosis of OCD (7–13). Current opinion holds that TS is a common neurobehavioral disorder with a heterogeneous clinical presentation (14). In addition, specific behavioral syndromes, such as OCD, are likely to co-occur with TS; however, whether TS with OCD is etiologically and, perhaps, genetically related to TS and OCD or is a more severe expression of the underlying neuropathology than either of the two, is a matter for debate (15).

This chapter focuses on the relationship between TS and OCD. The clinical features of OCD and TS and the assessment of these conditions are discussed, followed by a review of genetic evidence that supports the relationship between TS and OCD. The chapter also examines the neurobiologic correlates of OCD, including pathophysiologic and imaging studies. Finally, an overview of the treatment options for OCD in patients with TS are discussed.

OBSESSIVE–COMPULSIVE DISORDER

OCD is a psychiatric disorder characterized by recurrent obsessions, compulsions, or both, that are sufficiently severe as to interfere substantially with normal daily activity, school or occupational function, and social relationships (16).

Feelings of fear and anxiety typically accompany obsessive–compulsive symptoms (OCS). Obsessions and compulsions often cause marked distress and are time consuming. Obsessions are defined as recurrent ideas, thoughts, images, or impulses that intrude upon conscious thought and are persistent and unwelcome. Attempts are frequently made to ignore, suppress, or neutralize these thoughts with some other thoughts or actions. The person recognizes these symptoms to be a product of his or her own mind. Common obsessions typically include thoughts of violence, concern about germs, contamination, and illness, and repetitive doubts. Compulsions are defined as repetitive, purposeful behaviors usually performed in response to an obsession, according to certain rules, or in a stereotyped fashion and are designed to prevent psychological discomfort or some dreaded event or situation. The compulsive behavior is always excessive, not connected realistically to what it is designed to prevent, and the person recognizes that the behavior is unreasonable. More common compulsions typically involve hand washing, counting, checking, and touching (16).

CLINICAL FEATURES OF OCD IN TS

Epidemiology

OCD is reported to have a lifetime prevalence of between 1% and 2% (17,18). The disorder can have an onset in childhood; however, it typically occurs in late adolescence or early adulthood (19). Although it is commonly accepted that OCD is part of the TS clinical spectrum, whether patients with TS actually have OCD, or merely a continuum of OCB that may not be clinically important, remains unclear. Thus, although many patients with TS may exhibit obsessions and compulsions, these symptoms may not be severe enough to meet current psychiatric diagnostic criteria for OCD. In addition, many of the clinical features of OCD in patients with TS appear quite different from those observed in patients with psychiatric disorders or primary OCD. These factors, along with inconsistent methods, ascertainment bias (i.e., clinical versus nonclinical sampling), different diagnostic techniques, and age of the study population at the time of ascertainment, have hampered epidemiologic studies of OCD in TS.

Attempts to scientifically obtain prevalence estimates of OCD in TS date to the early 1960s. Torup (20) found in a sample of 237 children treated for tics between 1946 and 1947 in Denmark that 12% had evidence of OCB. Since then, many epidemiologic studies have reported that a relatively high percentage of TS populations have so-called "OCB phenomena" (21). However, this finding has been disputed. The early comprehensive textbook on TS by Shapiro et al. (4) argued strongly against drawing an association between OCD and TS. Shapiro and Shapiro (22) argue that OCB in patients with TS merely represents a type of a complex motor or sensory tic, a phenomenon they characterize as "impulsions." However, most studies provide rather compelling evidence that suggests that OCB does indeed occur in a large percentage of patients with TS and likely represents a true comorbid behavioral condition in this disorder. The percentage of OCB reported in TS ranges from 30% to 90% (23–26). Studies that have used standardized questionnaires or structured interviews have found that nearly 50% of patients with TS have features of either OCD or OCB (27,28).

Interestingly, studies of patients and families with primary OCD also report high rates of comorbid tic disorders. Rasmussen and Eisen (29) suggest that the lifetime occurrence of tics in patients with OCD is approximately 7%. Pittman et al. (30) reported that 6 of 16 patients (37%) with primary OCD also met criteria for tic disorder. Other studies of children with severe OCD have reported that 20% of these patients had simple motor tics (31,32). More compelling is the study by Leonard et al. (33), who reevaluated 54 children with OCD, 2 to 7 years after they had participated in various OCD treatment protocols (TS was an exclusionary diagnosis), with a neurologic examination and a structured interview to establish the absence of tics or TS. At the 2- to 4-year follow-up, eight subjects (15%) met criteria for TS, despite that fact that TS was an initial exclusionary criterion. The presentation and course of OCD in these subjects was indistinguishable from that of subjects with OCD who did not have TS.

More recently, Kurlan et al. (34) conducted a community-based study of school children to determine the true prevalence of tics in this sample. They also tested the children for behavioral disorders, such as OCD, to overcome past ascertainment bias and discern the true prevalence of these disorders in children with and without tics. They found that the children with tics were more likely to have OCD, further supporting the correlation between TS and OCD.

Phenomenology

Many clinical features between TS and OCD are shared. Both TS and OCD present episodically, wax and wane over time, or present in an unremitting fashion. Temporary remissions and improvement over time have been reported for both disorders (17,29,35). TS often presents with simple motor tics. Vocal tics often have a later onset, as does OCD when they co-occur. Patients with OCD may also present with a single obsession or compulsion and gradually progress to involve other thoughts or behaviors. Symptoms in both disorders are almost always exacerbated by physical and psychological stresses (e.g., acute illness, lack of sleep, anxiety, and depression), and patients often express a sense of relief upon completing a tic or a compulsive act. In both disorders, patients can exert some voluntary control, albeit variable, over their symptoms.

In addition to these general phenomenologic similarities, patients with TS and OCD and those with primary OCD also have other common clinical features. Frankel et al. (36) found that patients with TS and those with OCD but not TS endorsed fear of contamination and checking as their most frequent obsessions and compulsions. The authors also noted that such symptoms changed with age, with the younger patients exhibiting compulsive behavior related to impulse control, and the older patients manifesting behaviors more classically associated with OCD, such as checking, arranging, a need for order and routine, and fear of contamination.

Despite these similarities, differences have been reported in OCB among patients with TS and those with primary OCD. Pittman et al. (30) observed that certain kinds of compulsive behaviors, such as touching and a need for symmetry (e.g., "evening-up" rituals to ensure that the body was balanced or symmetric) occurred more often in the group with TS than in the group with primary OCD. Como and Kurlan (37) analyzed responses from the Leyton Obsessional Inventory-Child Version (LOI-CV) in 56 of 95 children with TS who scored above the cutoff on the LOI-CV, a score suggestive of OCD. They found that the most frequently endorsed items included a need for order and routine (72%), repetitive thoughts or indecision (68%), repetitive rituals (67%), and preoccupation with self-harm or injury to family (64%). The frequencies of these occurrences were different from those reported by Berg et al. (38), using the same inventory in a sample of children with OCD; these authors found that fear of contamination, checking rituals, and washing rituals were more common. A similar pattern was found in a study by George et al. (39) in which patients with TS and OCD (TS + OCD) had significantly more violent, sexual, and symmetric obsessions and more touching, counting, and self-damaging compulsions than the group with primary OCD, which had more dirt or contamination obsessions and cleaning or washing compulsions.

The severity of OCS symptoms is generally thought to be reduced in TS, a belief that is consistent with the current consensus that many patients with TS have OCB but not disabling OCD. Unfortunately, little data is available in the literature to support this claim. Psychometric studies comparing patients with TS + OCD and those with primary OCD have reported significantly lower mean scores in the groups with TS on various OCD inventories (30,40,41) than in the groups with primary OCD, even though the scores in both groups were significantly higher than those obtained in a healthy control population. However, these studies were limited by their relatively small sample sizes, inconsistent methods, and different diagnostic criteria for determining OCD.

More recent studies have attempted to address the issue of differences and similarities among TS, TS + OCD and OCD. However, many of these studies continue to by hampered by the same methodologic limitations. Most studies seem to agree that TS + OCD is more phenomenologically linked to TS than to primary OCD. Important differences in OCS have been found between patients with TS + OCD and those with only primary OCD. Typically, patients with TS + OCD are more likely to have violent images or impulses, concerns with illness or disease, concern with body or appearance, a need to know or remember, fear of saying or doing something wrong, mental play, self-injurious behaviors, touching, aggressive obsessions, and other ticlike or Tourette-related items (i.e., eye blinking) than patients with OCD alone. Patients with OCD usually reported more washing and contamination worries.

Patients with OCD typically experience more cognitive phenomena and autonomic anxiety along with their symptoms and not as much sensory phenomena as is observed in patients with TS or TS + OCD (42). A main difference between the patients with TS + OCD and those with primary OCD is the higher occurrence of nonanxiety-related stimulus-bound impulsions in TS + OCD, which has led several researchers to conclude that TS + OCD is more closely related to TS than to OCD and may represent a phenotypic expression of this disorder (12,13,43).

Assessment of OCD

The current diagnostic classification of OCD is detailed in the *The Diagnostic and Statistical Manual of Mental Disorders*, 4th edition (DSM-IV) (16). Unfortunately, the DSM-IV does not establish psychometric properties, such as reliability and validity, and it is not as useful as psychometric methods for rating symptom severity or response to treatment. In addition, given that many patients with TS exhibit OCB but typically do not meet DSM-IV criteria for OCD, a greater need exists to assess symptoms accurately in these patients. Until recently, accurate assessment of OCB was hampered by the limitations of existing rating instruments, such as lack of specificity for OCS, inadequate psychometric properties, and limiting examination to only certain types of obsessions and compulsions. Currently, no one scale has emerged as the most broadly accepted scale for an assessment of OCB. Nevertheless, several scales are widely available for assessing OCD.

The Leyton Obsessional Inventory (LOI) (44) and its associated child version (LOI-CV) (45) have been among the most widely used self-rating scales for OCD. The LOI is a 40-item scale in which the subject rates the occurrence of the symptom, ranging from never to frequently (36). The LOI-CV is a 44-item inventory typically administered to the child as a "yes/no" card-sorting task. Affirmative responses on the LOI-CV can be further analyzed to yield resistance and interference scores. Studies of the LOI and the LOI-CV have reliably identified OCD in TS populations (33,36,37,39,46). Inconsistent findings from drug trials, however, have raised questions regarding the use of the LOI to detect response to treatment (47).

The Maudsley Obsessional–Compulsive Inventory (MOCI), widely used in European studies, is a self-rating scale for OCD (48). The MOCI is short and easy to administer and is reported to have better psychometric properties than the LOI (47); however, there are no published studies of the MOCI specifically in TS populations.

Two commonly used observer-rated scales for OCD are the Comprehensive Psychopathological Rating Scale (CPRS), which has an eight-item OCD scale (49), and the National Institute of Mental Health (NIMH)-Global Obsessive–Compulsive Scale (50,51). Both scales are clinician-rated and are based on a structured or semistructured clinical interview. Psychometric studies of reliability and validity of these scales have been inconsistent (46) and relatively few studies have been conducted that include TS populations. Perhaps the major limitation of the observer-rated scales for OCD is the requirement that they be administered by a trained mental health clinician.

The Yale-Brown Obsessive–Compulsive Scale (Y-BOCS) and the corresponding children's Yale-Brown Obsessive–Compulsive Scale (CY-BOCS) have gained wide acceptance based upon their well-described psychometric properties (52,53) and their reported sensitivity to detect changes in OCD in placebo-controlled trials of antiobsessional drugs (54,55) in primary OCD patient populations. Open-label studies of fluoxetine have demonstrated the sensitivity of the Y-BOCS for detecting changes in patients with TS + OCD (56,57). Most treatment studies that use the Y-BOCS as the principal outcome variable suggest that a 35% decrease in Y-BOCS score from baseline indicates a clinically important improvement for both primary OCD and TS + OCD.

GENETICS

Twin studies of both OCD and TS report high concordance in monozygotic twins (58,59). In a study of 43 twin pairs in which one member of the pair had TS, 83% of the entire sample reported the presence of OCS (58). A higher rate of OCB is reported in monozygotic twin pairs with TS than in dizygotic twin pairs with TS (52% versus 15%) (58). In a follow-up evaluation of 14 monozygotic twin pairs with TS, Singer and Walkup (60) reported that at least one twin in nine pairs had OCD, whereas in seven of nine affected pairs, both twins had OCD.

Family studies of TS and OCD have reported strong familial patterns for both disorders (61,62), suggesting a possible genetic relationship between the two disorders (51,63). Data obtained from family studies of TS have found the prevalence of OCD among first-degree relatives to be significantly higher (9 to 13 times) than the prevalence of OCD estimated in the general population (58). Furthermore, rates of TS and OCD in families of TS probands with OCD were virtually the same as in the families of TS probands without OCD. Data from the Yale Family Study suggested that OCD alone could represent a variant expression of the TS gene (58). Other studies (61) have supported these findings. OCD by itself occurs more frequently in female relatives of TS probands than in male relatives (61), suggesting some sex-related expression of TS, with men being more likely to express the more classic clinical features of TS (i.e., motor and vocal tics), and women more likely to express OCD without any tics. This suggestion that OCD may be an alternative expression of the TS gene, especially in women, has hampered linkage analysis and gene localization studies (62). The original optimism regarding the well-defined "TS phenotype" has gradually been tempered, especially when associated behavioral symptoms such as OCD dominated the clinical picture (63).

Eapen et al. (8) showed that individuals with OCD who have similar OCS to those in individuals with TS + OCD are more likely to have a family history of OCD. This finding suggests that the familial form of OCD may be etiologically related to TS, whereas the nonfamilial form of OCD may derive from a different mechanism. Miguel et al. (13) also lend support to this idea with the suggestion that early-onset OCD is more frequently associated with tics, is typically more likely to be familial, and also seems to have a similar phenomenology to TS + OCD.

NEUROBIOLOGIC FEATURES OF TS AND OCD

Pathophysiology

Although the precise pathophysiology of both TS and OCD remains unknown, data suggest that both arise from dysfunction in the basal ganglia (60,64–66). Limbic circuitry is involved in TS, whereas the lateral prefrontal circuitry is involved in OCD. Although the pathogenesis of the two disorders does seem to differ, data seems to implicate basal ganglia thalamocortical components in both.

Clinical reports have been presented of "acquired tourettism" following neurologic insult to the basal ganglia (67), postencephalitic parkinsonism, tardive dyskinesia, and carbon monoxide poisoning (68). Further support for basal ganglia involvement in TS comes from the fact that dopamine-blocking agents (e.g., neuroleptics) suppress tics (69). Conversely, dopamine agonists can exacerbate tics.

The evidence implicating basal ganglia dysfunction in OCD comes from several lines of investigation. OCD has been reported in other movement disorders, including Sydenham's chorea (70), von Economo's encephalitis (71), Huntington's disease (72), and Parkinson's disease (73,74). Other support implicating the basal ganglia in the pathogenesis of OCD is derived from receptor studies and treatment studies. A high concentration of serotonin receptors is present in the basal ganglia of normal brains (75,76), and early pivotal clinical trials of first generation of selective serotonin reuptake inhibitors (SSRIs) such as fluoxetine and clomipramine showed that these agents significantly ameliorated OCD symptoms (77). Damage to regions of limbic or orbitofrontal basal ganglia thalamocortical circuits can result in acquired OCD (78).

The primary line of discordance with respect to a shared neurobiology between TS and OCD is the different neurochemical substrates postulated in the genesis of these two disorders. Although most of the literature has focused on dopaminergic mechanisms for TS and serotonergic mechanisms for OCD, evidence suggests that both transmitter systems may be involved in each disorder (60,79,80). Steingard and Dillon-Stout (66) have suggested that a subset of patients may present with either TS or OCD who have an abnormality or, perhaps, an imbalance, in both the serotonergic and dopaminergic systems. Given the known innervation of the basal ganglia by both neurotransmitter systems (64,65), this hypothesis remains compatible with neuroanatomic theories.

Leckman et al. (81) found that one difference among patients with OCD is that patients with no personal or family history of tic disorders had increased cerebrospinal fluid levels of oxytocin, compared with levels in patients with such a history, which were similar to those in patients with TS (without comorbid OCD) and in control subjects. Although this finding is based on a small subgroup (7 patients with OCD and a family history of tics), it suggests that oxytocin may play a role in the neurobiology of OCD unrelated to tics, but not of tic-related OCD.

Neuroimaging

The availability of high resolution scanners has also elucidated the neuroanatomic similarities between TS and OCD and lends further support to the known phenomenologic and neurochemical similarities. Several neuroimaging studies, including magnetic resonance imaging (MRI) and positron emission tomography (PET), have suggested that both TS and OCD are mediated by right frontal, orbitofrontal, and striatal mechanisms (82–84). Hypermetabolism of the orbitofrontal cortex and basal ganglia are also reported for both TS and OCD populations (85,86).

In a study by Breiter et al. (87), OCD subjects and age-matched controls were scanned using functional magnetic resonance imaging (fMRI) at baseline and while being presented with stimuli to provoke their OCD symptoms. They found that whereas controls showed no statistically significant brain activation changes, those with OCD exhibited lateral frontal, paralimbic (medial orbital gyrus, anterior cingulate, temporal cortex, and insular cortex), limbic (amygdala), and striatal (caudate and lenticulate) activation while being provoked with OCD-eliciting stimuli. However, these studies have not been conducted in patients with TS + OCD.

Peterson et al. (88) compared fMRI scans of patients with TS during periods of tic suppression and periods of spontaneous tic production. Of the 22 adult patients with TS, 10 also met criteria for comorbid OCD. During tic suppression, a wide range of neuronal activity was evident, including increases and decreases in activity in both subcortical and cortical areas. However, activation of subcortical regions was highly correlated with tic severity. Specifically, this study found decreased activation bilaterally in ventral globus pallidus and the putamen and midthalamic regions, and increased activation in the ventral head of the right caudate nucleus. These results were consistent in TS subjects with and without OCD.

An FDG-PET study by Braun et al. (89) suggested that patients with TS + OCD had higher rates of glucose use in the putamen than patients with the single diagnosis of OCD. Baxter et al. (86) reported that patients diagnosed with OCD, whether presenting with or without tics, had higher levels of orbitofrontal glucose use.

Meyer et al. (90) used PET type 2 vesicular monoamine transporter (VMAT2) binding to investigate presynaptic striatal dopamine terminal density. No difference was found either between TS and controls, or TS and TS + OCD, in striatal VMAT2 binding potential. However, the extent of these findings is limited by the small number of subjects in the study (5 with TS; 3 with TS + OCD).

The recent creation of a transgenic mouse model that might mimic TS + OCD has helped to expand our knowledge regarding the specific neuroanatomic regions that might be involved in patients with TS and comorbid OCD. Studies conducted with these mice suggest that TS + OCD symptoms arise from a hyperactive output of cortical–limbic glutamatergic neurons from somatosensory, orbitofrontal, and limbic regions (91,92).

TREATMENT OF OCD IN TS

The debilitating effect of OCD on social development, cognitive function, self-image, and family relations is well documented (93,94). In many patients with TS, symptoms of OCD, especially if severe, may be more disabling than tics or other TS-associated behavioral conditions such as attention-deficit hyperactivity disorder (ADHD) [see (105); Chapter 17 in this book]. In other cases, treating both tics and OCD may be necessary. The available psychopharmacologic agents well known to successfully treat primary OCD appear to have equivalent efficacy in patients with TS + OCD. In addition, previously established psychological treatment of OCD continues to be an effective option for patients and their families who are reluctant to take medications.

Careful and thorough clinical assessment of the patient is very important for determining proper treatment, particularly when the distinction between a compulsive ritual and a complex motor tic becomes blurred. In some patients, determining whether the behavior represents some type of compulsion or is merely an involuntary, albeit complex, motor tic is difficult. Similarly, the conscious awareness of somatosensory urges may be difficult to differentiate from obsessive thoughts. Leckman (95) has suggested that "obsessive thoughts" that are related to tics include recurrent, unwanted sensory urges or thoughts about tics, or thoughts that the sequence of tics must be "just right." On the other hand, true obsessions are intrusive, unwanted thoughts related to tics that lead to efforts to resist them and are associated with marked distress or interference with daily activity. Compulsive behaviors that may be more related to tics include stereotyped complex tics, such as tapping, picking, touching, kissing, copropraxia, hitting, biting, and "evening-up," whereas compulsions independent of tics include the more classic counting, checking, washing, and other repetitive rituals designed to prevent mental discomfort or a dreaded event. Response to pharmacologic treatment can be another helpful way to distinguish between tics and OCD.

Pharmacotherapy

The development of SSRIs, potent antidepressant medications, has revolutionized the pharmacotherapy of OCD [see (77) for an excellent review]. These agents have proven superior to placebo and other psychotropic drugs that have less effect on serotonin reuptake. Unfortunately, many of the original large, multicenter-controlled clinical trials of SSRIs have excluded patients with TS or tic disorders. Thus, fewer carefully controlled clinical trials of TS + OCD exist. The trials that have been conducted have relatively small sample sizes and have focused largely on clomipramine and fluoxetine. Other available SSRIs include sertraline, paroxetine, and fluvoxamine; Studies of these drugs in TS populations have not been published. More recently, citalopram, controlled-release paroxetine, and escitalopram have also become available; however, no clinical trials have been conducted using these agents for patients with TS + OCD.

Clomipramine has been reported in several small studies to be effective in treating TS + OCB and in some cases may reduce tic severity as well (96–98). This finding, however, has not been replicated reliably. Most patients with TS appear to tolerate clomipramine well, although increased tics have been reported in some studies (99). The side-effect profile of clomipramine resembles that of other tricyclic antidepressants and includes predominantly anticholinergic effects (dry mouth, constipation, sweating, and somnolence).

More trials of fluoxetine in patients with TS + OCD have been conducted, with mixed results. Riddle et al. (56,100) reported improvement in OCD in three of six children and in three men with TS. These findings were then replicated in an open-label study of 13 children and 13 adults with TS + OCD (101), which found a significant reduction on LOI scores. No substantial worsening or improvement in tics was found in this study, although tics were not systematically evaluated. A double-blind, placebo-controlled study of OCD in children with TS failed to demonstrate that fluoxetine was superior to placebo (102), although a trend was observed toward some improvement in tic severity, attentional abilities, and social functioning. However, this study was limited by a small sample size because of recruitment problems, which may have reduced its statistical power to detect a clinical effect. Most patients with TS, including children, tolerate fluoxetine well. Common side effects include nervousness, anxiety, insomnia, and restlessness. Given the activating properties of fluoxetine, morning dosing is usually recommended.

In a retrospective, case-controlled analysis of fluvoxamine response in patients with OCD, with and without comorbid tics, McDougle et al. (103) reported that although both groups demonstrated a statistically significant reduction in OCD, the frequency and magnitude of response in OCS differed significantly between the two groups. Improvement in OCD was found in 21% of patients with comorbid chronic tics, compared with 52% of patients with OCD who did not exhibit chronic tics. These data lend further support to the hypothesis that TS + OCD may represent a clinically meaningful subtype of OCD, both phenomenologically and in response to pharmacologic treatment.

Other medications used to treat OCD have included clonidine, a centrally acting α_2 noradrenergic agonist, buspirone, an anxiolytic agent that acts as a partial agonist at the serotonin receptor site, and clonazepam, a high-potency benzodiazepine that appears to increase synaptic serotonin. Of these drugs, clonidine is of particular interest, because it is reported to be effective in treating tics and symptoms of attention-deficit hyperactivity disorder (104). However, a double-blind study of clonidine failed to find a beneficial effect on severity of OCS in a subgroup of patients with TS and OCD (104). The more selective α_2 adrenergic agonist guanfacine has been shown to be effective in TS + ADHD (105); however, no studies in patients with TS + OCD have been conducted as yet.

γ-aminobutyric acid (GABA)-modulating agents (e.g., baclofen) have also been used to treat tics with some success (106); however, trials in patients with TS + OCD have not been conducted.

The emerging hypotheses that gonadal hormones may play a role in aggravating OCD symptoms (107) suggests another pharmacologic treatment strategy. Some open-label case studies of patients with OCD have reported temporary improvement from agents that produce nonspecific suppression of gonadal steroids. Although flutamide, a selective androgen antagonist, had beneficial effects on a patient with comorbid TS + OCD, when this approach was extended into a larger study, these benefits were not maintained (107–109). The results of this larger study suggest that the exacerbation of OCD symptoms may be mediated through estrogen receptors or some other receptor-independent mechanism (108).

More recent reports suggest that a subset of children may experience either abrupt onset or a dramatic exacerbation of tics, OCD associated with streptococcal infection, or both. These patients have been referred to by the acronym PANDAS (pediatric autoimmune neuropsychiatric disorders associated with streptococcal infections). Whether or not PANDAS is a true entity is currently being studied in large epidemiologic studies sponsored by the National Institutes of Health. Nonetheless, these children might respond to immunomodulatory treatments such as plasma exchange or intravenous immunoglobulin (IVIG). Treatment studies to date have been positive, with the reports of a recent study citing 14 out of 17 children (82%) showing improvement in tics, OCD, or both, lasting for 1 year (seven of eight for plasma exchange, seven of nine for IVIG) (110).

Augmentation techniques that combine SSRIs with other drugs such as anxiolytics and neuroleptics can be another treatment option for patients with TS and comorbid OCD. Delgado et al. (111) described a young man whose TS-related OCD responded to a combination of pimozide and fluvoxamine. Either agent used alone did not improve tics or OCD, and the use of fluvoxamine alone exacerbated his tics. These results support a previous finding that the addition of a neuroleptic enhanced the antiobsessional effect of fluvoxamine in 55% of patients with primary OCD (112). McDougle et al. (113) reported that the addition of haloperidol, a commonly used tic suppression medication, to fluvoxamine was beneficial for patients with comorbid OCD and tics.

Behavior Therapy

The effectiveness of behavioral therapy for treating OCD is well documented [see (114) for a comprehensive review]. Behavior therapy was one of the earliest effective treatments for OCD in the absence of any proven pharmacologic agents, before the advent of SSRIs. Various forms of behavior therapy successfully employed in the treatment of OCD have included thought stopping, systematic desensitization, exposure therapy, and response prevention (114). The use of behavioral techniques to treat tics is somewhat more controversial, because tics are considered neurologic involuntary movements, which occur randomly and are variably controlled by the patients. Nonetheless, Azrin and Peterson (115,116) reported considerable success reducing tics using a habit-reversal technique, which involves awareness training, self-monitoring, relaxation training, development of competing responses, and contingency management. Carefully controlled trials of behavior therapy with and without pharmacologic intervention are warranted to clarify the role of behavioral therapy in treating TS + OCD. Nonetheless, the use of various behavioral techniques remains a very effective treatment for patients and families who are reluctant to use medications.

Neurosurgical Treatment

The use of neurosurgical treatment for severe and treatment-resistant OCD dates back to the use of psychosurgery to treat a variety of psychiatric disorders (117). The large number of recent studies that document the putative neuroanatomic substrates of OCD makes neurosurgical therapy an intriguing treatment option. Surgical approaches to OCD include cingulotomy, subcaudate tractotomy, limbic leucotomy, and anterior capsulotomy. All of these approaches have produced improvement in OCD symptoms ranging from 50% to 100% (117). However, published studies of neurosurgical treatment of OCD in patients with TS are limited to case reports. Kurlan et al. (118) reported the results of neurosurgical treatment for severe OCD in two patients with TS. Both patients underwent anterior cingulotomy and achieved limited but sustained improvement in OCD symptoms and overall function. More recently, serious and irreversible disturbances in speech, swallowing, and gait were noted in a man with TS, who had severe self-injurious motor tics and OCD, following bilateral anterior cingulotomies and bilateral infrathalamic lesions placed stereotactically (119). Although improvement in OCD and transient improvement in tics were noted, this patient's neurologic deficits, including essentially unintelligible speech, persisted postoperatively. This study emphasizes the need for caution in applying surgical techniques for treating TS + OCD. However, neurosurgical therapy remains an option for patients with refractory symptoms who do not respond to SSRIs or behavioral therapy.

Two other more recent neural circuit–based therapies include deep brain stimulation (DBS) and transcranial magnetic stimulation (TMS). Both of these techniques are still quite experimental in treating OCD. DBS is minimally invasive and reversible. In this procedure, a small electrode is inserted directly into a targeted brain region (such as the subthalamic nucleus in patients with Parkinson's disease patients). Improvement in OCD symptoms has been reported after stimulation was applied to the anterior limb of the internal capsule (109). TMS, on the other hand, uses an electromagnet on the scalp to change the electrical activity in the cerebral cortex. To date, no studies have been reported of either DBS or TMS in patients with TS + OCD (109).

SUMMARY

A substantial body of scientific evidence suggests that obsessive–compulsive behavior occurs in a large percentage of patients with TS. Reliable estimates suggest that nearly 50% of patients with TS have some degree of obsessive–compulsive features. Most patients with TS have only mild OCB and thus would not meet the DSM-IV diagnostic criteria for OCD. Therefore, OCB is perhaps a more appropriate characterization of this behavioral phenomenon that occurs in TS. OCB in TS appears similar to the spectrum of the tic disorder in terms of its onset, severity, and course. As with tics, OCB is typically mild and not always substantially disabling. Although clinical features between TS + OCB and primary OCD overlap considerably, patients with TS + OCB appear to experience different types of obsessive thoughts and compulsive rituals. Compelling genetic evidence suggests that OCB may be an alternative expression of the TS phenotype, which may selectively affect female gene carriers. Identifying the TS gene in the future will substantially broaden our knowledge of this intriguing neurobehavioral disorder. Finally, neurobiologic evidence points to similar anatomic and chemical substrates in the pathogenesis of TS and OCD, suggesting that these two disorders share a common pathophysiology.

The clinical evaluation of patients with TS and their families should always include an assessment for OCB. Self-rated inventories of OCD such as the LOI, LOI-CV, and MOCI are useful screening scales. A more structured interview using the Y-BOCS (CY-BOCS) is useful for determining the degree and severity of OCB in TS as well as the response to therapy. Clinicians should keep in mind that OCB may be the most disabling feature of TS and may require treatment. Pharmacologic agents, such as SSRIs, and traditional behavioral therapy are proven effective treatments for OCB, which can substantially reduce the full effect of TS on patients and their families.

REFERENCES

1. Itard JMD. Memorie sur quelques forictions involuntaries des appareils de la locomotion de la prehension et de la voix. *Arch Genet Med* 1825;8:385–407.
2. Gilles de la Tourette G. Etude sur une affection nerveuse caractérisée par l'incoordination motrice accompagnée d'écholalie et de copralalie. *Arch Neurol* 1885;9:19–42.
3. Stevens H. The syndrome of Gilles de la Tourette and its treatment. *Med Ann Dist Columbia* 1964;33:277–279.
4. Shapiro AK, Shapiro E, Bruun RD, et al. *Gilles de la Tourette syndrome*. New York: Raven Press, 1978.
5. Murray TJ. Dr. Samuel Johnson's movement disorders. *Br Med J* 1979;1:1610–1614.
6. Robertson MM, Reinstein DZ. Convulsive tic disorder: Georges de la Tourette, Guinon, and Grasset on the phenomenology and psychopathology of Gilles de la Tourette syndrome. *Behav Neurol* 1991;4:29–56.
7. Coffey BJ, Miguel EC, Biederman J, et al. Tourette's disorder with and without obsessive–compulsive disorder in adults: are they different? *J Nerv Ment Dis* 1998; 186:201–206.
8. Eapen V, Robertson MM, Alsobrook JP II et al. Obsessive compulsive symptoms in Gilles de la Tourette syndrome and obsessive compulsive disorder: differences by diagnosis and family history. *Am J Med Genet (Neuropsychiatr Genet)* 1997;74:432–438.
9. Cath DC, Spinhoven P, van de Wetering BJM, et al. The relationship between types and severity of repetitive behaviors in Gilles de la Tourette's syndrome and obsessive–compulsive disorder. *J Clin Psychiatry* 2000; 61:505–513.
10. Cath DC, Spinhoven P, Hoogduin CAL, et al. Repetitive behaviors in Tourette's syndrome and OCD with and without tics: what are the differences? *Psychiatry Res* 2001;101:171–185.
11. Cath DC, Spinhoven P, van Woerkom TC, et al. Gilles de la Tourette's syndrome with and without obsessive–compulsive disorder compared with obsessive–compulsive disorder without tics: which symptoms discriminate? *J Nerv Ment Dis* 2001;189:219–228.
12. Miguel EC, Baer L, Coffey BJ. et al. Phenomenological differences appearing with repetitive behaviours in obsessive–compulsive disorder and Gilles de la Tourette's syndrome. *Br J Psychiatry* 1997;170:140–145.
13. Miguel EC, do Rosario-Campos MC, Shavitt RG, et al. The tic related obsessive–compulsive disorder phenotype and treatment implications. *Tourette Syndrome*. Philadelphia: Lippincott Williams &Wilkins, 2001.
14. Kurlan R. Tourette's syndrome: current concepts. *Neurology* 1989;39:1625–1630.
15. Sheppard DM, Bradshaw JL, Purcell R, et al. Tourette's and comorbid syndromes: obsessive compulsive and attention deficit hyperactivity disorder. A common etiology? *Clin Psychol Rev* 1999;19(5):531–552.
16. American Psychiatric Association. *Diagnostic and statistical manual of mental disorders*, 5th ed, (DSM-IV). Washington, DC: American Psychiatric Association, 1994.
17. Jenike M, Baer L, Minichello W. *Obsessive–compulsive disorder: theory and management*. Chicago: Year Book Medical Publishers, 1990.
18. Karno M, Golding JM, Sorenson SB, et al. The epidemiology of obsessive–compulsive disorder in five US communities. *Arch Genet Psychiatry* 1988;45:1094–1099.
19. Swedo SE, Rapoport JL, Leonard H, et al. Obsessive–compulsive disorder in children and adolescents. *Arch Genet Psychiatry* 1989;46:335–345.
20. Torup E. A follow-up study of children with tics. *Acta Paediatr Scand* 1962;51:261–268.
21. Robertson MM, Yakely JW. Obsessive–compulsive disorder and self-injurious behavior. In: Kurlan R, ed. *Handbook of Tourette's syndrome and related tic and behavioral disorders*. New York: Marcel Dekker Inc, 1992:45–87.
22. Shapiro AK, Shapiro E. Evaluation of the reported association of obsessive–compulsive symptoms or disorder with Tourette's disorder. *Compre Psychiatry* 1992; 33:152–165.
23. Jagger J, Prussoff BA, Cohen DJ, et al. The epidemiology of Tourette's syndrome: a pilot study. *Schizophr Bull* 1982;8:266–267.
24. Montgomery MA, Clayton PC, Freidhoff AJ. Psychiatric illness in Tourette syndrome patients and first

degree relatives. In: Freidhoff AJ, Chase TN, eds. *Gilles de la Tourette syndrome.* New York: Raven Press, 1982.
25. Nee LE, Polinsky RJ, Ebert MH. Tourette's syndrome: clinical and family studies. In: Freidhoff AJ, Chase TN, eds. *Gilles de la Tourette syndrome.* New York: Raven Press, 1982.
26. Pauls DL, Leckman JF. The inheritance of Gilles de la Tourette's syndrome and associated behaviors: evidence for autosomal dominant transmission. *N Engl J Med* 1986;315:993–997.
27. Caine ED, McBride MC, Chiverton P, et al. Tourette's syndrome in Monroe County school children. *Neurology* 1998;38:472–475.
28. Singer HS, Rosenberg LA. The development of behavioral and emotional problems in Tourette's syndrome. *Pediatr Neurol* 1989;5:41–44.
29. Rasmussen SA, Eisen JL. Epidemiology and clinical features of obsessive–compulsive disorder. In: Jenike M, Baer L, Minichello W, eds. *Obsessive compulsive disorder: theory and management.* Chicago: Year Book Medical Publishers, 1990.
30. Pittman RK, Green RC, Jenike MA, et al. Clinical comparison of Tourette's disorder and obsessive–compulsive disorder. *Am J Psychiatry* 1987;144:1166–1171.
31. Swedo SE, Rapoport JL, Leonard H, et al. Obsessive–compulsive disorder in children and adolescents: clinical phenomenology of 70 consecutive cases. *Arch Genet Psychiatry* 1989;46:335–341.
32. Rapoport JL. The neurology of obsessive–compulsive disorder. *J Am Med Assoc* 1988;260:2888–2890.
33. Leonard HL, Swedo SE, Rapoport JL, et al. Tourette syndrome and obsessive–compulsive disorder. In: Chase TN, Friedhoff AJ, Cohen DJ, eds. *Advances in neurology.* New York: Raven Press, 1992:83–93.
34. Kurlan R, Como PG, Miller B, et al. The behavioral spectrum of tic disorders: a community-based study. *Neurology* 2002;59:414–420.
35. Cohen DJ, Bruun RD, Leckman JF. *Tourette's syndrome and tic disorders: clinical understanding and treatment.* New York: John Wiley and Sons, 1988.
36. Frankel M, Cummings JL, Robertson MM, et al. Obsessions and compulsions in Gilles de la Tourette's syndrome. *Neurology* 1986;36:378–382.
37. Como PG, Kurlan R. Standardized assessment of attention deficit disorder and obsessive–compulsive disorder in a Tourette syndrome population. *J Clin Exper Neuropsychol* 1988;10:29.
38. Berg CZ, Rapoport JL, Whitaker A, et al. Childhood obsessive compulsive disorder: a two-year prospective follow-up of a community sample. *J Am Acad Child Adolesc Psychiatry* 1989;28:528–533.
39. George MS, Trimble MR, Ring HA, et al. Obsessions in obsessive–compulsive disorder with and without Gilles de la Tourette's syndrome. *Am J Psychiatry* 1993;150:93–97.
40. Stein DJ, Bruun RD, Josephson SC, et al. Obsessional severity in Tourette's syndrome. *J Clin Psychiatry* 1991;52:388.
41. Cath DC, Hoogduin CAL, van de Wetering BJM. Tourette syndrome and obsessive–compulsive disorder: analysis of associated phenomena. In: Chase TN, Friedhoff AJ, Cohen DJ, eds. *Advances in neurology.* New York: Raven Press, 1992:33–41.
42. Hanna GL, Piacentini J, Cantwell DP. Obsessive–compulsive disorder with and without tics in a clinical sample of children and adolescents. *Depress Anxiety* 2002;16:59–63.
43. Zohar AH, Pauls DL, Ratzoni G, et al. Obsessive–compulsive disorder with and without tics in an epidemiological sample of adolescents. *Am J Psychiatry* 1997;154:274–276.
44. Cooper J. The Leyton obsessional inventory. *Psychol Med* 1970;1:48–52.
45. Berg CZ, Rapoport JL, Flament M. The Leyton obsessional inventory-child version. *J Am Acad Child Adolesc Psychiatry* 1986;25:84–91.
46. Robertson MM, Gourdie A. Familial Tourette's syndrome in a large British pedigree: associated psychopathology, severity and potential for linkage analysis. *Br J Psychiatry* 1990;156:515–521.
47. Goodman WK, Price LH. Assessment of severity and change in obsessive–compulsive disorder. *Psychiatr Clin North Am* 1992;15:861–869.
48. Hodgson RJ, Rachman S. Obsessional compulsive complaints. *Behav Res Ther* 1977;15:389–395.
49. Asberg M, Montgomery SA, Perris C, et al. A comprehensive psychopathological rating scale. *Acta Psychiatr Scand Suppl* 1978; 271:529.
50. Insel TR, Murphy DL, Cohen RM, et al. Obsessive–compulsive disorder: a double-blind trial of clomipramine and clorgyline. *Arch Genet Psychiatry* 1983;40:605–612.
51. Rapoport J, Elkins R, Mikkelson E. Clinical controlled trial of chlorimipramine in adolescents with obsessive–compulsive disorder. *Psychopharmacol Bull* 1980;16:61–63.
52. Goodman WK, Price LH, Rasmussen SA, et al. The Yale-Brown obsessive compulsive scale: Part 1. Development, use and reliability. *Arch Genet Psychiatry* 1989;46:1006–1011.
53. Goodman WK, Price LH, Rasmussen SA, et al. The Yale-Brown obsessive compulsive scale: Part 11. Validity. *Arch Genet Psychiatry* 1989;46:1012–1016.
54. Goodman WK, Price LH, Rasmussen SA, et al. Efficacy of fluvoxamine in obsessive–compulsive disorder: a double-blind comparison with placebo. *Arch Genet Psychiatry* 1989;46:36–44.
55. Clomipramine Collaborative Group. Clomipramine hydrochloride in the treatment of patients with obsessive–compulsive disorder. *Arch Genet Psychiatry* 1991;48:730–738.
56. Riddle MA, Hardin MT, King R, et al. Fluoxetine treatment of children and adolescents with Tourette's syndrome and obsessive compulsive disorders: preliminary clinical experience. *J Am Acad Child Adolesc Psychiatry* 1990;29:45–48.
57. McDougle CJ, Goodman WK, Leckman JF, et al. The efficacy of fluvoxamine in obsessive–compulsive disorder: effects of comorbid chronic tic disorder. *J Clin Psychopharmacol* 1993;13:354–358.
58. Price RA, Kidd KK, Cohen DJ, et al. A twin study of Tourette syndrome. *Arch Genet Psychiatry* 1985;42:815–820.
59. Rasmussen SA, Tsuang MT. Clinical characteristics and family history in DSM-111 obsessive–compulsive disorder. *Am J Psychiatry* 1986;143:317–322.
60. Singer HS, Walkup JT. Tourette's syndrome and other tic disorders: diagnosis, pathophysiology and treatment. *Medicine* 1991;70:15–32.
61. Pauls DL, Pakstis AJ, Kurlan R, et al. Segregation and linkage analysis of Gilles de la Tourette's syndrome

and related disorders. *J Am Acad Child Adolesc Psychiatry* 1990;29:195–203.
62. Pauls DL, Raymond CL, Leckman JF, et al. A family study of Tourette's syndrome. *Am J Hum Genet* 1991; 48:154–163.
63. Heutink P, Breedveld GJ, van de Wetering BJM. Progress in gene localization. In: Kurlan R, ed. *Handbook of Tourette's syndrome and related tic and behavioral disorders*. New York: Marcel Dekker Inc, 1992: 317–335.
64. Haber SN, Lynd-Balta E. Basal ganglia-limbic systems interactions. In: Kurlan R, ed. *Handbook of Tourette's syndrome and related tic and behavioral disorders*. New York: Marcel Dekker Inc, 1992:243–266.
65. Haber SN, Kowall NW, Vonsattel JP, et al. Gilles de a Tourette syndrome: a postmortem neuropathological immunohistochemical study. *J Neurol Sci* 1986;75: 225–241.
66. Steingard R, Dillon-Stout D. Tourette's syndrome and obsessive–compulsive disorder. *Psychiatric Clin North Am* 1992;15:849–860.
67. Northan RS, Singer HS. Postencephalitic acquired Tourette-like syndrome in a child. *Neurology* 1991;41: 592–593.
68. Robertson MM. The Gilles de la Tourette syndrome: the current status. *Br J Psychiatry* 1989;154:147–169.
69. Luxenberg JS, Swedo DE, Flament MF, et al. Neuroanatomical abnormalities in obsessive–compulsive disorder. *Am J Psychiatry* 1988;145:1089–1093.
70. Rapoport JL. The biology of obsessions and compulsions. *Sci Am 1989*;3:83–89.
71. Jenike MA. Obsessive–compulsive disorder: a question of a neurologic lesion. *Compr Psychiatry* 1984;25: 298–304.
72. Cummings JL, Cunningham K. Obsessive–compulsive disorder in Huntington's disease. *Biol Psychiatry* 1992; 31:263–270.
73. Menza MA, Forman NW, Goldstein HS, et al. Parkinson's disease, personality, and dopamine. *J Neuropsychiatry Clin Neurosci* 1990;2:282–287.
74. Tomer R, Levin BE, Weiner WJ. Obsessive–compulsive symptoms and motor asymmetries in Parkinson's disease. *Neuropsychiatry Neuropsychol Behav Neurol* 1993;6:26–30.
75. Rapoport JL, Wise SP. Obsessive–compulsive disorder: evidence of basal dysfunction. *Psychopharmacol Bull* 1988;3:380–384.
76. Stuart A, Slater JM, Unwin HL, et al. A semiquantitative atlas of 5-hydroxytryptamine-I receptors in the primate brain. *Neuroscience* 1986;18:619–639.
77. Jenike M. Drug treatment of obsessive–compulsive disorder. In: Jenike M, Baer L, Minichello W, eds. *Obsessive–compulsive disorder: theory and management*. Chicago: Year Book Medical Publishers, 1990: 249–282.
78. Stein DJ. Obsessive–compulsive disorder. *The Lancet* 2002;360:397–405.
79. Goodman WK, McDougle CJ, Price LH, et al. Beyond the serotonin hypothesis: a role for dopamine in some forms of obsessive compulsive disorder? *J Clin Psychiatry* 1990;51:36–43.
80. Marazzitl D, Hollander E, Lensi P, et al. Peripheral markers of serotonin and dopamine function in obsessive–compulsive disorder. *Psychiatry Res* 1992; 42:41–51.
81. Leckman JF, Goodman WK, North WG, et al. Elevated cerebrospinal fluid levels of oxytocin in obsessive–compulsive disorder: comparison with Tourette's syndrome and healthy controls. *Arch Genet Psychiatry* 1994;54:782–792.
82. Baxter LR. Neuroimaging studies of obsessive compulsive disorder. *Psychiatric Clin North Am* 1993;15: 871–884.
83. Baxter LR, Schwartz JM, Guze BH, et al. PET imaging in obsessive compulsive disorder with and without depression. *J Clin Psychiatry* 1990;51:61–69.
84. George MS, Trimble MR, Costa DC, et al. Elevated frontal cerebral blood flow in Gilles de la Tourette syndrome: a 99Tcm-HMPAO SPECT study. *Psychiatr Res* 1993;5:143–151.
85. Chase TN, Foster NL, Fedio P, et al. Gilles de la Tourette syndrome: studies with fluorine-18-labeled fluorodeoxyglucose positron emission tomographic method. *Ann Neurol* 1984;15:175.
86. Baxter LR, Guze BH. Neuroimaging. In: Kurlan R, ed. *Handbook of Tourette's syndrome and related tic and behavioral disorders*. New York: Marcel Dekker Inc, 1992:289–304.
87. Breiter HC, Rauch SL, Kwong KK, et al. Functional magnetic resonance imaging of symptom provocation in obsessive–compulsive disorder. *Ar Genet Psychiatry* 1996;53:595–606.
88. Peterson BS, Skudlarski P, Anderson AW, et al. A functional magnetic resonance imaging study of tic suppression in Tourette's syndrome. *Arch Genet Psychiatry* 1998;55:326–333.
89. Braun AR, Stoetter B, Randolph C, et al. The functional neuroanatomy of Tourette's syndrome: An FDG-PET study. I. Regional changes in cerebral glucose metabolism differentiating patients and controls. *Neuropsychopharmacology* 1993;9:277–291.
90. Meyer P, Bohnen NI, Minoshima S, et al. Striatal presynaptic monoaminergic vesicles are not increased in Tourette's syndrome. *Neurology* 1999;53:371–374.
91. McGrath MJ, Campbell KM, Parks CR, Burton FH III. Glutamatergic drugs exacerbate symptomatic behavior in a transgenic model of comorbid Tourette's syndrome and obsessive–compulsive disorder. *Brain Res* 2000;877:23–30.
92. Nordstrom EJ, Burton FH. A transgenic model of comorbid Tourette's syndrome and obsessive–compulsive disorder circuitry. *Mol Psychiatry* 2002;7:617–625.
93. Flament MF, Koby E, Rapoport JL, et al. A childhood obsessive–compulsive disorder: a prospective follow-up study. *J Child Psychol Psychiatry* 1990;3:363–380.
94. King RA, Riddle MA. *Pathways of growth: essentials of child psychiatry*, Vol. 2. New York: Wiley; 1991.
95. Leckman JF. Tourette's syndrome. In: Hollander E, ed. *Obsessive compulsive-related disorders*. Washington, DC: American Psychiatric Press, 1993:113–137.
96. Ratzoni G, Hermesh H, Brandt N, et al. Clomipramine efficacy for tics, obsessions, and compulsions in Tourette's syndrome and obsessive–compulsive disorder: a case study. *Biol Psychiatry* 1990;27:95–98.
97. Yaryura-Tobias JA. Clomipramine treatment in. Gilles de la Tourette disease. *Am J Psychiatry* 1975; 132:1221.
98. Yaryura-Tobias JA, Neziroglu GA. Gilles de la. Tourette syndrome: a new clinico-therapeutic approach. *Prog Neuropsychopharmacol* 1977;1:355–358.

99. Caine ED, Polinsky RJ, Ebert MH, et al. Trial of chlorimipramine and desipramine for Gilles de la Tourette syndrome. *Ann Neurol* 1979;6:305–306.
100. Riddle MA, Leckman JF, Hardin MT, et al. Fluoxetine treatment of obsessions and compulsions In patients with Tourette's syndrome. *Am J Psychiatry* 1988;145:1173–1174.
101. Como PG, Kurlan R. An open-label trial of fluoxetine for obsessive–compulsive disorder in Gilles de la Tourette's syndrome. *Neurology* 1991;41:872–874.
102. Kurlan R, Como PG, Delley C, et al. A pilot controlled study of fluoxetine for obsessive–compulsive symptoms in children with Tourette's syndrome. *Clin Neuropharmacol* 1993;16:167–172.
103. McDougle CJ, Goodman WK, Leckman JF, et al. The efficacy of fluvoxamine in obsessive–compulsive disorder: effects of comorbid chronic tic disorder. *J Clin Psychopharmacol* 1993;13:354–358.
104. Leckman JF, Hardin MT, Riddle MA, et al. Clonidine treatment of Gilles de la Tourette's syndrome. *Arch Genet Psychiatry* 1991;48:324–328.
105. Scahill L, Chappell PB, Kim YS, et al. A placebo-controlled study of guanfacine in the treatment of children with tic disorders and attention deficit hyperactivity disorder. *Am J Psychiatry* 2001;158:1067–1074.
106. Singer HS, Wendlandt J, Krieger M, et al. Baclofen treatment in Tourette syndrome: a double-blind, placebo-controlled, crossover trial. *Neurology* 2001;56:599–604.
107. Greenberg BD, Altemus M, Murphy DL. The role of neurotransmitters and neurohormones in obsessive–compulsive disorder. *Int Rev Psychiatry* 1997;9:31–44.
108. Altemus M, Greenberg BD, Keuler D, et al. Open trial of Flutamide for treatment of obsessive–compulsive disorder. *J Clin Psychiatry* 1999;60:442–445.
109. Miguel EC, Shavitt RG, Ferrao YA, et al. How to treat OCD in patients with Tourette syndrome. *J Psychosom Res* 2003;55:49–57.
110. Perlmutter SJ, Leitman SF, Garvey MA, et al. Therapeutic plasma exchange and intravenous immunoglobulin for obsessive–compulsive disorder and tic disorder in childhood. *Lancet* 1999;354:1153–1158.
111. Delgado PL, Goodman WK, Price LH, et al. Fluvoxamine/pimozide treatment of concurrent Tourette's and obsessive compulsive disorder. *Br J Psychiatry* 1990;157:762–765.
112. McDougle CJ, Goodman WK, Price LH, et al. Neuroleptic addition in fluvoxamine-refractory obsessive–compulsive disorder. *Am J Psychiatry 1990*;147:652–654.
113. McDougle CJ, Goodman WK, Leckman JF, et al. Haloperidol addition in Fluvoxamine-refractory obsessive–compulsive disorder: a double-blind, placebo-controlled study in patients with and without tics. *Arch Genet Psychiatry* 1994;51:302–308.
114. Baer L, Minichello WE. Behavior therapy for obsessive–compulsive disorder. In: Jenike M, Baer L, Minichello W, eds. *Obsessive–compulsive disorder: theory and management*. Chicago: Year Book Medical Publishers, 1990:203–232.
115. Azrin NH, Peterson AL. Behavior therapy for Tourette's syndrome and tic disorders. In: Cohen DJ, Bruun RD, Leckman JF, eds. *Tourette's syndrome and tic disorders: clinical understanding and treatment*, New York: John Wiley and Sons, 1988.
116. Azrin NH, Peterson AL. An evaluation of behavioral treatments for Tourette's syndrome. *Behav Res Ther* 1992;30:167–174.
117. Mindus P, Jenike MA. Neurosurgical treatment of malignant obsessive compulsive disorder. *Psychiatric Clin North Am* 1992;15:921–938.
118. Kurlan R, Kersun J, Ballantine HT, et al. Neurosurgical treatment of severe obsessive–compulsive disorder associated with Tourette's syndrome. *Mov Disord* 1990;5:152–155.
119. Leckman JF, de Lotbinize AJ, Marek K, et al. Severe disturbances in speech, swallowing, and gait following stereotactic infrathalamic lesions in Gilles de la Tourette's syndrome. *Neurology* 1993;43:890–894.

19

Behavioral Abnormalities in Wilson's Disease

George J. Brewer

*Department of Human Genetics and Department of Internal Medicine,
University of Michigan Medical School, Ann Arbor, Michigan*

INTRODUCTION AND HISTORIC OVERVIEW

The main focus of this chapter is the behavioral abnormalities in Wilson's disease. However, to better understand how the behavioral abnormalities of this disorder fit into recognition, diagnosis, therapy, and prognosis, it is necessary to briefly review the fundamentals of the disease. Thus, we cover these areas before turning to the behavioral focus of this chapter in the final section.

Wilson first described this disorder, which bears his name, noting the association of liver disease with a neurologic movement disorder caused by pathology in various structures of the brain, such as the lenticular nucleus (1). Interestingly, with regard to the focus of this chapter, he also noted behavioral abnormalities in many patients with this disorder. Subsequently, other important discoveries were made, including the frequent presence of rings in the cornea of the eye, named after their codiscoverers, Kayser (2) and Fleischer (3). Gradually, the etiologic role of copper accumulation and copper toxicity was discovered (4–9). After biliary excretion of copper was found to be the mechanism for maintaining copper balance (10), the discovery was made that patients with Wilson's disease had defective biliary excretion of copper, which caused the copper accumulation (11). In other studies, the level of the copper-containing serum protein, ceruloplasmin, was found to be usually quite low in patients with Wilson's disease (12,13) and it was established that the disease was inherited as an autosomal recessive trait (14). Walshe developed two effective oral therapies for the disease, penicillamine (15) and trientine (16). Brewer and colleagues, in the United States, developed zinc for maintenance therapy (17–19), whereas Schouwink (20) and Hoogenraad (21) used zinc in patients with Wilson's disease in the Netherlands. The causative gene has been identified (22–24), leading to a discussion of molecular causation. Several monographs and reviews have been published on Wilson's disease and may be consulted for more background and details about the disease and its treatment (19,25–30).

MOLECULAR ETIOLOGY AND PATHOGENESIS

The causative gene is called *adenosine triphosphate 7B* (ATP7B) and codes for a copper-binding, membrane-bound ATPase. It bears a strong homology to the causative gene for Menke's disease, called ATP7A. The ATP7B protein is somehow involved in copper trafficking in the liver, and when both copies are defective, excess copper is not excreted into the bile. The protein also appears to be involved with ensuring that copper is incorporated normally into ceruloplasmin in the liver; defective ATP7B results in low secretion of mature ceruloplasmin into the blood.

Most diets contain about 1.0 mg of copper per day, which is about 0.25 mg more than required. Normally, this excess is excreted in the bile and lost in the stool. In patients with Wilson's disease, the failure to excrete this excess leads to a slow accumulation of copper. At first, the excess is stored in the liver, at least partially bound to metallothionein. After a time, the storage capacity of the liver is exceeded and liver damage begins. This damage probably begins in most patients during early childhood. In most patients, the liver damage is subclinical for a long time; that is, nothing is apparent to call attention to the underlying damage. With the liver unable to store more copper, circulating levels rise, and copper accumulates elsewhere in the body. The next most sensitive organ is the brain. About 50% of patients eventually present with clinically apparent liver disease at some point, whereas the remaining 50% present with brain manifestations. In about 50% of patients who develop brain manifestations, the symptoms are behavioral at first, preceding the onset of a neurologic movement disorder. In the remaining 50%, the onset of the movement disorder is often associated with concomitant behavioral disturbances.

The copper toxicity is oxidant in nature (25). Although the location of damage in the liver is no doubt related to the very high levels of copper in this organ, why certain areas of the brain are vulnerable is unclear. Copper levels are elevated in these areas, but they are not higher than in other parts of the brain that are unaffected. Nor are brain levels of copper any higher than similarly elevated levels of copper in organs that do not appear to be damaged. One can speculate either that the affected areas of the brain that produce symptoms are more sensitive to oxidant damage or that the oxidant defenses in these areas are not as good as in unaffected areas.

CLINICAL PRESENTATIONS

The hepatic presentations tend to occur in the teenage years or in the early twenties in Western countries. In India and other countries of the Far East, and perhaps in some populations of the Middle East, patients often present at a much earlier age (31–33). The hepatic presentation can take the form of an episode of hepatitis, with jaundice and other liver function test abnormalities. If undiagnosed, the hepatitis usually will resolve, only to recur. This cycle can go on for years, often leading to the misdiagnosis of chronic active hepatitis. In other patients, the liver damage results in cirrhosis severe enough to be discovered, either at the time of routine checkups, or perhaps because of a complication of the accompanying portal hypertension, such as bleeding esophageal or gastric varices. In some patients, the initial presentation is the development of hepatic failure, with ascites, peripheral edema, jaundice, and other symptoms of hepatic decompensation. This episode can be an explosive, fulminant event, in which case the only thing that will save the patient's life is hepatic transplantation. More mild to moderate hepatic failure can be treated effectively with medical therapy (34).

The last section of this chapter deals extensively with behavioral abnormalities, and thus they are not discussed any further here, except to point out that in some patients these abnormalities precede neurologic symptoms by a year or two, and that if the true cause were recognized, it could lead to an early diagnosis in many patients.

The neurologic presentation generally occurs in the late teenage years or in the twenties in most patients, although the age of presentation can be quite broad. Again, patients in the Far and Middle East tend to present with symptoms earlier. The neurologic symptoms result from damage in areas of the brain that coordinate movement; hence, Wilson's disease in these patients is a movement disorder. Table 19-1 presents a list of relatively common symptoms.

The abnormalities can be clustered under three major subheadings: tremor, incoordination, and dystonia. Dysarthria is the most common symptom (35). Commonly, patients' speech is hypophonic (low volume) and slurred because of incoordination or dystonia of the speech muscles. The dysarthria of Wilson's disease is nonspecific, meaning that not even experts can differentiate the dysarthria of Wilson's disease from that of other disorders. Several types of tremor are seen

TABLE 19-1. *Neurologic abnormalities often present in Wilson's disease*

Tremor, occasionally chorea
Dystonia
Incoordination
Dysarthria
Rigidity
Dysdiadochokinesia
Abnormal posture and/or gait
Drooling
Dysphagia
Eye movement abnormalities, diplopia

in Wilson's disease, none specific enough for this disease to allow it to be identified and differentiated from other diseases that cause tremor. Incoordination usually begins by involving fine movements, such as handwriting and buttoning buttons, but may progress to involve larger muscle groups of the hands, arms, and lower extremities. Dystonia may begin by muscle cramping in upper or lower extremities and then, in some patients, progress and gradually pull fingers, toes, hands, feet, arms, legs, neck, and trunk out of physiologic positions. This process is painful and may lead to irreversible contractures. In any given patient, the types and severity of these various disorders are quite variable.

A fairly large number of patients presenting neurologically have symptoms of autonomic nervous system dysfunction (36,37). These symptoms include postural hypotension, sexual problems, bladder or bowel malfunction, and others.

Motor and sensory systems are spared in Wilson's disease.

RECOGNITION OF AND SCREENING FOR WILSON'S DISEASE

A major problem in Wilson's disease is failure to recognize the disease, leading to long delays in diagnosis and further unnecessary, often irreversible, damage. Because the disease is treatable and treatment can arrest further damage, it is very important for a diagnosis to be made promptly. The three main problems that lead to a failure to recognize the possibility of Wilson's disease in a given patient are the rarity of the disease (about 1 in 40,000 in most populations), the wide variety of presenting symptoms, and the fact that the symptoms are not at all unique to Wilson's disease but occur in a variety of much more common diseases. Thus, the occasional patient with Wilson's disease tends to be hidden among hundreds of patients with viral hepatitis, alcoholic cirrhosis, essential tremor, and Parkinson's disease. Recommendations as to which patients should be screened for Wilson's disease are given in Table 19-2.

The screening tests recommended for Wilson's disease are listed in Table 19-3. The 24-hour urine copper test is the best overall screening test, because, in our experience, it is always greater than 100 µg per 24 hours (more than double the normal value) in symptomatic patients. The Kayser–Fleischer (KF) ring examination in patients with neurologic or behavioral symptoms is also very good, being positive in 99% or more of these patients. The serum ceruloplasmin test is useful as an index of suspicion, because levels are very

TABLE 19-2. *Types of patients that should be screened for Wilson's disease*

Viral negative hepatitis, chronic hepatitis, findings of persistently elevated transaminase enzymes
Cirrhosis under age 50 without a definitive diagnosis, patients under 50 with cirrhosis attributed to alcohol or hepatitis C
Hepatic failure patients under age 50
Patients with one or more symptoms of a movement disorder (see Table 19-1) under age 50
Diagnosis of Parkinson's disease, under age 50
Diagnosis of essential tremor, under age 50
Behavioral changes in a young person, such as loss of ability to focus, loss of emotional control, depression, accusations of substance abuse with little evidence

TABLE 19-3. *Recommended screening tests for Wilson's disease*

Test	Normal value	Symptomatic patients	Presymptomatic patients
24-h urine copper	20–50 µg	>100 µg	>65 µg
Kayser–Fleischer rings	Absent	Present in neurologic/psychiatric patients and in more than 50% of hepatic patients	30%–40%
Serum ceruloplasmin	20–35 mg/dL	Usually below 15. Low normal to normal in 15%	Same as symptomatic

low in a large proportion of patients. However, levels are normal or near normal in 10% to 20% of patients and are low in 10% of heterozygous carriers.

Screening tests that are not very useful include the so-called penicillamine provocative test, in which a dose of penicillamine is given to stimulate urine copper excretion. This test does not provide more information than the basic 24-hour urine copper excretion test and has not been standardized to determine if it separates heterozygous carriers from affected patients. Similarly, the 64 copper test, which evaluates incorporation of radiolabeled copper into ceruloplasmin over a 24- or 48-hour period, does not adequately separate carriers from affected persons. Mutation screening has not turned out to be generally useful because of the large number of causative mutations in ATP7B (38); the lack of a few mutations common enough to dominate the picture makes it impractical to screen patients (or diagnose them) in this manner in all but a few populations.

DEFINITIVE DIAGNOSIS OF WILSON'S DISEASE

In many patients, particularly in patients presenting with neurologic or behavioral symptoms, the screening tests provide adequate diagnostic certainty. For example, in such a patient, a 24-hour urine copper result greater than 100 μg and the presence of KF rings is adequate for diagnosis. A liver biopsy can be added for confirmation but is usually not necessary.

The diagnosis in the liver presentation is often a little more difficult, because KF rings are usually not present, and liver disease of other types, particularly those with an obstructive component, can elevate urine and even liver levels of copper. Usually, measuring liver copper levels quantitatively separates out the patients affected with Wilson's disease. In the most difficult cases, clues such as a low ceruloplasmin result can be very useful.

Full siblings of affected patients have a 25% risk of being affected but could still be asymptomatic. About 50% of such affected siblings have diagnostically elevated 24-hour urine copper, and about a third have KF rings. If both urine copper and KF rings are present, the diagnosis is established. If the urine copper is completely normal (less than 50 μg per 24 hours) after age 15 years, the patient may be unaffected. If the urine copper is intermediately elevated, the patient could be affected or be a carrier. Such a patient should have either a liver biopsy or a haplotype analysis. The haplotype analysis involves DNA studies to see if the sibling has inherited the same two chromosomes, containing a Wilson's mutation, that the index case has.

TREATMENT OF WILSON'S DISEASE

The treatment of Wilson's disease should be individualized (see Table 19-4), because simply using one drug to treat all phases and types of Wilson's disease is no longer reasonable. Initial therapy is designed to bring the acute copper toxicity under control, so that no further copper damage occurs. This phase generally requires a period of 8 to 16 weeks, depending on the drug used.

For maintenance (lifelong) therapy, to prevent reoccurrence of copper accumulation and copper toxicity, all three commercially available drugs (zinc, trientine, and penicillamine) are effective. We prefer zinc because of its superior safety profile, with trientine as second choice, because it is less toxic than penicillamine. Zinc

TABLE 19-4. *Treatment of Wilson's disease*

Type of therapy	1st choice	2nd choice
Maintenance	Zinc	Trientine
Presymptomatic	Zinc	Trientine
Pediatric	Zinc	Trientine
Pregnant	Zinc	Trientine
Initial—neurologic	Tetrathiomolybdate	Zinc or trientine
Initial—hepatic	Zinc plus trientine	Zinc plus penicillamine

TABLE 19-5. *Use of anticopper medications*

Medication	Adult dose	Monitoring
Zinc	50 mg t.i.d. separated from food by 1 h (pediatric dose: 25 mg bid until age 6, then 25 mg t.i.d. until age 16 or 125 pounds)	Urine copper every 3–6 mo, should be held below 125 μg/24 h Urine zinc done concomitantly should be above 2.0 mg/24 h
Trientine	500 mg bid separated from food, at least 1/2 h before and 2 h after	Early frequent monitoring of blood counts, chemistries, and urine Urine copper every 3–6 mo—see text
Penicillamine	Same as trientine	Same as trientine

acts by inducing intestinal cell metallothionein, which blocks copper absorption (39–42). Zinc regimens and monitoring methods are given in Table 19-5. Trientine and penicillamine are chelators that increase the urinary excretion of copper.

For presymptomatic patients, we use zinc from the beginning. For maintenance treatment of pediatric patients, we use zinc in reduced dosages (Table 19-5). During pregnancy, women should continue anticopper therapy to protect their own health. Zinc is our first choice (43), with trientine second. Penicillamine has some known teratogenicity (44–46). Our recommendation during pregnancy, irrespective of the drug used, is not to control copper levels too strongly so as to avoid copper deficiency, known to be teratogenic, in the fetus.

Initial treatment of patients with neurologic or psychiatric presentations is problematic, in that penicillamine has a 50% risk of worsening the neurologic condition, and 50% of those who worsen, or 25% of the original sample of patients, never recover their prepenicillamine baseline state (47). The mechanism probably involves mobilization of hepatic copper to the brain. On the basis of preliminary studies, trientine seems to have some risk of worsening the neurologic condition, but the risk appears to be less than with penicillamine (48). Zinc, we believe, is too slow acting for this type of patient.

The lack of a good treatment for this type of patient led us to evaluate tetrathiomolybdate (TM) (49–52). TM is a fast-acting, potent anticopper drug that quickly brings copper toxicity under control. Occasionally, patients (3.6% in our recent study) show worsening of neurologic symptoms while taking TM for initial treatment (52).

We believe that this occasional worsening during TM treatment is simply a part of the natural history of the disease, whereas the high frequency of worsening with penicillamine and to a lesser extent, trientine, is drug catalyzed.

Our recommendation for initial treatment of the neurologic presentation is to use TM for an 8- or 16-week program. Zinc can be started concomitantly and then continued when TM is stopped. The main problem with this recommendation is that TM is not yet commercially available and as of this writing is used only in a research protocol at the University of Michigan. As a second option, zinc alone can be useful, despite the possibility that the disease may progress until copper toxicity is controlled. An alternative option is to use trientine and accept the risk of worsening. If symptoms worsen, the trientine could be stopped.

In treating the hepatic failure presentation of Wilson's disease, one has to first consider the severity of the failure. If the patient's condition is too severe, the patient may have little chance of survival without hepatic transplantation. We use the Nazer index to triage these patients (53). The Nazer index combines three measures of liver status: bilirubin, prothrombin time, and serum aspartate aminotransferase (AST) levels. A score more than 6 indicates that the patient is unlikely to survive with only penicillamine medical treatment.

If medical therapy is used, we recommend a combination of 500 mg of trientine b.i.d. and 50 mg of zinc t.i.d. (34). This combination may provide better medical therapy than penicillamine alone, because we have had patients survive with Nazer scores as high as 9.

PROGNOSIS

Improvement in the neurologic disease after initiating treatment begins in about 5 to 6 months and continues for about 2 years. Disability after that is likely to be permanent, although the patient's status can be improved with physical therapy and so on. Our experience with drug treatment is that improvement is usually substantial. Remaining disability depends on the initial severity of the disease. Patients with mild to moderate disease often resume a relativity normal life. Improvement in behavioral symptoms generally follows the improvement in neurologic symptoms.

Improvement in the liver status after initiating treatment in patients with liver failure begins at about 2 to 4 months and continues for about a year. Generally, liver status tests normalize by 1 year. Of course, these patients, as well as most patients with neurologic symptoms and even those who are presymptomatic, have residual liver damage and often cirrhosis. However, in the absence of additional liver insults, residual liver damage in most patients will not affect lifespan.

One of the long-term risk factors is variceal bleeding from portal hypertension. Other patients may have the risk of aspiration as a result of dysphagia. A major problem is nonadherence to anticopper therapy. This therapy is lifelong, and many patients, particularly during their younger years, fail to adhere adequately, and their disease relapses as a consequence.

BEHAVIORAL ABNORMALITIES

The importance of the behavioral abnormalities in Wilson's disease has been underappreciated clinically throughout the history of the disease, with the hepatic and neurologic movement disorders taking center stage. However, the presence of behavioral abnormalities has been recognized from the very beginning. Wilson, in his article that initially defined this disease, reported substantial behavioral problems in 8 of his 12 cases (1). Since then, many authors have described various psychopathologic features, such as depression, anxiety, loss of emotional control, difficulty focusing on tasks, exhibitionism, antisocial behavior, and frank psychosis (54–75). Yet, these problems have not surfaced at the level of clinical awareness enough that they can be adequately used for diagnosis, prognosis, and treatment, or for providing an understanding of some of the problems the patient and the family may be facing.

In this section, we discuss three phases of behavioral abnormalities in Wilson's disease:

1. Behavioral abnormalities preceding or present at the time of clinical presentation, which are important in assisting early diagnosis of the disease.
2. Response of behavioral abnormalities to anticopper therapy; the prognosis for improvement.
3. Residual behavioral abnormalities in patients adequately treated with anticopper therapy.

Behavioral Abnormalities Preceding or Present at Diagnosis

Behavioral abnormalities are very common at diagnosis, particularly if the presentation is neurologic (58). Of the 31 patients who presented with neurologic symptoms in the Akil et al. series (58), 24 (about 75%) had psychiatric symptoms. These symptoms were primarily personality changes (in about 71% of the 24 patients), depression (in about 42%), and, occasionally, psychosis (in 8%). Personality changes included irritability, emotionality, bouts of anger or temper tantrums, anxiety, hypomania, sexual preoccupation or loss of sexual inhibition, excessive hand washing, and others. This list of abnormalities should not be considered exhaustive but rather illustrative of the types of behavioral manifestations. A given patient may have any combination of these symptoms.

Depression, found in 42% of patients, was felt to be underestimated, because only 50% of the patients were interviewed by a psychiatrist, and depression was probably underreported in the other patients (58). Suffice it to say that depression is quite common in these patients. To know whether depression in a given patient is primarily reactive—that is, whether it is a response to being ill or part of the copper toxicity syndrome—is difficult.

These abnormalities can precede the first neurologic symptoms by months or probably even a year or two. Our rule of thumb is that if the behavioral abnormalities were present three or more years before clinical presentation of neurologic disease, one should be skeptical of their relationship to Wilson's disease. They may simply be coincidental phenomena.

Cognitive changes are also quite common and were reported in 17% of the 24 patients in the study by Akil et al. (58). These changes are more often manifestations of an inability to focus on tasks, rather than true cognitive decline, although cognitive decline can also occur. The inability to focus causes drastic performance declines in school or at work and often leads to a misdiagnosis of substance abuse.

In my experience, patients with a purely hepatic presentation (no neurologic symptoms) rarely have obvious behavioral abnormalities (other than depression, which may be reactive) assignable to Wilson's disease. However, abnormalities may be present in some such patients but perhaps not as obvious as in patients with the neurologic presentation. The same may be said for patients diagnosed at the presymptomatic stage.

Dening and Berrios (65) reported retrospectively on psychiatric symptoms in 195 cases of Wilson's disease, all seen by John Walshe, the primary caregiver for Wilson's disease in Cambridge, England. The authors studied patients' first admissions, but many participants had apparently been previously treated for Wilson's disease, so the sample in fact appears to be a mixed population of untreated and previously treated patients. The data came primarily from the personal file that Dr. Walshe kept on each patient. The authors' analysis did not differentiate among patients with neurologic, hepatic, and presymptomatic presentations, although judging by one of their comments, patients with neurologic presentations were probably the most prevalent.

The authors found that 51% of the patients had some psychopathologic feature, and 20% were seen by psychiatrists before the diagnosis of Wilson's disease (65). Disorders of behavior, which included incongruous behavior, irritability, aggression, and personality change, were common. The authors paint a "typical" picture of odd, reckless, and disinhibited behavior, with loss of impulse control.

Although cognitive impairment initially seemed to be present in 45 cases, it was definitely present in only 11 (65). In many cases, the comment in the notes that indicated suspicion of impairment was based on the patients' appearance. The tests that were performed on a few patients may have produced poor scores because of diminished motor skills. Definite depression was found in 8 patients but was suspected in 33 others. Psychiatric symptoms (delusions and hallucinations) were rare, present in only 1% of patients.

Rathbun (62) reported on a series of 34 consecutive patients seen at the University of Michigan Medical Center, with myself as the primary caregiver for Wilson's disease; most patients were in the early stages of anticopper therapy. Of these patients, 22 presented with neurologic symptoms, 2 presented with liver disease, 1 presented with both neurologic and hepatic disease, and 9 were asymptomatic (presymptomatic, in our literature).

Of the 34 patients, 17 had histories of psychiatric disorders, including 7 patients with anxiety disorders (e.g., agoraphobia, conversion reaction, panic disorder), 9 patients with depression, and 1 patient with schizophrenia (62). Of these 17 patients, 10 had been hospitalized in a psychiatry facility from 2 weeks to several months before diagnosis.

The Michigan Neuropsychological Battery series of tests were conducted on these patients (62). The study design involved comparing scores of the 25 symptomatic patients to those of the 9 asymptomatic patients. In general, the mean scores of the symptomatic patients were lower than scores of the asymptomatic patients on almost all the tests, and the difference reached statistical significance on many tests. In particular, various aspects of IQ testing were consistently lower for the symptomatic patients, significantly so on one subtest. The symptomatic patients' performance was significantly poorer on the digit symbol substitution tests, one of which was oral and did not require motor skills. One test, the Purdue Pegboard Test, although showing severe deficits in symptomatic patients, also showed significant deficits in asymptomatic patients compared to the norm. The author suggests that this test may be of value diagnostically as showing an early abnormality in Wilson's disease (62).

Lauterbach et al. (75) reviewed the literature for neuropsychiatric abnormalities in "lenticular diseases," including Wilson's disease. They state that across studies, one fifth of Wilson's disease patients present initially with psychiatric features only, one-third present with predominantly psychiatric features, and two thirds eventually develop psychiatric abnormalities. They estimate that 50% of patients may undergo psychiatric hospitalization before the diagnosis of Wilson's disease is made.

The authors comment on the high rate of personality changes, typically manifesting as irritability or aggression, and on the relatively high rate of depression and the low rate of psychoses, which seem to be no more common than in the general population (75).

Many papers and books have been published that discuss psychiatric and behavioral disorders in Wilson's disease; some of these references are included here (54–75). From the publications that are cited above in some detail, and these other papers, a general picture of the behavioral abnormalities emerges, as presented in Table 19-6. Some numbers are provided to give a general picture of which abnormalities are the most prevalent, but these numbers should be recognized as estimates. A major problem with estimating prevalence is that patients in various studies are not always differentiated as to type of disease (neurologic, hepatic, asymptomatic) and may vary considerably in disease severity and other characteristics such as whether they had been diagnosed by a psychiatrist. In addition, in some studies, some of the patients had been treated for a time with anticopper agents.

The behavioral abnormalities in Wilson's disease may be summarized as follows. First, behavioral abnormalities are very common before and during presentation, particularly in patients who ultimately present with neurologic symptoms. Most of these patients see a psychiatrist or other behavioral health care worker long before the diagnosis is made. As we have emphasized, these early symptoms could be a diagnostic aid in Wilson's disease, but the true cause of these symptoms usually remains unrecognized until later, when neurologic symptoms develop. This situation results in delayed diagnosis and allows more injury to occur, some of which is likely to be irreversible. One estimate is that the diagnosis is missed in two thirds of patients who present with neurologic symptoms (most of whom have behavioral abnormalities), leading to a mean 13-month delay in diagnosis (76).

Second, the most common abnormalities are personality changes and mood disorders. The mood disorder is primarily depression, but the personality changes cover a wide variety of symptomatic expressions.

Third, cognitive impairment is often suspected in Wilson's disease, particularly in neurologically affected patients, but if present, impairment is usually mild. It is often probably more apparent than real and is suspected because of impaired motor function and because of difficulty focusing on tasks. As the tests performed by Rathbun (62) indicate, impairment (except on isolated tests) is quite mild.

The exact parts of the brain that are affected by copper toxicity to produce these behavioral abnormalities are difficult to ascertain. All parts of the brain have elevated copper levels in untreated Wilson's disease (55). In the areas involved in producing movement disorder neurologic symptoms, such as the basal ganglia, copper levels are not higher than in other parts of the brain (55). Thus, the assumption is that the basal ganglia and other areas damaged in the movement

TABLE 19-6. *Behavioral abnormalities in Wilson's disease at time of presentation*

Overall frequency	2/3 of neurologic patients 1/2 of mixed patients
Psychiatric treatment before diagnosis	2/3 of neurologic patients 1/3 of mixed patients

Common Abnormalities

Abnormality	Frequency
Personality changes	67% of neurologic patients 50% of mixed patients
Mood (primarily depression)	40% of neurologic patients 30% of mixed patients
Apparent significant cognitive impairment	20% of neurologic patients 10% of mixed patients

disorder presentation are simply more vulnerable to an elevated level of copper than other areas of the brain.

The same is probably true for areas affecting behavior; in some patients, these areas, which are probably multiple, are simply more sensitive to copper damage than other areas of the brain not affected, and more sensitive in these patients than in patients who do not show behavioral symptoms.

Some insight into the complicated interconnections in the brain that can affect behavior if injured can be found in the paper by Lauterbach et al. (75). From their review of "lenticulostriatal" diseases including Wilson's, I quote:

> The basal ganglia lenticulostriatal system is integral to processing cortical and limbic information. This system is composed of circuits communicating between the lenticular nucleus (putamen and globus pallidus) and the striatum (caudate nucleus and putamen). The lenticulostriatal system receives information from multiple limbic structures including the amygdala, cingulate gyrus, and nucleus accumbens (77). Projections to the thalamus and frontal lobe make the basal ganglia lenticulostriatal system of great importance in understanding behavior (78).
>
> The lenticulostriatal system is connected to the frontal cortex through five functionally segregated circuits implicated in motor, cognitive, and psychiatric manifestations of basal ganglia diseases (79,80). Three of these circuits—the dorsal prefrontal, orbitofrontal, and anterior cingulate—are implicated in primary psychiatric illnesses including depression, obsessive–compulsive disorder, and schizophrenia. Moreover, neurologic diseases involving these circuits carry an unusual proclivity for neuropsychiatric (81) and behavioral (82) disorders. Consequently, the basal ganglia lenticulostriatal system is one of the most important brain systems in neuropsychiatry.

The basic points to be made are

1. Patients with Wilson's disease often have both a neurologic movement disorder syndrome and numerous behavioral abnormalities.
2. Patients with Wilson's disease are known to have copper-induced damage to structures in the brain that affect movement control and behavior.

Response of Behavioral Abnormalities to Anticopper Therapy

The literature is rather meager on the response of Wilson's disease behavioral abnormalities to anticopper therapy. Only one study of any size has attempted to observe response to therapy, and it was retrospective. In 129 patients, Dening (64) noted that anticopper treatment significantly improved incongruous behavior and what he called cognitive impairment, usually during the first 3.5 years of treatment. However, symptoms such as irritability and depression tended to persist. Nonresponders were more likely than responders to have more dysarthria and hepatic involvement. Goldstein et al. (74) reported improved intellectual performance in eight patients after treatment. Other scattered case reports document improvements in hyperactivity, hypersexuality, disinhibition, aggressiveness, memory, IQ, and psychotic symptoms.

Our own experience with improvement in behavioral symptoms with treatment is anecdotal. Although we have seen and treated a very large number of newly diagnosed patients with the neurologic presentation, our scientific observations have been focused on neurologic improvement. Using a semiquantitative neurologic examination and a semiquantitative speech score, we have shown that most neurologic improvement occurs within 6 to 24 months after initiation of anticopper therapy (49–52).

A large proportion of these patients had behavioral abnormalities. Our experience has been that generally, considerable improvement in behavioral symptoms occurs during treatment, and the improvement follows the same time course as improvement in neurologic symptoms; that is, most of the improvement occurs during that 6- to 24-month window. Those patients that show neurologic improvement sufficient to resume a relatively normal life generally show comparable improvement in behavioral problems, such that the behavioral problems no longer are major impediments to living normal life. That is not to say that some abnormalities do not persist. Some abnormalities seem to be permanent residuals in patients treated for long periods. However, our impression is that those patients who recover the least neurologically also have the most residual behavioral problems, particularly depression. Of course, a good amount of the depression may be a reaction to the presence of continuing neurologic illness.

Residual Behavioral Abnormalities after Adequate Treatment with Anticopper Therapy

Certain abnormalities persist long enough after copper toxicity has been eliminated to be considered a relatively permanent part of the patient's damage. Generally, this damage is manifested as behavioral abnormalities that persist after 4 or 5 years of adequate anticopper therapy.

The group that has done the most work in this area is the team of Westermark, Portala, and others (69–73). Portala has done a dissertation (Ph.D. in Psychiatry) on this topic at Uppsala University in 2001 (73).

Twenty-nine patients who were treated for long periods were reported in the thesis (73). Two of the patients had received liver transplants; the rest were treated with anticopper drugs. Two patients never had symptoms, and four had primarily hepatic disease. Seven of the patients had a combination of hepatic disease and psychiatric symptoms. Eight patients had primarily neurologic symptoms. Four patients had a combination of neurologic and psychiatric symptoms. Three patients had a combination of hepatic, neurologic, and behavioral symptoms, and one had neurologic and hepatic symptoms.

Several components were present in the psychological assessment in the Portala thesis (73). One was a Comprehensive Psychopathological Rating Scale (CPRS) that was carried out by both self-assessment and by expert ratings (69,73). The main findings were that prominent psychopathology remained in these patients after long-term anticopper treatment. The mean score of the expert rating was 29.4, which is comparable to that of patients with moderate to severe depression (mean, 32.9) and is worse than that of patients with neurofibromatosis and psychiatric disease (mean, 16.1). By contrast, the mean score among healthy controls was 4.4. The authors found that the extent of psychiatric symptoms did not differ between patients presenting primarily with neurologic disease and those presenting primarily with hepatic disease.

The most common psychiatric symptoms were fatigability, difficulty concentrating, reduced sleep, muscular tension, sadness, and lack of appropriate emotion (69,73). The authors noted that women scored significantly higher (more abnormality) than men with respect to autonomic disturbances, rituals, feeling of being controlled, and labile emotional responses. Agreement between expert and self-ratings was low, with lower scores generally recorded in the self-assessment, a finding that indicates that patients underreport these symptoms. The authors suggest that expert evaluations ought to be part of the clinical assessment, to ensure that psychopathology is revealed and treated as necessary.

A study of personality traits was also carried out, using the Karolinska Scales of Personality (KSP) instrument, in which patients assess themselves (70,73). Female patients did not differ significantly from healthy female controls in any of the ratings, but male patients had less anxiety, suspicion, guilt, aggression, irritability, and hostility than healthy male controls. Further, male patients scored substantially lower (meaning they had less) than female patients in guilt, suspicion, and hostility. The opposite is usually found in healthy subjects.

The authors also studied sleep abnormalities in Wilson's disease (71,73). Forty-two percent of patients thought they had sleep problems, compared to the 25% in a control sample. No significant differences were observed in sleep time but patients took significantly longer to fall asleep and had greater numbers of nighttime awakenings correlated with nightmares. Patients also had significantly more episodes of a feeling of being temporarily paralyzed, either just before falling asleep or upon awakening. During the day, patients complained significantly more than controls of not being rested and of feeling fatigued. They took more naps during the day than controls.

The authors (72,73) also evaluated neuropsychological function using the Automated Psychological Test (APT). Patients with Wilson's disease performed more poorly than controls on all five finger-tapping tests, on simple reaction time, the simultaneous capacity background test, the short-term memory test, the index of word decoding speed, the grammatical reasoning test, and the perceptual maze test. They used a more global processing mode in selective attention. Simple reaction time varied considerably, and there was no significant correlation between simple and complex reaction time, whereas a strong correlation existed in healthy controls. Patients with hepatic and neurologic presentations had only minor differences and showed similar patterns.

In assessing the neuropsychological results, the authors comment that both simple and complex reaction times reflect important aspects of cognitive, executive, and behavioral functions, and that abnormalities seen in Wilson's disease are also seen in schizophrenia. The poor performance on the simultaneous capacity test illustrates the problems patients have in handling more than one task simultaneously. These patients use a more global strategy rather than a sequential strategy.

Portala et al. (69–73) have done an excellent job studying the residual abnormalities present in Wilson's disease after effective anticopper therapy. Although they studied a relatively small number of patients, much attention should be paid to their findings, and the study should be replicated as soon as possible with a larger number of patients. The following points are among the more important of their findings.

1. Extensive abnormalities are present in well-treated patients, suggesting that considerable permanent damage has been done to the circuits involved.
2. These abnormalities must have been present at time of presentation, suggesting that they are greatly underappreciated by clinicians diagnosing and treating these patients.
3. Anticopper treatment and great improvement in neurologic symptoms and liver function does not completely erase the psychological abnormalities.
4. These abnormalities are present to the same extent in patients with hepatic presentations (and probably also in presymptomatic patients) as they are in patients with neurologic presentations.

I feel some sense of discordance between the findings of Portala et al. (69–73) and my personal observations of patient recovery. The findings of Portala et al. (69–73) indicate very widespread and substantial behavioral and functional abnormalities and, if taken at face value, might suggest that patients with Wilson's disease remain very dysfunctional even after long-term anticopper treatment. On the other hand, my own experience is that when many of these patients initiate treatment, they are a psychiatric "mess," with all kinds of problems, including difficulties in interacting and functioning in society, but that 2 or 3 years later, they have resumed normal lives. Writers have resumed writing, editors have resumed editing, and doctors and nurses have resumed their medical careers. Looking at these patients after long-term anticopper treatment, I see them as functionally and psychologically normal. If my interpretations are valid, this psychological recovery is good news for patients. If they can feel and function normally, abnormal test results become less important.

Can these two seemingly conflicting observations both be valid? Perhaps, if in the process of healing, patients with Wilson's disease develop different coping mechanisms, as is suggested by Portala et al. (72,73) when they say the patients use a more global rather than a sequential strategy in solving problems. Perhaps defects persist and can be detected by tests, but they do not impair function substantially because the patients have developed compensatory mechanisms.

ACKNOWLEDGMENTS

The University of Michigan has filed a field of use patent for the antiangiogenic uses of TM. This property has been licensed to Attenuon LLC, a San Diego–based company. I have equity in and am a paid consultant to Attenuon.

REFERENCES

1. Wilson SAK. Progressive lenticular degeneration: a familial nervous disease associated with cirrhosis of the liver. *Brain* 1912;34:295–509.
2. Kayser B. Ueber einen Fall von angeborener grünlicher Verfärbung der kornea. *Klin Mbl Augenheilk* 1902;40:22–25.

3. Fleischer B. Zwei weitere Fälle von grünlicher Verfärbung der Kornea. *Klin Mbl Augenheilk* 1903;41:489–491.
4. Rumpel A. Ueber das wesen un die bedeutung der leberveränderungen und der pigmentierunen bei den damit verbundenen fällen von pseudosklerose, zugleich ein beitrag zur lehre von pseudosklerose (Westphal-Strümpell). *Dtsch Z Nervenheilk* 1913;49:54–73.
5. Vogt A. Kupfer und silber aufgespeichert in auge, leber, milz und nieren als symptoms der pseudosklerose. *Klin Mbl Augenheilk* 1929;83:417–419.
6. Haurowitz F. Ueber eine anomalie des kupferstoffwechsels. *Hoppe-Seviers Z Physiol Chem* 1930;190:72–74.
7. Glazebrook AJ. Wilson's disease. *Edinburgh Med J* 1945;52:83–87.
8. Cumings JN. The copper and iron content of brain and liver in the normal and in hepato-lenticular degeneration. *Brain* 1948;71:410–415.
9. Mandelbrote BM, Stanier MW, Thompson RHS, et al. Studies on copper metabolism in demyelinating disease of the central nervous system. *Brain* 1948;71:212–228.
10. Ravestyn AH. Metabolism of copper in man. *Acta Med Scand* 1944;118:163–196.
11. Frommer DJ. Defective biliary excretion of copper in Wilson's disease. *Gut* 1974;15:125–129.
12. Bearn AG, Kunkel HG. Biochemical abnormalities in Wilson's disease. *J Clin Invest* 1952;31:616.
13. Scheinberg IH, Gitlin D. Deficiency of ceruloplasmin in patients with hepatolenticular degeneration (Wilson's disease). *Science* 1952;116:484–485.
14. Bearn AG. A genetical analysis of thirty families with Wilson's disease (hepatolenticular degeneration). *Ann Hum Genet* 1960;24:33–43.
15. Walshe JM. Penicillamine. A new oral therapy for Wilson's disease. *Am J Med* 1956;21:487–495.
16. Walshe JM. Treatment of Wilson's disease with trientine (triethylene tetramine) dihydrochloride. *Lancet* 1982;1:643–647.
17. Brewer GJ, Hill GM, Prasad AS, et al. Oral zinc therapy for Wilson's disease. *Ann Intern Med* 1983;99:314–320.
18. Brewer GJ, Dick RD, Johnson VD, et al. Treatment of Wilson's disease with zinc: XV. Long-term follow-up studies. *J Lab Clin Med* 1998;132:264–278.
19. Brewer GJ. Recognition, diagnosis and management of Wilson's disease. *Proc Soc Exp Biol Med* 2000;223(1):39–49.
20. Schouwink G. De hepatocerebrale degeneratie, me een onderzoek naar de zinktofwisseling. MD Thesis, University of Amsterdam, 1961.
21. Hoogenraad TU, van Hattum J, van den Hamer CJA. Management of Wilson's disease with zinc sulphate. Experience in a series of 27 patients. *J Neurol Sci* 1987;77:137–146.
22. Bull PC, Thomas GR, Rommens JM, et al. The Wilson disease gene is a putative copper transporting P-type ATPase similar to the Menkes gene. *Nat Genet* 1993;5(4):327–337.
23. Tanzi RE, Petrukhin K, Chernov I, et al. The Wilson disease gene is a copper transporting ATPase with homology to the Menkes disease gene. *Nat Genet* 1993;5(4):44–50.
24. Yamaguchi Y, Heiny ME, Gitlin JD. Isolation and characterization of a human liver cDNA as a candidate gene for Wilson disease. *Biochem Biophy Res Commun* 1993;197:271–277.
25. Brewer GJ, Yuzbasiyan-Gurkan V. Wilson's disease. *Medicine* 1992;71:139–164.
26. Scheinberg IH, Sternlieb I. Wilson's disease. In: Smith LH Jr., ed. *Major problems in internal medicine*, Vol. 23. Philadelphia, PA: WB Saunders, 1984.
27. Hoogenraad TU. Wilson's disease. In: Warlow CP, Van Gijn J, eds. *Major problems in neurology*, Vol. 30. London: WB Saunders, 1996.
28. Brewer GJ. *Wilson's disease: a clinician's guide to recognition, diagnosis, and management.* Boston, MA: Kluwer Academic Publishers, 2001.
29. Brewer GJ. *Wilson's disease for the patient and family: a patient's guide to Wilson's disease and frequently asked questions about copper.* Philadelphia, PA: Xlibris, 2001.
30. Schilsky ML. Wilson disease: genetic basis of copper toxicity and natural history. *Semin Liver Dis* 1996;16:83–95.
31. Dastur DK, Manghani DK, Wadia NH. Wilson's disease in India I. Geographic, genetic, and clinical aspects in 16 families. *Neurology* 1968;18:21–31.
32. Bhave S, Bavdekar A, Pandit A. Changing pattern of chronic liver disease (CLD) in India. *Indian J Pediatr* 1994;61:675–682.
33. Bhave SA, Purohit GM, Pradhan AV, et al. Hepatic presentation of Wilson's disease. *Indian Pediatr* 1987;24:385–393.
34. Askari FK, Greenson J, Dick RD, et al. Treatment of Wilson's disease with zinc: XVIII. Initial treatment of the hepatic decompensation presentation with trientine and zinc. *J Lab Clin Med* 2003;142(6):385–390.
35. Starosta-Rubinstein S, Young AB, Kluin K, et al. Clinical assessment of 31 patients with Wilson's disease. Correlations with structural changes on MRI. *Arch Neurol* 1987;44:365–370.
36. Bhattacharya K, Velickovic M, Schilsky M, et al. Autonomic cardiovascular reflexes in Wilson's disease. *Clin Auton Res* 2002;12(3):190–192.
37. Meenakshi-Sundaram S, Taly AB, Kamath V, et al. Autonomic dysfunction in Wilson's disease—a clinical and electrophysiological study. *Clin Auton Res* 2002;12(3):185–189.
38. Cox DW, Roberts EA. Wilson disease. GeneClinics, University of Washington, Seattle, WA. Available: http://www.geneclinics.org/profiles/wilson/details.html.
39. Hall AC, Young BW, Bremmer I. Intestinal metallothionein and the mutual antagonism between copper and zinc in the rat. *J Inorg Biochem* 1979;11:57–66.
40. Menard MP, McCormick CC, Cousins RJ. Regulation of intestinal metallothionein biosynthesis in rats by dietary zinc. *J Nutr* 1981;111:1351–1361.
41. Oestreicher P, Cousins RJ. Copper and zinc absorption in the rat: mechanisms of mutual antagonism. *J Nutr* 1985;115:159–166.
42. Yuzbasiyan-Gurkan V, Grider A, Nostrant T, et al. The treatment of Wilson's disease with zinc: X. Intestinal metallothionein induction. *J Lab Clin Med* 1992;120:380–386.
43. Brewer GJ, Johnson VD, Dick RD, et al. Treatment of Wilson's disease with zinc: XVII. Treatment during pregnancy. *Hepatology* 2000;31:364–370.
44. Mjolnerod OK, Dommerud SA, Rasmussen K, et al. Congenital connective tissue defect probably due to D-penicillamine treatment in pregnancy. *Lancet* 1971;1:673–675.
45. Solomon L, Abrams G, Dinner M, et al. Neonatal abnormalities associated with D-penicillamine treatment during pregnancy. *N Engl J Med* 1977;296:54–55.
46. Rosa FW. Teratogen update: penicillamine. *Teratology* 1986;33:127–131.

47. Brewer GJ, Terry CA, Aisen AM, et al. Worsening of neurologic syndrome in patients with Wilson's disease with initial penicillamine therapy. *Arch Neurol* 1987; 44:490–493.
48. Brewer GJ, Schilsky M, Hedera P, et al. Double blind study of initial therapy of neurological Wilson's disease. *J Investig Med* 2003;51:2.
49. Brewer GJ, Dick RD, Yuzbasiyan-Gurkan V, et al. Initial therapy of patients with Wilson's disease with tetrathiomolybdate. *Arch Neurol* 1991;48:42–47.
50. Brewer GJ, Dick RD, Johnson V, et al. Treatment of Wilson's disease with ammonium tetrathiomolybdate: I. Initial therapy in 17 neurologically affected patients. *Arch Neurol* 1994;51:545–554.
51. Brewer GJ, Johnson V, Dick RD, et al. Treatment of Wilson disease with ammonium tetrathiomolybdate: II. Initial therapy in 33 neurologically affected patients and follow-up with zinc therapy. *Arch Neurol* 1996;53: 1017–1025.
52. Brewer GJ, Hedera P, Kluin KJ, et al. Treatment of Wilson's disease with tetrathiomolybdate: III. Initial therapy in a total of 55 neurologically affected patients and follow-up with zinc therapy. *Arch Neurol* 2003;60: 378–385.
53. Nazer H, Ede RJ, Mowat AP, et al. Wilson's disease: clinical presentation and use of prognostic index. *Gut* 1986;27:1377–1381.
54. Owen CA Jr. *Wilson's disease: the etiology, clinical aspects, and treatment of inherited copper toxicosis.* Park Ridge, NJ: Noyes Publications, 1981.
55. Brewer GJ, Fink JK, Hedera P. Diagnosis and treatment of Wilson's disease. *Semin Neurology* 1999;19(3): 261–270.
56. Williams DM, Lee GR. Hepatolenticular degeneration (Wilson's disease). In: Powell LW, ed. *Metals and the liver*. New York: Marcel Dekker Inc, 1978:241–311.
57. Brewer GJ. Yuzbasiyan-Gurkan V. Wilson's disease. *Medicine* 1992;71:139–164.
58. Akil M, Schwartz JA, Dutchak D, et al. The psychiatric presentations of Wilson's disease. *J Neurol Psychiatry Clin Neurosci* 1991;3:377.
59. Akil M, Brewer GJ. Psychiatric and behavioral abnormalities in Wilson's disease. In: Weiner WJ, Lang AE, eds. *Advances in neurology*, Vol. 65, *Behavioral neurology of movement disorders*. New York: Raven Press, 1995:171–178.
60. Jackson GH, Meyer A, Lippmann S. Wilson's disease: psychiatric manifestations may be the clinical presentation. *Postgrad Med* 1994;95:135–138.
61. Scheinberg IH, Sternlieb I, Richman J. Psychiatric manifestations in patients with Wilson's disease. *Birth Defects* 1968;4:85–99.
62. Rathbun JK. Neuropsychological aspects of Wilson's disease. *Int J Neurosci* 1996;85:221–229.
63. Knehr CA, Bearn AG. Psychological impairment in Wilson's disease. *J Nerv Ment Dis* 1956;124:251–255.
64. Dening TR. The neuropsychiatry of Wilson's disease: a review. *Int J Psychiatry Med* 1991;21:135–148.
65. Dening TR, Berrios GE. Wilson's disease: psychiatric symptoms in 195 cases. *Arch Gen Psychiatry* 1989;46: 1126–1134.
66. McDonald LV, Lake CR. Psychosis in an adolescent patient with Wilson's disease: effects of chelation therapy. *Psychosom Med* 1995;57:202–204.
67. Fink JK, Hedera P, Brewer GJ. Hepatolenticular degeneration (Wilson's disease). *Neurologist* 1999;5:171–185.
68. Oder W, Grimm G, Kollegger H, et al. Neurological and neuropsychiatric spectrum of Wilson's disease: a prospective study of 45 cases. *J Neurol* 1991;238: 281–287.
69. Portala K, Westermark K, von Knorring L, et al. Psychopathology in treated Wilson's disease determined by means of CPRS expert and self-ratings. *Acta Psychiatr Scand* 2000;101:104–109.
70. Portala K, Westermark K, Ekselius L, et al. Personality traits in treated Wilson's disease determined by means of the Karolinska scales of personality (KSP). *Eur Psychiatry* 2001;16:362–371.
71. Portala K, Westermark K, Ekselius L, et al. Sleep in patients with treated Wilson's disease. A questionnaire study. *Nord J Psychiatry* 2002;56(4):291–297.
72. Portala K, Levander S, Westermark K, et al. Pattern of neuropsychological deficits in patients with treated Wilson's disease. *Eur Arch Psychiatry Clin Neurol* 2001; 252(6):262–268.
73. Portala K. Psychopathology in Wilson's disease. Thesis, Acta Universitatis Upsaliensis, Uppsala, 2001.
74. Goldstein NP, Ewert JC, Randall RV, et al. Psychiatric aspects of Wilson's disease (hepatolenticular degeneration): results of psychometric tests during long-term therapy. *Am J Psychiatry* 1968;124:11.
75. Lauterbach EC, Cummings JL, Duffy J, et al. Neuropsychiatric correlates and treatment of lenticulostriatal diseases: a review of the literature and overview of research opportunities in Huntington's, Wilson's, and Fahr's diseases. A Report of the ANPA Committee on Research. *J Neuropsychiatry* 1998;10:249–266.
76. Walshe JM, Yealland M. Wilson's disease: the problem of delayed diagnosis. *J Neurol Neurosurg Psychiatry* 1992;55:692–696.
77. Nauta WJ. Limbic innervation of the striatum. *Adv Neurol* 1982;35:41–47.
78. Haber SN, Groenewegen HJ, Grove EA, et al. Efferent connections of the ventral pallidum: evidence of a dual striato pallidofugal pathway. *J Comp Neurol* 1985;235: 322–335.
79. Alexander GE, DeLong MR, Strick PL. Parallel organization of functionally segregated circuits linking basal ganglia and cortex. *Annu Rev Neurosci* 1986;9:357–381.
80. Cummings JL. Frontal subcortical circuits and human behavior. *Arch Neurol* 1993;50:873–880.
81. Robinson RG. In: Lauterbach EC, ed. *Psychiatric management in neurological disease*. Washington, DC: American Psychiatric Press, 2000.
82. Caplan LR, Schahmann JD, Kase CS, et al. Caudate infarcts. *Arch Neurol* 1990;47:133–143.

20
Hereditary Ataxia and Behavior

Nadejda Alekseeva,[1] Anita S. Kablinger,[1] James Pinkston,[2] Eduardo C. Gonzalez-Toledo,[3] and Alireza Minagar[2]

[1]Department of Psychiatry, Louisiana State University Health Sciences Center, Shreveport, Louisiana; [2]Department of Neurology, Louisiana State University Health Sciences Center, Shreveport, Louisiana; [3]Department of Radiology, Neurology, and Anesthesiology, Louisiana State University Health Sciences Center, Shreveport, Louisiana

The term "ataxia," derived from the Greek verb "tassein," means incapability to fine-tune posture and movement in a coordinated fashion. Neuropathologic processes that involve the cerebellum and its afferent and efferent connections cause ataxia. Ataxic syndromes may be hereditary or acquired. Hereditary ataxias are a diverse group of neurogenetic disorders, which share ataxia as their most prominent clinical feature. Autosomal dominant ataxias are a heterogeneous group, recognized by the presence of progressive truncal and limb ataxia. They include the spinocerebellar ataxias (SCAs), dentatorubral–pallidolusian atrophy (DRPLA), and episodic ataxias (EAs). The estimated prevalence of autosomal dominant cerebellar ataxias is 5 in 100,000 (1,2). Other hereditary ataxias show autosomal recessive (including Friedreich's ataxia) or X-linked inheritance. SCAs are similar to Huntington's disease (HD) and are caused by expanding CAG repeats that code for polyglutamines. As with HD, expansions of the repeat may occur in successive generations, leading to earlier onset of disease. All of the SCAs with already discovered genetic abnormality are caused by abnormal CAG repeats, which manifest as an expansion of polyglutamine "dose" above the threshold necessary to cause disease. A summary of SCA types, with the chromosomes and abnormal mutations involved, is presented in Table 20-1. Common brain areas affected include basal ganglia, brainstem nuclei, cerebellum, and spinal motor nuclei, along with distinct regions in each condition.

With more research into the clinical features of the autosomal dominant cerebellar ataxias, a clearer picture of the cognitive impairment and behavioral abnormalities associated with them is emerging. With each discovery, the role of normal cerebellar function and its connection with cerebral cortex in human behavior becomes better understood. Despite the presence of certain genetic and pathologic similarities among autosomal dominant hereditary ataxias, rates of behavioral abnormalities and cognitive impairment vary among these patients. At this time, no treatment is available to slow progression or to prevent onset of motor or behavioral symptoms in any of the hereditary ataxias.

SPINOCEREBELLAR ATAXIA 1

Spinocerebellar ataxia 1 (SCA1) is caused by an expansion of a CAG repeat within the SCA1 gene on chromosome 6p. It is the most common autosomal dominant ataxia worldwide, accounting for one third of cases (3). Patients with SCA1 present with increasing cerebellar and noncerebellar manifestations usually after age 20; however, a juvenile form has been described. Cerebellar manifestations of SCA1 include ataxia, gaze-evoked nystagmus, hypermetric saccades, decreased optokinetic nystagmus, and inability to suppress vestibule–ocular reflex. Noncerebellar neurologic symptoms consist of dysarthria, dysphagia, ophthalmoparesis, pyramidal tract abnormalities, muscle atrophy,

TABLE 20-1. Classification of hereditary spinocerebellar ataxic disorders

Disease	Chromosome	Gene product	Genetic mutation
Autosomal dominant SCA			
SCA1	6p22	Ataxin-1	Expansion of CAG repeat
SCA2	12q24.1	Ataxin-2	Expansion of CAG repeat
SCA3	14q32.1	Ataxin-3	Expansion of CAG repeat
SCA4	16q22.1	—	—
SCA5	11q13	—	—
SCA6	19p13.1	Calcium channel CACNLA1	Expansion of CAG repeat
SCA7	3p14	Ataxin-7	Expansion of CAG repeat
SCA8	13q21	Expansion of CTA/CTG repeat	—
SCA10	22q13	Expansion of ATTCT repeat	—
SCA11	15q14–q21.3	—	—
SCA12	5q31	Phosphatase 2A	Expansion of CAG repeat
SCA13	19q13.3–4	—	—
SCA14	19q13.4	—	—
SCA15		—	—
SCA16	8q22.1–24.1	—	—
SCA17		TATA-binding protein	Expansion of CAG/CAA repeat
SCA19	1p21–q12	—	—
SCA20	7p21.3–p15.1	—	—
SCA21	7p21.3–p15.1	—	—
DRPLA	12p13.31	Atrophin-1	Expansion of CAG repeat
Episodic ataxia 1	12p13	K channel (KCNA1)	Missense mutations
Episodic ataxia 2	19p13.1	Calcium channel (CACNLA1)	Truncating missense, or expansion of CAG repeat

loss of vibratory sensation, optic disc pallor, and bladder dysfunction.

Dementia is not reported to occur in SCA1, but mild cognitive impairment and mental deterioration is seen in 5% to 25% of patients in the advanced stages of the disease (4–10). Prominent impairment of verbal memory and fronto-executive tasks has been reported in SCA1 patients (11–13). Burk et al. (12) performed a detailed neuropsychological study of 15 SCA1 patients and 11 matched controls, including tests for IQ, attention, verbal and visuospatial memory, and executive functions. These tests revealed verbal memory and executive function abnormalities in SCA1 patients, whereas visuospatial memory and attention were not significantly impaired compared to that in healthy controls. The authors concluded that cognitive impairment seen in SCA1 patients corresponds to the concept of "frontal–subcortical" dementia, reflecting disruption of afferent and efferent pathways of the prefrontal cortex and subcortical structures, including the cerebellum. Certain features such as aphasia, agnosia, and apraxia, which occur in patients with cortical dementias (i.e., Alzheimer's disease) do not manifest in SCA1 patients. On the basis of anatomic studies, prefrontal association areas are known to be connected to the cerebellum by pons, and the efferent links originate from the dentate nucleus and project to the prefrontal cortex (14,15). These anatomic findings further lend support to the close functional relationship between the cerebellum and prefrontal cortex. Genis et al. described two types of behavioral changes in a large SCA1 kindred: a frontal-like syndrome with euphoria and emotional lability was seen in some patients, but in most patients, psychiatric symptoms appeared late in the disease, manifesting as nocturnal shouting and crying, irritability, and aggression (16).

SPINOCEREBELLAR ATAXIA 2

The onset of SCA2 may be in childhood, adolescence, or adulthood. Symptoms consist of worsening ataxia, action or postural tremor, absence of reflexes, slow saccades, dysarthria, and ophthalmoplegia (17). The childhood form of SCA2 is characterized by bradykinesia and rigidity (18). Payami et al. (19) reported a form of SCA2 that presented as levodopa-responsive familial parkinsonism. SCA2 is associated with cognitive impairment. Storey et al. (20) studied 8 affected members of an Australian pedigree of northern Italian origin who had SCA2. Neurologic and neuropsychological assessment of these subjects revealed frontal-executive dysfunction in most of them. Le Pira et al. (21) evaluated cognitive impairment in 18 SCA2 patients to verify the role of different disease-related factors such as age of onset, disease duration, and clinical severity on intellectual abilities. Compared to healthy controls, SCA2 patients showed impaired verbal memory, executive function, and attention. SCA2 patients also had defective attention skills and performed significantly worse than controls on a nonverbal intelligence task. Developmental delay has also been reported in SCA2 (22).

SPINOCEREBELLAR ATAXIA 3 (MACHADO–JOSEPH DISEASE)

Patients with spinocerebellar ataxia 3 (SCA3) develop ataxia, external ophthalmoplegia, pyramidal and extrapyramidal disorders, and amyotrophic muscle wasting as well as neuropathy. SCA3 is classified into three forms: (a) early onset SCA3 (type 1), characterized by rigidity and dystonia; (b) late-onset SCA3 (type 2), in which patients develop peripheral neuropathy with mild ataxia; and (c) the most common form of SCA3 (type 3), which begins in the third decade of life and is characterized by progressive ataxia. Various neuroophthalmologic abnormalities develop, including supranuclear ophthalmoparesis, decreased blinking, diplopia, impaired smooth visual pursuit, and nystagmus. A number of brainstem symptoms may occur, such as dysarthria, dysphonia, facial weakness, and facial fasciculations (23). Most clinical studies of SCA3 patients have reported either absence of cognitive impairment (24–27) or mild loss of memory (28). Although dementia is uncommon in SCA3 patients (29, 30), Lokkegaard et al. (31) studied two large Danish and one Norwegian family with SCA3 and reported dementia among these patients. Recent studies have found impaired executive function and visual processing in SCA3 patients (32–34). Sleep disturbances such as rapid eye movement (REM) behavior disorder and restless legs syndrome have also been reported in some patients with Machado–Joseph disease (MJD) (35–37). Psychiatric symptoms including depression, apathy, and anxiety also occur (34,36,38). However, some groups have found that SCA3 patients are less likely to be depressed than nonaffected family members once they develop florid symptoms of the illness (32).

SPINOCEREBELLAR ATAXIA 4

The clinical manifestations of this rare form of hereditary ataxia include worsening ataxia, pyramidal tract abnormalities, and sensory axonal neuropathy. SCA4 symptoms develop during adulthood. One family with SCA4, but without neuropathy or pyramidal tract involvement, has been reported. Behavioral symptoms have not been reported in SCA4 (39).

SPINOCEREBELLAR ATAXIA 5

SCA5 is more slowly progressive than the other SCAs, and patients with adult onset disease generally have a normal lifespan. Dementia has not been reported in this condition (40).

SPINOCEREBELLAR ATAXIA 6

Progressive cerebellar ataxia is the main feature of SCA6 (41). Other neurologic manifestations consist of dysarthria, nystagmus, saccadic intrusions in smooth pursuit, gaze palsy, vertigo, and sensory loss (42). Globas et al. (43) evaluated cognitive status in 12 patients with genetically confirmed SCA6 and 12 matched control subjects, using a battery of neuropsychological tests to assess general intellectual abilities, attention, verbal and visuospatial memory, and executive functions. Only mild deficits in executive tasks, without general intellectual impairment, were detected in these patients as compared to control subjects.

SPINOCEREBELLAR ATAXIA 7

Spinocerebellar ataxia 7 (SCA7), also known as hereditary ataxia with retinal degeneration, is characterized by progressive cerebellar ataxia, dysarthria, dysphagia, retinal degeneration, optic atrophy, pigmentary retinopathy, cone-red dystrophy, and visual loss (44). In cases with disease onset in infancy or childhood, patients have a rapidly progressive course with failure to thrive and regression from motor milestones. Behavioral disorders have not been reported in these patients.

SPINOCEREBELLAR ATAXIA 8

Spinocerebellar ataxia 8 (SCA8) is usually a slowly progressive disease that manifests in adulthood, at a mean age of 40 to 50 years. The clinical picture of SCA8 consists of slowly worsening dysarthria, dysphagia, ataxia of trunk and extremities, hyperreflexia, and mild sensory loss (45); occasionally nystagmus and dysmetric saccades; and rarely, ophthalmoplegia. Behavioral abnormalities have not been reported in these patients (46).

SPINOCEREBELLAR ATAXIA 10

Spinocerebellar ataxia 10 (SCA10) is characterized by ataxia and seizures. Other clinical features associated with SCA10 include dysarthria, tremor, mild mental retardation, gaze-evoked nystagmus, and fragmented smooth visual pursuit. A high prevalence of psychiatric symptoms was found in a study of 18 affected individuals, over 50% of whom had psychiatric disorders, including mood disturbance, aggression, or both of these conditions together (47). Personality evaluation of these patients detected depressive, aggressive, and irritable traits. Low intelligence was seen in the group overall, with IQ scores ranging from 61 to 94; EEGs commonly showed slow, fused, and disorganized activity, suggesting widespread cerebral dysfunction (47).

SPINOCEREBELLAR ATAXIA 11

Spinocerebellar ataxia 11 (SCA11) is a slowly progressive disease that manifests between the third and fourth decades of life. Clinical manifestations consist of ataxia, gait disorder, and hyperreflexia, with no extrapyramidal, motor, or sensory deficits (48). Psychiatric and cognitive changes have not been reported in these patients.

SPINOCEREBELLAR ATAXIA 12

The age of onset for spinocerebellar ataxia 12 (SCA12) varies from 8 to 55 years, with a mean age of onset in the fourth decade. SCA12 is the only form of SCA that can initially present with head and arm tremor. Typical clinical manifestations consist of ataxia, parkinsonism, dysmetria, hyperreflexia, dementia, and abnormal ocular movements (49). Peripheral nervous system involvement manifests with focal myokymia and polyneuropathy. Magnetic resonance imaging (MRI) of the brain reveals prominent cerebellar and cortical atrophy.

SPINOCEREBELLAR ATAXIA 13

Spinocerebellar ataxia 13 (SCA13) was initially reported in a French family (50). In almost all the affected family members, the neurologic deficits began in childhood, and progression was slow. Clinical manifestations consist of ataxia and moderate mental retardation (IQ, 62–76), along with dysarthria, nystagmus, and delay in achieving motor and cognitive milestones.

SPINOCEREBELLAR ATAXIA 14

Spinocerebellar ataxia 14 (SCA14), which was reported in a Japanese family, may develop at any age, with a mean age of onset between the 4th and 5th decades. Age of onset in the Japanese family ranged from 10 to 59 years (51). Clinical manifestations of SCA14 consist of slowly progressive ataxia, with axial myoclonus and tremor. Other associated neurologic deficits include gaze-evoked nystagmus and decreased tendon reflexes. Behavioral disorders, including cognitive decline, have not been reported among these patients.

SPINOCEREBELLAR ATAXIA 15

Pure cerebellar ataxia [spinocerebellar ataxia 15 (SCA15)] has been reported in an Australian Anglo-Celtic family (52). Neurologic manifestations of SCA15 are impaired handwriting, dysarthria, dysphagia, and ocular movement abnormalities. Most of these patients are only mildly affected and remain ambulatory. Cognitive decline in SCA15 has not been reported.

SPINOCEREBELLAR ATAXIA 16

Miyoshi et al. (53) described a Japanese family with spinocerebellar ataxia 16 (SCA16), characterized by truncal ataxia, speech ataxia, and head tremor. The symptoms develop in the 2nd to 6th decades of life. Other neurologic deficits include nystagmus and impaired smooth visual pursuit. Cognitive decline has not been reported.

SPINOCEREBELLAR ATAXIA 17

A CAG/CAA repeat expansion in the TATA box-binding protein gene causes spinocerebellar ataxia 17 (SCA17). Onset of SCA17 usually occurs in the 3rd to 5th decades of life. Clinical manifestations of SCA17 consist of progressive cerebellar ataxia, dementia, and psychosis (54). Numerous psychiatric symptoms in SCA17 have been reported, and some patients present with pure psychiatric symptoms in the absence of a movement disorder (55). De Michele et al. (56) reported two Italian families with SCA17 in whom the ataxia was followed by dementia, psychiatric symptoms, seizures, and extrapyramidal features. Brain MRI of affected individuals from both families revealed marked cerebral and cerebellar atrophy. Rolfs et al. (55) reported clinical and neuropathologic features of SCA17. The neuropsychiatric features of the 15 patients in this series consisted of schizophrenia, aggression, paranoia, mania, constructive apraxia, depression, aggressive behavior, mutism, and self-mutilation. Dementia was seen in more than 50% of cases. Only three of the patients showed no behavioral changes. In another report, Bruni et al. (57) described the clinical and neuropathologic features of SCA17 in four generations of a family with 16 affected individuals. Behavioral abnormalities such as lack of insight, anxiety, depression, delusional thoughts, auditory hallucinations, loss of personal hygiene, distractibility, loss of interest, and irritability, as well as frontal-type dementia, preceded ataxia in these patients. Toyoshima et al. (58) recently reported a case of a patient homozygous for SCA17 whose phenotype was similar to HD. This patient had rapidly progressive dementia, emotional incontinence, and chorea.

SPINOCEREBELLAR ATAXIA 19

Spinocerebellar ataxia 19 (SCA19) was initially described in one Dutch family with mild progressive ataxia (59), peripheral neuropathy, postural tremor, myoclonus, and cognitive impairment. Cognitive impairment in these patients consists of a mild disturbance of abstract reasoning with poor performance on executive tasks such as the Wisconsin Card Sorting Test (59).

SPINOCEREBELLAR ATAXIA 21

Vuillaume et al. (60) reported a French family with slowly progressive gait and limb ataxia, associated with akinesia, rigidity, hyporeflexia, and tremor. Some of these patients demonstrate mild cognitive decline.

DENTATORUBRAL–PALLIDOSYLVIAN ATROPHY

Dentatorubral–pallidosylvian atrophy is caused by an expanded CAG repeat on chromosome 12. DRPLA clinically manifests with a wide range of neurologic deficits including ataxia, choreoathetosis, dystonia, ballismus, myoclonus, epilepsy, and severe dementia (61,62). It accounts for 20% of autosomal dominant cerebellar ataxias seen in people of Japanese descent and is seen less commonly in other ethnic groups (40). Patients with early onset DRPLA, who experience extremely rapid disease progression, show mental retardation (63). Recently, Munoz et al. (64) reported a 62-year-old female patient with DRPLA, who at the time of genetic diagnosis manifested severe ataxia, dysarthria, and cognitive decline. Brain MRI revealed remarkable cerebellar and brainstem atrophy, with hyperintensities of the periventricular white matter. Adachi et al. (65) describe four patients with DRPLA who presented with delusions and psychosis. Potter et al. (66) describe a family with prominent psychiatric symptoms, mental retardation, and a movement disorder in affected individuals. These patients carried the diagnosis of HD until genetic testing revealed they had DRPLA.

EPISODIC ATAXIAS

Autosomal dominant episodic ataxia is identified by childhood or adolescent onset of episodic ataxia, vertigo, dysarthria, and nystagmus. Episodic ataxia type 1 is characterized by clinically brief attacks (usually minutes) of ataxia; on neurophysiologic evaluation, myokymia may be observed. The clinical attacks are precipitated by sudden changes in body position, emotional stress, and vestibular stimulation. This form of hereditary ataxia is caused by a missense mutation in the potassium channel gene (KCNA1), which is located on chromosome 12p13. Episodic ataxia type 2 is characterized by longer-lasting attacks (hours and even days) of ataxia, which are accompanied by vertigo, nausea, and vomiting. This condition is caused by a mutation in the gene for voltage-dependent P/Q-type calcium channel (CACNA1A). The gene locus has been mapped to chromosome 19. The mutation can be an expansion of CAG repeat or a missense mutation that causes truncation of the gene product (67). Cognitive decline and behavioral abnormalities have not been reported in patients with episodic ataxias type 1 and 2.

STUDIES OF COGNITION AND PSYCHIATRIC SYMPTOMS IN CEREBELLAR DEGENERATION

Most of the autosomal dominant forms of hereditary ataxias are newly described disorders and our data about the clinical features of these patients is limited. Perhaps the best-studied ataxias of this type are SCA1, SCA2, and SCA3. Comparative neuropsychological studies that address the differences among these disorders are rare. Burk et al. (13) performed a comparative study of intellectual function in patients with SCA1, SCA2, or SCA3. The authors found subtle executive deficits and mildly impaired verbal memory and concluded that because SCA1, SCA2, and SCA3 all share severe cerebellar degeneration, the differences in severity of cognitive impairment among these three groups should be attributed to disruption of the cerebro–cerebellar circuitry.

Leroi et al. (68) compared a group of 31 patients with degenerative cerebellar disease to 21 HD patients. The cerebellar group included patients with sporadic and hereditary cerebellar disease. The cerebellar group comprised 20 patients with SCA, including 11 sporadic cases and 9 with a familial pattern of inheritance. The remaining patients with cerebellar degeneration had either multisystem atrophy (5 patients) or SCA of unknown etiology. Almost 80% of the patients with cerebellar degeneration had psychiatric disorders, a prevalence similar to that seen in the HD group, although the symptoms tended to be less severe in the cerebellar patients. Mood disorders and personality change were prominent symptoms in both groups. Cognitive impairment, including dementia, was seen in almost 20% of patients with cerebellar degeneration and in more than 70% of HD patients. Mild dementia, resembling that seen in HD, has been reported in other work with hereditary ataxia patients (33). Psychotic disorders were seen in 10% of patients with cerebellar degeneration but were not observed in the HD group. The authors comment that animal and human data suggest that the cerebellum may modulate both cognitive and emotional behavior (69,70). These data confirm results from an older study of hereditary ataxia of all types, which found psychiatric disorders in 23% of patients (71). A recent study of patients with cerebellar degeneration found that more than 50% of all patients displayed psychopathology, including depression, personality change, cognitive impairment, anxiety, and psychosis (72). Thus, although research has not yet focused specifically on the SCAs, data suggest that, at the very least, mild psychiatric symptoms and cognitive impairment occurs in a substantial number of these patients.

GENETIC TESTING FOR HEREDITARY ATAXIAS

Commercial testing is now widely available for many of the hereditary ataxias. The psychosocial effects of testing have received little study. Genetic counseling for autosomal dominant SCAs should follow a model similar to that described for HD, with the understanding that genetic tests have limited ability to predict disease course for any individual patient (73). Ethical, emotional, and social issues raised by genetic testing for hereditary ataxias are similar to those seen for HD, a disease with more established genetic testing protocols (74). Little is known regarding predictive testing for those who are at risk for a hereditary ataxia. Smith et al. (75) studied 50 people at risk for hereditary ataxias, along with others at risk for muscular dystrophy and hereditary neuropathy, who underwent genetic testing for these disorders. The authors found that most of these individuals felt that genetic testing was beneficial. Anxiety and depression were seen in some of those whose genetic tests were positive and in a few individuals with negative test results. Because predictive genetic test results can have a long-range effect on family planning and relationships, it should be done in the context of supportive counseling by experienced professionals.

SUMMARY

Recognizing cognitive deficits and psychiatric disorders in patients with autosomal dominant ataxias is relatively new. At this time, the percentage of patients with these disorders who experience changes in cognition or psychiatric symptoms is unknown. Cognitive impairment, when seen, is often found on tests of executive function, probably reflecting disruption of afferent and efferent pathways of the prefrontal cortex and subcortical structures, including the cerebellum. Widespread global dysfunction does occur in some cases, especially later in the disease course. Psychiatric symptoms including depression, aggression, irritability, and psychosis have all been reported. As these behavioral changes receive further study, one hopes that guidelines for treating these symptoms will emerge. Clinicians should be mindful of the psychosocial effects that genetic testing for the hereditary ataxias may have, especially in cases of predictive testing for those who are asymptomatic but at risk because of family history. Guidelines established for genetic testing in HD may be helpful when approaching these cases.

REFERENCES

1. Konigsmark BW, Weiner LP. The olivopontocerebellar atrophies: a review. *Medicine (Baltimore)* 1970;49: 227–241.
2. Harding AE. The clinical features and classification of the late onset autosomal dominant cerebellar ataxias: a study of families, including descendants of "the Drew family of Walworth." *Brain* 1982;105:1–28.
3. Campanella G, Filla A, De Michele G. Classifications of hereditary ataxias. A critical overview. *Acta Neurol (Napoli)* 1992;14(4-6):408–419.
4. Goldfarb LG, Chumakov MP, Petrov PA, et al. Olivopontocerebellar atrophy in a large Iakut kinship in eastern Siberia. *Neurology* 1989;39(11):1527–1530.
5. Spadaro M, Giunti P, Lulli P, et al. HLA-linked spinocerebellar ataxia: a clinical and genetic study of large Italian kindreds. *Acta Neurol Scand* 1992;85:257–265.
6. Dubourg O, Durr A, Cancel G, et al. Analysis of the SCA1 CAG repeat in a large number of families with dominant ataxia: clinical and molecular correlations. *Ann Neurol* 1995;37:176–180.
7. Sasaki H, Fukazawa T, Yanagihara T, et al. Clinical features and natural history of spinocerebellar ataxia type 1. *Acta Neurol Scand* 1996;93:64–71.
8. Giunti P, Sweeney MG, Spadaro M, et al. The trinucleotide repeat expansion on chromosome 6p (SCA1) in autosomal dominant cerebellar ataxias. *Brain* 1994; 117(Pt 4):645–449.
9. Kameya T, Abe K, Aoki M, et al. Analysis of spinocerebellar ataxia type 1 (SCA1)-related CAG trinucleotide expansion in Japan. *Neurology* 1995;45: 1587–1594.
10. Ranum LP, Chung MY, Banfi S, et al. Molecular and clinical correlations in spinocerebellar ataxia type I: evidence for familial effects on the age at onset. *Am J Hum Genet* 1994;55:244–252.
11. Burk K, Bosch S, Globas C, et al. Executive dysfunction in spinocerebellar ataxia type 1. *Eur Neurol* 2000; 46:43–48.
12. Burk K, Bosch S, Globas C, et al. Executive dysfunction in spinocerebellar ataxia type 1. *Eur Neurol* 2001; 46:43–48.
13. Burk K, Globas C, Bosch S, et al. Cognitive deficits in spinocerebellar ataxia type 1, 2, and 3. *J Neurol* 2003; 250:207–211.
14. Middleton FA, Strick PL. Anatomical evidence for cerebellar and basal ganglia involvement in higher cognitive function. *Science* 1994;266(5184):458–461.
15. Middleton FA, Strick PL. Dentate output channels: motor and cognitive components. *Prog Brain Res* 1997; 114:553–566.
16. Genis D, Matilla T, Volpini V, et al. Clinical, neuropathologic, and genetic studies of a large spinocerebellar ataxia type 1 (SCA1) kindred: (CAG)n expansion and early premonitory signs and symptoms. *Neurology* 1995;45:24–30.
17. Wadia N, Pang J, Desai J, et al. A clinicogenetic analysis of six Indian spinocerebellar ataxia (SCA2) pedigrees. The significance of slow saccades in diagnosis. *Brain* 1998;121(Pt 12):2341–2355.
18. Schols L, Gispert S, Vorgerd M, et al. Spinocerebellar ataxia type 2. Genotype and phenotype in German kindreds. *Arch Neurol* 1997;54:1073–1080.
19. Payami H, Nutt J, Gancher S, et al. SCA2 may present as levodopa-responsive parkinsonism. *Mov Disord* 2003; 18:425-429.

20. Storey E, Forrest SM, Shaw JH, et al. Spinocerebellar ataxia type 2: clinical features of a pedigree displaying prominent frontal-executive dysfunction. *Arch Neurol* 1999;56:43–50.
21. Le Pira F, Zappala G, Saponara R, et al. Cognitive findings in spinocerebellar ataxia type 2: relationship to genetic and clinical variables. *J Neurol Sci* 2002;201(1-2):53–57.
22. Moretti P, Blazo M, Garcia L, et al. Spinocerebellar ataxia type 2 (SCA2) presenting with ophthalmoplegia and developmental delay in infancy. *Am J Med Genet* 2004;124A(4):392–396.
23. Paulson H, Ammache Z. Ataxia and hereditary disorders. *Neurol Clin* 2001;19:759–782.
24. Burt T, Blumbergs P, Currie B. A dominant hereditary ataxia resembling Machado-Joseph disease in Arnhem Land, Australia. *Neurology* 1993;43:1750–1752.
25. Coutinho P, Andrade C. Autosomal dominant system degeneration in Portuguese families of the Azores Islands. A new genetic disorder involving cerebellar, pyramidal, extrapyramidal and spinal cord motor functions. *Neurology* 1978;28:703–709.
26. Fowler HL. Machado-Joseph-Azorean disease. A ten year study. *Arch Neurol* 1984;41:921–925.
27. Rosenberg RN, Nyhan WL, Bay C, et al. Autosomal dominant striatonigral degeneration. A clinical, pathologic, and biochemical study of a new genetic disorder. *Neurology* 1976;26:703–714.
28. Sequeiros J, Coutinho P. Epidemiology and clinical aspects of Machado-Joseph disease. *Adv Neurol* 1993;61:139–153.
29. Barbeau A, Roy M, Cunha L, et al. The natural history of Machado-Joseph disease. *Can J Neurol Sci* 1984;11:510–512.
30. Ishikawa K, Mizusawa H, Saito M, et al. Autosomal dominant pure cerebellar ataxia. A clinical and genetic analysis of eight Japanese families. *Brain* 1996;119:1173–1182.
31. Lokkegaard T, Nielsen JE, Hasholt L, et al. Machado-Joseph disease in three Scandinavian families. *J Neurol Sci* 1998;156(2):152–157.
32. Radvany J, Camargo CH, Costa ZM, et al. Machado-Joseph disease of Azorean ancestry in Brazil: the Catarina kindred. Neurological, neuroimaging, psychiatric and neuropsychological findings in the largest known family, the "Catarina" kindred. *Arq Neuropsiquiatr* 1993;51(1):21–30.
33. Kish SJ, El-Awar M, Stuss D, et al. Neuropsychological test performance in patients with dominantly inherited spinocerebellar ataxia. Relationship to ataxia severity. *Neurology* 1994;44:1738–1746.
34. Zawacki TM, Grace J, Friedman JH. Sudarsky. Executive and emotional dysfunction in Machado-Joseph disease. *Mov Disord* 2002;17:1004–1010.
35. Syed BH, Rye DB, Singh G. REM sleep behavior disorder and SCA-3 (Machado-Joseph disease). *Neurology* 2003;60(1):148.
36. Fukutake T, Shinotoh H, Nishino H, et al. Homozygous Machado-Joseph disease presenting as REM sleep behaviour disorder and prominent psychiatric symptoms. *Eur J Neurol* 2002;9(1):97–100.
37. Schols L, Haan J, Riess O, et al. Sleep disturbances in spinocerebellar ataxias: is the SCA3 mutation a cause of restless legs syndrome? *Neurology* 1998;51:1603–1607.
38. Takei A, Honma S, Kawashima A, et al. Beneficial effects of tandospirone on ataxia of a patient with Machado-Joseph disease. *Psychiatry Clin Neurosci* 2002;56(2):181–185.
39. Nagaoka U, Takashima M, Ishikawa K, et al. A gene on SCA4 locus causes dominantly inherited pure cerebellar ataxia. *Neurology* 2000;54:1971–1975.
40. Koeppen AH. The hereditary ataxias. *J Neuropathol Exp Neurol* 1998;57(6):531–543.
41. Matsumura R, Futamura N, Fujimoto Y, et al. Spinocerebellar ataxia type 6. Molecular and clinical features of 35 Japanese patients including one homozygous for the CAG repeat expansion. *Neurology* 1997;49:1238–1243.
42. Sinke RJ, Ippel EF, Diepstraten CM, et al. Clinical and molecular correlations in spinocerebellar ataxia type 6. *Arch Neurol* 2001;58:1839–1844.
43. Globas C, Bosch S, Zuhlke CH, et al. The cerebellum and cognition. Intellectual function in spinocerebellar ataxia type 6 (SCA6). *J Neurol* 2003;250:1482–1487.
44. Aleman TS, Cideciyan AV, Volpe NJ, et al. Spinocerebellar ataxia type 7 (SCA7) shows a cone-rod dystrophy phenotype. *Exp Eye Res* 2002;74:737–745.
45. Day JW, Schut LJ, Moseley ML, et al. Spinocerebellar ataxia type 8: clinical features in a large family. *Neurology* 2000;55:649–657.
46. Ikeda Y, Dalton JC, Moseley ML, et al. Spinocerebellar ataxia type 8: molecular genetic comparisons and haplotype analysis of 37 families with ataxia. *Am J Hum Genet* 2004;75:3–16.
47. Rasmussen A, Matsuura T, Ruano L, et al. Clinical and genetic analysis of four Mexican families with spinocerebellar ataxia type 10. *Ann Neurol* 2001;50:234–239.
48. Worth PF, Giunti P, Gardner-Thorpe C, et al. Autosomal dominant cerebellar ataxia type III: linkage in a large British family to a 7.6-cM region on chromosome 15q14-21.3. *Am J Hum Genet* 1999;65:420–426.
49. Holmes SE, O'Hearn EE, McInnis MG, et al. Expansion of a novel CAG trinucleotide repeat in the 5' region of PPP2R2B is associated with SCA12. *Nat Genet* 1999;23:391–392.
50. Herman-Bert A, Stevanin G, Netter JC, et al. Mapping of spinocerebellar ataxia 13 to chromosome 19q13.3-q13.4 in a family with autosomal dominant cerebellar ataxia and mental retardation. *Am J Hum Genet* 2000;67:229–235.
51. Yamashita I, Sasaki H, Yabe I, et al. A novel locus for dominant cerebellar ataxia (SCA14) maps to a 10.2-cM interval flanked by D19S206 and D19S605 on chromosome 19q13.4-qter. *Ann Neurol* 2000;48:156–163.
52. Storey E, Gardner RJ, Knight MA, et al. A new autosomal dominant pure cerebellar ataxia. *Neurology* 2001;57:1913–1915.
53. Miyoshi Y, Yamada T, Tanimura M, et al. A novel autosomal dominant spinocerebellar ataxia (SCA16) linked to chromosome 8q22.1-24.1. *Neurology* 2001;57:96–100.
54. Fujigasaki H, Martin JJ, De Deyn PP, et al. CAG repeat expansion in the TATA box-binding protein gene causes autosomal dominant cerebellar ataxia. *Brain* 2001;124(Pt 10):1939–1947.
55. Rolfs A, Koeppen AH, Bauer I, et al. Clinical features and neuropathology of autosomal dominant spinocerebellar ataxia (SCA17). *Ann Neurol* 2003;54:367–375.
56. De Michele G, Maltecca F, Carella M, et al. Dementia, ataxia, extrapyramidal features, and epilepsy: phenotype spectrum in two Italian families with spinocerebellar ataxia type 17. *Neurol Sci* 2003;24:166–167.

57. Bruni AC, Takahashi-Fujigasaki J, Maltecca F, et al. Behavioral disorder, dementia, ataxia, and rigidity in a large family with TATA box-binding protein mutation. *Arch Neurol* 2004;61:1314–1320.
58. Toyoshima Y, Yamada M, Onodera O, et al. SCA17 homozygote showing Huntington's disease-like phenotype. *Ann Neurol* 2004;55(2):281–286.
59. Verbeek DS, Schelhaas JH, Ippel EF, et al. Identification of a novel SCA locus (SCA19) in a Dutch autosomal dominant cerebellar ataxia family on chromosome region 1p21-q21. *Hum Genet* 2002;111:388–393.
60. Vuillaume I, Devos D, Schraen-Maschke S, et al. A new locus for spinocerebellar ataxia (SCA21) maps to chromosome 7p21.3-p15.1. *Ann Neurol* 2002;52:666–670.
61. Takahashi H, Ohama E, Naito H, et al. Hereditary dentatorubral-pallidoluysian atrophy: clinical and pathologic variants in a family. *Neurology* 1988;38:1065–1070.
62. Yabe I, Sasaki H, Kikuchi S, et al. Late onset ataxia phenotype in dentatorubro-pallidoluysian atrophy (DRPLA). *J Neurol* 2002;249:432–436.
63. Koide R, Ikeuchi T, Onodera O, et al. Unstable expansion of CAG repeat in hereditary dentatorubral-pallidoluysian atrophy (DRPLA). *Nat Genet* 1994;6(1):9–13.
64. Munoz E, Campdelacreu J, Ferrer I, et al. Severe cerebral white matter involvement in a case of dentatorubropallidoluysian atrophy studied at autopsy. *Arch Neurol* 2004;61:946–949.
65. Adachi N, Arima K, Asada T, et al. Dentatorubral-pallidoluysian atrophy (DRPLA) presenting with psychosis. *J Neuropsychiatry Clin Neurosci* 2001;13(2):258–260.
66. Potter NT, Meyer MA, Zimmerman AW, et al. Molecular and clinical findings in a family with dentatorubral-pallidoluysian atrophy. *Ann Neurol* 1995;37(2):273–277.
67. Guida S, Trettel F, Pagnutti S, et al. Complete loss of P/Q calcium channel activity caused by a CACNA1A missense mutation carried by patients with episodic ataxia type 2. *Am J Hum Genet* 2001;68:759–774.
68. Leroi I, O'Hearn E, Marsh L, et al. Psychopathology in patients with degenerative cerebellar diseases: a comparison to Huntington's disease. *Am J Psychiatry* 2002;159:1306–1314.
69. Berman AJ. Amelioration of aggression: response to selective cerebellar lesions in the rhesus monkey. *Int Rev Neurobiol* 1997;41:111–119.
70. Liotti M, Mayberg HS, Brannan SK, et al. Differential limbic-cortical correlates of sadness and anxiety in healthy subjects: implications for affective disorders. *Biol Psychiatry* 2000;48:30–42.
71. Skre H. A study of certain traits accompanying some inherited neurological disorders. *Clin Genet* 1975;8:117–135.
72. Liszewski CM, O'Hearn E, Leroi I, et al. Cognitive impairment and psychiatric symptoms in 133 patients with diseases associated with cerebellar degeneration. *J Neuropsychiatry Clin Neurosci* 2004;16:109–112.
73. Tan E, Ashizawa T. Genetic testing in spinocerebellar ataxias: defining a clinical role. *Arch Neurol* 2001;58:191–195.
74. International Huntington Association and the World Federation of Neurology Research Group on Huntington's Chorea. Guidelines for the molecular genetics predictive test in Huntington's disease. *J Med Genet* 1994;31(7):555–559.
75. Smith CO, Lipe HP, Bird TD. Impact of presymptomatic genetic testing for hereditary ataxia and neuromuscular disorders. *Arch Neurol* 2004;61:875–880.

21

Behavioral Symptoms Associated with Essential Tremor

Elan D. Louis

Department of Neurology, Columbia University, New York, New York

Essential tremor (ET) is a chronic, progressive neurologic disease. The motor feature that is the hallmark of the illness is a 4- to 12-Hz kinetic tremor that may involve several regions of the body, including the arms and head but rarely the legs (1–6). When the tremor involves multiple body regions, it usually occurs gradually, in stages, and the disease-specific pattern of spread is typically from the arms to cranial structures (e.g., the head). As with other progressive conditions (e.g., motor neuron disease and parkinsonism), ET may represent a family of related diseases rather than a single disease, and the neurologic manifestations exhibited by any one patient may depend on the location of the disease pathology or pathologies within the nervous system. Thus, although the kinetic tremor in ET may be the result of an abnormality in an olivo–cerebellar–thalamic pathway, patients with ET often have signs of more widespread cerebellar involvement (e.g., intention tremor, ataxia, and eye motion abnormalities) (7–10), abnormalities attributable to basal ganglia dysfunction (e.g., rest tremor and subclinical bradykinesia) (11,12), and cognitive–neuropsychiatric manifestations that may result from abnormalities in pathways that involve connections between subcortical or cerebellar structures and higher cortical centers (13,14). Also, as with several of the other progressive conditions, olfactory dysfunction and loss of body mass index may accompany ET (15,16). The cognitive–neuropsychiatric manifestations of ET, which have received relatively little attention until recently, are the focus of this chapter. The "old view" of ET is that it is a monosymptomatic condition, but our understanding of the illness has advanced so that we now realize that, as in other progressive movement disorders like Parkinson's disease (PD) and Huntington's disease (HD), ET is characterized by both motor and nonmotor manifestations. A broader understanding of the clinical picture of ET, encompassing both motor and nonmotor deficits, would be beneficial, not just in understanding the pathophysiology of the disease but also as an aid to understanding patient motivations and perceptions during treatment.

COGNITION

Clinical anecdote suggests that dementia is no more prevalent in patients with ET than in age-matched healthy controls; however, this observation has not been substantiated with either cross-sectional data that compares the prevalence of dementia in patients with ET or longitudinal data that assesses the relative risk of dementia in patients with ET compared with that of controls. On the basis of anecdotal observation, James Parkinson declared that the intellect was "uninjured" (17) in patients with PD, whereas we know that dementia affects between 10% and 40% of patients with PD (18–22). The potential association between ET and dementia, however, remains an essentially unstudied area.

In the last several years, four studies of cognition in ET (13,23–26) have been conducted. Several of these studies were motivated by the need to perform neuropsychological evaluations on patients with ET before deep brain stimulation surgery. The basic characteristics of these studies are outlined in Table 21-1. The studies each

TABLE 21-1. *Studies of cognition in ET*

Authors	Number of cases with ET	Normal control group?	Other comparison group?	Normative data?
Gasparini et al. 2001 (13)	27	15	15 with PD	No
Lombardi et al. 2001 (23)	18	No	18 with PD	Yes
Lacritz et al. 2002 (24)	13	No	13 with PD	Yes
Duane et al. 2002 and Vermilion et al. 2001 (25,26)	55	No	No	No

enrolled between 13 and 55 patients with ET. Of the four studies, one enrolled a group of healthy controls. Two of the studies enrolled patients with PD as a comparison group and also used published normative data, whereas one of the studies did neither. In several of the studies, patients were taking medications for ET, which might have had cognitive effects, whereas in other studies, patients were not taking such medications. The selection criteria for patients are not entirely clear in all studies, but some patients were selected on the basis of presurgical evaluations, which raises the issue of selection bias. More specifically, because the selection was not random, was the selection of patients with ET related in some way to their cognitive state? The selected sample may not have been representative of the source population. A second concern with many of the studies is that data on the severity of tremor are not reported, and results are not stratified on the basis of disease duration or tremor severity. The presence and the severity of cognitive deficits may have been related to tremor severity or duration. We describe each of these four studies in greater detail.

Gasparini et al. (13) studied 27 patients with ET, including 15 with a family history of ET and 12 with a family history of PD. These patients were compared to 15 normal controls and 15 patients with PD. The patients with ET and PD were presumably selected from a clinical setting in Italy, but the selection criteria for both groups are not specified, nor are details provided about the number of cases from which the study sample was selected. The mean duration of disease for patients with ET was 17.8 years, although there was a wide range, and data are not stratified by duration or severity. The severity of tremor is not reported; however, none of the patients was medicated for tremor. The authors found that the patients with ET performed more poorly than the controls in the Stroop test and the Wisconsin Card Sorting Test, indicating impairments in both attentional and conceptual thinking. None of the patients with ET had cognitive complaints, making these findings subclinical.

Lombardi et al. (23) studied 18 patients with ET who were evaluated with a presurgical neuropsychological assessment and were compared to 18 patients with PD and to normative data. The mean duration of disease was 36.3 years, which was approximately double that noted in the patients in the Gasparini study (13). Some of the patients were medicated for tremor. This study used a larger battery of tests than the Gasparini study (13), with tests of working memory and attention, language, visuospatial processes, reasoning and conceptualization, memory, executive functions, and mood. The study showed that in comparison with normative data, patients with ET had cognitive impairments, including deficits in verbal fluency, naming, recent memory, working memory, and mental set shifting. The largest deficits occurred in verbal fluency and mental set shifting, followed by naming, memory, and working memory. On average, the magnitude of the cognitive deficits was mild but ranged from unnoticeable to severe. The mean Mini-Mental State Examination score was high (26.9 ± 2.0), indicating that dementia was not an issue for the most part. No correlation was seen between tremor scores and performance on any of the cognitive and affective measures in the battery (all p greater than 0.10).

Lacritz et al. (24) studied 13 patients with ET and compared them to 13 patients with PD and to normative data. All were seen for neuropsychological assessment as part of their evaluations before surgery for ET. Of the 13 patients, 4 were taking medication for tremor. All subjects scored 25 or higher on a Mini-Mental State Examination (mean, 27.5). Mild cognitive impairment (e.g., forgetfulness or word-finding difficulties) was reported in 54% of the patients with ET but was not thought to be severe enough to affect daily function. None of the patients met criteria for dementia. Fifty percent of patients with ET demonstrated evidence of at least mild impairment (defined as performing at least 1 standard deviation (SD) below the normative mean) on at least 5 of 10 measures. As a whole, the ET group performed at least one SD below the normative mean on measures of cognitive flexibility, figural fluency, and selective attention. Of the 13 patients with ET, 12 demonstrated at least mild impairment on one or more cognitive measures.

In the final study (25,26), 55 patients with ET were examined, but not compared with a control group, with another comparison group, or with any normative data. No information was available on how these 55 patients were selected. Problems with attention were more prevalent in this study than were memory or perceptual motor deficits.

In summary, the few studies to date, although methodologically dissimilar in some respects, all point to some degree of impairment of cognition in patients with ET, compared with either normative control data or enrolled control subjects. Impairment is generally mild and subclinical. The pattern of neuropsychological deficits in each of these studies suggests an abnormality either in frontal–subcortical (basal ganglia and thalamus) pathways or a cerebellar cognitive syndrome resulting from an abnormality in cerebellar–frontal circuitry. Selection bias is a concern, and the ability to extend these findings to a randomly selected group of patients with ET is uncertain and is an area that will require further study. In addition, cross-sectional and longitudinal studies are needed to examine any possible associations between ET and dementia.

DEPRESSION

Few data address the possibility of an association between ET and mood disorders. Given the propensity for tremor to result in functional disability (1), one could hypothesize that depressive symptoms and depression might be more prevalent among patients with ET than controls and that the more severe the tremor, the more prevalent the depressive symptoms or depression. Conversely, a mood disorder may be part of the underlying disease process rather than a response to the tremor and may further contribute to the functional disability.

Lombardi et al. (23) reported significantly higher levels of depressive symptoms in patients with ET being evaluated for surgery compared to normative data. They used the Geriatric Depression Scale to assess depressive symptoms. Data, however, are not provided. Lacritz et al. (24) noted that 3 of 13 patients with ET evinced mild depressive symptoms on the Beck Depression Inventory (scores, 12–14) and one showed moderate symptoms (score, 20). Selection bias is a concern for both of these studies in which patients were being evaluated for surgery, and the ability to extend these findings to a randomly selected group of patients with ET is uncertain.

Louis et al. (1) conducted a case-control study of functional disability, comparing two groups of patients with ET (cases) to two groups of control subjects. The cases with ET were either ascertained from a community-based study of ET in northern Manhattan, New York (n = 37) or from a tertiary referral center, Columbia-Presbyterian Medical Center (n = 52). Current major depressive disorder was assessed using the depression module of the Structured Clinical Interview for *The Diagnostic and Statistical Manual of Mental Disorders*, 4th edition (DSM-IV). Current major depression was present in 5.4% of patients in the community, compared with 2.7% of community controls, and in 10.8% of tertiary referral patients versus 5.4% of their controls. Although the proportion of patients who were depressed was twice as high as that among controls, the proportions themselves were low (5.4%–10.8%) and, given the modest sample size, the difference between cases and controls was not statistically significant. Interestingly, though, these data suggest that patients seen in a tertiary referral center (i.e., those with more severe tremor) were more likely to be depressed than were their counterparts in the community. In another ongoing study of patients with ET, ascertained from the same tertiary referral center, and controls ascertained by random digit dialing (27), current antidepressant medication use was reported in 9.5% of 147 patients with ET compared to 6.7% of 210 controls (difference not significant; data unpublished).

Overall, these data suggest that the prevalence of depressive symptoms, depression, and use of antidepressant medications was relatively low in patients with ET (less than 10%). Further studies are needed to compare the prevalence of depressive symptoms and the types of these symptoms in patients with ET and in controls.

ANXIETY AND SOCIAL PHOBIA

Embarrassment can be a major issue for patients with ET and this aspect of the illness, rather than functional disability, is often the main reason why patients want to be treated (6). Several studies have provided data on anxiety and social phobia in patients with ET. Louis et al. (1), in their case–control study of functional disability, compared anxiety in two groups of patients with ET (cases) with that in two groups of controls. Anxiety was assessed with a Hamilton Anxiety Rating Scale. Mean ratings were generally low but were higher for patients with ET than for controls (8.0 in patients with ET versus 4.8 in controls, $p < 0.001$). As part of the framework of this study, social phobia was also assessed in 94 patients with ET and in 85 controls (28). Both current and lifetime social phobia were assessed with the Liebowitz Social Anxiety Scale. Whereas the likelihood of a history of lifetime social phobia was comparable in the two groups (21.6% of patients with ET versus 15.5% of controls, p = 0.31), current social phobia was significantly more common among patients with ET (14.8%) than among controls (3.6%, p = 0.01). At a tertiary referral center, lifetime social phobia was present in one third (32.7%) of patients with ET. The study reported that patients with social phobia reported greater fear than controls did and avoided eating, drinking, and writing in public more often. The severity of social phobia symptoms and that of tremor each independently contributed to functional disability.

In summary, anxiety and social phobia can occur in patients with ET, with current social phobia affecting approximately one in six patients with ET and a history of lifetime social phobia affecting as many as one in three of these patients. Fear, embarrassment, and the desire to avoid eating, drinking, and writing in public often motivate patients' desire for treatment.

PERSONALITY

The presence of cognitive deficits in ET in several reports raises the question as to whether other nonmotor domains may also be affected in patients with ET. Characteristic personality traits have been associated with several other movement disorders, including HD (29) and PD (30). Chatterjee et al. (14) conducted a case–control study of personality in ET, using a commonly employed self-reported measure of personality, the Tridimensional Personality Questionnaire (TPQ). The goal of this study was to determine whether patients with ET differed from controls in any of the three main dimensions of personality. Patients with ET and controls underwent the same evaluation. All the patients with ET, who lived in the New York tristate region, were cared for at the Neurological Institute of New York, Columbia-Presbyterian Medical Center. The control subjects were recruited from the same set of zip codes as the patients in the New York, New Jersey, and Connecticut region by random digit dialing and were frequency matched to patients with ET by age, sex, and race. The TPQ is a 98-item, self-administered true or false instrument. It measures personality traits across three higher-order dimensions. These dimensions are harm avoidance (HA) (HA, anxiety prone vs. risk taking), novelty seeking (NS) (NS, anger prone vs. docile), and reward dependence (RD) (RD, sentimental vs. aloof). Each dimension can be evaluated with a subscale score (HA, NS, RD subscale scores), which can be summed to yield a TPQ score. The mean HA subscale score was significantly higher in the 55 patients with ET than in the 61 controls (15.5 ± 8.1 versus 11.6 ± 7.2, p = 0.005). Mean RD and NS subscale scores did not differ between patients and controls. In a linear regression analysis that adjusted for age, presence or absence of ET remained significantly associated with the HA subscale score (p = 0.009). When the model was expanded to include age, sex, race, and years of education, the association with the HA subscale score remained significant (p = 0.005). A high HA score defines a person who is pessimistic, fearful, shy, anxious, and easily fatigued. It is unclear whether the higher HA subscale score in ET patients reflects functional disability caused by the tremor or whether it is a manifestation of the disease pathology. HA scores did not correlate with the patients' own assessment of disability or with several measures of tremor severity, suggesting that the personality profile was not entirely the result of tremor-related disability, although longitudinal studies are needed to fully examine this issue.

In summary, distinctive personality characteristics might be associated with ET. This potential association requires further study. Whether these characteristics predate the illness, accompany the onset of illness, or are the result of the effects of the illness is not clear at this time.

SUBSTANCE ABUSE AND ALCOHOLISM

Given the fact that sedatives, and particularly ethanol, are known to diminish the amplitude of tremor (31,32), patients with ET might use more ethanol than others do and perhaps even abuse ethanol. Few studies have actually attempted to quantify ethanol intake in patients with ET compared with that in controls. Louis et al. (33) quantified current daily intake of ethanol in patients with ET and in controls. Patients with ET were seen by neurologists at the Neurological Institute of New York, Columbia-Presbyterian Medical Center. Controls were identified from the New York Metropolitan area using random digit dialing. These controls were frequency matched to cases on 5-year age strata, gender, and ethnicity. Data about diet were collected in person by a trained tester using a Semi-Quantitative Food-Frequency Questionnaire. This 20-minute questionnaire included questions on frequency of consumption of 61 foods, including alcoholic beverages (beer, wine, and liquor). The questionnaire has shown good reliability and validity related to recent nutrient intake. The study included 130 patients with ET and 175 control subjects. The mean daily ethanol intake in patients with ET was 8.2 ± 13.9 gm versus 6.2 ± 9.3 gm in controls; medians were 2.4 versus 1.9 gm (Mann–Whitney z score = 0.14, p = 0.89) (Table 21-2). Older individuals might refrain from the use of ethanol because of contraindications or interactions with medications, so a difference in ethanol consumption between cases and controls might only be apparent in younger persons. Therefore, the sample was stratified into those who were younger than 50 years of age and those older than 50. In the 18 patients with ET who were younger than 50, the mean daily ethanol intake was 11.6 ± 18.3 gm, compared with 4.8 ± 6.6 gm in the 18 controls of the same age; medians were 5.8 versus 2.5 gm (Mann–Whitney z score = 0.36, p = 0.37). In summary, ethanol consumption appeared to be low in most of the patients with ET and in controls, but whether it might be higher in young patients with ET compared to young controls remains to be determined. In the subanalysis of younger individuals, the median daily ethanol intake in these patients with ET was more than twice as high as that in controls, but the sample size was small, and the difference was not significant. In

TABLE 21-2. *Ethanol consumption in ET cases and controls*

Beverage	Cases with ET	Controls
Beer		
<1/mo	89 (68.5%)	121 (69.1%)
<1/d	36 (27.7%)	53 (30.3%)
1/d	2 (1.5%)	1 (0.6%)
2–3/d	1 (0.8%)	0
≥4/d	2 (1.5%)	0
Wine		
<1/mo	63 (48.5%)	69 (39.4%)
<1/d	50 (38.5%)	89 (50.9%)
1/d	12 (9.2%)	13 (7.4%)
2–3/d	4 (3.1%)	3 (1.7%)
≥4/d	1 (0.8%)	1 (0.6%)
Liquor		
<1/mo	81 (62.3%)	108 (61.7%)
<1/d	38 (29.2%)	53 (30.3%)
1/d	8 (6.2%)	11 (6.3%)
2–3/d	3 (2.3%)	3 (1.7%)
≥4/d	0	0

All p ≥0.05.

other case–control studies of ethanol consumption in ET, ethanol was examined in small numbers of patients and was not quantified in grams (34,35) or studied in men only (34,35). In one other study (36), data on monthly consumption were presented in three groups (less than 200 gm, 200 gm, or greater than 200 gm). Although the proportion of participants who consumed more than 200 grams of ethanol per month was "somewhat greater" among the 115 patients with ET than among the 76 controls, this difference did not reach significance. Despite some early reports of alcoholism in patients with ET (34,37), most case–control studies have not found a higher proportion of alcoholics among patients with ET than among controls (35,36).

In summary, young patients with ET might be more prone than their control counterparts to use ethanol in excess, but little evidence exists to suggest that older patients with ET overuse or abuse ethanol.

SUMMARY

As the complexity and heterogeneity of ET emerge, greater interest has been taken in the nonmotor manifestations of this disease. The fact that the motor manifestations reflect widespread anatomic pathology (e.g., cerebellum, basal ganglia) suggests that the nonmotor aspects might be a manifestation of an illness that affects multiple areas of the nervous system. Therefore, nonmotor aspects of the disease might reflect the presence of disease pathology in a particular area of the brain. Alternatively, nonmotor aspects could be the result of the tremor itself and the effects that it has on disability, mood, and personality. Finally, some of the nonmotor aspects could reflect the possibility that individuals with these disorders have a shared predisposition for ET and that a common mechanism underlies both. Further work is needed to define the extent of the nonmotor manifestations, their presence or absence in the predisease state, and their progression over time. These studies will further our insights into the mechanisms and anatomic pathology of ET and help us to develop a broader understanding of issues that are important in treating the individuals with this disease.

ACKNOWLEDGMENTS

Dr. Louis is supported by R01 NS39422 and R01 NS42859 (National Institutes of Health, Bethesda, MD).

REFERENCES

1. Louis ED, Barnes L, Albert SM, et al. Correlates of functional disability in essential tremor. Mov Disord 2001;16:914–920.
2. Louis ED, Greene P. Essential tremor. In: Rowland. LP, ed. Merritt textbook of neurology, 10th ed. Philadelphia, PA: Lea & Febiger, 2000:678–679.
3. Hubble JP, Busenbark KL, Koller WC. Essential tremor. Clln Neuropharm 1989;12:453–482.
4. Findley LJ, Koller WC. Essential tremor: a review. Neurology 1987;37:1194–1197.
5. Critchley M. Observations on essential tremor (heredofamilial tremor). Brain 1949;72:113–139.
6. Louis ED. Essential tremor. N Engl J Med 2001;345:887–891.
7. Stolze H, Petersen G, Raethjen J, et al. Gait analysis in essential tremor—further evidence for a cerebellar dysfunction. Mov Disord 2000;15(Suppl. 3):87.
8. Deuschl G, Wenzelburger R, Loffler K, et al. Essential tremor and cerebellar dysfunction. Clinical and kinematic analysis of intention tremor. Brain 2000;123:1568–1580.
9. Singer C, Sanchez-Ramos J, Weiner WJ. Gait abnormality in essential tremor. Mov Disord 1994;9:193–196.
10. Helmchen C, Hagenow A, Miesner J, et al. Eye movement abnormalities in essential tremor may indicate cerebellar dysfunction. Brain 2003;126:1319–1332.
11. Rajput AH, Rozdilsky B, Ang L, et al. Significance of Parkinsonian manifestations in essential tremor. Can J Neurol Sci 1993;20:114–117.
12. Cohen O, Pullman S, Jurewicz E, et al. Rest tremor in essential tremor patients: prevalence, clinical correlates, and electrophysiological characteristics. Arch Neurol 2003;60:405–410.
13. Gasparini M, Bonifati V, Fabrizio E. et al. Frontal lobe dysfunction in essential tremor. A preliminary study. J Neurol 2001;248:399–402.
14. Chatterjee A, Jurewicz EC, Applegate LM, et al. Personality in essential tremor. Mov Disord JNNP 2004;75:958–961.
15. Louis ED, Bromley SM, Jurewicz EC, et al. Olfactory dysfunction in essential tremor: a deficit unrelated to disease duration or severity. Neurology 2002;59:1631–1633.
16. Louis ED, Marder K, Jurewicz EC, et al. Body mass index in essential tremor. Arch Neurol 2002;59:1273–1277.
17. Louis ED. The shaking palsy. The first forty-five years. A journey through the British literature. Mov Disord 1997;12:1068–1072.
18. Celesia GG, Wanamaker WM. Psychiatric disturbances in Parkinson's disease. Dis Nerv Syst 1972;33:577–583.
19. Lieberman A, Dziatolowski M, Kupersmith M, et al. Dementia in Parkinson's disease. Ann Neurol 1979;6:355–359.
20. Martilla RJ, Rinne UK. Dementia in Parkinson's disease. Acta Neurol Scand 1976;54:431–441.

21. Mayeux R, Stern Y, Rosenstein R, et al. An estimate of the prevalence of dementia in idiopathic Parkinson's disease. *Arch Neurol* 1988;45:260–263.
22. Mayeux R, Chen J, Mirabello E, et al. An estimate of the incidence of dementia in patients with idiopathic Parkinson's disease. *Neurology* 1990;40:1513–1517.
23. Lombardi WJ, Woolston DJ, Roberts JW, et al. Cognitive deficits in patients with essential tremor. *Neurology* 2001;57:785–790.
24. Lacritz LH, Dewey R Jr, Giller C, et al. Cognitive functioning in individuals with "benign" essential tremor. *J Int Neuropsychol Soc* 2002;8:125–129.
25. Duane DD, Vermilion KJ. Cognitive deficits in patients with essential tremor. *Neurology* 2002;58:1706.
26. Vermilion K, Stone A, Duane D. Cognition and affect in idiopathic essential tremor. *Mov Disord* 2001;16:S30.
27. Louis ED, Zheng W, Jurewicz EC, et al. Elevation of blood β-carboline alkaloids in essential tremor. *Neurology* 2002;59:1940–1944.
28. Schneier FR, Barnes LF, Albert SM, et al. Characteristics of social phobia among persons with essential tremor. *J Clin Psychiatry* 2001;62:367–372.
29. Bolt JM. Huntington's chorea in the West of Scotland. *Br J Psychiatry* 1970;116:259–270.
30. Menza M. The personality associated with Parkinson's disease. *Curr Psychiatry Rep* 2000;2:421–426.
31. Growden JH, Shahani BT, Young RR. The effect of alcohol on essential tremor. *Neurology* 1975;25:259–262.
32. Koller WC, Biary N. Effect of alcohol on tremors: comparison with propranolol. *Neurology* 1984;34:221–222.
33. Louis ED, Jurewicz EC, Applegate L, et al. Semiquantitative study of current coffee, caffeine and ethanol intake in essential tremor cases and controls. *Mov Disord* 2004;19:499–504.
34. Schroeder D, Nasrallah HA. High alcoholism rate in patients with essential tremor. *Am J Psychiatry* 1982;139:1471–1473.
35. Koller WC. Alcoholism in essential tremor. *Neurology* 1983;33:1074–1076.
36. Rautakorpi I, Martilla RJ, Rinne UK. Alcohol consumption of patients with essential tremor. *Acta Neurol Scand* 1983;68:177–179.
37. Nasrallah HA, Schroeder D, Petty F. Alcoholism secondary to essential tremor. *J Clin Psychiatry* 1982;43:163–164.

22

Behavioral and Psychiatric Manifestations in Dystonia

Marjan Jahanshahi

Sobell Department of Motor Neuroscience and Movement Disorders, Institute of Neurology, London, United Kingdom

Dystonia is a movement disorder associated with basal ganglia dysfunction (1–3), in which sustained muscle contractions give rise to abnormal postures or involuntary movements (4,5). Dystonia can affect one part of the body (focal dystonia), two or more adjacent parts (segmental dystonia), or many parts (generalized). Multifocal dystonia affects more than one site of the body, and hemidystonia affects two or more sites on one side of the body. Focal dystonia affecting the neck muscles is known as *spasmodic torticollis*. Spasmodic dysphonia affects the muscles involved in speech. Dystonia involving the periorbital muscles of the eyes is called *blepharospasm*. Oromandibular dystonia affects the muscles of the jaw. In writer's cramp, the muscles involved in writing undergo spasm during writing. Blepharospasm and oromandibular dystonia occurring together is labeled *Meige's syndrome*. From a clinical perspective, another important factor in the classification of dystonia is the distinction between primary and secondary dystonia. In the primary form of the disorder, dystonia is the main clinical feature, and tremor can also be present, but there is no evidence of neurodegeneration. A large proportion of patients with primary dystonia exhibit the *DYT1* gene mutation associated with the GAG deletion in the *DYT1* gene on chromosome 9 (6). *DYT1* dystonia has autosomal dominant inheritance with low penetrance, and only 30% to 40% of the carriers develop dystonia (7,8). Secondary or symptomatic dystonia develops following brain injury or chronic use of dopamine receptor–blocking drugs, such as neuroleptic medication, or in association with degenerative disorders such as Wilson's disease or Huntington's disease. A new class of "dystonia plus syndromes" has also been identified, which includes dopa-responsive dystonia and myoclonic dystonia. Investigation into the genetic causes of dystonia has progressed during the past two decades, and 13 different dystonia genes have been mapped to various forms of dystonia [for review, see (7,8)]. In addition to the *DYT1* gene, genes have been mapped for dopa-responsive dystonia, myoclonic dystonia, and paroxysmal or the episodic form of dystonia. In primary dystonia, age of onset is an important factor in determining the progression of dystonia to other anatomic sites, and a distinction is made between young and adult-onset dystonia. When the onset of dystonia is before the age of 28, and if the legs are affected first, it is likely to affect other parts of body. In contrast, in adult-onset dystonia, the sustained muscle contractions are first seen after the age of 28 and are likely to remain focal.

Epidemiologic studies in the United States, China, Egypt, Japan, northeast England, and seven European countries have investigated the prevalence of dystonia (9–14). In the study from northeast England, the prevalence of generalized and focal dystonia was 1.42 and 12.86 cases per 100,000 population, respectively (11). Because the methods adopted for each study differ, the exact prevalence rates differ across studies. Nevertheless, the studies agree in two respects: first, that focal dystonia is more prevalent than generalized dystonia, and second, that dystonia is more prevalent than had been previously presumed and more prevalent than neurologic disorders such as motor neuron disease, myasthenia gravis, and muscular dystrophy.

This chapter considers the nature and prevalence of psychiatric illness in primary dystonia and the wider effect of dystonia on daily activities, psychological well-being, social functioning, and quality of life (QOL) of patients. The origins of psychiatric morbidity in dystonia are discussed. Diagnostic considerations about less common cases of psychogenic dystonia are also considered before reviewing the management and therapeutic approaches adopted in optimally dealing with concomitant psychiatric illness and psychosocial dysfunction in patients with dystonia.

THE CONVOLUTED HISTORY OF THE PSYCHIATRIC APPROACH TO DYSTONIA

Although the view of dystonia as an organic neurologic disorder gained prominence in the 1900s when Oppenheim (15) described the disorder, this view coexisted with psychogenic causal models of the disorder from the 1940s to the 1960s, and even into the 1970s. Several features of dystonia contributed to the persistence of psychogenic causal models. The bizarre nature of the postural abnormalities; relief of some forms of dystonia by the geste antagoniste (16); improvement of the dystonic postures and movements through relaxation, sedation, and hypnosis and, conversely, the sensitivity of the postures and movements to social and mental stress (17); the occurrence of spontaneous remission in cervical dystonia (18); the task specificity of some forms of dystonia such as simple writer's cramp; and a failure to find any anatomic, physiologic, or biochemical abnormality in these disorders provided fuel for psychogenic models (4). Psychogenic causal models of dystonia have ranged from the psychoanalytic to the behavioral. In the case of torticollis, for example, psychoanalytic formulations emphasized the symbolic meaning of the head turn as "representing a looking away from adult responsibilities," "having significance of a phallic nature," "symbolizing of hanging one's head in shame, due to guilt and shame over past transgressions,"

"a turning away from something painful or intolerable," and "a regressive phenomenon representing the infant's seeking of the mother's breast" (19). At the other extreme, behavioral causal models of torticollis proposed that the muscle spasms were "a drive-reducing avoidance response, which is repeatedly conditioning itself" (20) or "an anxiety-reducing response which is reinforced as it allows escape from an anxiety-provoking work situation" (21).

Two lines of argument were used to support the psychogenic models of dystonia. The first suggested that patients with dystonia had abnormal personalities; specifically, that they were neurotic and obsessional (22) or that their personality was characterized by the "conversion V" profile typical of hysteria. The second proposal to support psychogenic models was that psychological trauma—for example, a major life event, marital discord, job instability, or general stress—preceded the onset of dystonia. Because torticollis is the most prevalent focal dystonia, these proposals have been most extensively investigated in people with this form of cervical dystonia. Many studies relied only on personal impressions of the personality of the patient with torticollis (22–25), whereas other studies combined interviews with unstandardized personality tests such as the Rorschach test (19,26,27). Although of all the studies reported abnormal personality traits in a proportion of patients with torticollis, and some studies identified psychological factors preceding the onset of torticollis (22,24,26), these studies were largely unsystematic. Since the 1970s, other investigators have examined the assumptions of the psychogenic model of torticollis in a more systematic manner (28–35) and have used standardized personality measures; some investigators have even included control groups of patients with other chronic disorders (29,30,31–35). Of these more systematic studies, some (29,31,32) did not find any evidence of abnormal personality profiles in patients with torticollis, whereas other studies (28,30,34) reported that neurotic personality traits and increased obsessionality characterized a proportion of patients with torticollis. In the study by Jahanshahi and Marsden (34), however, a similar proportion of patients with cervical spondylosis, who were assessed as a control group, also had personality profiles with high neuroticism and obsessionality, and the mean scores of the two groups did not differ on any of the dimensions assessed. Furthermore, similar personality profiles are found in other patient groups with chronic neurologic disorders. Consequently, Jahanshahi and Marsden (34) proposed that the presence of neurotic and obsessional profiles in a small proportion of patients with torticollis does not support a psychogenic causal model but represents a form of "reactive neuroticism" similar to depression, and that the destabilization of personality in a subgroup of patients is a reaction to the onset of or experience of living with a disabling, deforming, and chronic neurologic illness.

Psychogenic formulations have also been applied to other focal dystonias, such as writer's cramp (36–38), and suggest that muscle cramps represent a neurotic disorder or a dysfunctional grip of writing instruments, which could be appropriately treated with behavioral methods that aim to reverse the dysfunctional habit (39–41). The association of writer's cramp and focal hand dystonia with psychopathology has been investigated to refute such formulations. Harrington et al. (42) and Grafman, Cohen, and Hallett (43) used standardized scales to measure neuroticism, depression, and anxiety and correlated the responses with measures of writing speed and manual dexterity (finger tapping) and with performance on a serial reaction-time task. Harrington et al. (42) reported no differences between 22 patients and controls on the anxiety scales, and although writing speed was slower in the patients with writer's cramp, no significant association was found between writing speed and anxiety. Grafman, Cohen, and Hallett (43) found that 4 patients in their sample of 20 patients with focal hand dystonia, either writer's cramp or musician's palsy, had mild depression but that for the sample as a whole, performance on all motor tasks, the Minnesota Multiphasic Personality Inventory (MMPI), Beck Depression Inventory (BDI), and Spielberger Trait Anxiety Scale was within normal limits. The authors did not find any association between motor performance and measures of psychopathology other than a correlation between depression scores on the MMPI and reaction times.

On the MMPI, the conversion V pattern— high scores on the hypochondriasis and hysteria scales, coupled with low scores on the depression scale—is considered to be characteristic of patients with conversion disorder, in which the patient converts personally distressing psychological problems into more socially acceptable somatic complaints (44). To test for the presence of such conversion V profiles, Jahanshahi and Marsden (45) administered a short version of the MMPI to 61 patients with adult-onset idiopathic torticollis. Thirty-six percent of the patients had normal MMPI profiles, only 5 patients (9%) had a conversion V profile, and most patients had higher scores on the depression scale than on the hysteria or hypochondriasis scales, indicating the presence of mild depression. The fact that 22.5% of low-back pain sufferers with organic neurologic evidence of their complaint have a conversion V profile on the MMPI test suggests that it may represent factors other than the presence of a conversion disorder. Items of the hysteria and hypochondriasis scales have been selected to measure concern with the body and physical health. Patients with genuine neurologic disorders who may be preoccupied with controlling their symptoms, can also achieve high scores on these tests. Patients with spasmodic dysphonia exhibit similar results on the MMPI. Aronson et al. (46) found that 62% of the patients with dysphonia who were studied exhibited some neurotic symptoms, whereas 38% of patients had normal profiles. The profiles of patients with dysphonia showed higher scores on the scales for depression and social introversion. The emotional traits most commonly exhibited by the patients with dysphonia included compulsiveness, suppressed anger, and verbal repression. However, these patients scored considerably lower on the hysteria and hypochondriasis scales, which differentiated their MMPI profiles from those of patients with psychogenic aphonia.

The second assumption of the psychogenic model of dystonia, that psychological trauma such as occurrence of a major life event, marital discord, job instability, or general stress precedes the onset of dystonia, has also been examined in a number of studies on torticollis (30,31,34,35). In these studies, about 50% of the patients with torticollis identified psychosocial or physical trauma as events preceding the onset of their head deviation. However, in the study by Jahanshahi and Marsden (34), a similar proportion of the patients with cervical spondylosis in the control group also reported similar events preceding their illness. In a questionnaire study of 200 patients with spasmodic dysphonia, Izdebski and Dedo (47) found that 15% of the patients associated their voice problems with stress, 2.6% associated their problems with psychological disorder, and 5.6% associated them with emotional trauma. On the basis of these data, the authors concluded that no specific indication of a psychogenic etiology could be identified in these patients. In some cases, the events reported might have acted as precipitating factors or triggers for the onset of dystonia in already predisposed individuals (48,49), whereas in others these events may have represented "causal attributions" made by patients retrospectively attempting to make sense of a relatively rare disorder (34).

Some patients with dystonia report experiencing psychiatric illness before the onset of their neurologic illness. For example, 2 of the 29 patients (6.5%) studied by Mathews et al. (31) received psychiatric treatment for depression before the onset of torticollis. Similarly, 6.3% of the patients with torticollis studied by Cockburn (29) had an earlier psychiatric history. In the sample of 85 patients with adult-onset idiopathic torticollis studied by Jahanshahi and Marsden (35), 5 patients (5.9%) had a prior psychiatric history, compared with 7 of 49 (14.3%) in the control group (patients with cervical spondylosis). Therefore, about 6% of patients with torticollis seem to have a psychiatric history, most commonly depression or anxiety disorders, before the onset of neurologic illness. Although psychogenic formulations suggest that a high prevalence of psychiatric morbidity preceding the onset of the motor symptoms indicates the psychogenic etiology of the movement disorder, it is evident from the results of these studies, which included control groups, that the prevalence of prior psychiatric illness is no higher in dystonia than in other chronic disorders.

The evidence reviewed demonstrates that neurotic and obsessional personality traits, conversion V profiles, and traumatic events before onset of torticollis are present in only a small proportion of patients rather than in all cases and are typical of a similar proportion of patients with other chronic disorders. This evidence refutes the psychogenic causal model of dystonia. The advances made in identifying the genetic forms of the disorder and the functional anatomic evidence for altered striatofrontal processing in idiopathic dystonia have undoubtedly played a more important role than the studies cited above in dispensing with the psychogenic model of dystonia (50–52). Nevertheless, because the psychogenic causal model coexisted with the view of dystonia as a neurologic disorder, even as recently as a decade ago, initial misdiagnosis of idiopathic dystonia as a psychogenic disorder was quite common and was reported in 52% (53), 43% (4), 24.7% (54), 44% (55), and 50% (56) of cases in various neurology clinics. In a survey of 100 patients with adult-onset torticollis in 1989, 60% of patients reported that they had been told that their problem was "all in their mind" at some stage before it was diagnosed as a neurologic disorder (Jahanshahi and Marsden, unpublished observations). In a subsequent survey of 705 people with dystonia in the United Kingdom, 37% of patients reported that a doctor had suggested that their condition was "all in the mind" before they received their neurologic diagnoses of dystonia (57). Compared to the earlier estimate of 60% reported by Jahanshahi and Marsden, the more recent finding, that 37% of patients were erroneously told by doctors that their problem was "all in the mind," suggests that medical familiarity with and recognition of dystonia has improved and that such misdiagnosis of idiopathic dystonia as a psychogenic disorder has been reduced. Probably the foremost historic reason for this improved diagnostic ability is the gradual emergence and increasing prominence, since the mid-1970s, of movement disorders as an important specialty in neurology. This development has led to a burgeoning of research and publications on dystonia, which has in turn increased awareness of the disorder as a neurologic entity among non-neurologists such as general practitioners and psychiatrists.

We have now come full circle. Almost 100 years after dystonia was first described by Oppenheim (15), most cases are considered to be neurologic, and only a very few of the cases are considered psychogenic.

Dystonia, as a disabling, deforming, and chronic neurologic disorder, is associated with psychiatric complications that are now considered to be multifactorially determined, with both biochemical and psychosocial factors contributing to their development.

PREVALENCE AND NATURE OF PSYCHIATRIC ILLNESS IN DYSTONIA

Compared to other movement disorders associated with basal ganglia dysfunction, such as Parkinson's disease (PD) or Huntington's disease (HD), in which psychiatric morbidity has been extensively examined, dystonia has been the subject of relatively few studies investigating the prevalence and nature of coexisting psychiatric illness. Most of the existing literature has focused on torticollis.

Patterson and Little (23) conducted a psychiatric evaluation in 83 of their 103 patients with torticollis and identified psychiatric disorder in 21 cases (25.3%). Early studies mainly relied on standardized self-reported measures to examine the extent of psychopathology in dystonia. Jahanshahi and Marsden (34,35) administered the BDI, Beck Hopelessness Scale, the Spielberger Trait Anxiety Scale, and the Leyton Obsessional Inventory to 100 patients, 85 of whom had adult-onset idiopathic torticollis, and a control group of 49 patients with cervical spondylosis. They also used questionnaires to obtain information about the presence or absence of psychiatric disorder and the nature of the diagnoses and corroborated this information by checking the patients' hospital records. Twenty-three patients with torticollis (17%) had a past or current history of psychiatric disorder, compared to 13 of the controls (26.5%), a nonsignificant difference. In both groups, depression and anxiety prevailed as the most common class of psychiatric disorder, present in 21 of the 23 patients with torticollis who had a psychiatric history. Of the remaining two patients with torticollis, one was diagnosed with obsessive–compulsive disorder (OCD), and the other with personality disorder. Mean scores on the BDI were significantly higher in the patients with torticollis than in the control group, and twice as many patients with torticollis (28.6%) were moderately to severely depressed, according to the BDI, than were controls (15.4%). The two groups did not differ in scores on the measures of hopelessness, trait anxiety, or obsessionality. Ideally, interview schedules should have been used instead of self-reported measures, because the aim was to survey a large sample of patients; however, this approach was deemed impractical, and using questionnaires of proven reliability and validity, corroborated by review of the hospital records, was instead considered the most pragmatic method. Nevertheless, the large sample size and the inclusion of a disease control group make the studies by Jahanshahi and Marsden (34,35) important in the investigation of psychopathology in torticollis.

A number of subsequent studies relied on structured interview schedules. Naber et al. (58) used structured interviews and the criteria from the *The Diagnostic and Statistical Manual of Mental Disorders*, 3rd edition (DSM-III) to assess psychiatric morbidity in 32 patients with torticollis and a control group of patients with PD. Current psychiatric disorder was found in 2 of the 32 patients (6.25%). This low rate may partly reflect a sampling bias, because the patients for this study were recruited through a patient association or by advertisement. Wenzel et al. (59) used the Structured Clinical Interview for DSM-III-R (SCID) to diagnose lifetime and current psychiatric illness in 44 patients (20 women and 24 men) with spasmodic torticollis consecutively referred to a neurology clinic. A current or lifetime psychiatric diagnosis was found in 29 patients (65.8%), of whom 13 (29.5%) had a past history of psychiatric illness, and all others (16 patients, 36.4%) had at least one current diagnosis. Eighteen patients (40.8%) had more than one diagnosis. Panic disorder with or without agoraphobia in 13 patients (29.5%) and major depressive disorder in 11 patients (25%) were the most common single lifetime or current diagnostic categories. Past or current alcohol or substance abuse was found in six patients (13.6%), and OCD was noted in three patients (6.8%). In a later report by the same group, Moraru et al. (60) also administered the SCID and DSM-III-R criteria together with two self-rated scales, the BDI and the Symptom Check List (SCL-90), to 40 patients with cervical dystonia. A subgroup of the patients (12%) was found to have high levels of psychopathology, with concomitant levels of depression and anxiety on the BDI and SCL-90. When both previous and current episodes of psychiatric illness were considered, 22 of the 40 patients (55%) met the criterion of at least one psychiatric disorder, with anxiety and depression being the most common diagnostic categories.

Gundel et al. (61) compared psychiatric morbidity in 48 patients with torticollis and 48 patients with alopecia areata (controls). The SCID-I and DSM-IV were used, together with the SCL-90, the Freiburger Coping Strategies Scale, and the Social Phobia Scale. Current psychiatric morbidity was more common among the patients with torticollis (77.1%) than among the controls (41.7%). Of the 48 patients with torticollis, 33 (68.8%) met the DSM-IV criteria for current anxiety disorder, and 9 (18.8%) met the criteria for mood disorders. In contrast, 16 (33.3%) and 6 (12.5%) of the 48 controls had current anxiety and mood disorders, respectively. The lifetime prevalence of psychiatric disorder was also significantly higher among the patients with torticollis (91.7%) than among the controls (60.4%). Psychiatric morbidity in both groups was significantly higher than in a representative German population. Compared to normative data for the SCL-90, general psychopathology was more common in the torticollis and alopecia groups, and the two groups did not differ significantly from each other. In contrast, social phobia ratings were significantly higher in the patients with torticollis than in the controls. Risk for current psychiatric morbidity was 3.7 times higher among patients with torticollis than among controls. Although the duration of illness was longer in the patients with torticollis (12.5 years) than in the patients with alopecia (8.7 years), the authors concluded that higher prevalence of psychiatric morbidity in torticollis could not be simply secondary to altered physical appearance or chronic disease, because alopecia is also a visible illness that alters physical appearance. However, the greater psychiatric morbidity in dystonia may arise from the fact that patients with alopecia develop ways of hiding their altered physical appearance, a coping mechanism that is not possible in dystonia. Using the same methods and measures, the same group also investigated psychiatric disorder, and specifically social phobia, in a consecutive series of 116 patients with torticollis (61). Current psychiatric disorder was found in 75.9% of these patients, with 16.4% of patients exhibiting mood disorder, 50% exhibiting anxiety disorders, and 7.8% exhibiting adjustment disorders. Social phobia, the most common anxiety disorder, was found in 41.3% of patients. The prevalence of mood disorders in the patients with torticollis was 2.4 times higher, and prevalence of social phobia was 10 times higher, than in a representative population of 483 Germans aged 45 to 65. Measures of torticollis severity on the Tsui scale did not show any association with the DSM-IV psychiatric diagnoses, which was correlated with the use of maladaptive depressive coping strategies as measured on the Freiburger scale. To account for the high rate of social phobia in torticollis, Gundel et al. (61) point to the key role played by low self-esteem, caused by a sense of disfigurement and disturbed body image, which was previously described as the cornerstone of self-related negative cognitions (35) and shown to be the major predictor of depression in these patients (62,63).

Psychiatric morbidity in other forms of dystonia has been investigated. Among the 22 patients with writer's cramp studied by Harrington et al. (42), 4 patients had a psychiatric history: 2 of depression and 2 of anxiety disorder. On the basis of brief psychiatric interviews, none of the 20 patients with writer's cramp or musician's palsy studied by Grafman, Cohen, and Hallett (43) reported a remarkable psychiatric history. Three of these 20 patients had scores on the MMPI, the BDI, and the Spielberger Trait Anxiety Scale that suggested mild clinical disorder, 1 of whom also had multiple somatic complaints.

Although the association between OCD and dystonia was originally reported in an unsystematic fashion, it has long been noted. Bindman and Tibbets (37) described 9 of 10 patients with writer's cramp as having obsessional personalities, and patients with torticollis were also noted to have obsessional personalities (22). Subsequent studies used more systematic approaches and found that patients with blepharospasm and those with torticollis have significantly more obsessive–compulsive symptoms than healthy controls (64,65). Brooks et al. (66) used the SCID and DSM-III-R, the SCL-90-R, and the Hamburg Obsession–Compulsion Inventory to compare 13 patients with blepharospasm to 13 patients with hemifacial spasm. The two groups were matched in terms of age, sex ratio, and duration of illness. The patients with blepharospasm had higher scores on the obsessional–compulsive inventory, but none of the patients met the DSM-III-R criteria for OCD. In each group, four patients had a lifetime diagnosis of major depressive illness but were not depressed at the time of study. Among the 13 patients with blepharospasm, 3 had simple phobias, 1 had a social phobia, and 2 had histories of alcohol or analgesic abuse. Two of the 13 patients with hemifacial spasm had panic disorder. In both groups, scores on the SCL-90-R scale did not differ from normative data for eight of the categories. With the aim of examining the occurrence of OCD and its familial prevalence in idiopathic dystonia, Cavallaro et al. (67) studied 76 patients with idiopathic focal dystonias (50% with blepharospasm, 36.8% with torticollis, 9.2% with dysphonia, 1.3% with oromandibular dystonia, and 2.7% with writer's cramp) and a control group of 129 surgical patients, using scores on the Yale-Brown Obsessive–Compulsive Scale and DSM-IV criteria for lifetime and current OCD. Fifteen (19.7%) of the patients with dystonia met the criteria for OCD, two (3.5%) met criteria for obsessive–compulsive spectrum disorders, and eight (10.5%) were diagnosed as having subclinical OCD, because they not did report any distress or interference associated with their symptoms. In the control group of surgical patients, the prevalence of OCD was 0.77%, which was significantly lower than in the dystonia group. The risk for OCD was significantly higher among first-degree relatives of patients with dystonia and OCD than among first-degree relatives of patients with dystonia but no OCD; it was also higher than risk among first-degree relatives of control patients. To investigate the presence of obsessive–compulsive characteristics, Kubota et al. (68) compared scores on the Yale-Brown Obsessive–Compulsive Scale among 12 patients with writer's cramp, patients with writing impairment caused by peripheral nerve lesions, and age and sex-matched healthy controls. The patients with writer's cramp had significantly higher scores than patients with writing impairment or healthy controls, and their compulsive symptoms were mainly related to cleaning and ordering. Psychiatric symptoms, such as OCD, are commonly reported in patients with myoclonic dystonia. Saunders-Pullman et al. (69) reported a higher rate of OCD, anxiety disorders, and alcohol dependence in people carrying the mutation associated with inherited myoclonic dystonia.

The available evidence indicates that psychiatric morbidity is higher in patients with dystonia than in community samples or in patients with other forms of chronic disease. Depression, anxiety, and OCD are the most common psychiatric diagnoses in dystonia. The focus of the literature has been mainly on torticollis and some other forms of focal dystonia. Age of onset is likely to be an important determinant of susceptibility to psychiatric morbidity in dystonia. Future studies should consider focusing on the prevalence of psychiatric problems among patients with childhood-onset generalized dystonia compared to those with adult-onset dystonia.

EFFECT OF DYSTONIA ON PSYCHOSOCIAL FUNCTIONING, PERCEIVED STIGMA, AND QUALITY OF LIFE

When considering the consequences of a chronic illness such as dystonia, a useful distinction between impairment, disability (or activity), and handicap (or participation) has been proposed by the World Health Organization (WHO). Impairment is the combined effect of all the symptoms of the illness. Disability refers to the way in which the impairment affects the patients' daily activities. Handicap reflects the effect of the disease in its widest personal and social sense and the restrictions experienced by the individual because of the illness. The handicap associated with a chronic illness and its effect on QOL are considered in broad domains of life and or social roles such as mobility, work, social and leisure activities, relationships with others, physical independence, and economic self-sufficiency. Impairment and disability are measured against some general reference of normality. In contrast, handicap and QOL can be adequately evaluated only in relation to each individual's life circumstances, immediate social context, and future expectations, that is, in terms of how that person functioned, worked, and engaged in social and leisure activities before the onset of the illness; the QOL they would have expected to have if the illness had not occurred. Thus, the effect of a chronic neurologic disorder such as dystonia is considered in terms of the associated disability and handicap and the influence of these drawbacks on the patient's QOL. Dystonia is not only a disabling disorder, but also often a deforming one. In addition to patients' individual characteristics and circumstances, which play a key role in determining the extent of disability and handicap, other factors in the wider social context (such as social prejudice) and environmental obstacles (such as inadequate transport facilities and lack of access to public buildings) can also contribute to perceived stigma and create further handicap. Dystonia has a major effect on daily activities, social functioning, perceptions of stigma, and QOL. This evidence is reviewed in the following sections. For the sake of clarity, this body of empirical evidence has been divided into three categories: psychosocial functioning, stigma, and QOL.

Psychosocial Functioning

Dystonia affects the ability of patients to develop or continue many of their key social roles, such as marital and employment status. The sample of 100 patients with torticollis and the control group of 49 patients with cervical spondylosis studied by Jahanshahi and Marsden (34,35) differed substantially in terms of marital status. Similar percentages of patients in the two groups were married or divorced, and for those who were married, no differences were reported between groups in marital satisfaction or discord.

However, a larger percentage of patients with torticollis (20%) than of patients with cervical spondylosis (4.1%) were single. Further analysis established that this difference was not attributable simply to the older age and the later age of disease onset in the cervical spondylosis group, and that the postural deviation of the head and its concomitant social avoidance and social stigma was perhaps an obstacle to marriage in those patients with torticollis. The proportion of patients who were employed was similar in the torticollis and control groups (about 41% in both groups), but five times as many of the patients with torticollis (22.2%) were "permanently sick" and unemployed for longer than 6 months, compared with the controls (4.2%). The negative effect of adult-onset dystonia on employment is confirmed by later studies. In a large survey of 641 patients with dystonia in northern England, Butler et al. (70) confirmed the negative effect of dystonia on employment status and annual income. At the start of the study, only 32.4% of the patients surveyed were either working or available for work. Over the next 3 years, this figure reduced to 25.5%. Among the sample patients, 13.3% were permanently sick, and 11.8% had retired because of ill health. Patients' mean annual income in 1993 or 1996 was approximately £7,400, and 50% of them had an income of less than £6,000 (i.e., $9,700). These data clearly demonstrate the economic hardship experienced by people with dystonia and their families.

Dystonia can occur as an occupational palsy, particularly in musicians or singers, affecting the muscles of the neck, hands, or larynx. Five such cases of musicians and singers with dystonia were described by Butler et al. (71). These case histories demonstrate two things. First, that there can be a prolonged period between development of symptoms and medical diagnosis of dystonia. In one case, there was a delay of 14 years. Second, that when symptoms are severe, the onset of dystonia can put an end to the occupational life of musicians, as illustrated by a singer who developed spasmodic dysphonia.

Jahanshahi and Marsden (35) compared quantitative and qualitative features of depression in 85 patients with torticollis and in a control group of 49 patients with cervical spondylosis. The patients with torticollis not only had significantly higher scores than the control group on the BDI, but also showed qualitatively distinct features of depression. Qualitative analyses showed that the group differences on the BDI were related to the patients with torticollis scoring higher than the patients with cervical spondylosis on the cognitive and affective items (e.g., "I feel I am a complete failure as a person" or "I feel that there are permanent changes in my appearance that make me look unattractive"), but no differences were seen on the physical somatic aspects of depression (e.g., "I don't sleep as well as I used to" or "I get tired more easily than I used to"). A subsequent item-by-item analysis of the BDI revealed that the patients with torticollis had significantly higher scores on the lack of satisfaction, sense of punishment, self-blame, self-accusation, self-punitive or suicidal thoughts, body image, and work inhibition items of the BDI relative to the controls. Thus, negative self-referent cognitions emerged as the main qualitative feature of depression in torticollis. A negative view of the self, the world, and the future constitute what has been labeled the cognitive triad in Beck's (72) theory of depression. Jahanshahi and Marsden (35) suggest that depression in torticollis is primarily characterized by a negative view of the self, probably relating to the disturbed body image and low self-esteem associated with the head deviation. Jahanshahi and Marsden (62,63) also provided evidence for this hypothesis by examining the possible role of disability and negative body image on development of depression in torticollis. To assess the effect of torticollis on daily activities and body concept, Jahanshahi and Marsden (62) developed and validated a 27-item Functional Disability Questionnaire (FDQ) and a 22-item Body Concept Scale. According to the FDQ and the Body Concept Scale, the patients with torticollis were more disabled than the controls; these findings were significant for the social disability and leisure activities subscales but not for the physical activity or self-care subscales of the FDQ. Further analysis showed that disfigurement and depression accounted for the differences between the groups in leisure activities. In contrast, the higher social disability of the patients with torticollis could not be fully explained by these variables, suggesting that in the course of their illness, the patients with torticollis develop well-established patterns of social avoidance, which have become partly dissociated from and independent of their postural abnormality and mood state. The patients with torticollis had a substantially more negative body concept and rated themselves as being more disfigured than the control group patients. Stepwise regression analyses showed that depression had different determinants in the two groups. For the patients with torticollis, self-rated disfigurement was the most important predictor of depression, accounting for 14% of its variance. Together with extraversion, neuroticism, disability, body concept, pain, self-rated disease severity (indexed by ratings of perceived control over head position and movement), duration of illness, and age of onset, self-rated disfigurement accounted for 63% of the variance of depression scores. These results suggest that higher rates of depression in patients with torticollis may be partly a function of low self-esteem resulting from the disfigured body. Depression may also represent mourning the loss of the old and "unflawed" body. The effects of disfigurement on psychological well-being and social adjustment may be understood in light of evidence that physical appearance has profound implications for interpersonal interaction and that attractiveness has a "halo" effect of social perception, such that what is beautiful is also perceived as good (73). The primary role of disfigurement in causing depression in patients with torticollis, together with previous research demonstrating the major psychosocial effect of physical deformity on the individual (74,75), suggests that such a halo effect of physical appearance also extends to self-perception.

In a chronic illness such as dystonia, the association between impairment, disability, and handicap is not necessarily direct or one to one. Not all impairments result in disability, and not all disabilities cause handicaps. Each individual copes with the stress of chronic illness in a different manner. The association between impairment, disability, and handicap varies across patients. Some people with dystonia may be greatly disabled and may restrict their lives although impairment is mild, whereas others may not be handicapped despite severe impairment and disability. A host of mediating factors, including the personal characteristics and resources of the individual, play a key role in determining how impairment is translated into disability or handicap. Research on a spectrum of chronic disorders has established that a number of factors influence how well people adjust to and cope with chronic illness (62,63,76–79). Table 22-1 provides a summary of the personal characteristics, life circumstances, and social and environmental factors in the setting in which each individual lives that play a part in preventing or producing handicap. The important contribution of these other factors means that although the degree of impairment and disability is undoubtedly important, these factors do not inevitably lead to handicap. Instead, individuals have the opportunity to use their personal and social resources to prevent impairment and disability from producing handicap. The psychological makeup of the individual, his or her appraisal of a situation, and the coping strategies used by each individual are important in determining handicap.

TABLE 22-1. *Some of the main factors that can influence adjustment to and coping with chronic illness*

Disease-related factors
   Age of onset
   Duration of illness
   Progression
   Extent of control over symptoms
Personal Characteristics
   Gender
   Age
   Beliefs about control
   Appraisal of illness
   Self-esteem
   Perceived self-efficacy
   Coping styles and strategies
Life Circumstances
   Marital status
   Employment status and nature of work
   Financial situation
Social and Environmental Factors
   Type and suitability of accommodation
   Living alone or with others
   Social support

[From Jahanshahi M. The psychosocial impact of Parkinson's disease and its clinical management. In: Playford D, ed. *Neurological rehabilitation of Parkinson's disease*. London: Martin Dunitz, Taylor and Francis Group, Elsevier, 2003:25–47, with permission (80)].

Against this framework, Jahanshahi (78) investigated the role of a number of mediating variables such as coping strategies, social support, self-esteem (self-worth and self-deprecation), and locus of control to identify other personal or social factors that contribute to depression in patients with torticollis. Of 67 patients, 24% were moderately to severely depressed. Cognitive and emotion-focused strategies were more frequently used than instrumental ways of coping. Female patients used both adaptive and maladaptive coping strategies more frequently than male patients. The number of individuals who were potential sources of support was not large (mean 2.7), but the patients were generally satisfied with the available social support. Stepwise regression analysis established that of the mediating variables, self-deprecation was the most significant single predictor of depression and accounted for 59% of its variance. Disability, disease severity (as measured by self-ratings of the degree of control over head position or movement), extent of satisfaction with available social support, and use of maladaptive coping strategies accounted for a further 18% of variance of depression. A further regression analysis established that body concept ($R^2 = 0.52$) and maladaptive coping strategies (R^2 change 7%) were the main predictors of self-deprecation, together accounting for 58% (adjusted R^2) of the variance of this negative component of self-esteem in torticollis. These results confirmed that depression in torticollis is centered around self-deprecation, which is in turn predicted by the negative body concept associated with the postural abnormality of the head. Although depression and self-deprecation were selected as dependent variables of interest in the regression analyses, the direction of causality cannot be established from such cross-sectional data, and the relationship of these variables is best considered to be reciprocal. Although longitudinal analysis has identified low self-esteem as a vulnerability factor for depression (81), self-deprecation can also be a consequence of depression. Nevertheless, these results have established the close associations between depression and key psychosocial variables in torticollis, and the precise nature and direction of these associations require further evaluation through longitudinal follow-up in future studies.

Spasmodic dysphonia affects the voice and impairs speech, which makes communication, particularly use of the telephone, difficult and has work-related implications (82). A number of studies investigated the psychological and social effects of spasmodic dysphonia. In 11 patients with spasmodic dysphonia, Ginsberg et al. (83) reported anxiety and depression secondary to vocal symptoms. Ewing (84) found that patients with spasmodic dysphonia express feelings of social isolation. Cannito (85) assessed 18 female patients with spasmodic dysphonia on several standardized measures of psychological function: the Zung Depression Scale, the Spielberger State-Trait Anxiety Inventory, and the Somatic Complaints Checklist. The patients with spasmodic dysphonia showed significant differences from a healthy control group on all measures. Using available cutoffs, 39% of the patients with dysphonia were considered "clinically" depressed. In a later study, Murry et al. (86) assessed 32 patients with dysphonia on the same measures as in the Cannito (85) report and compared them to a sample of 18 healthy individuals in that study. As in the earlier study, the authors found that scores on depression and anxiety scales were significantly elevated in the dysphonia group, compared with scores for healthy individuals, although the differences on the Somatic Complaints Checklist did not reach significance. In a third study by the same group (87), a shortened version of the Erickson Scale of Communication Attitudes was added to the measures of depression and anxiety previously used and administered to 20 patients with dysphonia who were compared with 20 healthy controls. The patients with dysphonia expressed substantially more negative attitudes about communication. Whurr et al. (88) assessed aspects of psychosocial functioning in 46 patients with spasmodic dysphonia using the BDI, Mood Adjective Checklist (MACL), and the Crown-Crisp Experiential Index. Speech samples from a subgroup of 16 patients were assessed for voice quality and fluency. On the BDI, mild-to-moderate self-reported depression was present in 37% of the patients. Mean dysphonia patient scores on the Crown-Crisp Index were lower than previous data for patients with primary psychiatric illness and were similar to those for other patient groups with chronic physical illnesses such as arthritis. On the MACL, the spasmodic dysphonia group had scores similar to those previously reported for patients with other neurologic disorders.

Given the beneficial effect of botulinum injections in reducing muscle contractions, normalizing postural abnormality, and relieving pain, the effect of this treatment on psychosocial functioning has been investigated. In the first such study, Jahanshahi and Marsden (89) assessed specific aspects of psychosocial functioning, namely depression, disability, body concept, and self-esteem, in 26 patients with adult-onset idiopathic torticollis before and after one or more botulinum injections. Following botulinum injections, 85% of the patients and 88% of their relatives reported improvements in symptoms of torticollis. The symptomatic improvement of torticollis with botulinum was associated with significant improvement of depression and disability. In contrast, the changes in positive self-esteem, self-deprecation, and body concept were not significant. Because the muscle contractions and head deviation return as the toxin wears off, the "normalization" of the postural abnormality is neither complete nor permanent, which probably accounts for the absence of a significant effect on body concept and self-esteem. In the study by Whurr et al. (88), various dimensions of mood, speech quality, and fluency were assessed in patients with spasmodic dysphonia before and after botulinum injections. After treatment with toxin, voice quality and fluency improved. Following the injections, specific aspects of mood also improved significantly, particularly anxiety and phobia for the male patients, whereas self-reported depression, levels of which were relatively low in the sample, remained unchanged. Similar findings have been reported by Murry et al. (86) and Liu et al. (90). In these studies, depression and anxiety were assessed before and after botulinum injections in patients with spasmodic dysphonia. Self-reports of specific aspects of mood differed significantly between patients and controls; these aspects were improved for the patients treated with botulinum.

Stigma

Goffman (91) used the term *stigma* to describe any condition, behavior, trait, or attribute that marks an individual as "unacceptable" or "inferior." Goffman considered that the term "discredited" reflected the experiences of those individuals who feel stigmatized. This term refers to the stigmatized individual's assumption that his or her "being different" is already known about. Goffman suggests that a major problem confronting such a person is that of controlling the internal tension experienced during social interaction, to change the impression of others, while attempting to manage a "spoiled identity." Stereotype, prejudice, and bias, based on inappropriate concepts of "what constitutes normality," all play a role in determining societal reactions to physical disability and disfigurement. The investigation of perceived stigma in patients with physical or neurologic disorders, such as those with rectal cancer and colostomy (92), epilepsy (93), or dystonia (94,95) considers illness within a wider social context (i.e., in terms of the reactions of others to the patients' disorders as well as the patients' perceptions of these reactions). Such perceptions may in turn influence the patients' subsequent social interactions and psychological well-being.

Torticollis and spasmodic dysphonia, which affect physical appearance and the patients' ability to communicate verbally, are the most socially "visible" of the focal dystonias and are likely to affect social interaction and give rise to perceptions of stigma. Using the Stigma Scale, Papathanasiou et al. investigated perceived stigma in 63 patients with spasmodic dysphonia (94) and in 73 patients with spasmodic torticollis. Patients with spasmodic dysphonia or torticollis experienced considerable stigma. For both groups of patients, perceived stigma was not associated with gender, marital status, employment status, or duration of illness. For the patients with spasmodic dysphonia, "self-consciousness," "feeling apologetic," and "feeling odd and different" were the main components of stigma, reported by 89%, 86%, and 80% of the sample, respectively. In this study, 67% of the patients reported that dysphonia had an effect on their working lives, 74% reported an effect on their private lives, and 79% reported an effect on their social lives. In the patients with torticollis, most of the 73 participants had felt "some" or "severe" stigma. For the torticollis group, perceived stigma was negatively correlated with age. The main components of perceived stigma in torticollis were "self-consciousness," "feeling odd and different," and "feeling unattractive," which were reported by 93%, 91%, and 86% of patients, respectively. Therefore, in patients with torticollis, perceived stigma was mainly focused on physical appearance and attractiveness. In this group, perceived stigma is clearly related to the postural deviation of the head, which affects physical appearance. This observation is consistent with the finding that negative self-referent cognitions and negative body image were the prominent components of depression in one study of torticollis (35). In torticollis, the involuntary movements and postural abnormality of the head can give the patients a "bizarre" appearance. The resulting embarrassment can lead patients to avoid social activities and eventually result in social isolation.

In a study conducted on behalf of the Epidemiological Study of Dystonia in Europe (ESDE) Collaborative Group, Ben-Shlomo, Camfield, and Warner (96) used the Stigma Scale to investigate the psychosocial factors that influenced QOL in 289 patients with dystonia. Perceived stigma was significantly associated with both the physical and mental summary scores on the SF36, with higher stigma predicting worse QOL. However, when the contribution of other demographic, disease-related, or psychosocial mediating factors were taken into account, the contribution of stigma to the physical and mental components of QOL on the SF36 was no longer significant. This finding suggests that the influence of stigma on QOL may be mediated through psychological distress, such as depression and anxiety.

Quality of Life

Under normal circumstances, an individual's QOL is related to how he or she functions and feels, as evidenced by indicators such as physical and mental health, social activities and relationships, work, financial situation, and living circumstances. When a person develops dystonia, "health-related QOL" encompasses the total effect, as perceived by the person, of the illness and its treatment on the individual's physical, psychological, social, and occupational functioning. For persons who are chronically ill, the term "QOL" incorporates the way in which they react personally and emotionally to the illness and the differences they perceive between their actual and desired activities and life styles. As with handicap, QOL varies among individuals. For this reason, many of the factors outlined in Table 22-1 are likely to influence the effect of chronic illness on an individual's QOL. QOL measures are now considered better indices of the effect of chronic illness than measures of impairment or disability. QOL measures rely on self-report by the patients because their primary purpose is to assess the effect of illness as perceived by the person who is ill.

Unlike the explosion of QOL research in many neurologic disorders, including movement disorders such as PD, relatively little research has been performed on QOL in dystonia. The first study to examine QOL in dystonia was by Gudex et al. (101), who administered the generic SF36 and EuroQol to 130 adults with various forms of dystonia. On the EuroQol, the scores of both groups of patients with dystonia indicated significantly worse QOL on the mobility, self-care, usual activities, pain or discomfort, and anxiety–depression subscales, compared with normative data from the general population. Patients with nonfocal dystonia (n = 37) had more problems on the mobility, self-care, and usual activities subtests than those with focal dystonia (n = 93), but only differences on usual activities were significant. Similarly, on the SF36, the scores of patients with dystonia indicated poorer QOL than norms for the general population, although the differences were not significant. Where the comparison of the patients with dystonia with the normative data from the general population is informative, it should be interpreted with caution because demographic details differed between the groups, a circumstance that could have been overcome by including a control group. Employment status and age affected QOL scores—the unemployed patients with dystonia had poorer QOL than the employed patients, and the younger patients had poorer QOL than the older patients. Following administration of botulinum injections, nonsignificant improvements were noted in several of the EuroQol and SF36 dimensions.

Muller et al. (102) used the SF36 and the BDI to assess QOL and depression in 89 patients with blepharospasm and 131 patients with cervical dystonia. Both groups of patients with dystonia scored significantly worse than an age-matched community sample on all eight domains of the SF36. With the exception of pain, which was significantly worse for the cervical dystonia group, no differences were found between the two dystonia groups in any of the QOL domains. On the BDI, 47% of the patients with cervical dystonia and 37% of those with blepharospasm reported some level of depression, with moderate to severe depression reported by 13.7% of the patients with cervical dystonia and 15.2% of the patients with blepharospasm. In the cervical dystonia group, pain was associated with QOL and was considered to contribute to depression. Gender differences were found in the blepharospasm group but not in the cervical dystonia group. Women with blepharospasm scored significantly lower on all SF36 scales and were more depressed than male patients. The patients with blepharospasm, particularly the men with a long duration of illness, had a significantly better QOL, perhaps suggesting some form of adaptation to the illness over time.

The beneficial effect of botulinum injections on measures of QOL in dystonia noted by Gudex et al. (101) has been confirmed. In 64 patients with cervical dystonia, Brans et al. (103) found that performance on the pain and disability subtests of the Toronto Western Spasmodic Torticollis Rating Scale (TWSTRS) and on the handicap and general health perception subscales of the medical outcome study scale improved following botulinum injections in the 54 patients who continued treatment. In a pharmacoeconomic evaluation of botulinum, Brefel-Courbon et al. (104) established that although botulinum increased the cost of treating the 21 patients with torticollis in their sample from a mean of $97 to $228, it significantly decreased the clinical symptoms and improved the emotional, social, and pain-related domains of QOL. Hogikyan et al. (105) assessed voice-related QOL (V-RQOL) in 27 patients with spasmodic dysphonia. At baseline assessment, patients had very low V-RQOL scores, both for the social–emotional and physical functioning domains. Botulinum injections produced dramatic and significant improvements in the V-RQOL scores. The magnitude of the treatment effect appears to change across injections. The EuroQoL and the SF36 were used by Hilker et al. (106) to assess QOL in 50 patients with cranial (blepharospasm, n = 20; Meige's syndrome, n = 5), and cervical dystonia (n = 25) and to determine how botulinum injections influenced QOL in these patients. At baseline assessment, the scores of the patients with dystonia on the SF36 were lower than normative data from the German general population, particularly on the physical functioning, emotional limitations of role, and mental health dimensions. Whereas the patients with cranial dystonia were characterized by restricted physical and social functioning, those with cervical dystonia complained of pain. As expected, with effective toxin treatment, scores on the EuroQol and SF36 improved, particularly those for social functioning, mental health, physical limitation of role, and pain. In their study, Muller et al. (102) also examined the effect of botulinum treatment of blepharospasm and cervical dystonia on QOL. In contrast to previous studies, the authors found that despite significant clinical improvement of the dystonia symptoms following treatment with botulinum, the injections did not produce a significant change in QOL measured on the SF36 in the patients with blepharospasm, and only two of the eight domains, including pain, improved for the patients with cervical dystonia. In contrast, other studies have demonstrated that following botulinum injections in cervical dystonia, measures of QOL are more sensitive indices of functional change than clinical impairment scales (107,108).

Two large-scale studies of QOL in cervical dystonia have been conducted by the ESDE Collaborative Group. In the first study by Camfield et al. (109), the SF36 was administered to 289 patients with cervical dystonia across seven European countries. Compared to a cross section of the general population of similar age, the patients with cervical dystonia had scores that indicated worse QOL in all eight domains of the SF36. QOL scores of these patients showed significant effects of age, gender, and education. QOL related to physical functioning and general health with age worsened significantly. For the energy or vitality, pain, and physical function domains, male patients had significantly better scores than female patients. Patients with lower education had worse QOL scores, but this difference was significant only for the domains of social functioning and emotional role limitation. When the scores of the patients with cervical dystonia were compared with similar data previously reported for patients with other neurologic disorders such as PD, multiple sclerosis, or stroke, the patients with dystonia notably had the best scores on physical function but the worst scores for mental health and emotional role limitation. Although this comparison should be interpreted with caution because of age and sex differences between the samples in these studies, it nevertheless suggests that despite being the least physically disabling disorder, cervical dystonia has the greatest effect on the mental health and emotional and social functioning of the patients. In a second study by the ESDE Group, Ben-Shlomo et al. (96) assessed a number of mediating variables, including many of the measures used by Jahanshahi (78), to further investigate the determinants of the negative effect of cervical dystonia on QOL. Gender, educational level, social support, and response to botulinum treatment, which were significant individual predictors of the physical summary score of the SF36, were no longer significant in multivariate analyses that adjusted for the contribution of other factors. Positive self-esteem and self-deprecation, retired status, duration of illness, and severity of torticollis remained significant predictors of physical summary scores, even in multivariate analyses. However, severity of anxiety and depression, measured on the Beck Anxiety Scale and the BDI, emerged as the most important predictors of the physical summary score on the SF36. For the mental summary score on the SF36, disease duration and severity, cohabitating status, self-deprecation, and social support were important predictors, with anxiety and depression showing the largest effects. Several features of these results are particularly interesting. First, they establish that dysfunctional mood (e.g., depression and anxiety) is the most important predictor of QOL in dystonia, as it is in other movement disorders, such as PD (110). Second, severity and duration of illness, self-deprecation, and social support have emerged as important predictors of both depression (62,78) and QOL (96) in torticollis, because of the close association between depression and QOL.

To date, all studies of QOL in dystonia have employed generic QOL measures, such as the EuroQol or the SF36. The advantage of relying on such generic QOL measures is that these measures enable us to contrast QOL in dystonia with the normative data for the general population and enable us to compare the effect of dystonia with the effect of other neurologic disorders, such as PD, multiple sclerosis, and stroke. However, the lack of disease-specific QOL measures might also mean that disease-specific effects of dystonia on the lives of patients, such as the disfigurement, negative body image, and self-deprecation associated with the postural abnormality, which have been shown to be a central feature of the patients' emotional reactions (33,62,78,96), are being missed when using such generic measures. To overcome this problem, Muller et al. (111) developed a disease-specific QOL measure for patients with craniocervical dystonia and assessed its reliability and validity. The final questionnaire, the craniocervical dystonia questionnaire (CDQ-24), has 24 items belonging to five subscales: stigma, emotional well-being, pain, activities of daily living, and social and family life. Factor analysis confirmed the domain structure of the CDQ-24 and showed that the five factors accounted for 68% of the total variance. The convergent validity of the CDQ-24 was established in relation to the SF36. Its internal consistency was satisfactory for all subscales, and the scale had good test–retest reliability. Its sensitivity to change was shown in reflecting significant improvement following treatment with botulinum injections. Thus, the CDQ-24 has proven reliability and validity, and its use in future studies will provide information about disease-specific features of the effect of craniocervical dystonia on QOL. Undoubtedly, other disease-specific measures of QOL for other forms of dystonia will be developed in due course.

ORIGINS OF PSYCHIATRIC MORBIDITY AND PSYCHOSOCIAL DYSFUNCTION IN DYSTONIA

Psychiatric morbidity in dystonia is likely to have a multitude of etiologies, from biological to functional to psychosocial. Genetic studies revealed an association between dystonia and dopamine. In *DYT1* dystonia, the torsin A protein is expressed at high levels in the substantia nigra pars compacta, a structure that is rich in dopamine-producing cells (112,113). Cervical dystonia and blepharospasm are associated with polymorphisms in dopamine receptor genes (114,115). In dopa-responsive dystonia, patients' symptoms improve dramatically with levodopa therapy. Furthermore, the presence of parkinsonism and dystonia in several syndromes, and the mutation in the D_2 dopamine receptor in myoclonic dystonia, also suggest an anatomic and functional linkage between dystonia and the dopaminergic system (8). Because dopamine is important in psychiatric disorders such as depression, dystonia and other aspects of psychiatric morbidity such as depression might have a common biologic basis.

The striatofrontal circuits implicated in the regulation of mood and motivation, such as the limbic circuit between the ventral striatum and the anterior cingulate or the orbitofrontal circuit between this area of the frontal cortex and the caudate (116), might play a role in the genesis of psychiatric morbidity in dystonia. In dystonia, functional imaging demonstrated altered activation of the cortical targets of the limbic and dorsolateral circuits. For example, during freely selected joystick movements, patients with dystonia showed greater activation than control subjects in the lateral premotor cortex, Brodmann area 8, anterior cingulate area, ipsilateral dorsolateral prefrontal cortex, rostral supplementary motor area, and bilateral lentiform nuclei (51). Functional imaging studies demonstrated that there is striatofrontal involvement in OCD (117,118). Thus, the high prevalence of OCD in dystonia may relate to dysfunction of the limbic or orbitofrontal circuits. There is also evidence of a possible shared genetic predisposition to OCD and dystonia (67) and of an association between myoclonic dystonia with OCD and mutation of the *DYT11* M-D gene (8).

A variety of factors, including initial contacts of patients with the medical profession and their psychological and behavioral reactions to disfigurement and to perceived societal stigma, probably contribute considerably to psychiatric morbidity, impaired psychosocial function, and poor QOL in patients with dystonia. Even today, when the view of dystonia as an organic neurologic disorder has been well established, patients usually undergo a lengthy and distressing experience of multiple referrals to medical services before a diagnosis of dystonia as a neurologic disorder is made (34,35,57,70). A survey by the members of the Dystonia Society revealed that 67% of patients had at least five or more medical consultations before diagnosis (57). This prolonged route to diagnosis is frequently traumatic and tinged with self-blame, because patients have been led to believe that their condition has a psychological origin (34,35,57,70). Once diagnosis is made, patients have to face a new form of despair—spontaneous remissions are rare (18), and available treatments—such as anticholingergic medication, botulinum injections, and surgery—are suitable only for some patients and do not result in complete relief of symptoms. In some forms of dystonia, muscle cramps are associated with pain, which can be distressing. Dystonia can interfere with performance of daily activities and can result in functional disability. In the dystonias in which the postural abnormality is visible (e.g., torticollis, oromandibular dystonia, and generalized dystonia) or audible (e.g., spasmodic dysphonia), the associated embarrassment can lead to the patient avoiding social activities and can eventually cause social isolation. In dystonia, the visible or audible nature of the postural abnormality can make others perceive the patients as bizarre or odd. This aspect of the disorder can have a profound effect on the patient's "body concept," which denotes the feelings and attitudes that individuals have towards their bodies. Besides being affected by objective information obtained from inspecting the body, the development of body concept is highly influenced by the prevailing cultural norms and reactions of others to the individual's appearance (73). Body concept plays a fundamental role in the earliest foundations of self-esteem. Available evidence points to the personal and emotional costs of alterations in the body caused by disease or accidental injury (74,75). Conversely, in a study of 250 patients with congenital or acquired craniofacial deformities, Lefebvre and Barclay (119) reported that the improved physical appearance and more positive body concept that resulted from reconstructive surgery were associated with concomitant emotional improvement and better QOL. It is known from studies of people with facial disfigurement that perceived stigma and embarrassment are associated with social avoidance (120). Even minor deformities such as a prominent nose have been found to be associated with psychological disturbance (121), with rhinoplastic operation resulting in improved psychological functioning (122). From this literature, and from the evidence of the fundamental role played by disfigurement and self-deprecation in causing depression in patients with dystonia (62,78), it has been proposed that disfigurement leads to poor body concept and self-image, which in turn give rise to self-deprecation and low self-esteem, which sets the stage for depression, social avoidance, and isolation (78).

The secondary nature of disability, depression, and impaired QOL in dystonia is revealed by the fact that they improve following successful treatment of dystonia, for example, with botulinum injections (86,88–90,101–108), or after peripheral denervation (123) or deep brain stimulation (124). Furthermore, longitudinal follow-up of patients with torticollis over a 2-year period has established that changes in the clinical severity of dystonia are associated with significant alteration of depression, disability, and body concept (63). This evidence clearly indicates that the psychosocial sequelae of dystonia are closely related to the clinical severity of the illness.

PSYCHOGENIC DYSTONIA

All forms of dystonia, particularly the focal dystonias such as torticollis, blepharospasm, spasmodic dysphonia, and writer's cramp, were at various times erroneously considered to be psychogenic, representing some form of neurotic, conversion, somatization, or factitious disorder. Dystonia is now well established as a neurologic disorder, although rare cases of psychogenic dystonia exist. Psychogenic movement disorders have been defined as those "which cannot be fully accounted for by any known organic syndrome and which appear as based on available clinical evidence to have significant psychological and/or psychiatric contributants" (125).

Rates of Psychogenic Dystonia in Movement Disorder Clinics

Cases of psychogenic dystonia constitute a few patients seen in movement disorders clinics. Table 22-2 shows the rate of psychogenic movement disorders in large series of patients in specialist movement disorder clinics. The rates of psychogenic illness among the variety of movement disorders seen at these clinics range from 1% (56,99) to 3.3% (100). Psychogenic dystonia was present in 1% of Marsden's (99) patients and 2.5% of Fahn's (98) patients. Factor et al. (100) studied a series of 28 cases of psychogenic disorder among the consecutive referrals of 842 patients with movement disorders and found that tremor was most common (n = 14, 50%), followed by dystonia (n = 5, 18%), myoclonus (n = 4, 14%), and parkinsonism (n = 2, 7%). Sa and Lang (126) reported 33 patients diagnosed with psychogenic movement disorders at the Toronto Western Hospital between July 2000 and June 2001. Among these patients, psychogenic tremor was the most common symptom (n = 13, 39.5%), followed by psychogenic dystonia (n = 10, 30.3%). Whereas the series of cases studied by Factor et al. (100) and Sa and Lang (126) suggest that psychogenic tremor is more common than psychogenic dystonia, Williams, Ford, and Fahn (125) reported, from a series of cases with psychogenic movement disorders at the Colombia Presbyterian Medical Center that the reverse is true, with psychogenic dystonia found in 82 of the 131 cases (62.6%) and psychogenic tremor in only 21 patients (16%). This finding may reflect a referral bias, however, because the Movement Disorders Center at Colombia is a major specialist center for dystonia.

Diagnosis of Psychogenic Dystonia

In the absence of biologic markers for dystonia, differentiating psychogenic from idiopathic dystonia depends on careful history taking and clinical observation of the symptoms. Table 22-3 lists a number of criteria for the differential diagnosis of psychogenic dystonia from the classic neurologic illness (97,98). The central criterion for documentation of psychogenic dystonia is relief of symptoms by psychotherapy, suggestion, or placebo (125). Some additional specific features of psychogenic dystonia outlined by Williams, Ford, and Fahn (125) include onset of dystonia at rest; onset of dystonia in the foot of adult patients; incongruous features such as absence of dystonic tremor, absence of null point, and absence of sensory tricks; spontaneous pain with passive movement; startle-induced elaboration of dystonic postures; and abrupt changes in dystonia. Patients with psychogenic movement

TABLE 22-2. *Rates of psychogenic movement disorders in a number of specialist movement disorders clinics across the world*

Authors/centers	Total sample size	Type of MD	Percent psychogenic MD
Lesser and Fahn (55)	85	All	n = 1, 1.2%
Marsden (56)	400	All	n = 5, 1.25%
Fahn and Williams (97)	814	All	n = 21, 2.6%
Fahn (98)	2,715	dystonia	n = 67, 2.5%
Marsden (99)	2,221	dystonia	n = 21, 1%
Factor et al. (100)	842	All	n = 28, 3.3%

MD, movement disorder.

TABLE 22-3. *Clinical features that suggest psychogenic dystonia*

Abrupt onset
Dystonia beginning as a fixed posture or as a paroxysmal dystonia
Inconsistency of dystonic movements across time
Incongruous dystonic movement and postures
Other movement disorders, usually presenting as bizarre movements including bizarre gait, and often as a paroxysmal disorder
Movements and postures disappear with distraction
False weakness
False sensory complaints
Multiple somatizations
Self-inflicted injuries
Obvious psychiatric disturbance
Spontaneous remissions
Responsive to placebo, suggestion, or psychotherapy

[From Fahn S, Williams DT Psychogenic dystonia. In S Fahn et al. (Eds) Dystonia 2. Advances in Neurology, Raven Press, New York, 1988, 431–455 and Fahn S. Psychogenic movement disorders. In: Marsden CD, Fahn S, eds. *Movement disorders 3.* Oxford: Butterworth-Heinemann, 1994:359–372, with permission.]

disorders are often employed in the health professions, are involved in some form of litigation or compensation claim, or exhibit evidence of anticipating secondary gain, such as avoiding undesirable employment or expecting continued attention and care from a devoted spouse (99).

The diagnosis of psychogenic dystonia is based on evidence from clinical observation and the patient's history. On the basis of this information, Fahn and Williams have proposed four levels of certainty in the diagnosis (97). Diagnosis of documented psychogenic dystonia depends on two criteria. First, because spontaneous remissions are relatively rare in dystonia but occur in a small percentage of patients with torticollis (18,127,128), the dystonic movements and postures should be permanently relieved by suggestion, placebo, or psychotherapy. Second, when left alone and supposedly unobserved, the patient should be free of symptoms. In clinically established psychogenic dystonia, the movements and postures are inconsistent over time or incongruent with classic neurologic dystonia, and other features such as false weakness, false sensory deficits, presence of multiple somatizations, and psychiatric disturbance provide confidence in the diagnosis of psychogenic disorder. When the movements and postures are inconsistent or incongruous but no additional signs are observed, or when the movement disorder is consistent with organic disease but the patient shows multiple somatizations or additional neurologic signs such as false weakness or self-inflicted injury, a diagnosis of probable psychogenic dystonia is appropriate. In possible psychogenic dystonia, obvious emotional disturbance is present in a patient whose movement disorder is consistent and congruent with organic disease. Because psychiatric disturbance and emotional morbidity can occur in organic dystonia, caution is necessary in diagnosing and managing cases of probable or possible psychogenic dystonia (129). A factor that can render diagnosis difficult is that a patient may present with both organic and psychogenic symptoms. Factor et al. (100) and Sa et al. (126) reported concomitant organic and psychogenic movement disorders in 25% and 9% of their samples, respectively. In a family with genetically confirmed *DYT1* dystonia, Bentivoglio et al. (130) reported that the mother of the most severely affected individual presented with a clinically established psychogenic movement disorder resembling dystonia, which had been originally misdiagnosed as severe generalized dystonia. Despite the fact that four family members had *DYT1* dystonia and the woman in question was a carrier of the *TOR1A* mutation of the *DYT1* gene, the authors proposed a diagnosis of clinically established psychogenic dystonia on the basis of clinical observations in her case.

Unlike epilepsy, in which the electroencephalogram (EEG) can help establish the diagnosis of pseudoseizures, in the case of dystonia, differentiating psychogenic from idiopathic dystonia largely relies on clinical observation and expertise. Nevertheless, other tests may provide further evidence to support the diagnosis of psychogenic dystonia. In dystonia, a reduction of reciprocal inhibition of the H reflex by electrical stimulation (131) and abnormal recovery of the blink reflex in blepharospasm (3) have been described, and these phenomena may prove helpful in differential diagnosis in some cases. In contrast, co-contraction of antagonist muscles, characteristic of organic dystonia, can also be present in psychogenic dystonia, and the electromyogram (EMG) therefore cannot be used as a diagnostic aid. Functional imaging may be valuable in differentiating psychogenic from organic dystonia. In a recent study, 85 patients with psychogenic nonepileptic seizures had a greater degree of personality abnormality than 63 patients with epilepsy and 100 healthy controls. Borderline personality disorder and overly controlled and avoidant personality were the most characteristic profiles in the psychogenic-seizure group (132). Similar comparison of psychogenic and idiopathic dystonia using personality scales such as the MMPI may reveal characteristic personality profiles for the psychogenic group, which may be valuable in differentiating them from the organic group (43,45,46) on this scale.

Features of Psychogenic Dystonia and Common Types of Psychiatric Disturbance in Psychogenic Dystonia

The largest series of patients with psychogenic dystonia have been investigated by Fahn and Williams (97). All but 2 of these 21 cases with documented or clinically established psychogenic dystonia were women. The median age at onset was 23 years for the patients with dystonia (n = 14) and 33 years for those with paroxysmal dystonia (n = 7). The feet were common sites of first onset of dystonia both for those patients with childhood-onset and atypically for patients with adult-onset dystonia (4). The duration of illness, that is, the time between the first onset of symptoms and diagnosis as psychogenic dystonia, ranged from 1 month to 15 years. The five patients with a duration of illness of 2 months or less had complete and persistent remissions. Because of the initial misdiagnosis of organic disease, several patients received inappropriate treatments, including a right thalamotomy in one patient and casting of the involved foot in two patients.

Eighteen patients with documented or clinically established psychogenic dystonia were reviewed (133). Most patients (14 out of 18) had a clear precipitating event before onset, which was abrupt in most patients, with rapid progression commonly to fixed dystonia. Even in patients with adult-onset dystonia, involvement of the legs was common (12 out of 18 patients). Most patients had other psychogenic movement disorders or neurologic signs and multiple somatizations. Outcomes varied: symptoms resolved completely in a number of patients, whereas in others, the psychogenic symptoms and associated disability persisted.

Factor et al. (100) described the characteristics of 28 cases with documented or clinically established psychogenic movement disorders, 5 of whom (18%) had psychogenic dystonia. The patients had many clinical features suggesting that their problems had psychogenic origins, including abrupt onset (54%), a precipitating event (61%), improvement or disappearance of symptoms with distraction (86%, more evident in cases with tremor than in those with dystonia), selective disabilities (39%), and multiple somatizations (36%). Secondary gain, including compensation and litigation, was present in 18 patients (64%). Half of the patients had been previously diagnosed with psychiatric disorders: nine with depression, five with alcohol abuse, three with anxiety disorders, two with posttraumatic stress disorder, and two with paranoid schizophrenia. Crimlisk et al. (134) conducted a neurologic and psychiatric follow-up study of 64 of 73 patients who had been admitted to the National Hospital for Neurology and Neurosurgery between 1989 and 1991 with medically unexplained motor symptoms, of whom 35 (48%) had no motor function and 38 (52%) had abnormal motor activity (e.g., tremor, dystonia, and ataxia). Of these patients, 96% were white. Only 11% of patients were employed at follow-up, and 22% of patients worked in medical or paramedical fields. Among 64 patients contacted at follow-up, 3 patients had new organic neurologic disorders that fully or partly explained their previous symptoms. Psychiatric disorders were observed in 44 of 59 patients (75%), which in 33 patients (75%) coexisted with unexplained motor symptoms. Depression was the most common diagnosis in these patients (n = 24, 41%). Anxiety disorder or phobia was present in nine patients (15%). Psychotic symptoms were rare (n = 4, 7%). Personality disorder was diagnosed in 31 of 59 patients (45%). At follow-up, 23 of 64 patients (36%) had a current psychiatric diagnosis, commonly a continuation or relapse of previous disorders, with only 3 patients developing a new psychiatric disorder. Patients with abnormal motor activity in the follow-up period were more likely to have a current psychiatric disorder than those with absence of motor function.

Feinstein et al. (135) followed, either in person or by telephone interview, 42 of 85 patients with documented or clinically established psychogenic movement disorders who were seen at the Movement Disorders Clinic of the Toronto Western Hospital. Although only 52% of the original patients were followed, no demographic or illness-related differences were found between participants and the patients who refused follow-up. SCID-I and II interviews were conducted to establish DSM-IV diagnoses. Ten of the 42 patients (10.8%) had psychogenic dystonia, and 26 patients (61.9%) had psychogenic tremor. There were more women (61.9%) than men (38.1%) in the sample; most patients were married (64.3%), unemployed (76.2%), and obtaining disability or social security benefits (59.5%). Seven patients (16.7%) were pursuing litigation in relation to their movement disorder. Only two patients had no psychiatric problems at the time of assessment, and an Axis I diagnosis of mental illness was made in 40 patients (95.3%), with about 35% of the patients having two diagnoses, for example, conversion disorder plus depression or anxiety. Conversion disorder was the most common current diagnosis, present in 85.7% of patients, followed by anxiety (38.1%), major depression (19.1%), anxiety and depression (11.9%), and other somatoform disorders (7.1%). One patient suffered from schizoaffective disorder, and personality disorder was present in 45% of the patients.

The most consistent finding across samples was a sex bias, with a higher proportion of women than men having psychogenic dystonia or other movement disorders (97,99,100,135). As expected from the nature of psychogenic movement disorders, another consistent finding is the presence of high levels of coexistent psychiatric disorders in these patients, with depression being the most common disorder across studies, with the exception of the study by Feinstein et al. (135) that found anxiety disorders to be more prevalent than psychiatric disorders. Sudden onset preceded by a specific triggering event and onset in the feet of an adult are other characteristic features of psychogenic dystonia (97,133).

Prognosis and Treatment of Psychogenic Dystonia

Fahn and Williams (97) used DSM-III criteria to classify patients with psychogenic dystonia into three categories: somatoform disorder, factitious disorder, or malingering. In somatoform disorder, physical symptoms are caused by unconscious psychological factors not under the patient's direct, voluntary control. The fact that psychological factors play a primary etiologic role can be ascertained from the close timing of the development or worsening of the physical symptoms and the occurrence of an event that triggers the unconscious psychological conflict or need. Alternatively, the symptom may free the patient from an undesirable activity or support that would otherwise not be possible. Conversion disorder and somatization disorder (also called hysteria or Briquet's syndrome) are the two main forms of somatoform disorder. In contrast, in a factitious disorder such as Münchausen's syndrome, the physical symptoms are under voluntary control and are intentionally produced because of some unknown psychological need. Factitious disorder indicates a mental disorder. In malingering, the physical symptoms are deliberately produced to attain a specific goal, such as achieving financial gain through compensation or avoiding work or school, or to evade prosecution for a crime. Malingering is not considered to be a mental disorder. From clinical experience, an estimated quarter of the patients with psychogenic dystonia, particularly those with conversion reactions and depression, can be restored to normal health, whereas those with factitious disorders or malingering are rarely helped by medical professionals (99). Although differentiating between somatoform or factitious disorder and malingering in cases of psychogenic dystonia has prognostic value and implications for choosing appropriate management and treatment, doing so is difficult, because a patient's volitional intent cannot be established (97).

Sa and Lang (126) believe that in psychogenic movement disorders, the prognosis for resolving the movement disorder and the psychiatric illness is poor. Nevertheless, intensive and focused management and treatment can be of value in many patients. A series of 21 patients with documented or clinically established psychogenic dystonia was admitted to a hospital (97). Following assessment, they were informed by a neurologist and psychiatrist that their illness had emotional origins. A combination of suggestion that the symptoms would improve, placebo therapy, psychotherapy, physiotherapy, and antidepressant medication was used. Nine of the 21 patients (42.9%) showed complete and permanent relief, and 4 (19%) had moderate but permanent relief of their symptoms.

Of the 28 patients with psychogenic movement disorders investigated by Factor et al. (100), the symptoms resolved in 10 patients and persisted in 10 patients; 8 patients were unavailable for follow-up. Of the ten recovered cases, five occurred spontaneously (three with suggestion), two after psychotherapy and physical treatment, one after placebo therapy, one following improvement of psychosis, and one after the personal injury claim had been settled. Those patients whose psychogenic movement disorder resolved had shorter duration of illness at the time of initial visit (22 months) than patients whose symptoms persisted (42 months). Among the 64 patients with unexplained motor symptoms followed by Crimlisk et al. (134), the index symptom had completely resolved in 18 patients (28%), had improved in 13 patients (20%), was unchanged in 9 patients (14%), and worsened in 24 patients (38%). When patients were classified into two groups of 31 improved and 33 not improved patients, the factors that emerged as prognostic of good outcome in a regression analysis were the presence of symptoms for less than 1 year, comorbid psychiatric disorder, and change in marital status in the follow-up period. In contrast, receipt of financial benefits at first admission or pending litigation indicated poor prognosis.

Feinstein et al. (135) described 42 of 85 patients with documented or clinically established psychogenic movement disorders who were followed either in person or by telephone interview to establish psychiatric diagnoses. The average duration of follow-up was 3.2 years (range, 1–7 years). Ten of the forty-two patients (23.8%) had psychogenic dystonia. At follow-up, the psychogenic movement disorder was present in all but 4 of the 42 patients (90.5%), and in 2 of the 4 patients, the psychogenic movement disorder had been replaced with another somatoform disorder. Fourteen patients (33.3%) thought that their movement disorder had improved, 10 (23.8%) patients thought that their disorder was stable, and 14 (33.3%) patients considered that their disorder had worsened. The patients whose movement disorder had remitted or improved were classified as having good outcomes (42.9%), and those who considered themselves to be stable or worse were considered as having a poor outcome. Only 2 of the 42 patients (4.8%) had no psychiatric diagnosis at follow-up. In a further follow-up study (136), a detailed neurologic examination was completed on 23 of the 85 patients with psychogenic movement disorders, most of whom had been psychiatrically interviewed by Feinstein et al. (135). All of this subgroup of patients still had a psychogenic movement disorder at follow-up. For 82.6% of these patients, daily activities such as self-care, dressing, and eating were impaired. For patients whose symptoms had remained stable or had improved, this change occurred within the first year of illness. The results of these two studies indicate that in most patients, neither the psychogenic movement disorder nor the underlying psychiatric illness resolve over time. However, a number of factors were found to predict better course, outcome, or both (135). Significant correlations between disease course and the duration of symptoms, mode of onset, and extent of psychiatric comorbidity (number of Axis I diagnoses) indicated that shorter duration, a more sudden onset, and fewer comorbid psychiatric diagnoses were associated with better course and outcome. Similar associations have been previously reported in conversion disorder, in which a short duration of illness, presence of an emotional trigger or precipitant, and absence of long-standing psychopathology predict a good outcome (137). In the study by Feinstein et al. (135), age, years of education, employment status, involvement in litigation, and type of movement disorder did not show any significant correlations with the course of the psychogenic movement disorder. Regression analyses showed that marital status was the only predictor of major depression, whereas duration of illness (significant) and depression (nonsignificant trend) were the main predictors of outcome of the psychogenic movement disorder.

Several strategies have been recommended for managing patients with psychogenic dystonia (97). First, patients should preferably be admitted to the hospital for assessment and initial phases of treatment because if they are informed about the diagnosis in an outpatient setting, many patients do not return for appropriate treatment. Second, in addition to neurologic clinical examination and observation, tests such as EEG or videotaping during sleep, which may be helpful in confirming the diagnosis of psychogenic dystonia, should be completed. A psychiatric consultation may help identify the psychodynamics of the psychogenic symptoms. Third, the diagnosis of psychogenic dystonia should be thoroughly discussed with the patient once it is established. Although the absence of a progressive neurologic disorder should be communicated to the patient, the patient's symptoms and the distress they are causing should not be dismissed as unimportant. Providing an explanation of the patient's symptoms within a neurobehavioral framework and highlighting the close association between the mind and the body may be more acceptable to the patient. Fourth, the treatment approach must be individually tailored to the needs of each patient. Medical treatment of psychiatric illness with antidepressants and anxiolytic medication may be necessary. Some patients may be prone to suicide and may require close observation. All patients should be provided with psychotherapy. Suggestion, placebo therapy, positive reinforcement, and physiotherapy are other approaches that may prove valuable.

Duration of illness and presence and extent of psychopathology are factors that have emerged as major prognostic factors for resolving psychogenic movement disorders (100,134,135). Direct early treatment of psychiatric disorders in these patients is more likely to result in resolution of the movement disorder. In contrast, financial gain or pending litigation predict poor outcome (134), and there is some indication that once outstanding litigation or compensation claims have been sorted, financial gain may no longer act as motivation for the psychogenic symptoms to persist, and they may resolve [e.g., (100)]. Encouraging speedy settlement of claims may prove of clinical value.

MANAGEMENT OF PSYCHIATRIC DISORDERS AND PSYCHOSOCIAL DYSFUNCTION IN DYSTONIA

Dystonia is associated with considerable disability in activities of daily living, depression, anxiety, and OCD; perceptions of stigma by a proportion of patients; and poor QOL. In managing psychiatric and psychosocial sequela of dystonia, two general approaches can be recommended. The first is to pursue effective medical treatment of the dystonia, which may improve some aspects of psychosocial functioning. The second approach is to treat the comorbid psychiatric disorders directly and manage the psychosocial dysfunction. Each of these approaches are considered in the following sections.

Improvement of Comorbid Psychiatric Disorders and Psychosocial Sequelae with Effective Medical Treatment of Dystonia

In a 2-year follow-up study of 67 patients with torticollis, Jahanshahi and Marsden (63) found that change in the clinical severity of torticollis during the follow-up period had a considerable effect on psychological adjustment. Those patients whose torticollis improved were less depressed and less disabled and had a more positive body concept than the patients whose torticollis had worsened during the follow-up period. This finding indicates that the psychosocial sequelae of dystonia is related to the clinical severity of the illness and suggests that successful medical management of dystonia is likely to benefit the mood and psychosocial status of the patient. The reduction of the clinical severity of dystonia with standard medical management or specific treatments such as botulinum injections, peripheral denervation, or deep brain stimulation is associated with improvement in daily functioning, mood, and some aspects of psychosocial functioning.

Before the mid-1980s, when botulinum injections were first used to treat dystonia, anticholinergics were the main medical treatment option available. A variety of other approaches from alternative or complementary medicine such as acupuncture, relaxation therapy, and biofeedback, were also tried by a relatively large proportion of patients with dystonia, with varying degrees of perceived efficacy (33,94,95,138). Among these alternative therapies, the efficacy of biofeedback for treatment of writer's cramp (139) and torticollis (140) has been shown to be equivalent to that of control therapies such as relaxation training and habit reversal or relaxation therapy and graded neck exercises, both of which produce a few improvements. However, relaxation therapy and biofeedback, as therapeutic procedures that involve direct involvement and participation of the patient, are likely to enhance perceived self-efficacy and have been shown to significantly reduce disability and depression in torticollis (140)

From the mid-1980s until recently, when the new surgical approaches (141–143) for treatment of dystonia were introduced, botulinum injections in affected muscles was the main medical and peripheral method of denervation and the sole surgical treatment option for focal dystonia. Successful treatment of focal dystonias (86,88–90) with botulinum improves depression, anxiety, and disability in daily activities. Similarly, using a variety of QOL measures, researchers have demonstrated that improvement of the clinical features of dystonia is associated with significant improvement in QOL, particularly social functioning, mental health, physical limitation of role, and pain for patients with torticollis (101–104,106–108); spasmodic dysphonia (105); blepharospasm; or Meige's syndrome (102,106). In a prospective study of selective peripheral denervation in 37 patients with botulinum-resistant torticollis, Munchau et al. (123) assessed psychosocial function including QOL (EuroQoL), depression and anxiety (Beck scales), pain (McGill Pain Questionnaire), and a number of mediating variables (self-esteem, body concept, acceptance of illness, perceived stigma) in a subgroup of 12 patients. Twelve months after surgery, the TWSTRS global outcome score indicated functionally significant improvement in 68% of the patients. More importantly, in the representative subgroup of 12 patients, the symptomatic improvement was accompanied by considerable amelioration of psychosocial function and QOL, as shown by significant change in the measures of QOL, stigma, perceived disfigurement, and body concept. Improvement of depression was transient, considerable at 16 weeks after surgery but not 2 years postoperatively. Self-esteem and acceptance of illness were not altered by surgery. These results indicate that although not all facets of psychological adjustment are improved by peripheral denervation, nevertheless, in torticollis this surgical treatment can benefit various aspects of psychosocial functioning, such as perceived disfigurement and body concept, that are not altered by botulinum injections (89). In five patients with segmental (n = 1) or generalized (n = 4) dystonia who had deep-brain stimulation of the internal segment of the globus pallidus (GPi), Kupsch et al. (124) reported that 3 to 12 months postoperatively, optimal stimulation at 130 Hz significantly improved symptoms by 40%, and QOL (measured with the EuroQol and the PDQ39) improved by 60%.

Direct Treatment of Comorbid Psychiatric Disorders

Effective medical treatment of dystonia will reduce the effect of the illness on daily activities and is likely to be valuable in managing the psychosocial sequelae of the illness. However, such a purely medical approach is unlikely to be completely effective as the sole course of action in preventing disability and depression and in promoting QOL, for several reasons. First, despite substantial improvement of muscle contractions and postural abnormality with medical treatments such as botulinum toxin, certain aspects of the negative psychological effect of the illness such as the sense of disfigurement and the negative body concept do not improve in every patient (89). Second, the relation between the degree of impairment associated with the symptoms and the resulting disability and depression is not necessarily direct (78). Third, evidence exists that besides the severity of the symptoms, a multitude of person-related social and environmental factors operate to influence an individual's adjustment to dystonia (78,96). For these reasons, direct management of the psychosocial sequelae of the illness is very important, and it cannot be assumed that disability, anxiety, and depression in patients would simply disappear with medical treatment of dystonia. Various approaches may prove valuable in the direct treatment and management of psychiatric disorder and psychosocial dysfunction in dystonia. These approaches include direct drug therapy for depression and anxiety, informing and educating the patient, ensuring access to adjunct therapy and to key workers, and providing cognitive-behavioral therapy. In addition, because evidence exists that depression and other mood disorders are not reliably diagnosed by neurologists in the course of consultations (144), neurologists as well as general practitioners must be educated about the common occurrence of psychiatric morbidity in dystonia.

Major depression and anxiety in dystonia require direct treatment with medication. However, the emergence of negative self-related cognitions centered around disfigurement and poor self-image as the distinguishing feature of depression in torticollis, and the fact that the biologic symptoms of depression were much less salient in this group of patients (35,62,63), have implications for the treatment of depression in "visible" dystonias that affect self-image, such as torticollis, blepharospasm, Meige's syndrome, or generalized dystonia, or that influence communication with others, such as spasmodic dysphonia. Antidepressant medication is unlikely to be a sufficient therapy for depression in dystonia and should be complemented with cognitive-behavioral treatment focusing on modifying the negative body image, self-deprecation, and low self-esteem. Both depression and anxiety can be successfully treated with cognitive-behavioral techniques (72,145). The first step is for patients to accept the reality of their chronic illness, come to terms with the limitations imposed by it, and find ways of working around these limitations. For example, patients can schedule important activities after a course of botulinum injections, when their dystonia is at its best, or use alternative methods to achieve goals, such as typing instead of writing in cases with writer's cramp. Second, in the course of cognitive-behavioral therapy, patients come to appreciate the close relation between their thoughts, feelings, and behavior. They also learn to monitor their thoughts to establish that what they think affects the way they feel and behave. The negative thinking style in depression is characterized by the way these individuals perceive themselves, the world, and the future in negative terms (72,145). To counteract self-deprecation and to protect their sense of positive self-esteem, patients need to realize that despite the visible disfigurement produced by dystonia, their past achievements have not been altered and that dystonia is no obstacle to reaching new and realistic goals. Similarly, in anxiety, the thinking style is focused on a sense of threat and danger. In the course of therapy, depressed and anxious patients learn to identify and challenge their negative thoughts and thinking errors, such as overgeneralization, disqualifying the positive, or personalizing, which result in biased interpretations of reality. Anxious patients are also provided with relaxation training to counteract any physical symptoms of anxiety and arousal that can act to magnify anxiety or fear. With those anxious patients with dystonia who have developed severe avoidance or restriction of social activity, desensitization or "graded exposure" to the feared situations is employed. Given that psychosocial factors also contribute to depression and QOL in dystonia (63,78,96), patients should also be encouraged to remain socially involved and active and not to give up professional or social roles because of embarrassment. Because practical and emotional social support is important in protecting individuals emotionally against the stress of chronic illness (78,146), patients should be encouraged to maintain their social ties with friends and family. Other than reports of perceived efficacy by patients (33,94,95,138), there is no evidence regarding the value of cognitive-behavior therapy or psychosocial intervention in dystonia. Well-designed studies are clearly required.

Whereas the course of childhood-onset dystonia is more difficult to map, cases of adult-onset dystonia are likely to remain focal. In adult-onset cases, providing patients with information about the illness, its likely course, and medical treatment options may prepare them for what to expect in the coming years and allow them to recruit the personal, social, and financial resources necessary for coping with the effect of the illness on their daily activities, work, and social relationships. Marshaling these resources promotes a greater sense of personal control and overcomes feelings of helplessness. The patients can also be educated about the key role played by psychosocial factors, such as social support and coping strategies, in determining how well they adjust to life with dystonia. Patients should be encouraged to recruit a network of relatives and friends who can provide them with emotional and practical support at times of need. Patients should be educated about adaptive ways of coping, such as seeking information about the illness and treatment options, recruiting social support and practical help, and discouraging reliance on maladaptive strategies. Communication with doctors is a two-way process, and patients need to become aware that they can play an active role in managing their dystonia by explicitly telling their neurologist about any anxiety or depression they may be feeling, so that such symptoms can be directly treated. Although all these procedures for informing and educating patients are likely to be valuable to patients with dystonia, little evidence-based information exists about their efficacy.

Some patients benefit from access to adjunct therapy, such as physiotherapy. Physiotherapy exercises may be helpful in increasing the range of joint movements, promoting muscle relaxation, and easing pain. Graded neck exercises and relaxation therapy reduced disability and improved depression in a small sample of patients with torticollis (140). In 1990, the Royal College of Physicians of the United Kingdom noted that in standard neurologic practice the psychosocial needs of patients with chronic neurologic disorders were rarely addressed. The report recommended that "some districts should appoint and evaluate the effectiveness of 'key workers' assigned to individual patients." Access to key workers, such as specialist nurses, may be a good approach for management of dystonia. Such contact will ensure that following diagnosis, patients and families are not left to their own devices to cope with the implications of the illness and its effects on their lives. In dystonia, the value of access to a nurse specialist has been evaluated by Jahanshahi et al. (147). They conducted a controlled study in which 24 patients with dystonia were randomly allocated to "intervention" or "control" groups. The two groups were matched on important demographic and illness-related variables. To assess mood and psychosocial function, all patients completed a set of questionnaires twice, at baseline and 6 months later. In the intervening period, those patients allocated to the intervention group received two home visits and five telephone calls from the nurse specialist. This contact was not provided to the control group. The nurse specialist had a major effect on the intervention group by providing information and facilitating referral of patients to other health care agencies. The patients in the intervention program found access and contact with a nurse specialist to be of great value, and they particularly appreciated the "opportunity to talk to someone about the illness and the problems caused by it" and "knowing that the nurse practitioner could be contacted if problems arose." However, the intervention group did not show any significant changes on measures of psychosocial function. The fact that all patients had chronic disease, the brevity of the contact with the nurse specialist, and the short duration of follow-up were factors that could have influenced the absence of statistically significant change on the psychosocial measures employed. Future studies should establish whether more intensive contact with a nurse specialist immediately after diagnosis or early in the course of illness would produce significant improvement of disability, mood, psychosocial functioning, and QOL in dystonia.

Dystonia has a major psychological and social effect on the patient. Successful clinical management of psychiatric morbidity and negative psychosocial consequences of dystonia require a variety of approaches that can help the patient adjust and live well with this chronic disorder.

REFERENCES

1. Marsden CD. The problem of adult-onset idiopathic torsion dystonia and other isolated dyskinesias in adult life (including blepharospasm, oromandibular dystonia, dystonic writer's cramp, and torticollis, or axial dystonia). *Adv Neurol* 1976a;14:259–276.
2. Marsden CD. Dystonia: the spectrum of the disease. *Res Publ Assoc Res Nerv Ment Dis* 1976b;55:351–367.
3. Berardelli A, Rothwell JC, Hallett M, et al. The pathophysiology of primary dystonia. *Brain* 1998;121 (Pt 7):1195–1212.
4. Marsden CD, Harrison MJG. Idiopathic torsion dystonia (dystonia musculorum deformans) A review of forty-two patients. *Brain* 1974;97:793–810.
5. Fahn S, Marsden CD, Calne DB. Classification and investigation of dystonia. In: Marsden CD, Fahn S, eds. *Movement disorders 2*. London: Butterworths, 1987: 332–358.
6. Ozelius LJ, Kramer PL, de LD, et al. Strong allelic association between the torsion dystonia gene (DYT1) and loci on chromosome 9q34 in Ashkenazi Jews. *Am J Hum Genet* 1992;50(3):619–628.
7. Klein C, Ozelius LJ. Dystonia: clinical features, genetics and treatment. *Curr Opin Neurol* 2002;15:491–497.
8. Nemeth AH. The genetics of primary dystonia and related disorders. *Brain* 2002;125:695–721.
9. Nutt JG, Muenter MD, Melton LJ, et al. Epidemiology of dystonian Rochester, Minnesota. *Advances Neurology* 1988;50:365–361.
10. Nakashima K, Rothwell JC, Day BL, et al. Reciprocal inhibition between forearm muscles in patients with writer's cramp and other occupational cramps, symptomatic hemidystonia and hemiparesis due to stroke. *Brain* 1989;112:681–697.
11. Duffy PO, Butler AG, Hawthorne MR, et al. The epidemiology of the primary dystonias in the North of England. *Adv Neurol* 1998;78:121–125.
12. Epidemiological Study of Dystonia in Europe Collaborative Group. A prevalence study of primary dystonia in eight European countries. *J Neurol* 2000;24:787–793.
13. Li S, Scoenberg BS, Wang C et al. A prevalence study of Parkinson's disease and other movement disorders in the People's Republic of China. *Arch Neurol* 1985; 42:655–657.
14. Kandil MR, Tohamy SA, Fattah MA, et al. Prevalence of chorea, dystonia and athetosis in Assiut, Egypt: a clinical and epidemiological study. *Neuroepidemiology* 1994;13(5):202–210.
15. Oppenheim H. Uber eine eigenartige Krampfkrankheit des kindleichen und jugenlichen alters (dys deformans) *Neural Centralbl* 1911;30:1090–1107.
16. Filipovic S, Jahanshahi M, Viswanathan SR, et al. Clinical features of the geste antagoniste in cervical dystonia. In: Fahn S, Hallett M, De Long M, eds. *Dystonia 4. Advances in neurology*, Vol. 94. Philadelphia, PA: Lippincott Williams & Wilkins, 2003:191–203.
17. Jahanshahi M. Factors that ameliorate or aggravate spasmodic torticollis. *J Neurol Neurosurg Psychiatry* 2000;68:227–229.
18. Jahanshahi M, Marion M-H, Marsden CD. Natural history of adult-onset idiopathic torticollis. *Arch Neurol* 1990;47:548–552.
19. Cleveland SE. Personality dynamics in torticollis. *J Nerv Mental Diseases* 1961;129:150–161.
20. Meares R. Behavior therapy and spasmodic torticollis. *Arch Gen Psychiat* 1973;28:104–107.
21. Brierly H. The treatment of spasmodic torticollis by behaviour therapy. *Behav Res Ther* 1967;5:139–142.
22. Tibbetts RW. Spasmodic torticollis. *J Psychosom Res* 1971;15:461–469.
23. Patterson RM, Little SC. Spasmodic torticollis. *J Nerv Ment Dis* 1942;98:571–599.
24. Patterson MT. Spasmodic torticollis. Results of psychotherapy in 21 cases. *Lancet* 1945;III:556–559.
25. Rondot P, Jedynak CP, Ferey G. *Le torticolis spasmodique*. Paris: Masson, 1981.
26. Herz E, Glaser GH. Spasmodic torticollis. II. Clinical evaluation. *Arch Neurol Psychiatry* 1949;49:381–389.
27. Kaste M, Iiavanainen M, Juntunen J, et al. Brain involvement in spasmodic torticollis. *Am Acta Neurol Scand* 1981;63:373–380.
28. Meares R, Lader M. Electromyographic studies in patients with spasmodic torticollis. *J Psychosom Res* 1971;15:13–18.
29. Cockburn JJ. Spasmodic torticollis: a psychogenic condition? *J Psychosom Res* 1971;15:471–477.
30. Choppy-Jacolin M, Ferry G, Demaria C. A psychometric study of 34 patients afflicted with spasmodic torticollis. *Acta Neurol Scand* 1977;55:483–492.
31. Mathews WB, Beasley P, Parry-Jones W, et al. Spasmodic torticollis: a combined clinical study. *J Neurol Neurosurg Psychiatry* 1978;41:485–492.
32. van Hoof JJM, Horstink MWI, Berger HJC, et al. Spasmodic torticollis: the problem of pathophysiology and assessment. *J Neurol* 1987;234:322–327.
33. Jahanshahi M, Marsden CD. Treatments for torticollis. *J Neurol Neurosurg Psychiatry* 1989;52:1212–1220.
34. Jahanshahi M, Marsden CD. Personality in torticollis: a controlled study. *Psychol Med* 1988a;18:375–387.
35. Jahanshahi M, Marsden CD. Depression in torticollis: a controlled study. *Psychol Med* 1988b;18:925–933.
36. Crisp AH, Moldofsky H. A psychosomatic study of writer's cramp. *Br J Psychiatry* 1965;111:841–858.
37. Beech HR. The symptomatic treatment of writer's cramp. In: Eysenck HJ, ed. *Behaviour therapy and the neuroses: readings in modern methods of treatment derived from learning theory*. Oxford: Pergamon Press, 1960:349–372.
38. Bindman E, Tibbets RE. Writer's cramp, a rational approach to treatment. *Br J Psychiatry* 1977;131:143–148.
39. Sylvester JD, Liversedge LA. Conditioning and the occupational cramps. In: Eysenck HJ, ed. *Behaviour therapy and the neuroses: readings in modern methods of treatment derived from learning theory*. Oxford: Pergamon Press, 1960:334–347.
40. Liversedge LA, Sylvester JD. Conditioning techniques in the treatment of writer's cramp. In: Eysenck HJ, ed. *Behaviour therapy and the neuroses: readings in modern methods of treatment derived from learning theory*. Oxford: Pergamon Press, 1960:327–333.
41. Condrau G. Analytic therapy with a patient suffering from compulsion neurosis and writer's cramp. *Am J Psychiatry* 1988;3:211–220.
42. Harrington R, Wieck A, Marks I, et al. Writer's cramp: not associated with anxiety. *Mov Disord* 1988;3: 195–200.
43. Grafman J, Cohen L, Hallett M. Is focal hand dystonia associated with psychopathology? *Mov Disord* 1991; 6:29–35.

44. Green RL. *The MMPI: an interpretive manual.* New York: Grune & Stratton, 1980.
45. Jahanshahi M, Marsden CD. Conversion "V" profiles in torticollis. *Behav Neurol* 1989;2:219–225.
46. Aronson AE, et al. Spastic dysphonia. I. Voice, neurologic and psychiatric aspects. *J Speech Hear Disord* 1968;33:203–218.
47. Izdebski K, Dedo H. Spastic dysphonia: a patient profile of 200 cases. *Am J Otolaryngol* 1984;5:7–14.
48. Sheehy M, Marsden CD. Trauma and pain in torticollis. *Lancet* 1990;I:77–78.
49. Schott G. The relationship of peripheral trauma and pain to dystonia. *J Neurol Neurosurg Psychiatry* 1985;48:698–701.
50. Tempel LW, Perlmutter JS. Abnormal cortical responses in patients with writer's cramp. *Neurology* 1993;43(11):2252–2257 [published erratum appears in *Neurology* 1994;44(12):2411]
51. Ceballos-Baumann A, Passingham RE, Warner T, et al. Overactive prefrontal and underactive motor cortical areas in idiopathic dystonia. *Ann Neurol* 1995;37(3):363–372.
52. Ibanez V, Sadato N, Karp B, et al. Deficient activation of the motor cortical network in patients with writer's cramp. *Neurology* 1999;53(1):96–105.
53. Herz E. Dystonia. III. Pathology and conclusions. *Arch Neurol Psychiatry* 1944;51:20–26.
54. Cooper IS, Cullinan T, Riklan M. The natural history of dystonia. *Adv Neurol* 1976;14:157–169.
55. Lesser DP, Fahn S. Dystonia: a disorder often misdiagnosed as a conversion reaction. *Am J Psychiatry* 1978;135:349–352.
56. Marsden CD. Hysteria: a neurologist's view. *Psychol Med* 1986;16:277–288.
57. Dystonia Society. *Diagnostic survey.* London: The Dystonia Society, 1993.
58. Naber D, Winberger DR, Bullionger M, et al. Personality variables, neurological and psychopathological symptoms in patients suffering from spasmodic torticollis. *Compr Psychiatry* 1988;29:182–187.
59. Wenzel T, Schnider P, Wimmer A, et al. Psychiatric comorbidity in patients with spasmodic torticollis. *J Psychosom Res* 1998;44:687–690.
60. Moraru E, Schnider P, Wimmer A, et al. Relation between depression and anxiety in dystonic patients. Implications for clinical management. *Depress Anxiety* 2002;16:100–103.
61. Gundel H, Wolf A, Xidara V, et al. Social phobia in spasmodic torticollis. *J Neurol Neurosurg Psychiatry* 2001;71:499–504.
62. Jahanshahi M, Marsden CD. Body concept, disability and depression in torticollis. *Behav Neurol* 1990a;3:117–131.
63. Jahanshahi M, Marsden CD. A longitudinal follow-up study of depression, disability, and body concept in torticollis. *Behav Neurol* 1990b;3:233–246.
64. Bihari K, Pigott TA, Hill JL, et al. Blepharospasm and obsessive–compulsive disorder. *J Nerv Ment Dis* 1992a;180:130–132.
65. Bihari K, Hill JL, Murphy DL. Obsessive–compulsive characteristics in patients with idiopathic torticollis. *Psychiatry Res* 1992b;42:267–272.
66. Brooks A, Thiel A, Angerstein D, et al. Higher prevalence of obsessive–compulsive symptoms in patients with blepharospasm than in patients with hemifacial spasm. *Am J Psychiatry* 1998;155:555–557.
67. Cavallaro R, Galardi G, Cavallini CM, et al. Obsessive compulsive disorder among idiopathic focal dystonia patients: an epidemiological and family study. *Biol Psychiatry* 2002;52:356–361.
68. Kubota Y, Murai T, Okada T, et al. Obsessive–compulsive characteristics in patients with writer's cramp. *J Neurol Neurosurg Psychiatry* 2001;71:413–414.
69. Saunders-Pullman R, Shriberg J, Heimann G, et al. The spectrum of myolconus dystonia: possible association with OCD and alcohol dependence. *Neurology* 2002;58:242–245.
70. Butler AG, Duffey PO, Hawthorne MR, et al. The socioeconomic implications of dystonia. In: Fahn S, Marsden CD, DeLong M, eds. *Advance in neurology*, Vol. 78: *Dystonia 3.* Philadelphia, PA: Lippincott Williams & Wilkins, 1998:349–358.
71. Butler AG, Duffey PO, Hawthorne MR, Barnes MP The impact of focal dystonia on the working life of musicians in the United Kingdom. In: Fahn S, Hallett, M, De Long, M (Eds.), *Advance in neurology*, Vol. 94: *Dystonia 4.* Philadelphia, PA: Lippincott Williams & Wilkins, 2004:257–259.
72. Beck AT. *Depression: causes and treatment.* Philadelphia, PA: University of Pennsylvania Press, 1972.
73. Lacey JH, Birtchnell SA. Body image and its disturbances. *J Psychosom Res* 1986;30:623–631.
74. Harris DL. The symptomatology of abnormal appearance: an anecdotal survey. *Br J Plast Surg* 1982;35:312–323.
75. Green BC, Pratt CC, Grisby TE. Self-concept among patients with long-term spinal cord injury. *Arch Phys Med Rehabil* 1984;65:751–754.
76. Felton BJ, Revenson TA. Coping with chronic illness: a study of illness controllability and the influence of coping strategies on psychological adjustment. *J Consult Clin Psychol* 1984;52:343–353.
77. MacCarthy B, Brown R. Psychosocial factors in Parkinson's disease. *Br J Clin Psychol* 1989;28:41–52.
78. Jahanshahi M. Psychosocial correlates of depression in torticollis. *J Psychosom Res* 1991;35:1–15.
79. Folkman S, Lazarus RS. If it changes it must be a process: study of emotion and coping during three stages of a college examination. *J Pers Soc Psychol* 1985;48:150–170.
80. Jahanshahi M. The psychosocial impact of Parkinson's Disease and its clinical management. In: Playford D, ed. *Neurological rehabilitation of Parkinson's disease.* London: Martin Dunitz, Taylor and Francis Group, Elsevier, 2003:25–47.
81. Brown GW, Andrews B, Harris T, et al. Social support, self-esteem, and depression. *Psychol Med* 1986;16:813–831.
82. Smith E, Taylor M, Mendoza M, et al. Spasmodic dysphonia and vocal fold paralysis: outcome of voice problems and work-related functioning. *J Voice* 1998;12:223–232.
83. Ginsberg G, Wallack J, Strain J, et al. Defining the psychiatric role in spastic dysphonia. *Gen Hosp Psychiatry* 1968;10:132–137.
84. Ewing S. Coming to grips with spasmodic dysphonia. National Spasmodic dysphonia Newsletter, Spring/Summer, 1993.
85. Cannito MP. Emotional considerations in spasmodic dysphonia: psychometric quantification. *J Commun Disord* 1991;24:313–329.

86. Murry T, Cannito MP, Woodson GE. Spasmodic dysphonia: emotional status and botulinum toxin treatment. *Arch Otolaryngol Head Neck Surg* 1994;120:310–316.
87. Cannito MP, Murry T, Woodson G. Attitudes toward communication in adductor spasmodic dysphonia before and after botulinum toxin injection. *J Med Speech-Lang Pathol* 1994;2:125–133.
88. Whurr R, Lorch M, Lindsay M, et al. Psychological function in spasmodic dysphonia before and after treatment with botulinum toxin. *J Med Speech-Lang Pathol* 1998;6:81–91.
89. Jahanshahi M, Marsden CD. Psychological functioning before and after treatment of torticollis with botulinum toxin. *J Neurol Neurosurg Psychiatry* 1992;55:229–231.
90. Liu CY, Yu JM, Wang NM, et al. Emotional symptoms are secondary to the voice in patients with spasmodic dysphonia. *Gen Hosp Psychiatry* 1998;20:255–259.
91. Goffman E. *Stigma: notes on the management of spoiled identity.* London: Penguin, 1963.
92. MacDonald, L. The experience of stigma: living with rectal cancer. In: Anderson R, Bury M, eds. *Living with chronic illness: the experience of patients and their families.* London, Allen and Unwin, 1988.
93. Scambler G, Hopkins A. Being epileptic: coming to terms with stigma. *Sociol Health Illn* 1986;8:26–43.
94. Papathanasiou I, MacDonald L, Whurr R, et al. Perceived stigma among patients with spasmodic dysphonia. *J Med Speech-Lang Pathol* 1997;5:251–261.
95. Papathanasiou I, MacDonald L, Whurr R, et al. Perceived stigma in spasmodic torticollis. *Mov Disord* 2001;16:280–285.
96. Ben-Shlomo Y, Camfield L, Warner T, The Epidemiological Study of Dystonia in Europe Collaborative Group. What are the determinants of quality of life in people with cervical dystonia? *J Neurol Neurosurg Psychiatry* 2002;72:608–614.
97. Fahn S, Williams DT. Psychogenic dystonia. In: Fahn S et al., eds. *Dystonia 2. Advances in neurology.* New York: Raven Press, 1988:431–455.
98. Fahn S. Psychogenic movement disorders. In: Marsden CD, Fahn S, eds. *Movement disorders 3.* Oxford: Butterworth-Heinemann, 1994:359–372.
99. Marsden CD. Psychogenic problems associated with dystonia. In: Weiner WJ, Lang AE, eds. *Behavioural neurology of movement disorders, Advances in neurology.* New York: Raven Press, 1995:319–326.
100. Factor SA, Podskalny GD, Molho ES. Psychogenic movement disorders: frequency, clinical profile and characteristics. *J Neurol Neurosurg Psychiatry* 1995;59:406–412.
101. Gudex CM, Hawthorne MR, Butler AG, et al. Effect of dystonia and botulinum toxin treatment on health-related quality of life. *Mov Disord* 1998;13:941–946.
102. Muller J, Kemmler G, Wissel J et al., The Austrian Botulinum Toxin and Dystonia Study Group. The impact of blepharospasm and cervical dystonia on health-related quality of life and depression. *J Neurol* 2002;249:842–846.
103. Brans JWM, Lindeboom RL, Aramideh M, et al. Long-term effect of botulinum toxin on treatment and functional health in cervical dystonia. *Neurology* 1998;50:1461–1463.
104. Brefel-Courbon C, Simonetta-Moreau M, More C, et al. A pharmacoeconomic evaluation of botulinum toxin in the treatment of spasmodic torticollis. *Clin Neuropharmacol* 2000;23:203–207.
105. Hogikyan ND, Wodchis WP, Spak C, et al. Longitudinal effects of botulinum toxin injections on voice-related quality of life (V-RQOL) for patients with adductory spasmodic dysphonia. *J Voice* 2001;15:576–586.
106. Hilker R, Schischniaschvili M, Ghaemi M, et al. Health related quality of life is improved by botulinum neurotoxin type A in long-term treated patients with focal dystonia. *J Neurol Neurosurg Psychiatry* 2001;71:193–199.
107. Odergren T, Tollback A, Borg RPT, et al. Efficacy of botulinum toxin for cervical dystonia. A comparison of the methods for evaluation. *Scand J Rehabil Med* 1994;26:191–195.
108. Lindeboom RL, Brans JWM, Aramideh M, et al. Treatment of cervical dystonia: a comparison of measures for outcome assessment. *Mov Disord* 1998;13:706–712.
109. Camfield L, Ben-Shlomo Y, Warner T. The Epidemiological Study of Dystonia in Europe Collaborative Group. Impact of cervical dystonia on quality of life. *Mov Disord* 2002;17:838–841.
110. Schrag A, Jahanshahi M, Quinn NP. What contributes to quality of life in patients with Parkinson's disease? *J Neurol Neurosurgery Psychiatry* 2000;69:308–312.
111. Muller J, Wissel J, Kemmler G et al., The Austrian Botulinum Toxin and Dystonia Study Group. Craniocervical dystonia questionnaire (CDQ-24): development and validation of a disease-specific quality of life instrument. *J Neurol Neurosurg Psychiatry* 2004;75:749–753.
112. Augood SJ, Penny JB, Friberg IK, et al. Expression of the early-onset torsion dystonia gene (DYT1) in human brain. *Ann Neurol* 1998;43:669–673.
113. Augood SJ, Martin DM, Ozelius LJ, et al. Distribution of the mRNAs encoding torsion A and torsin B in the normal adult human brain. *Ann Neurol* 1999;46:761–769.
114. Placzek MR, Misbahuddin A, Chaudhuri KR, et al. Cervical dystonia is associated with polymorphism in the dopamine (D5) receptor gene. *J Neurol Neurosurg Psychiatry* 2001;71:262–264.
115. Misbahuddin A, Placzek MR, Chaudhuri KR, et al. A polymorphism in the dopamine receptor DRD5 is associated with blepharospasm. *Neurology* 2002;58:124–126.
116. Cummings JL. Frontal-subcortical circuits and human behaviour. *J Psychosom Res* 1998;44:627–628.
117. McGuire PK, Bench CJ, Frith CD, et al. Functional anatomy of obsessive–compulsive phenomena. *Br J Psychiatry* 1994;164:459–468.
118. Rauch SL, Jenike MA, Alpert NM, et al. Regional cerebral blood flow measured during symptom provocation in obsessive–compulsive disorder using oxygen 15-labelled carbon dioxide and positron emission tomography. *Arch Gen Psychiatry* 1994;51:62–70.
119. Lefebvre A, Barclay S. Psychosocial impact of craniofacial deformities before and after reconstructive surgery. *Can J Psychiatry* 1982;27:579–583.
120. McGrouther DA. Facial disfigurement. *Br Med J* 1997;314:991–992.
121. Hay GG. Psychiatric aspects of cosmetic nasal operations. *Br J Psychiatry* 1970;116:85–97.

122. Hay GG, Heather BB. Changes in psychometric test results following cosmetic nasal operations. *Br J Psychiatry* 1973;122:89–90.
123. Münchau A, Palmer JD, Dressler D, et al. Prospective study of selective peripheral denervation for botulinum-toxin resistant patients with cervical dystonia. *Brain* 2001;124:769–783.
124. Kupsch A, Klafke S, Kuhn AA, et al. The effects of frequency in pallidal deep brain stimulation for primary dystonia. *J Neurol* 2003;250:1201–1205.
125. Williams DT, Ford B, Fahn S. Phenomenology and psychopathology related to psychogenic movement disorders. In: Weiner WJ, Lang AE, eds. *Advances in neurology*. New York: Raven Press, 1995:231–257.
126. Sa DS, Lang AE. Psychogenic parkinsonism and dystonia. In: Bedard M-A et al., eds. *Mental and behavioural dysfunction in movement disorders*. Totowa, NJ: Humana Press, 2003:399–408.
127. Jayne D, Lees A, Stern G. Remission in spasmodic torticollis. *J Neurol Neurosurg Psychiatry* 1984;47:1236–1237.
128. Friedman A, Fahn S. Spontaneous remissions in spasmodic torticollis. *Neurology* 1986;36:398–400.
129. Miyasaki JM, Sa DS, Galvez-Jimenez N, et al. Psychogenic movement disorders. *Can J Neurol Sci* 2003;30(Suppl. 1):S94–100.
130. Bentivoglio AR, Loi M, Valenta EM, et al. Phenotypic variability of DYT1-PTD: Does the clinical spectrum include psychogenic dystonia? *Mov Disord* 2002;17:1058–1063.
131. Panizza M, Lelli S, Nilsson J, et al. H-reflex recovery curve and reciprocal inhibition of H-reflex in different kinds of dystonia. *Neurology* 1990;40:824–928.
132. Reuber M, Pukrop R, Bauer J, et al. Multidimensional assessment of personality in patients with psychogenic non-epileptic seizures. *J Neurol Neurosurg Psychiatry* 2004;75:743–748.
133. Lang AE. Psychogenic dystonia: a review of 18 cases. *Can J Neurol Sci* 1995;22:136–143.
134. Crimlisk HL, Bhatia K, Cope H, et al. Slater revisited: 6 year follow-up study of patients with medically unexplained motor symptoms. *Br Med J* 1998;316:582–586.
135. Feinstein A, Stergiopolous V, Fine J, et al. Psychiatric outcome in patients with a psychogenic movement disorder. *Neuropsychiatry Neuropsychol Behav Neurol* 2001;14:169–176.
136. Fine J, Stergiopolous V, Nieves A, et al. Long-term follow-up of psychogenic movement disorders. *Neurology* 2000;54(Suppl. 3):A50–A51.
137. Couprie W, Wijdicks EFM, Roojmans HGM, et al. Outcome in conversion disorder: a follow-up study. *J Neurol Neurosurg Psychiatry* 1995;58:750–752.
138. Junker J, Oberwittler C, Jackson D, et al. Utilization and perceived effectiveness of complementary and alternative medicine in patients with dystonia. *Mov Disord* 2004;19:158–1611.
139. Wieck A, Harrington R, Marks I, et al. Writer's cramp: a controlled trial of habit reversal treatment. *Br J Psychiatry* 1988;153:111–115.
140. Jahanshahi M, Sartory G, Marsden CD. A controlled evaluation of the efficacy of EMG biofeedback treatment of spasmodic torticollis. *Biofeedback Self Regul* 1991;16:413–448.
141. Vitek JL, Zhang J, Evatt M, et al. GPi pallidotomy for dystonia: clinical outcome and neuronal activity. *Adv Neurol* 1998;78:211–219.
142. Kumar R, Dagher A, Hutchison W-D, et al. Globus pallidus deep brain stimulation for generalized dystonia: clinical and PET investigation. *Neurology* 1999;53(4):871–874.
143. Coubes P, Roubertie A, Vayssiere N, et al. Treatment of DYT1-generalised dystonia by stimulation of the internal globus pallidus. *Lancet* 2000;355(9222):2220–2221.
144. Bridges KW, Goldberg DP. Psychiatric illness in inpatients with neurological disorders: patients' views on discussion of emotional problems with neurologists. *Br Med J* 1982;289:656–658.
144. Beck AT. *Cognitive therapy and the emotional disorders*. New York: International Universities Press, 1976.
146. Siegal BR, Calsyn RJ, Cuddihee RM. The relationship of social support to psychological adjustment in endstage renal disease patients. *J Chronic Dis* 1987;40:337–344.
147. Jahanshahi M, Brown RG, Whitehouse C, et al. Contact with a nurse practitioner—a short-term evaluation study in Parkinson's disease and dystonia. *Behav Neurol* 1994;7:189–196.

23

Autoaggressive Immune-Mediated Movement Disorders

Davide Martino and Gavin Giovannoni

Institute of Neurology, Departments of Neuroimmunology and Neuroinflammation, University College London, London, United Kingdom

The clinical picture in disturbances of the basal ganglia is often characterized by the coexistence of three clinical features: motor disturbances (hypokinetic or hyperkinetic disorders), psychiatric disturbances, and varying degrees of cognitive impairment (1). This characteristic triad is compatible with the complex role played by the basal ganglia in the normal functioning of the cerebral cortex. Patients with different disorders of the basal ganglia, such as neurodegenerative conditions (e.g., Parkinson's disease and Huntington's disease), primary central nervous system (CNS) infections, tumors, vascular lesions, abnormal copper load (i.e., Wilson's disease), progressive calcium deposition (i.e., Fahr's disease), neurodevelopmental diseases [e.g., tic disorders, Tourette's syndrome, childhood-onset obsessive–compulsive disorder (OCD), and Attention-Deficit Hyperactivity Disorder (ADHD)], all exhibit both extrapyramidal movement disorders and psychiatric features, although presentations vary. Immune-mediated or inflammatory disorders that affect the basal ganglia are no exception. Sydenham's chorea (SC), the first putative autoimmune movement disorder to be described, exhibits a similar spectrum of clinical features (2). Over the last two decades, the spectrum of putative immune-mediated basal ganglia disorders has widened, and in this chapter, we demonstrate that the full spectrum of basal ganglia dysfunction has now been observed. A better understanding of the complexities of autoimmune disorders has provided us with both a new perspective on basal ganglia disease and the potential to treat some of these disorders with immunomodulatory therapies.

BASIC PRINCIPLES OF AUTOIMMUNITY

The concept of autoimmunity has recently been redefined in view of the emerging evidence that autoimmune reactions are not all harmful and that some may be beneficial in playing a role in tissue repair and homeostasis (3). A preferable term, therefore, to describe pathologic autoimmunity is autoaggressive immune-mediated disorders (AAIMDs), which can be defined as immunologic disorders characterized by the breakdown of self-tolerance to healthy tissues.

Lymphocytes (the principal "conductors" of adaptive or specific immunity), during their development, express receptors, which bind specifically to an undefined number of self-antigens, therefore carrying a natural autoimmune potential (4). The physiologic process meant to eliminate or downregulate these autoreactive cells is called *tolerance*. Tolerance involves both B and T lymphocytes. B cells mediate specific humoral immunity through the synthesis of specific antibodies (4). In humans, these cells develop in the bone marrow from pluripotent stem cells to mature naive B cells in an antigen-independent process; mature naive B lymphocytes gain specific antigen reactivity in the periphery, recirculating through secondary lymphoid tissues (i.e., spleen, lymph nodes, and tonsils), where they may encounter a wide variety of self-antigens and non–self-antigens (5). Such encounters with antigens drive B-cell differentiation, generating B-cell clones and producing highly specific antibodies against defined antigens. If one of these antigen happens to be a self-antigen or a foreign antigen that mimics a self-antigen, the potential for AAIMD is established. Additionally, B cells are also capable of binding, internalizing, and processing antigens and hence are included among the professional antigen-presenting cells (APC). T cells, on the other hand, are responsible for specific cell-mediated immunity, controlling (T-helper and T-regulatory lymphocytes) the activation and differentiation of immune-competent cell types, including T-cell subsets, or directly killing (cytotoxic T cells) infected cells. T lymphocytes coordinate the immune response against pathogens whose peptide fragments have been displayed on the surface of APCs, such as B lymphocytes and dendritic cells (5). As soon as the peripheral B lymphocyte meets a recognizable antigen, the antigen is internalized by the B cell and presented on its surface to a T-helper cell. The interaction between the two lymphocytes results in proliferation and differentiation of the T cell, which in turn will stimulate and support B-cell development (4). Through the process of affinity maturation, the B cells produce high-affinity antibodies, which are specific to the inciting antigen.

B-cell tolerance operates through deletion of self-reactive B cells within the bone marrow and the secondary lymphoid organs (6,7) or through their functional inactivation in the periphery (anergy) (8). Autoreactive T cells are largely deleted in the thymus by negative selection and a process called *thymic education* (9). T cells with autoreactive potential that escape this process are maintained in an anergic state by a process called *peripheral tolerance* (9). Several mechanisms that result in a loss of tolerance to self have been hypothesized, and include (a) primary T-cell autoimmune deviation (insufficient intrathymic deletion of self-reactive clones and dysfunction of T-suppressor or regulatory cells), (b) primary B-cell autoimmune deviation, and (c) autoimmunity induced by environmental factors acting on an apparently normal immune system (4). As mentioned previously, the "normal immune system" contains autoreactive lymphocytes, which can cause AAIMD if they escape the mechanisms that maintain peripheral tolerance. Immune dysregulation or an environmental trigger can result in the peripheral activation of these autoreactive cells and can trigger the development of an AAIMD. Environmental triggers include a wide variety of infectious agents (10), which can accidentally activate B or T cells by producing superantigens. Superantigens are groups of proteins or peptides that are capable of activating a large number of lymphocytes in an antigen-independent manner (5). If one of these lymphocytes happens to be autoreactive, an AAIMD could be triggered. A second mechanism occurs through the process of "molecular mimicry" (4,5,11). Molecular mimicry occurs when sufficient structural similarity exists between a microbial antigen and a self-antigen or between the complexes formed by a microbial antigenic epitope and a specific major histocompatability complex MHC molecule. The final common pathway, however, is the activation of self-reactive B or T lymphocytes, which can then result in an AAIMD (12). These activated lymphocytes then migrate through the body, and if they encounter the specific cross-reactive self-antigen, they initiate an autoaggressive cascade of events (Fig. 23-1). These events damage healthy tissue through well-defined cell-mediated or autoantibody-mediated mechanisms.

Molecular mimicry occurs in several AAIM neurologic diseases and is also thought to play a crucial role in the pathogenesis of SC (13), in which an autoaggressive immune response is triggered by infection with Group A β-hemolytic streptococci (GABHS). The principle of molecular mimicry might also explain the pathogenesis of the expanding spectrum of poststreptococcal movement disorders.

Neoplastic processes are also capable of triggering autoaggressive immune responses. The expression of onconeural antigens by specific peripheral tumors results in an appropriate peripheral antitumor immune response. However, because these antigens also are expressed normally within the CNS, when activated T cells primed against the onconeural antigens perceive this antigen in the appropriate context within the

```
                           Infection
                               │
                               ▼
         Exposure to microbial antigens mimicking self-antigens
        ┌──────────────┬─────────────────┬──────────────┐
        │              ▼                 ▼              │
        │    Activation of antigen-   Activation of antigen-
        │     specific T cells         specific B cells
        │    (potentially autoreactive) (potentially autoreactive)
        │              │                 │              │
        │              ▼                 ▼              │
        │    Migration of autoreactive  Migration of autoreactive
        │     T-cell clone into CNS    B-cell clone into CNS
        │              │                 │              │
        │              ▼                 ▼              │
        │    Local cell-mediated       Production of autoreactive
        │     immune reaction           immunoglobulins
        │              ╲                 ╱              │
        │               ▼               ▼               │
        │        Ig-mediated immunological cascade,     │
        │        e.g., complement and microglial activation
        │                      │                        │
        │                      ▼                        │
        │              Neuronal damage                  │
        │                      │                        │
        │                      ▼                        │
        └──────────── Neoantigen release ───────────────┘
                      and spread
                  of antigenic determinant
```

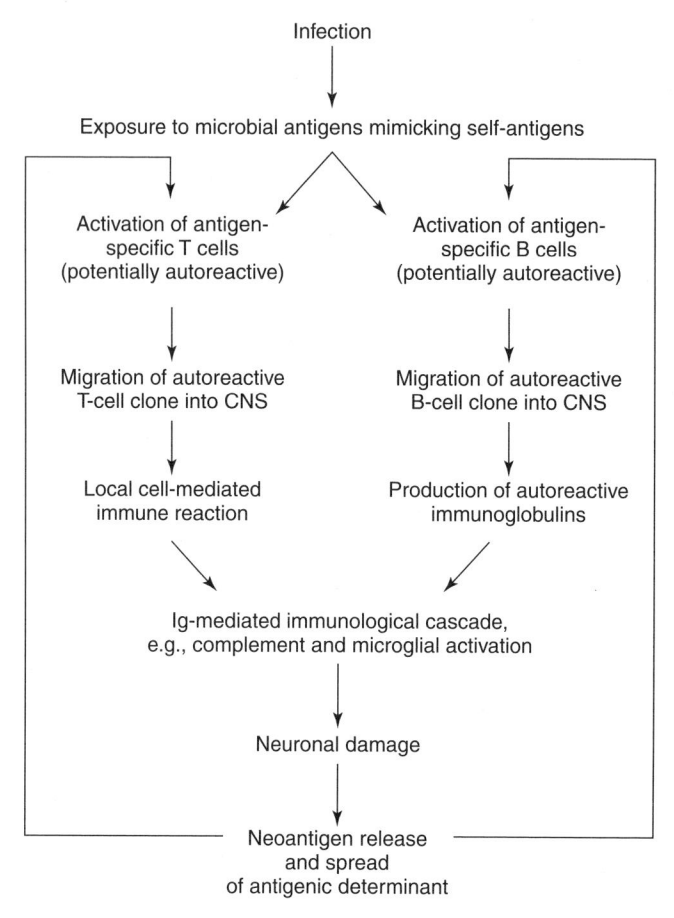

FIG. 23-1. Schematic representation of the mechanisms potentially involved in molecular mimicry triggered by an infectious agent.

CNS, an autoaggressive immune reaction is initiated in the CNS. This phenomenon gives rise to the relatively rare group of paraneoplastic autoaggressive immune-mediated disorders (14).

AAIMD can be a multisystem disease but is often organ specific or tissue specific, the CNS being no exception. The CNS is constantly under immunologic surveillance, and activated T lymphocytes are capable of entering the CNS without disrupting the blood–brain barrier (BBB). The perivascular areas of the CNS are the proposed sites where migrating lymphocytes are most likely to encounter self-antigens in the correct context and to induce an AAIMD (15). The self-antigens have to be presented to T cells in the context of a specific MHC class I, or possibly class II, molecule and must receive the obligatory costimulatory signal. Once activated, the T cell proliferates and produces a cocktail of proinflammatory cytokines, which in turn activates local effector cells, which, in this case, includes astrocytes, microglia, and endothelial cells. These cells in turn produce numerous inflammatory mediators, which recruit circulating leukocytes to establish a local inflammatory reaction. As part of this cascade, T-cell–dependent B-cell activation occurs, with the consequent production of specific autoantibodies (15). These autoantibodies are capable of amplifying the inflammatory response if they are able to recognize their targets by either complement-mediated damage or antibody-mediated cytotoxicity. The local inflammatory response disrupts the integrity of the BBB.

Another possibility in an AAIMD of the CNS is that the initial pathologic event is antibody-mediated complement activation, followed by secondary recruitment of T cells, which then initiate a typical T-cell–mediated inflammatory reaction (4). Autoantibodies, which passively cross either an intact or a damaged BBB, have been hypothesized to activate the complement system after reacting with their target autoantigen. Local astrocytes and microglia are then activated by components of the complement cascade, through their Fc receptors, or by both mechanisms. These local effector cells, once activated, produce cytokines, for example, tumor necrosis factor-α (TNF-α), interleukin-1 (IL-1), and other inflammatory mediators, such as reactive oxygen and nitrogen species. As part of this local inflammatory reaction, the endothelium is activated, and a second wave of leukocyte recruitment occurs, which includes autoreactive T lymphocytes that have been primed in the periphery. These lymphocytes then trigger a typical cell-mediated inflammatory cascade, which results in tissue damage and clinical disease.

Another hypothesis suggests that autoimmunity may be induced by traumatic, inflammatory, or ischemic processes that expose hidden or cryptic self-antigenic determinants to autoreactive lymphocytes. These activated T cells then initiate or amplify the local immune response, extending tissue damage. The inflammatory response damages the structure or function (or both) of the anatomic areas targeted by the process. This general scheme, summarized in Fig. 23-1, is theoretically applicable to all areas of the CNS, including the basal ganglia.

POSTINFECTIOUS (POSTSTREPTOCOCCAL) DISORDERS

Recently, postinfectious AAIMDs, particularly poststreptococcal disorders, have captured the interest of specialists in the field of neuropsychiatry and movement disorders. GABHS infection has been related to several different neurologic and psychiatric signs and symptoms, all characterized by basal ganglia dysfunction. GABHS is an important gram-positive bacterial pathogen; humans seem to be its only biologic host (16). It mainly colonizes the throat or the skin and is responsible for several well-defined suppurative infections, reactions to bacterial toxins, and postinfectious autoaggressive immune-mediated sequelae. Among these sequelae, the most well recognized are rheumatic fever (RF) and acute glomerulonephritis (17). There is no evidence that GABHS directly enters the brain. Acute rheumatic fever (ARF) is preceded by a streptococcal infection of the upper respiratory tract and results in a multiorgan inflammatory response directed at the heart, joints, and brain (16). GABHS is a versatile pathogen, and many strains have been identified (17). These strains vary considerably in their potential to cause RF (18). Outbreaks of specific rheumatogenic strains may account for the marked temporal and geographic fluctuations in the incidence of ARF (19,20). A genetic predisposition might be involved in the development of this condition because only 2% to 3% of subjects affected by a GABHS throat infection develop ARF, and ARF occurs frequently in familial form (18). In addition, ARF has been linked, in some population groups, to HLA subtypes (21–23).

Starting with the neuropsychiatric manifestation of ARF, namely SC, we review the clinical features and the pathophysiology of the poststreptococcal neuropsychiatric disorders. Observations during the last 10 years have suggested a much broader spectrum for this group of disorders than had been identified in the past.

SYDENHAM'S CHOREA

SC is considered the prototypic poststreptococcal autoimmune neuropsychiatric disorder. The immunologic hallmark of SC is the presence of antineuronal antibodies, which are thought to arise in response to an infection with GABHS and then cross-react with antigens in the basal ganglia (24). SC is still prevalent in developing countries, and particularly in developing communities (13,25), and occurs in 10% to 40% of the patients affected by RF, mainly children 5 to 15 years old (26). SC recurs in 10% to 25% of cases (13). Chorea is clearly the predominant feature of SC, involving the face and extremities, but a constellation of neurologic signs, including hypotonia, dysarthria, and gait disturbances, is generally present. For a more detailed overview of the neurologic features of SC, consult some of the comprehensive reviews on this topic (13, 26,27).

Psychiatric symptoms have been described in patients with SC since the initial work by Thomas Sydenham in 1686. The first behavioral features to be reported were emotional lability, regressive exaggeration of normal emotions, fidgeting, anxiety, night terrors, and inattention (2). These features were initially called *choreic temperament* and constituted a "fairly uniform picture" (28). Their spectrum has been redefined, thanks to recent prospective observational studies. Interestingly, considerable psychiatric comorbidity has also been observed in patients with RF who did not have SC (29). In the past decades, tics have been reported in patients with SC (30). More recently, Mercadante et al. assessed neuropsychiatric symptoms in RF and SC (29) and found that 73% of the children with SC had a tic disorder, whereas tic disorders occurred in only 20% of the children affected by RF without chorea. Because of the difficulty in differentiating between motor tics and choreic movements, vocal tics have been more readily described in SC; clicking sounds, smacking sounds, whistling, throat clearing, sniffing, word repetition, and palilalia have been reported in this condition (31). In another group of patients described by Swedo et al., other types of tics, such as simple motor tics and dystonic tics, have been observed (32). A high prevalence of emotional disorders (i.e., obsessive–compulsive neurosis, anxiety, and depression) in SC was reported for the first time by a case series published in the 1960s, which did not use standardized methods of assessment (33, 34). In more recent years, Swedo et al. conducted a comprehensive examination of 11 children with SC, during which emotional symptoms were evaluated; 9 children without a previous history of obsessionality developed acute-onset obsessive–compulsive symptoms (OCS), and 4 of them fulfilled criteria from *The Diagnostic and Statistical Manual of Mental Disorders*, 3rd edition, Revised (DSM III-R) for OCD (35). The symptoms of these children were similar to the symptoms of OCD in children and adults: they included obsessional fears of germ contamination and of doing something wrong; worry about harm to self or their mothers; washing, counting, checking, and hoarding rituals; and the need to do or say things "just right." Such symptoms preceded abnormal movements by about 2 to 4 weeks and tended to disappear before remission of chorea. Even if the physician noticed the chorea in these children, OCS were of greater concern to some of them, who kept these symptoms hidden for fear of being considered "bad" or "crazy." Interestingly, in a 4-year prospective study on the occurrence of OCS and OCD in SC, Asbahr et al. observed that the incidence and severity of OCS increased with every relapse of SC (36). These authors suggested that recurrent GABHS infections and the subsequent basal ganglia dysfunction might have a cumulative effect. Other authors (29) have reported lower percentages of obsessive–compulsive features than that reported by Swedo et al.; group sizes, differences in assessment methods, lack of prospective follow-up, and referral bias might account for such discrepancies. Separation anxiety, generalized anxiety, social phobia, and enuresis have been observed in 9% to 13% of patients with SC, whereas Mercadante et al. found that major depressive disorder was present in 9 of 22 (40.9%) patients with SC (29). Difficulties in sustaining attention are common during the acute phase of SC (2). Attention disorders in SC, however, were never assessed properly until a decade ago (32). This issue is of major interest because the pathophysiology of ADHD involves dysfunction in neural pathways connecting the deep gray matter, mainly the basal ganglia, to frontal cortical areas (1). Swedo et al. (32) reported that one third of the patients with SC in their study had symptoms consistent with ADHD. At times, episodes of chorea exacerbated existing ADHD symptoms, whereas, in other cases, ADHD symptoms arose *de novo* in association with the movement disorder. Mercadante et al. (29) reported a strikingly extensive comorbidity of ADHD and SC (i.e., 45.5% of patients with SC were also affected by ADHD). In contrast to children with other psychiatric features, a child with RF and an antecedent history of ADHD, combined type, had a markedly higher risk of developing SC (95%) than did patients who had RF but no history of ADHD (36%). In the past, nonaffective psychoses, closely resembling schizophrenia, have been associated with rheumatic chorea, identifying a subtype of SC called *chorea insaniens* (2,26,37). Delirium, unstructured delusions, and hallucinations were considered the most common hallmarks of chorea insaniens. Recent literature has not confirmed this observation (29), and the incidence of clearly psychotic symptoms in SC might be considerably lower than was thought in the past.

Imaging studies reveal a predominant involvement of the basal ganglia in SC. Giedd et al. described selective increases in the volumes of the caudate, putamen, and globus pallidus in patients with SC compared with healthy controls (38). Pathologic changes in other brain structures have been reported, particularly in the cerebral cortex and thalamus, but the extent of the lesions was smaller (38). Striatal neuronal dysfunction or loss has also been indicated by a reduction of the N-acetyl-aspartate peak, detected by magnetic resonance proton spectroscopy (39). Postmortem studies suggest that inflammation is the main pathologic change in SC (40,41), and the structural changes detected by magnetic resonance imaging (MRI) are edematous swelling of the striatum and high-signal lesions of the basal ganglia, mainly on T2-weighted images (42–44). These findings are seen in only a few patients with SC, however, and are generally reversible with the clinical picture; their volume and signal intensity are not related to the severity of symptoms. However, permanent striatal changes were documented in some patients with persistent SC (45). Contrast enhancement on MRI is a very rare finding (42). Single photon emission computed tomography (SPECT) and positron emission tomography (PET) studies revealed hyperperfusion and hypermetabolism of the striatum and thalamus compatible either with an active inflammatory process in these structures or with enhanced striatal activity related to increased corticostriatal inputs (46,47). Therefore, even if imaging studies suggest an inflammatory process in only a few patients with SC, they confirm a selective, and generally transient, involvement of the basal ganglia that is consistent with the clinical features.

Cross-reactivity between GABHS and host tissues (i.e., molecular mimicry) promotes an autoimmune response in RF. Rheumatic carditis is caused by a cell-mediated and antibody-mediated immune attack, and evidence of a similar pathophysiology in SC is growing. Autoantibodies cross-reacting between streptococcal and brain epitopes is thought to be the mechanism causing the brain damage. Ideally, five criteria have to be fulfilled to prove that a disorder is induced by autoantibodies (see Table 23-1). Antineuronal antibodies (criterion 1) have been found in the serum and cerebrospinal fluid (CSF) of most patients with SC (24,48–51). All studies in human post-mortem and rat brain have reported that these anti-basal ganglia antibodies (ABGA) are IgG directed, in a relatively selective fashion, against basal ganglia structures, and that large striatal neurons are the most frequently targeted structure. ABGA are also present in healthy individuals, as part of their natural autoantibody repertoire, but in substantially smaller proportions. The selective immune response against basal ganglia tissue suggests that the autoantigens in SC are restricted to, or at least most abundant in, the basal ganglia, particularly in the striatum, and recent evidence demonstrates recurrent reactivity of ABGA to striatal antigens that have a molecular weight of 40,

TABLE 23-1. *Criteria for establishing the causal role of antibodies in the pathogenesis of autoantibody-mediated disorders*

1. Autoantibodies should be present or should be abundant in serum or cerebrospinal fluid of most patients compared with that of healthy individuals.
2. Immunoglobulins bound to target antigen at the key site of pathology should be detectable immunohistochemically by light or electron microscopy.
3. Plasma exchange, which removes immunoglobulins from circulation, should have a therapeutic effect.
4. Injection of serum or purified immunoglobulin should transfer the disease phenotype to experimental animals.
5. An experimental disease homologous to the human disorder should be inducible by sensitizing susceptible animals with the corresponding target antigen.

(From Archelos JJ, Hartung HP. Pathogenetic role of autoantibodies in neurological diseases. *Trend Neurosci* 2000;23:317–327, with permission.)

45, or 60 kDa (49). An animal model of SC, induced by passive transfer of antibody (criterion 5), was never obtained, although infusing the sera of patients with SC into rodent subthalamic nucleus has been shown to increase apomorphine-stimulated ipsilateral circling (52). In a small trial, plasma exchange (PE) (criterion 3) improved clinical symptoms in four of five children with SC, and chorea did not recur in any of these children during the following 10 months (53). What is the pathogenic role of ABGA, and what is their molecular target? The ideal targets of these autoantibodies are evolutionarily conserved molecules that have a high degree of homology between the streptococcal and human isoforms. Streptococcal cell wall antigens were the first antigens to be considered responsible for molecular mimicry. Brain-specific antibody reactivity of sera from SC patients was removed by absorption using cell wall preparations of rheumatogenic streptococcal strains (54), and attention was focused on specific serotypes of the M protein (M6 in particular), one of the major streptococcal virulence factors. Recently, investigators have suggested that other surface antigens capable of inducing an autoantibody-mediated response against neuronal cells might be present (55). Current hypotheses about the direct pathogenic effect of ABGA include antibody-dependent complement-mediated cytotoxicity, and ganglioside-mediated modulation of neuronal intracellular signaling and neurotransmitter release (55). Overall, however, antibody-mediated damage directly caused by ABGA must be distinguished from an alternative pathogenetic mechanism, in which ABGA might be a mere epiphenomenon, secondary to basal ganglia damage. Ongoing research is focusing on defining the precise anatomic and molecular targets of ABGA, their pathogenic effects, and their diagnostic validity.

PEDIATRIC AUTOIMMUNE NEUROPSYCHIATRIC DISORDERS ASSOCIATED WITH STREPTOCOCCAL INFECTIONS

In the 1990s, a tenfold increase in the number of children presenting with new-onset tics was reported in association with a community outbreak of GABHS infections in the state of Rhode Island, USA (56). Soon after, the clinical picture of pediatric autoimmune neuropsychiatric disorders associated with streptococcal infections (PANDAS) was documented by a group led by Susan Swedo, from the National Institutes of Mental Health, Bethesda, MD, USA (57). The cohort described by this group comprised 50 children who satisfied the DSM-IV criteria for OCD, tic disorder, or both and shared specific features of age and type of onset, time-course, association with GABHS infections, and associated neurologic comorbidity. The five clinical criteria used to define the PANDAS subgroup are listed in Table 23-2. Inclusion in this subgroup implied that these children did not have "overt" chorea, which would have suggested a diagnosis of SC; moreover, they apparently neither exhibited any of the major clinical manifestations of RF (particularly carditis and arthritis) nor presented with a family history of RF. The identification of PANDAS as a distinct nosologic entity is still a matter of debate (58). In fact, the five diagnostic criteria were originally formulated as working criteria, with the objective of defining a homogenous subgroup of patients with OCD and tic disorder. In addition, PANDAS have strong clinical similarities to SC, and the link with recent GABHS infection suggests a similar inflammatory or autoaggressive immune-mediated pathogenesis. OCD symptoms in the PANDAS cohort strongly resemble those

TABLE 23-2. *Operative criteria for the diagnosis of pediatric autoimmune neuropsychiatric disorders associated with streptococcal infections (PANDAS)*

1. Presence of obsessive–compulsive disorder or tic disorder or both (meeting DSM-IV criteria)
2. Prepubertal onset of symptoms
3. Episodic course characterized by acute, severe onset and dramatic symptom exacerbations
4. Neurologic abnormalities (e.g., choreiform movements) present during symptom exacerbations
5. Temporal relation between GABHS infections and symptom exacerbations

[Swedo SE, Leonard HL, Garvey M, et al. Pediatric autoimmune neuropsychiatric disorders associated with streptococcal infections: clinical description of the first 50 cases. *Am J Psychiatry* 1998;155(2):264–271.]

documented in SC (32,57)—fear of contamination, fear of harm to self or others, religious ideation, and violent images were the most common obsessions in the affected children, whereas checking, washing, repeating, counting, and ordering were the most common compulsive actions documented. Psychiatric comorbidity was common in children with PANDAS. ADHD, affective disorders, and anxiety disorders were the most prevalent (40%, 42%, and 32%, respectively). In addition, the onset of a number of behavioral symptoms coincided with the onset of the OCD and tics and displayed the same relapsing–remitting course of tics and OCS. The most notable of these behavioral features were emotional lability, change in school performance, personality change, bedtime fears and rituals, and fidgeting. Such symptoms occur also in patients with SC; they are distressing to the children and are clearly distinguishable from the patients' premorbid state. As in SC, PANDAS have an episodic course, characterized by abrupt onset (symptoms are often said to appear "overnight," or "out of the blue") and dramatic or sudden exacerbations. The younger age at onset (6.3 + 2.7 years for tics and 7.4 + 2.7 years for OCD) and the male preponderance in PANDAS suggest that neurodevelopmental maturation of the basal ganglia at the time of exposure to GABHS, together with hormonal factors, modulates the phenotype of poststreptococcal disorders toward either chorea or tics and OCS. Interestingly, Murphy and Pichichero, through prospective PANDAS case identification and follow-up, showed that patients with the most recurrences of GABHS infection developed more prominent behavioral symptoms than other patients and that their OCD symptoms became more chronic and persistent (59). This finding is highly reminiscent of the observations of Asbahr et al. on the behavioral symptoms of patients with SC (36) and might be explained by more widespread immune-mediated damage of the basal ganglia following repeated infection. Murphy and Pichichero have also shown that the time lag between subsequent infections and symptom exacerbation becomes briefer, often less than a week. This finding has also been described in patients with SC and suggests that the exacerbations may be triggered by a secondary or recall immunologic response. The temporal association between a GABHS infection and onset of tics and OCD is essential for the definition of PANDAS (criterion 5). Unfortunately, confirming such an association in PANDAS is often as difficult as it is in SC, but for different reasons. In SC, the long latency between the throat infection and the onset of chorea increases the chances that GABHS will have cleared from the pharynges by the time of examination and that antistreptococcal antibody titers will have normalized. The clinical picture, the association with other rheumatic elements, and the response to antibiotics help confirm the diagnosis. In PANDAS, diagnosis requires that some exacerbations are associated with serologic evidence of recent streptococcal infection, such as positive antistreptococcal titers, a positive GABHS throat culture, or an episode of scarlet fever, within the month before presentation. However, because positive throat cultures in asymptomatic carriers and a positive single antistreptolysin O (ASO) or anti-DNAseB determination are quite common in the general population, the authors state that not only must rising titers coincide with symptom exacerbation, but falling titers must coincide with clinical remissions (57). Therefore, the difficulty of obtaining longitudinal laboratory data increases the chance of making an incorrect diagnosis of PANDAS. However, as in SC, not all exacerbations have to be associated with GABHS infections, and some recurrences can be triggered by other infectious or noninfectious immunologic responses. Swedo et al. propose a minimum of two exacerbations clearly related to GABHS infections in order to confirm the diagnosis, but this cut-off requires validation (57). A double-blind, crossover trial of penicillin prophylaxis in patients with PANDAS yielded inconclusive results because of failure in achieving adequate streptococcal prophylaxis in both arms of the study (60). Conversely, evidence from the 12 patients followed by Murphy and Pichichero suggests that rapid resolution of symptoms can be achieved with antibiotic treatment. The MRI findings documented previously in SC have been reproduced by Giedd et al. in the same cohort described by Swedo et al.; children with PANDAS were found to have larger caudate, putamen, and globus pallidus volumes than healthy children (61).

Although the comparison between PANDAS and SC reinforces the concept that PANDAS could be a distinct poststreptococcal disorder, at least two points of ambiguity exist in their clinical definitions. The first is represented by criterion 4, which refers to the presence of neurologic abnormalities during exacerbations. Even if such a criterion includes a very wide array of neurologic signs, the authors report moderate or minimal "choreiform movements" as the most common feature, specifying that none of these patients had "overt" chorea. Such terminology seems confusing and suggests that some of these patients might have an atypical form of SC (58). Moreover, these children were not screened for heart involvement (the second point of ambiguity) using sensitive methods (i.e., echocardiography). RF is known to be associated with a higher risk of developing neuropsychiatric disorders, especially OCD and tic disorders. Preliminary evidence shows echocardiographic abnormalities in a subgroup of patients with possible streptococcal-related tic disorder (62). Accurate cardiologic assessment should be introduced in the prospective follow-up of patients who fulfill the PANDAS criteria in order to better evaluate the degree of overlap between PANDAS and RF. Because of the rigidity of the working diagnostic criteria for PANDAS, identifying large cohorts of patients with this syndrome has been difficult; hence, few studies have been performed to confirm its autoimmune pathogenesis, and most have given preliminary and inconsistent results. Mittleman has found similarities in the cytokine profiles of patients with PANDAS, suggesting a possible role for cytokine dysregulation (63). As in SC, ABGA were also detected in PANDAS, and the targeted antigens corresponded to those identified in subjects with SC (i.e., those with molecular weights of 40, 45, or 60 kDa) (64). ABGA are therefore potentially good surrogate markers in poststreptococcal neurologic disorders. Another evidence for the autoimmune nature of PANDAS comes from a double-blind randomized trial of immunomodulatory therapies (65). This study compared PE with intravenous immunoglobulin (IVIG) and sham IVIG for treating tics and OCS in 29 children with PANDAS. Both treatments significantly improved emotional symptoms and global functioning. PE improved symptoms near the end of the first week of treatment, whereas the beneficial effect of IVIG was not usually seen before the third week of treatment; moreover, PE (the only treatment that fulfills criterion 3 for autoantibody-mediated pathophysiology shown in Table 23-1) produced greater symptom relief, especially with OCS.

IMPLICATIONS FOR THE PATHOGENESIS OF TOURETTE'S SYNDROME, OBSESSIVE–COMPULSIVE DISORDER, AND ATTENTION-DEFICIT HYPERACTIVITY DISORDER

The diagnoses of Tourette's syndrome and OCD fulfill the first diagnostic criterion of PANDAS (57). Streptococcal infections might, therefore, be relevant in a subgroup of patients with Tourette's syndrome (TS) or OCD. The etiology of these disorders is probably multifactorial, with a strong genetic component, but also involves several environmental factors, including infections, potentially altering the presentation and exacerbation of tics and OCS. Moreover, as in PANDAS, TS and OCD often present with comorbidity and exhibit a fluctuating temporal pattern. A direct relation between streptococcal infections and TS and OCD has been observed in several cross-sectional studies, which reported higher levels of antistreptococcal antibodies in patients with these conditions than in age-matched healthy or diseased controls (66–69). These findings, however, have not always been reproduced (70). Many studies report a higher incidence of ABGA in patients with chronic tic disorder, TS, and OCD. Most of these studies report that these antibodies bind to antigens with specific molecular weights, most frequently 40, 45, 60, 67, or 83 kDa (69,71–75). Evidence for the possible autoimmune nature of TS comes from recent experiments in rat models, in which a dose-related increase in stereotypies and vocalizations was observed after striatal infusion of serum or isolated IgG from patients with TS (76,77). Rat brain immunofluorescence revealed binding of human IgG to striatal neurons (76). A recent study, however, failed to reproduce these findings (78). Occasionally, a postinfectious Tourettism may be caused by other infectious agents (e.g., herpes simplex virus, varicella zoster virus, and human immunodeficiency virus), and notably, in these cases, ABGA were absent from both serum and CSF, suggesting the involvement of a predominantly cell-mediated immune response (79) and further confirming the possibility that a TS-like syndrome might have an infectious origin.

The relation between poststreptococcal autoimmunity and ADHD also deserves further investigation. Peterson et al. found a significant association between antibody titers and a DSM-IV diagnosis of ADHD (80). Moreover, higher antibody titers in patients with ADHD or OCD were associated with larger putamen and globus pallidus volumes, suggesting that recurrent GABHS infections might be associated with basal ganglia enlargement (80). In addition, sporadic cases of an ADHD-like syndrome, secondary to a GABHS infection (81) or a parainfectious viral encephalitic illness (79), have been recently reported.

POSTSTREPTOCOCCAL NEUROPSYCHIATRIC DISORDER: WIDENING THE SPECTRUM

Since the first description of PANDAS, the array of poststreptococcal neuropsychiatric disorders has been widened further to include new elements (82–86). A prospective study of 40 children from the United Kingdom, who presented with movement disorders following streptococcal pharyngitis, has been recently published (87). Streptococcal infection was defined by pharyngeal culture, streptococcal serology, or both. Their neurologic and psychiatric features are listed in Table 23-3. Points of major interest in the case series are the remarkable variety of the reported movement disorders and the associated behavioral features. Several factors may account for the different phenotypes of the *poststreptococcal neuropsychiatric disorders*, which include age at onset, sex, and family history of neuropsychiatric or motor disorders. Ninety-three percent of the patients with dyskinesia were found to be ABGA-positive using the methods described above, reinforcing the link between this wide clinical spectrum and ABGA (64).

Other well-defined postinfectious CNS diseases may present with inflammatory lesions of the basal ganglia. Because GABHS infections may contribute to the pathogenesis of some of these illnesses, including them within the spectrum of poststreptococcal neuropsychiatric disorders is tempting. In a report on 10 cases of poststreptococcal acute disseminated encephalomyelitis (ADEM), Dale et al. showed that this subtype exhibited a clinical phenotype that was different from classic ADEM and similar to other poststreptococcal disorders (88).

TABLE 23-3. *The extended spectrum of poststreptococcal neuropsychiatric disorders in 40 children*

Movement disorders: number of patients (%)		Psychiatric symptoms: number of patients (%)	
Chorea	20 (50%)	Aggressive, oppositional or disruptive behavior	14 (35%)
Vocal tics	17 (42.5%)		
Motor tics	16 (40%)	Emotional lability	13 (32.5%)
Dystonia	5 (12.5%)	Anxiety	11 (27.5%)
Tremor	3 (7.5%)	Obsessive–compulsive behavior	9 (22.5%)
Stereotypy	2 (5%)		
Opsoclonus	2 (5%)	Sleep disorders	9 (22.5%)
Myoclonus	1 (2.5%)	Depression	7 (17.5%)
Paroxysmal dystonic choreoathetosis	1 (2.5%)	Attention deficit	7 (17.5%)
		Echolalia	4 (10%)
		Visual hallucinations	2 (5%)
		Social disinterest	2 (5%)

Numbers are taken largely from a prospective study of 40 UK children presenting with movement disorders following streptococcal pharyngitis (see References 82–87 for details).
[From Dale RC, Heyman I, Surtees RAH, et al. Dyskinesias and associated psychiatric disorders following streptococcal infections. *Arch Dis Child* 2004 *(in press)*, with permission.]

Dystonia, behavioral symptoms, and a direct involvement of basal ganglia (demonstrated by MRI) were the predominant features. Similarly, an encephalitis lethargica (EL)-like syndrome might also be related to GABHS infections. Its clinical picture is characterized by sleep disorders, lethargy, parkinsonism, hyperkinesias (including tics), psychiatric symptoms, and eye movement abnormalities (i.e., external and internal ophthalmoplegia, nystagmus, and oculogyric crises). Psychiatric disease in EL comprises OCD, catatonia, mutism, apathy, and conduct disorders (see Fig. 23-2). Figure 23-2 shows an abnormal dopamine transporter (DAT) study using SPECT and an abnormal MRI study in a 47-year-old woman with EL. The patient presented with double vision and headache, followed by the rapid development of behavioral disorder. These symptoms were followed within hours by increasing confusion and reduced level of consciousness. She was admitted to the intensive care unit and was found to be hypersomnolent. During her admission, she notably exhibited oculogyric crises and persistent hiccuping. On recovering from the acute encephalitic illness, she developed parkinsonism, characterized by rigidity and bradykinesia, with superimposed tics and dystonic posturing of the right arm. In addition to the movement disorder, she developed a chronic psychiatric disorder characterized by obsessive–compulsive behavior, chronic anxiety, panic attacks, and dysthymia. The MRI study during the acute encephalitic crisis showed bilateral swelling of the striatum, with associated signal change on the T2- (left) and proton density-weighted images (center). These areas were shown to enhance diffusely after the administration of gadolinium (right). The abnormal signal change was also noted to extend into the posterior hypothalamus and midbrain (not shown). The DAT scan shows bilaterally reduced and asymmetric dopamine transporter density in the striatum. This patient's serum was positive for ABGA. A recent case series of 20 patients with an EL-like syndrome confirmed an association with previous upper respiratory tract infections and ABGA in the serum and CSF (89).

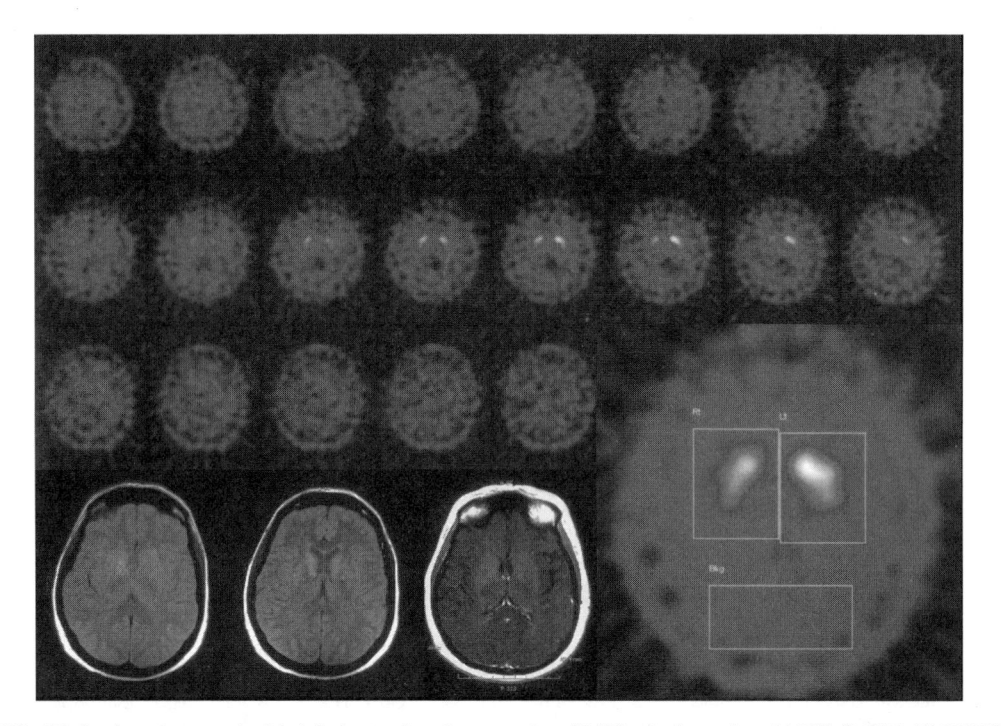

FIG. 23-2. An abnormal striatal dopamine transporter (DAT) study, using [123I] β-CIT ([123I]2β-carbomethoxy-3β-(4-iodophenyl)tropane) single photon emission computed tomography (SPECT) and an abnormal MRI study in a 47-year-old woman with encephalitis lethargica.

SYSTEMIC AUTOIMMUNE DISORDERS

Systemic autoimmune diseases involve the CNS with a highly variable spectrum of manifestations. The broadest spectrum of CNS manifestations is observed in systemic lupus erythematosus (SLE). As in other immune-mediated disorders, basal ganglia involvement in neuropsychiatric lupus (NPL) is typically expressed with a comorbid movement disorder (i.e., chorea, hemiballism, parkinsonism, and cranial–cervical dystonia) and behavioral features (90,91). Chorea has been described in association with many other systemic immune disorders, such as primary antiphospholipid syndrome (PAPS), autoimmune thyroiditis, rheumatoid arthritis, Sjögren's syndrome, Behçet's syndrome, Henoch–Schönlein syndrome, periarteritis nodosa, and Churg–Strauss syndrome (92). Parkinsonian signs occur very rarely in SLE or in other systemic immune disorders and can manifest in association with psychiatric features, which include mutism, depression, anorexia, memory disturbances, and psychosis (93). Overall, the exact degree of comorbidity of movement disorders and psychiatric impairment in NPL is unknown. Further investigations are warranted to identify a subgroup with predominant neuropsychiatric features and its underlying pathophysiology.

In SLE, autoimmunity against the CNS seems to be mainly caused by autoantibodies (94,95), although the contribution of a cell-mediated mechanism should be thoroughly assessed. NPL chorea has often been related to the presence of antiphospholipid antibodies (aPL) in the patients' sera. Whether aPL simply increase the risk for ischemic lesions, through their prothrombotic effect, or whether they also have a direct effect on neural cells is not clear. In more than one third of patients with NPL and with chorea, CT scan and MRI reveal cerebral infarcts of the striatum (96). On the other hand, a direct effect of aPL on neural cells has also been proposed. In this respect, during the acute phase of chorea different studies have notably reported striatal hypermetabolism associated with SLE or PAPS on fluorodeoxyglucose (FDG)-PET, similar to what is found in SC (97,98), although this result was not confirmed by other authors (99). Such a finding is clearly not compatible with a hypoxic-ischaemic process. *In vitro* and *in vivo* models have shown that aPL binds to neural cells of different brain areas, but direct binding to basal ganglia has not been reported (100). Other families of autoantibodies, and cell-mediated mechanisms, may be involved in basal ganglia dysfunction during systemic autoimmune diseases, but evidence in favor of a predominant mechanism is currently lacking.

Autoimmune mechanisms have been observed to influence the course of movement disorders linked to female sex hormones, such as chorea gravidarum (CG) and oral contraceptive–induced chorea. Patients with CG present with a sudden onset of chorea, generally in the course of an otherwise uncomplicated pregnancy (101). CG is generally considered to result from a combination of an underlying CNS disorder and the peculiar hormonal status during gestation (101). Among these underlying conditions, autoimmune causes play a primary role. CG more frequently manifests in women with a past history of SC (102–105) or an underlying SLE or PAPS (106–109). Interestingly, psychiatric symptoms, such as depression and psychosis, may precede the movement disorder, which, particularly in autoimmune subtypes of CG, occurs in the second or third trimester (101). Likewise, oral contraceptive–induced chorea has been hypothesized to be caused, at least in a subgroup of patients, by reactivation of SC (110–112) or by the development of other autoimmune disorders, such as SLE (96,113). In this respect, a recent case report described a 19-year old woman with oral contraceptive–induced chorea, who did not have a past history of SC but had ABGA in her serum (114). Some researchers have suggested that states characterized by high estrogen levels can cause hypersensitivity to dopamine by modifying postsynaptic dopamine receptors (115); further work is, nevertheless, needed to better understand the complex relation between estrogens, autoimmunity, and basal ganglia dysfunction.

PARANEOPLASTIC DISORDERS

Involvement of the basal ganglia occurs in only a few patients with a paraneoplastic syndrome of the CNS. These patients generally exhibit a movement disorder, typically chorea, parkinsonism, or dystonia, which is usually not associated with psychiatric comorbidity. The current view of paraneoplastic neurologic disorders is that most, if not all, of them are immune-mediated syndromes triggered by the expression of a constitutive CNS antigen by a peripheral tumor (14). Paraneoplastic chorea (PC) has always been considered extremely rare; nevertheless, the number of patients with chorea induced by an underlying, and often occult, neoplastic process has increased during the last 10 years, probably because of advancing knowledge about the pathophysiology of paraneoplastic syndromes. In most of the cases reported in the literature, chorea has been associated with lung cancer, usually a small cell lung carcinoma (SCLC) (116–122), and with presence of an antibody against a 66-kDa neuronal cytoplasmic protein, related to the collapsin response-mediator protein (CRMP-5) family, in the sera and CSF (119). PC is usually subacute in onset, often presents in the elderly, and is mostly accompanied by encephalopathy, visual loss, ataxia, polyneuropathy, abrupt loss of smell and taste, and limbic encephalitis. The latter presents with prominent psychiatric features and cognitive impairment. Basal ganglia alterations compatible with inflammation are often seen on MRI; they are transient and tend to revert after 3 to 4 months. Postmortem examination, reported in a few cases (118,121), reveals paraneoplastic inflammation of the basal ganglia, with marked neuronal loss, microglial activation, and perivascular lymphocytic infiltration, mainly by T lymphocytes. PC seems to improve after treating the underlying tumor and with immunotherapy (120).

Paraneoplastic dystonia and parkinsonism have been rarely associated with gynecologic tumors (particularly breast cancer), but in almost all of these cases, psychiatric comorbidity was absent, and pathologic findings revealed predominant involvement of the brainstem, with sparing of the basal ganglia, except the substantia nigra (116,123,124).

SUMMARY

Poststreptococcal disorders exhibit a remarkable comorbidity of neurologic and psychiatric features. A similar combination of symptoms is also described in other conditions, such as connective tissue or paraneoplastic disorders, albeit less frequently. A better understanding of the underlying mechanisms associated with autoaggressive immune-mediated attack on the basal ganglia is required. This understanding will ideally aid clinicians in diagnosing these conditions and lead to appropriate clinical trials, for example, of chemoprophylaxis strategies to prevent recurrent streptococcal infection and of the use of immunosuppressive treatments.

ACKNOWLEDGMENTS

We would like to acknowledge and thank the European Union for generously supporting Dr. Davide Martino through a Marie Curie Training Fellowship. We also thank the Tourette Syndrome Associations of the United Kingdom and United States for funding our research and Janet Alsop for her precious help in editing the manuscript.

REFERENCES

1. Ring HA, Serra-Mestres J. Neuropsychiatry of the basal ganglia. *J Neurol Neurosurg Psychiatry* 2002; 72(1):12–21.
2. Moore DP. Neuropsychiatric aspects of Sydenham's chorea: a comprehensive review. *J Clin Psychiatry* 1996; 57(9):407–414.
3. von Herrath MG, Harrison LC. Antigen-induced regulatory T cells in autoimmunity. *Nat Rev Immunol* 2003; 3(3):223–232.
4. Hartung HP, Toyka KV, Kieseier BC. Immune mechanisms in neurological disease. In: Asbury AK, McKhann GM, McDonald WI et al., eds. *Diseases of the nervous system*. 3rd ed, Vol. 2. Cambridge, UK: Cambridge University Press, 2002:1501–1526.
5. Salmi M, Jalkanen D. How do lymphocytes know where to go: current concepts and enigmas of lymphocyte homing. *Adv Immunol* 1997;64:139–218.
6. Nemazee DA, Burki K. Clonal deletion of B lymphocytes in a transgenic mouse bearing anti-MHC class I antibody genes. *Nature* 1989;337:562–565.
7. Rathmell JC, Thompson SE, Xu JC, et al. Expansion or elimination of B cell in vivo: dual roles for CD40- and Fas (CD95)-ligands modulated by the B cell antigen receptor. *Cell* 1996;87:319–329.
8. Goodnow CC, Crosbie J, Adelstein S, et al. Altered immunoglobulin expression and functional silencing of self-reactive B lymphocytes in transgenic mice. *Nature* 1988;334:676–682.
9. Van Parijs L, Abbers AK. Homeostasis and self-tolerance in the immune system: shutting lymphocytes off. *Science* 1998;280:243–248.
10. Pleister A, Eckels DD. Cryptic infection and autoimmunity. *Autoimmun Rev* 2003;2:126–132.

11. Brocke S, Hausmann S, Steinmann L, et al. Microbial peptides and superantigens in the pathogenesis of autoimmune diseases of the central nervous system. *Semin Immunol* 1998;10:57–67.
12. Karlsen AE, Dryberg T. Molecular mimicry between non-self, modified self and self autoimmunity. *Semin Immunol* 1998;10:25–34.
13. Marques-Dias MJ, Mercadante MT, Tucker D, et al. Sydenham's chorea. *Psychiatr Clin North Am* 1997;20(4):809–820.
14. Darnell RB, Posner JB. Paraneoplastic syndromes involving the nervous system. *N Engl J Med* 2003;349:1543–1554.
15. Archelos JJ, Hartung HP. Pathogenetic role of autoantibodies in neurological diseases. *Trend Neurosci* 2000;23:317–327.
16. Cunningham MW. Pathogenesis of group A streptococcal infections. *Clin Microbiol Rev* 2000;13:470–511.
17. Bisno AL, Brito MO, Collins CM. Molecular basis of group A streptococcal virulence. *Lancet Infect Dis* 2003;3:191–200.
18. Stollerman GH. Rheumatic fever in the 21st century. *Clin Infect Dis* 2001;33:806–814.
19. Smoot JC, Korgenski EK, Daly JA, et al. Molecular analysis of group A Streptococcus type emm18 isolates temporally associated with acute rheumatic fever outbreaks in Salt Lake City, Utah. *J Clin Microbiol* 2002;40:1805–1810.
20. Smoot JC, Barbian KD, Van Gompel JJ, et al. Genome sequence and comparative microarray analysis of serotype M18 group A Streptococcus strains associated with acute rheumatic fever outbreaks. *Proc Natl Acad Sci USA* 2002;99:4668–4673.
21. Olmez U, Turgay M, Ozenirler S, et al. Association of HLA class I and class II antigens with rheumatic fever in a Turkish population. *Scand J Rheumatol* 1993;22:49–52.
22. Hafez M, Chakravarti A, el-Shennawy F, et al. HLA antigens and acute rheumatic fever: evidence for a recessive susceptibility gene linked to HLA. *Genet Epidemiol* 1985;2:273–282.
23. Visentainer JE, Pereira FC, Dalalio MM, et al. Association of HLA-DR7 with rheumatic fever in the Brazilian population. *J Rheumatol* 2000;27:1518–1520.
24. Husby G, Van de Rijn I, Zabriskie JB, et al. Antibodies reacting with cytoplasm of subthalamic and caudate nuclei neurons in chorea and acute rheumatic fever. *J Exp Med* 1976;144:1094–1110.
25. Carapetis JR, Currie BJ, Mathews JD. Cumulative incidence of rheumatic fever in an endemic region: a guide to the susceptibility of the population? *Epidemiol Infect* 2000;124(2):239–244.
26. Nausieda PA, Grossman BJ, Koller WC, et al. Sydenham chorea: an update. *Neurology* 1983;30:331–334.
27. Cardoso F, Eduardo C, Silva AP, et al. Chorea in fifty consecutive patients with rheumatic fever. *Mov Disord* 1997;12:701–703.
28. Bleuler E, Brill AA. *Textbook of psychiatry*. New York: Arno Press, 1976.
29. Mercadante MT, Busatto GF, Lombroso PJ, et al. The psychiatric symptoms of rheumatic fever. *Am J Psychiatry* 2000;157:2036–2038.
30. Creak M, Guttmann E. Chorea, tics, compulsive utterances. *J Ment Sci* 1935;81:834–839.
31. Mercadante MT, Campos MC, Marques-Dias MJ, et al. Vocal tics in Sydenham's chorea. *J Am Acad Child Adolesc Psychiatry* 1997;36:305–306.
32. Swedo SE, Leonard HL, Schapiro MB, et al. Sydenham's chorea: physical and psychological symptoms of St Vitus dance. *Pediatrics* 1993;91(4):706–713.
33. Freeman JM, Aron AM, Collard JE, et al. The emotional correlates of Sydenham's chorea. *Pediatrics* 1965;35:42–49.
34. Aron AM, Freeman JM, Carter S. The natural history of Sydenham's chorea: review of literature and long-term evaluation with emphasis on cardiac sequelae. *Am J Med* 1965;38:83–95.
35. Swedo SE, Rapoport JL, Cheslow DL, et al. High prevalence of obsessive–compulsive symptoms in patients with Sydenham's chorea. *Am J Psychiatry* 1989;146:246–249.
36. Asbahr FR, Ramos RT, Negrao AB, et al. Case series: increased vulnerability to obsessive–compulsive symptoms with repeated episodes of Sydenham chorea. *J Am Acad Child Adolesc Psychiatry* 1999;38(12):1522–1525.
37. Diefendorf AR. Mental symptoms of acute chorea. *J Nerv Ment Dis* 1912;39:161–172.
38. Giedd JN, Rapoport JL, Kruesi MJ, et al. Sydenham's chorea: magnetic resonance imaging of the basal ganglia. *Neurology* 1995;45:2199–2202.
39. Castillo M, Kwock L, Arbelaez A. Sydenham's chorea: MRI and proton spectroscopy. *Neuroradiology* 1999;41:943–945.
40. Greenfield JG, Wolfsohn JM. The pathology of Sydenham's chorea. *Lancet* 1922;2:603–606.
41. Colony HS, Malamud N. Sydenham's chorea. A clinicopathologic study. *Neurology* 1956;6:672–676.
42. Kienzle GD, Breger RK, Chun RW, et al. Sydenham chorea: MR manifestations in two cases. *Am J Neuroradiol* 1991;12(1):73–76.
43. Ju TH, Kao KP, Chen CC. Sydenham chorea. *Am J Neuroradiol* 1993;14(5):1265.
44. Heye N, Jergas M, Hotzinger H, et al. Sydenham chorea: clinical, EEG, MRI and SPECT findings in the early stage of the disease. *J Neurol* 1993;240(2):121–123.
45. Emery ES, Vieco PT. Sydenham Chorea: magnetic resonance imaging reveals permanent basal ganglia injury. *Neurology* 1997;48(2):531–533.
46. Lee PH, Nam HS, Lee KY, et al. Serial brain SPECT images in a case of Sydenham chorea. *Arch Neurol* 1999;56(2):237–240.
47. Goldman S, Amrom D, Szoliwowski HB, et al. Reversible striatal hypermetabolism in a case of Sydenham's chorea. *Mov Disord* 1993;8:355–358.
48. Kotby AA, El Badawy N, El Sokkary S, et al. Antineuronal antibodies in rheumatic chorea. *Clin Diagn Lab Immunol* 1998;5:836–839.
49. Church AJ, Cardoso F, Dale RC, et al. Anti-basal ganglia antibodies in acute and persistent Sydenham's chorea. *Neurology* 2002;59:227–231.
50. Church AJ, Dale RC, Cardoso F, et al. CSF and serum immune parameters in Sydenham's chorea: evidence of an autoimmune syndrome? *J Neuroimmunol* 2003;136:149–153.
51. Singer HS, Loiselle CR, Lee O, et al. Anti-basal ganglia antibody abnormalities in Sydenham chorea. *J Neuroimmunol* 2003;136:154–161.
52. Loiselle CR, Singer HS. Genetics of childhood disorders: XXXI. Autoimmune disorders, part 4: is Sydenham chorea an autoimmune disorder? *J Am Acad Child Adolesc Psychiatry* 2001;40(10):1234–1236.
53. Garvey MA, Swedo SE, Shapiro MB, et al. Intravenous immunoglobulin and plasmapheresis as effective

treatments of Sydenham's chorea [Abstract]. *Neurology* 1996;46:A147.
54. Bronze MS, Dale JB. Epitopes of streptococcal M proteins that evoke antibodies that cross-react with human brain. *J Immunol* 1993;151:2820–2828.
55. Kirvan CA, Swedo SE, Heuser JS, et al. Mimicry and autoantibody-mediated neuronal cell signaling in Sydenham chorea. *Nat Med* 2003;9(7):914–920.
56. Kiessling LS, Marcotte AC, Culpepper L. Antineuronal antibodies in movement disorders. *Pediatrics* 1993;92:39–43.
57. Swedo SE, Leonard HL, Garvey M, et al. Pediatric autoimmune neuropsychiatric disorders associated with streptococcal infections: clinical description of the first 50 cases. *Am J Psychiatry* 1998;155(2):264–271.
58. Singer HS, Loiselle C. PANDAS: a commentary. *J Psychosom Res* 2003;55(1):31–39.
59. Murphy ML, Pichichero ME. Prospective identification and treatment of children with pediatric autoimmune neuropsychiatric disorder associated with group A streptococcal infection (PANDAS). *Arch Pediatr Adolesc Med* 2002;156(4):356–361.
60. Garvey MA, Perlmutter SJ, Allen AJ, et al. A pilot study of penicillin prophylaxis for neuropsychiatric exacerbations triggered by streptococcal infections. *Biol Psychiatry* 1999;45:1564–1571.
61. Giedd JN, Rapoport JL, Garvey MA, et al. MRI assessment of children with obsessive–compulsive disorder or tics associated with streptococcal infection. *Am J Psychiatry* 2000;157:281–283.
62. Cardona F, Romano A, Ventriglia, F, et al. Defining streptococcal-related tic disorders: contribution of echocardiography [Abstract]. *Eur Child Adolesc Psychiatry* 2003;12(Suppl. 2):I-29–I-30.
63. Mittleman BB. Cytokine networks in Sydenham's chorea and PANDAS. *Adv Exp Med Biol* 1997;418:933–935.
64. Church AJ, Dale RC, Giovannoni G. Anti-basal ganglia antibodies: a possible diagnostic utility in idiopathic movement disorders? *Arch Dis Child* 2004;89:611–614.
65. Perlmutter SJ, Leitman SF, Garvey MA, et al. Therapeutic plasma exchange and intravenous immunoglobulin for obsessive–compulsive disorder and tic disorders in childhood. *Lancet* 1999;354:1153–1158.
66. Muller N, Riedel M, Straube A, et al. Increased anti-streptococcal antibodies in patients with Tourette's syndrome. *Psychiatry Res* 2000;94:43–49.
67. Muller N, Kroll B, Schwarz MJ, et al. Increased titers of antibodies against streptococcal M12 and M19 proteins in patients with Tourette's syndrome. *Psychiatry Res* 2001;101:187–193.
68. Cardona F, Orefici G. Group A streptococcal infections and tic disorders in an Italian pediatric population. *J Pediatr* 2001;138:71–75.
69. Church AJ, Dale RC, Lees AJ, et al. Tourette's syndrome: a cross sectional study to examine the PANDAS hypothesis. *J Neurol Neurosurg Psychiatry* 2003;74(5):602–607.
70. Loiselle CR, Wendlandt JT, Rohde CA, et al. Anti-streptococcal, neuronal, and nuclear antibodies in Tourette syndrome. *Pediatr Neurol* 2003;28:119–125.
71. Singer HS, Giuliano JD, Hansen BH, et al. Antibodies against human putamen in children with Tourette syndrome. *Neurology* 1998;50:1618–1624.
72. Trifiletti RR, Bandele AN. Antibodies to the calpain-calpastatin complex in patients with tics, Tourette syndrome, or obsessive–compulsive disorder [Abstract]. *Ann Neurol* 2000;48:542.
73. Wendlandt JT, Grus FH, Hansen BH, et al. Striatal antibodies in children with Tourette's syndrome: multivariate discriminant analysis of IgG repertoires. *J Neuroimmunol* 2001;119:106–113.
74. Hoekstra PJ, Horst G, Limburg PC, et al. Increased seroreactivity in tic disorder patients to a 60 kDa protein band from a neuronal cell line. *J Neuroimmunol* 2003;141:118–124.
75. Dale RC, Church AJ, Giovannoni G, et al. Obsessive–compulsive disorder: cross-sectional study for recent streptococcal infection and anti-basal ganglia antibodies [Abstract]. *Eur Child Adolesc Psychiatry* 2003; 12(Suppl. 2):I/24.
76. Hallett JJ, Harling-Berg CJ, Knopf PM, et al. Antistriatal antibodies in Tourette syndrome cause neuronal dysfunction. *J Neuroimmunol* 2000;111:195–202.
77. Taylor JR, Morshed SA, Parveen S, et al. An animal model of Tourette's syndrome. *Am J Psychiatry* 2002; 159:657–660.
78. Loiselle CR, Lee O, Moran TH, et al. Striatal microinfusion of Tourette syndrome and PANDAS sera: failure to induce behavioral changes. *Mov Disord* 2004;19:390–396.
79. Dale RC, Church AJ, Heyman I. Striatal encephalitis after varicella zoster infection complicated by Tourettism. *Mov Disord* 2003;18:1554–1556.
80. Peterson BS, Leckman JF, Tucker D, et al. Preliminary findings of antistreptococcal antibody titers and basal ganglia volumes in tic, obsessive–compulsive, and attention deficit/hyperactivity disorders. *Arch Gen Psychiatry* 2000;57:364–372.
81. Waldrep DA. Two cases of ADHD following GABHS infection: a PANDAS subgroup? *J Am Acad Child Adolesc Psychiatry* 2002;41:1273–1274.
82. Dale RC, Heyman I, Surtees RAH, et al. Dyskinesias and associated psychiatric disorders following streptococcal infections. *Arch Dis Child* 2004;89:604–610.
83. Dale RC, Church AJ, Benton S, et al. Post-streptococcal autoimmune dystonia with isolated bilateral striatal necrosis. *Dev Med Child Neurol* 2002;44:485–489.
84. DiFazio MP, Morales J, Davis R. Acute myoclonus secondary to group A beta-hemolytic streptococcus infection: a PANDAS variant. *J Child Neurol* 1998;13:516–518.
85. Martinelli P, Ambrosetto G, Minguzzi E, et al. Late-onset PANDAS syndrome with abdominal muscle involvement. *Eur Neurol* 2002;48:49–51.
86. Smyth P, Sinclair DB. Multifocal myoclonus following group A streptococcal infection. *J Child Neurol* 2003; 18:434–436.
87. Dale RC, Church AJ, Surtees RAH, et al. Post-streptococcal autoimmune neuropsychiatric disease presenting as paroxysmal dystonic choreoathetosis. *Mov Disord* 2002;17:817–820.
88. Dale RC, Church AJ, Cardoso F, et al. Poststreptococcal acute disseminated encephalomyelitis with basal ganglia involvement and auto-reactive antibasal ganglia antibodies. *Ann Neurol* 2001;50:588–595.
89. Dale RC, Church AJ, Surtees RAH, et al. Encephalitis lethargica syndrome: 20 new cases and evidence

of basal ganglia autoimmunity. *Brain* 2003;127: 21–33.
90. Jennekens FGI, Kater L. The central nervous system in systemic lupus erythematosus. Part 1. Clinical syndromes: a literature investigation. *Rheumatology* 2002; 41:605–618.
91. Cervera R, Munther A, Khamashta MA, et al. Systemic lupus erythematosus: clinical and immunologic patterns of disease expression in a cohort of 1000 patients. *Medicine* 1993;72:113–124.
92. Valldeoriola F. Movement disorders of autoimmune origin. *J Neurol* 1999;246:423–431.
93. Garcia-Moreno JM, Chacon J. Juvenile parkinsonism as a manifestation of systemic lupus erythematosus: case report and review of the literature. *Mov Disord* 2002;17:1329–1335.
94. Jennekens FGI, Kater L. The central nervous system in systemic lupus erythematosus. Part 2. Pathogenetic mechanisms of clinical syndromes: a literature investigation. *Rheumatology* 2002;41:619–630.
95. Arbuckle MR, McClain MT, Rubertone MV, et al. Development of autoantibodies before the clinical onset of systemic lupus erythematosus. *N Engl J Med* 2003;349:1526–1533.
96. Cervera R, Asherson RA, Font J, et al. Chorea in the antiphospholipid syndrome. Clinical, radiologic, and immunologic characteristics of 50 patients from our clinics and the recent literature. *Medicine* 1997;76:203–212.
97. Furie R, Ishikawa T, Dhawan V, et al. Alternating hemichorea in primary antiphospholipid syndrome: evidence for contralateral striatal hypermetabolism. *Neurology* 1994;44:2197–2199.
98. Sunden-Cullberg J, Tedroff J, Aquilonius SM. Reversible chorea in primary antiphospholipid syndrome. *Mov Disord* 1998;13:147–149.
99. Guttman M, Lang AE, Garnett ES, et al. Regional cerebral glucose metabolism in SLE chorea: further evidence that striatal hypometabolism is not a correlate of chorea. *Mov Disord* 1987;2:201–210.
100. Chapman J, Cohen-Armon M, Shoenfeld Y, et al. Antiphospholipid antibodies permeabilize and depolarize brain synaptoneurosomes. *Lupus* 1999;8:127–133.
101. Golbe LI. Pregnancy and movement disorders. *Neurol Clin* 1994;12(3):497–508.
102. Wilson P, Preece AA. Chorea gravidarum. *Arch Int Med* 1932;471:671–697.
103. Lewis BV, Parsons M. Chorea gravidarum. *Lancet* 1966; 1:284–286.
104. Zegart KN, Schwartz RH. Chorea gravidarum. *Obstet Gynecol* 1968;32:24–27.
105. Cardoso F. Chorea gravidarum. *Arch Neurol* 2002;59: 868–870.
106. Donaldson IM, Espiner EA. Disseminated lupus erythematosus presenting as chorea gravidarum. *Arch Neurol* 1971;25:240–244.

107. Ichikawa K, Kim RC, Givelber H, et al. Chorea gravidarum—report of a fatal case with neuropathological observations. *Arch Neurol* 1980;37:429–432.
108. Lubbe WF, Walker EB. Chorea gravidarum associated with lupus anticoagulant—successful outcome of pregnancy with prednisone and aspirin therapy. Case report. *Br J Obstet Gynaecol* 1983;90:487–490.
109. Lubbe WF, Butler WS, Palmer SJ, et al. Lupus anticoagulant in pregnancy. *Br J Obstet Gynaecol* 1984;91: 357–363.
110. Nausieda P, Koller W, Weiner W, et al. Chorea induced by oral contraceptives. *Neurology* 1979;29:1605–1609.
111. Dove DJ. Chorea associated with oral contraceptives. *Am J Obstet Gynecol* 1980;137:740–742.
112. Greene PM. Chorea induced by oral contraceptives. *Neurology* 1980;30:11.
113. Mathur AK, Gatter RA. Chorea as the initial manifestation of oral contraceptives induced lupus erythematosus. *J Rheumatol* 1988;6:1042–1043.
114. Miranda M, Cardoso F, Giovannoni G, et al. Oral contraceptive induced chorea: another condition associated with anti-basal ganglia antibodies. *J Neurol Neurosurg Psychiatry* 2004;75:327–328.
115. Nausieda PA, Koller WC, Weiner WJ, et al. Modification of postsynaptic dopaminergic sensitivity for female sex hormones. *Life Sci* 1979;25:521–526.
116. Albin RL, Bromberg MB, Penney JB, et al. Chorea and dystonia: a remote effect of carcinoma. *Mov Disord* 1988;3:162–169.
117. Heckmann JG, Lang CJ, Druschky A, et al. Chorea resulting from paraneoplastic encephalitis. *Mov Disord* 1997;12:464–466.
118. Tani T, Piao Y, Mori S, et al. Chorea resulting from paraneoplastic striatal encephalitis. *J Neurol Neurosurg Psychiatry* 2000;69:512–515.
119. Yu Z, Kryzer TJ, Griesmann GE, et al. CRMP-5 neuronal autoantibody: marker of lung cancer and thymoma-related autoimmunity. *Ann Neurol* 2001;49:146–154.
120. Vernino S, Tuite P, Adler CH, et al. Paraneoplastic chorea associated with CRMP-5 neuronal antibody and lung carcinoma. *Ann Neurol* 2002;51:625–630.
121. Tremont-Lukats IW, Fuller GN, Ribalta T, et al. Paraneoplastic chorea: case study with autopsy confirmation. *Neuro-oncol* 2002;4:192–195.
122. Kinirons P, Fulton A, Keoghan M, et al. Paraneoplastic limbic encephalitis (PLE) and chorea associated with CRMP-5 neuronal antibody. *Neurology* 2003;61: 1623–1624.
123. Pittock SJ, Lucchinetti CF, Lennon VA. Anti-neuronal nuclear antibody type 2: paraneoplastic accompaniments. *Ann Neurol* 2003;53:580–587.
124. Fahn S, Brin MF, Dwork AJ, et al. Case 1, 1996: rapidly progressive parkinsonism, incontinence, impotency, and levodopa-induced moaning in a patient with multiple myeloma. *Mov Disord* 1996;11:298–310.

24
Psychopathological and Cognitive Correlates of Tardive Dyskinesia in Patients Treated with Neuroleptics

Ikwunga Wonodi,[1] L. Elliot Hong,[2] and Gunvant K. Thaker[2]

[1]Maryland Psychiatric Research Center, Motor Disorders Clinic,
University of Maryland School of Medicine, Baltimore, Maryland;
[2]Department of Psychiatry, Maryland Psychiatric Research Center,
University of Maryland School of Medicine, Baltimore, Maryland

Tardive dyskinesia (TD) is a neurologic syndrome consisting of abnormal involuntary movements of the tongue, mouth, face, trunk, and extremities that affects 20% to 40% or more of patients treated chronically with neuroleptic drugs (1–3) and is recognized as one of the most debilitating adverse effects of treatment with these agents (4–6). Oral-facial movements are found in most patients with TD and may include lip smacking, puckering, sucking movements, vermiform and lateral tongue movements, facial pouting, grimacing, and lateral jaw movements. Other movements include slow writhing movements of the trunk; irregular limb movements, especially choreoathetoid movements of the fingers and toes; and lordotic posturing. In severe cases, the diaphragmatic, esophageal, and pelvic muscles may be involved, resulting in grunting (glottal dyskinesia) and breathing difficulties; problems with swallowing, including risk for aspiration; and thrusting pelvic movements; respectively (7). The dyskinetic movements are usually worsened by emotional arousal and are typically absent during sleep. Patients may attempt to suppress some of the involuntary movements for varied periods and may even incorporate them into volitional movements. Commonly, the patient is either not aware of the involuntary movements of TD or does not present with subjective complaints of involuntary movements, except in severe cases (8). The topography of the observed involuntary movements has been used to characterize the syndrome into two subtypes: orofacial dyskinesia and limb-trunkal dyskinesia. Evidence suggests that these two subtypes may be pathophysiologically distinct (9,10).

The wide variation in the reported prevalence of TD, which ranges from 2% to 65%, can be attributed to the varied definitions of TD, the use of different assessment methods, and the lack of control of predictor variables (11,12). TD, in its severest form, interferes with purposeful activities, speech, and respiration and can result in secondary injuries (e.g., bruises, lip ulceration, dental damage, and joint inflammation), which impede socialization (6). Most cases of TD are mild and display temporal fluctuations over time (13).

The serendipitous discovery of the psychotropic properties of chlorpromazine (14) was a historic event in medicine and marked a revolutionary change in the pharmacologic treatment of psychiatric disorders. Five years after chlorpromazine was introduced as a neuroleptic agent (15), the first report of TD was published. It described three elderly women who developed lip-smacking dyskinetic movements 2 to 8 weeks after initiation of chlorpromazine treatment. Shortly after this report, Kruse (16) published the first report of TD in the American literature (16). Subsequently, this hitherto unknown medication-induced adverse effect was increasingly observed in children and adults (17–20). Early observations of TD stressed its potential irreversibility (21). However, it is now known that many mild to moderately severe cases can improve if chlorpromazine is withdrawn. The clinical conundrum in managing TD is that most patients who develop TD require continued treatment with antipsychotic medications. However, most cases of TD are mild and are not necessarily progressive, even with continued exposure to antipsychotics (22).

The reported incidence of TD in patients treated with neuroleptics is 5% per treatment year for the first 5 years (1), and the cumulative 5-year incidence rate is 20% to 26% (1,2,23). Several risk factors for developing TD have been consistently identified, including advanced age, cumulative exposure to neuroleptic drugs, intermittent exposure to antipsychotics, a diagnosis of an affective disorder, female sex, and being of black ancestry (2,5,24–30), though the risk of female sex seems to be related to age and estrogen levels rather than to a specific effect of sex. Other risk factors include a history of alcohol abuse or dependence, diabetes mellitus, extrapyramidal syndrome, and structural brain abnormalities (31–37). With the advent of the new generation of antipsychotic agents, which are less liable to induce involuntary movements, TD is likely to be less of a public health issue in the future (38). However, the prevalence of TD continues to increase, even in patients treated with atypical antipsychotic agents who may have had prior treatment with typical antipsychotic drugs (39).

NEUROLEPTICS, ANTIPSYCHOTIC AGENTS, AND ATYPICALITY

The term *neuroleptic* was coined following the introduction of the new drug chlorpromazine by Delay, Deniker, and Harl (14) as a treatment for patients with chronic schizophrenia (14). Chlorpromazine effectively reduced delusions, hallucinations, and excitement and was described as inducing tranquilization in hospitalized patients without producing the severe treatment-related depression associated with reserpinelike drugs that was the mainstay of antipsychotic treatment at the time (40,41). This quality was ascribed to the drug's ability to reduce rather than paralyze nerve activity. Subsequently, other members of what was later called the classic neuroleptic family were developed and introduced into the psychopharmacologic armamentarium, including phenothiazines (e.g., fluphenazine, perphenazine, and thioridazine), butyrophenones (e.g., haloperidol and pimozide), and thioxanthines (e.g., thiothixene). These agents differed in their potency and adverse effects—the most common and bothersome of which were the extrapyramidal side effects (EPS). However, they all shared similar efficacy.

Current antipsychotic treatment of psychotic disorders is based on antidopaminergic agents. Nevertheless, manipulation of dopamine transmission alone fails to alleviate some positive and most negative symptoms completely and has minimal effect on preexisting cognitive impairment. Atypical antipsychotic agents that manipulate D_1/D_2 and 5HT2 receptors offer little advantage over the older generation antipsychotics for treating positive and primary negative symptoms. The newer agents may have an advantage, however, in ameliorating depression and hostility and in reducing rates of suicide, hospital readmission, and motor side effects, because their improved tolerability—they do not cause EPS or related motor dysphoric effects—can increase adherence to treatment. Unfortunately, the atypical antipsychotics are associated with serious side effects, including weight gain, cardiac conductivity problems, increased cardiovascular stress, and risk of diabetes.

PATHOPHYSIOLOGY OF TARDIVE DYSKINESIA

Theories on the Pathophysiology of Tardive Dyskinesia

Several theories on the etiopathophysiology of TD have been advanced to better comprehend the nature of the disorder and to guide treatment interventions in patients with this disabling neurologic condition. Abnormalities in several neurotransmitter pathways have been implicated in the pathophysiology of TD including dopamine, γ-aminobutyric acid (GABA), acetylcholine, serotonin, norepinephrine, and the opiod enkephalin (ENK).

Dopamine Supersensitivity Hypothesis

Klawans and Rubovits (42) first proposed the hypothesis implicating striatal dopamine supersensitivity in the pathogenesis of TD in 1970, on the basis of observed similarities between L-dopa–induced dyskinesia (LID) and TD. The theory stated that prolonged blockade of striatal dopamine receptors induced supersensitivity of these receptors analogous to the denervation-induced supersensitivity observed in peripheral muscles. The supporting evidence for this hypothesis is predominantly pharmacologic: dopamine antagonists (e.g., haloperidol) and dopamine depleters (e.g., reserpine) ameliorate dyskinesia; dopamine agonists exacerbate dyskinesia (as in LID); and withdrawal of conventional antipsychotics *unmasks* supersensitive dopamine receptors and temporarily exacerbates dyskinesia (*withdrawal dyskinesia*). Cholinergic stimulation, thought to oppose dopaminergic signaling in the basal ganglia, reduces dyskinesia in some patients.

Dopamine supersensitivity alone cannot account for the pathophysiology of TD. Pharmacologic studies provide evidence that dopamine receptor supersensitivity occurs early (by 2 to 3 weeks) in the course of treatment with antipsychotics and in tandem with the synaptic phenomenon of depolarization blockade. However, TD is a chronic adverse event that manifests in months to years. All rats and humans who receive chronic treatment with conventional antipsychotics develop dopamine receptor supersensitivity in dopamine terminal brain areas, but not all of the humans express TD, nor do the rats express what is considered to be an animal analog of TD, that is, vacuous chewing movements (VCM). Furthermore, at least one neuroreceptor imaging study showed no difference in D_2 receptor binding between equally treated patients with and without TD (43), and no differences have been demonstrated in levels of dopamine metabolites in the cerebrospinal fluid (CSF) (44). Postmortem brain tissue analyses in equally antipsychotic-exposed patients do not reveal more striatal dopamine receptors in patients with schizophrenia who had TD than in patients without TD (45). Finally, dopamine receptor supersensitivity occurs acutely to subacutely when dopamine antagonist treatment is initiated and reverses within a few weeks after the medication is discontinued, whereas TD occurs after chronic exposure and persists for months to years. The current revision to the dopamine supersensitivity hypothesis suggests that although dopamine supersensitivity might not lead to TD, it might be a necessary first step in the pathophysiologic process that eventually results in medication-induced dyskinesias. This revision of the supersensitivity hypothesis has gained strong support from research showing that clozapine, a medication not known to cause TD, does not induce the dopamine supersensitivity found with conventional antipsychotics.

GABA Dysfunction Hypothesis

A modification to the dopamine supersensitivity hypothesis, which implicates GABA dysfunction, was introduced to incorporate the deficiencies of the dopamine theory (6,46–48). Normally, transient and controlled inhibition of neurons in the substantia nigra pars reticulata (SNr) results in a pause in the tonic inhibition of the projection regions, thereby enabling normal body or saccadic eye movements (49,50). The GABA hypothesis of TD suggests that abnormal basal ganglia function arising from diminished GABAergic–enkephalinergic transmission results in an imbalance between the direct and indirect striatal output pathways, whereby inhibitory stimulation to the thalamus decreases overall, leading to increased activity of the excitatory glutamatergic thalamocortical pathway and, ultimately, increased neuronal activity in the premotor—motor–supplementary motor cortex, resulting in dyskinesia (51–53).

Additional neurophysiologic evidence that implicates GABA hypofunction was found in data obtained from oculomotor studies: patients with schizophrenia and TD showed a twofold increase in abnormal saccadic eye movements when compared with a group of patients without TD, and these saccadic abnormalities predicted which patients with TD would display improvement in dyskinetic movements when treated with GABA agonists (54,55). Furthermore, saccadic abnormalities in patients with TD persist even after TD symptoms improve following discontinuation of the offending conventional antipsychotic drug (56). On the basis of this evidence, our group has proposed that hypofunction in the GABAergic efferent neurons of the SNr occurs as a consequence of chronic neuroleptic treatment and that this step is also essential in the development of TD.

Enkephalin Modulation of GABAergic Function

The opiod peptide ENK coexists with GABA in the projection neurons of the striatum, forming an "indirect" pathway, which is implicated in the pathophysiology of dyskinesia. Within the basal ganglia, ENK is integral to the dopamine D_2 receptor–containing indirect pathway, which inhibits the projection neurons in the globus pallidus externa (GPe) and excites those in the SNr. Experimental evidence suggests a functional negative interaction of ENK cotransmission in GABAergic striatal efferents to the globus pallidus (57,58). An increase in ENK activity in pathologic conditions results in disinhibition of projection regions, resulting in VCM in laboratory animals or dyskinesia in humans. This evidence is supported by findings that repeated administration of ENK in rat striatum produces abnormal movements (59,60). Chronic treatment with antipsychotic agents results in increased ENK activity; interestingly, such increases occur in only those rats that develop VCM (61).

The therapeutic role of ENK antagonism in dyskinesia is suggested by laboratory findings that it dramatically reduces chronic neuroleptic–induced VCM (60), and modulating ENK activity by antagonizing glutamatergic N-methyl-D-aspartate (NMDA) transmission may hold promise in treatment of dyskinesias (62,63). Clinical trials have been carried out using opiate antagonists to treat TD and LID, with poor results (64,65). We have used a combination of a GABA mimetic drug and an ENK antagonist to treat neuroleptic-induced dyskinesia, with encouraging results that provide the first evidence that this strategy is effective (30).

Oxidative Stress, Free Radicals, and Tardive Dyskinesia

Several reports implicate striatal neurotoxicity, arising from damage by free radicals, in the pathogenesis of TD (66–69). Prolonged dopamine receptor blockade by antipsychotic medications is hypothesized to cause secondary damage by increasing dopamine turnover and metabolism, which leads to the formation of free radicals (67,70,71). Dopamine is metabolized by membrane-bound monoamine oxidase (MAO) to dihydrophenylacetic acid and subsequently to homovanillic acid (HVA). Further oxidation by MAO produces hydrogen peroxide, which forms free radicals. Convergent with this process, blockade of D_2 receptors also increases the synaptic release of aspartate and glutamate in the striatum, leading to oxidative damage caused by activation of glutamatergic transmission (72,73). The increased oxidative stress and generation of free radicals from these reactions damage cellular proteins, lipid membranes, and other cellular constituents and cause cumulative damage to neurons. This hypothesis has formed the basis of the attempts to prevent or treat TD with antioxidant medications that act as free radical scavengers, such as vitamin E and prostaglandin, though the results have been mixed (74–79).

Phenylalanine and Tardive Dyskinesia

Phenylalanine is a large neutral amino acid that acts as a precursor to tyrosine. Abnormality in the metabolism of phenylalanine may be associated with TD, particularly in men. Male patients with TD show an increased availability of phenylalanine in the brain in response to high protein or oral phenylalanine challenge (80). The greater availability of phenylalanine is likely to increase dopamine synthesis or may have direct neurotoxic effect. The role of phenylalanine in TD is further supported by the finding that administration of branched chain amino acids results in a considerable decrease in TD (80).

NEUROBEHAVIORAL CORRELATES OF TARDIVE DYSKINESIA

Considerable evidence supports the role of the basal ganglia and the cortico–striato–pallido–nigro–thalamocortical tract in both motor and cognitive function (52,81,82). Five frontosubcortical circuits connect regions of the frontal lobe (i.e., dorsolateral prefrontal, orbitofrontal, anterior cingulate cortex, supplementary motor area, and the frontal eye fields) with the striatum, globus pallidus, and thalamus in a functional network that mediates volitional motor activity, saccadic eye movements, emotion, motivation, cognition, and social behavior (see Fig. 24-1) (81,83). Alexander et al. (81,84) further proposed that these frontal–striatal–thalamic circuits are anatomically segregated. For example, they hypothesize a relatively pure motor circuit that maintains somatotopic organization throughout the loop, terminating in the supplementary motor area (81,84). Furthermore, they describe oculomotor, dorsolateral prefrontal, lateral orbitofrontal, and anterior cingulate loops. Though they propose a network that would explain pure motor dysfunction, pathophysiologic processes that affect one system (e.g., chronic dopamine receptor blockade with consequent changes in neighboring structures), might potentially also disrupt the dorsolateral and orbitofrontal circuits and might be expected to result in substantial consequences to higher cognitive processes.

In patients with Parkinson's disease, brain pathology is not confined to the nigrostriatal dopaminergic system but also involves the mesocortical and mesolimbic pathways described above, causing substantial impairment in cognitive functions and emotion (85–87). Extrapolating from this observation, investigators have posited that TD may also result in complex aberrations in this neuronal circuit, causing disturbances of perception, mood, cognition, and volitional movements.

TARDIVE DYSKINESIA IN THE SCHIZOPHRENIA SPECTRUM

Although the bulk of TD literature originates from patient populations that have schizophrenia,

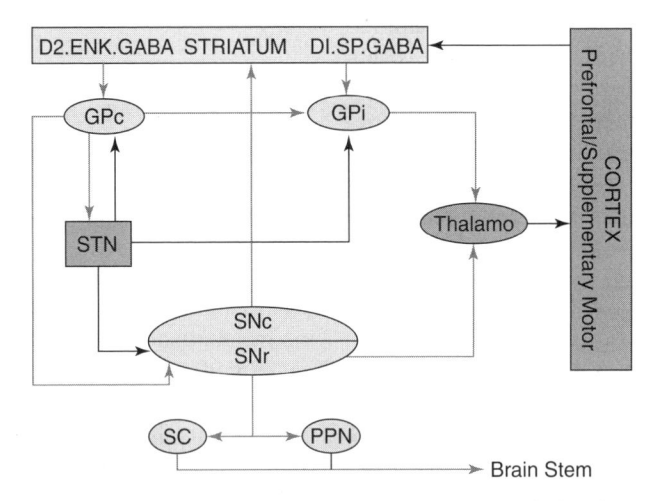

FIG. 24-1. Model of the cortico–striato–pallido–thalamocortical circuit that loops through the basal ganglia. The loop is involved in the generation and control of motor behavior and several cognitive functions. The inhibitory GABAergic (Grey broken line) pathways are shown with the excitatory glutamatergic (Black line) pathways. The inhibitory indirect pathways is illustrated as originating from D2 receptor or enkephalinergic or GABAergic expressing striatal spiny neurons to relay in the globus pallidus externa (GPe) and subsequently project to the subthalamic nucleus (STN) and the substantia nigra pars reticulata (SNr). The main output nuclei of the basal ganglia, the GPi and the SNr, are illustrated. SC, superior colliculus; PPN, pedinculopontine nucleus; SNc, substantia nigra pars compacta; Gpi, globus pallidus interna; SP, substance P; ENK, enkephalin.

the occurrence of TD is well described in all disorders for which antipsychotic medications are clinically indicated or symptomatically effective, including schizophrenia, psychotic affective disorders (PAD) (unipolar and bipolar), mental retardation, pervasive developmental disorders, neurodegenerative disorders, and gastrointestinal or labyrinthine dysfunction (88,89). Indeed, TD occurs in patients inappropriately treated with chronic neuroleptic therapy.

Schizophrenia, Tardive Dyskinesia, and Psychopathology

Though the syndrome of TD in schizophrenia is widely believed to be a consequence of prolonged exposure to dopamine-blocking medications, descriptions of choreiform and orofacial dyskinesias in patients with schizophrenia predate the introduction of antipsychotic medications (90–92). Reports of prevalence rates of 15% to 23% of spontaneous dyskinesia and dyskinetic-like movements among patients with chronic schizophrenia who have never been treated with antipsychotics have suggested that the motor disorder and the schizophrenia disease process are intrinsically related (93–95). Interestingly, individuals with schizophrenia-spectrum personality disorder (i.e., schizotypal, schizoid, and paranoid personality disorders), a disorder defined by its phenomenological and, perhaps, genetic relatedness to schizophrenia but lacking the confounding effects of florid psychosis, history of neuroleptic exposure or institutionalization, and medical comorbidity, also have a higher prevalence of spontaneous dyskinesia than healthy controls (96).

No consistent pattern of TD vulnerability has been found in patients with schizophrenia who have anxiety or depressive symptoms. However, some investigators have posited that patients with schizophrenia and TD are more vulnerable to display nonspecific "activation or affectivity" symptoms, such as tension, excitability, hostility, mannerisms, and posturing, interspersed with periods of apathy (97–100), which may become more pronounced upon withdrawal of neuroleptics (101), a syndrome called *tardive dysmentia*.

The phenomenon of lack of awareness of abnormal movements in schizophrenia closely parallels the lack of insight these patients have about their illness, although lack of awareness also commonly occurs in patients with abnormal movements (e.g., patients with Parkinson's or Huntington's disease) who are not schizophrenic. Furthermore, patients with psychiatric disorders, such as bipolar affective psychosis, seem to be more aware of their neuroleptic-induced movements than patients with schizophrenia (8,102). Investigators (8,103) have argued that this lack of awareness of TD and lack of insight into illness are aspects of the same neuronal dysfunction. Further evaluation of patients with schizophrenia with the "deficit syndrome" (104) reveals a considerably reduced awareness of TD than in patients without the syndrome (8,102). This finding of lack of awareness or denial of TD by patients is important in treating the disorder. Increased training of clinicians in recognizing and documenting dyskinesia would translate into more effective clinical care through the identification of at-risk patients, early detection of involuntary movements, and the institution of therapeutic measures (105).

Cognitive Dysfunction and Tardive Dyskinesia

Well-documented evidence suggests that organic or developmental brain pathology is a risk factor for TD (106,107). Cognitive dysfunction is considered to be at the core of the pathophysiology of schizophrenia (108,109) and is believed to result from frontal lobe pathology (110–112). Psychopharmacological studies suggest that the basal ganglia are sites of action for antipsychotics (113–115). The correlation between cognitive dysfunction and TD has been a topic of active debate among researchers of schizophrenia (116). There is a wealth of information on the high prevalence of TD in patients with cognitive impairments. The association of cognitive impairments with TD has substantially favored patients with schizophrenia who display deficits in global measures of cognitive status such as the Mini-Mental Status Examination (MMSE) (117,118). However, many of the patients in these studies were severely demented or were mute (119). Additionally, no specific or localizing cognitive deficits were reported in these patients, most of whom were from cohorts of elderly and chronically ill patient populations. Other neuropsychological measures of impairment used in these early studies include the Paired Associate Learning Test, Wechsler Adult Intelligence Scale, and the Ray-Auditory Verbal Learning Test (120,121). In contrast, other studies have failed to find an association between TD and cognitive impairments in older patient populations (121–123). Interestingly, at least one prospective study of patients with mixed psychiatric diagnoses observed that patients who later developed TD demonstrated poorer premorbid performance than other patients on a test of reasoning ability (124).

The findings that clinical correlates and associations with particular symptom domains differ between orofacial and limb-trunkal TD suggest that these two TD subtypes may be pathophysiologically distinct (10,125). More detailed studies now note a correlation between TD with orofacial topography and cognitive impairments (88,89,126). Myslobodsky (127) noted impaired performance on recall tasks but not on the recognition tasks by patients with TD, compared with patients without TD, which was in accord with findings in patients with basal ganglia disorders. Another study observed that poor procedural learning correlated with both TD severity (128) and imaging abnormalities in the caudate nuclei, further implicating basal ganglia pathology.

Pantelis et al. have previously concurred with the body of evidence suggesting that frontal–striatal–thalamic circuits are disrupted in schizophrenia, that deficits in executive function (including some memory functions) result from disruption of these neural networks (129–131), and that this disruption may explain the high incidence of TD in schizophrenia. Furthermore, they have provided supporting evidence that in patients with schizophrenia, the pattern of neurocognitive deficits observed in patients with TD and negative symptoms is similar to that found in patients with basal ganglia pathology. This evidence suggests a shared underlying pathology for negative symptoms and orofacial dyskinesia, and for neurocognitive impairments, involving frontal–striatal–thalamic circuits.

Tardive Dyskinesia and Negative versus Positive Symptoms

Patients with schizophrenia who have predominantly negative symptoms (e.g., poverty of speech, alogia, avolition, curbing of interests, diminished sense of purpose, and blunted affect), particularly those with poverty of speech and blunted affect, have been observed to be at increased risk of developing TD (132). The weight of evidence supports the proposal that the pathological process responsible for negative symptoms can contribute to the genesis of both orofacial and limb-trunkal dyskinesia but that the contribution to orofacial dyskinesia is weak in the absence of age-related brain changes (133). Barnes and Liddle (134) have argued that in certain patients with schizophrenia who have relatively marked signs of organic brain disruption, movements disorders are more likely to develop in response to antipsychotic drug administration and that these patients also have poorer prognoses (135). Interestingly, both orofacial and limb-trunkal dyskinesia are associated with negative symptoms in schizophrenia. However, unlike limb-trunkal dyskinesia, orofacial dyskinesia tends to occur earlier in neuroleptic-treated patients with prominent negative symptoms than in patients without prominent negative symptoms (136,137). Orofacial dyskinesia is therefore thought to arise from a complex interaction between the effects of dopamine blockade and age-related changes in relevant brain systems, probably the nigrostriatal dopamine system. Thus, the relation between global negative symptoms and TD occurs most prominently in older, more chronically ill patient populations, particularly in patients with a mean age of 55 years (89,137). Findings also suggest that neuroleptic-treated patients with prominent negative symptoms are more likely to develop tardive akathisia than orofacial dyskinesia (135,138).

This body of evidence contrasts with attempts to correlate positive symptoms of schizophrenia (i.e., delusions, hallucinations, disorganized speech, and grossly disorganized or catatonic behavior) with TD. Several studies performed in more acutely psychotic and younger patient populations with schizophrenia who had more prominent positive symptomatology have failed to show a consistent correlation of these symptoms with TD (93,116,139–141). However, associations between TD and global positive symptoms have been reported, predominantly with thought disorder and disorganization symptoms (100,142, 143). Investigators disagree about the specific neuronal substrates of thought disorder and of hallucinations and delusions. For example, one hypothesis states that "reality distortion" (i.e., delusions and hallucinations) and "disorganization" (i.e., inappropriate affect and thought disorder) are two discrete domains of what have been grouped together as positive symptoms (144). Thus, investigators who have reported correlations between positive symptoms and TD may have been interpreting the independent loading of thought disorder with hallucinations and delusions, rather than with inappropriate affect (145). Furthermore, the lack of correlation with positive symptoms may be partly accounted for by the confounding effects of masking of involuntary movements by vigorous treatment of acute positive symptoms with antipsychotics. This hypothesis is further supported by at least one report of a positive but nonsignificant correlation between drug-induced parkinsonism and positive symptomatology (146).

Tardive Dyskinesia and Oculomotor Dysfunction

Basal ganglia form critical components of the cortical–subcortical–cortical oculomotor loop, which, as suggested by recent data, consists of two parallel but distinct smooth-pursuit and saccadic pathways (81,147). Classic studies by Hikosaka and Wurtz (148) demonstrated that basal ganglia provide tonic inhibition of the superior colliculus (SC) and thus control saccade generation (148). More recently, Pokorny and Basso (149) showed that SNr neurons are modulated during pursuit (149). Thus, diseases of basal ganglia are associated with abnormalities both in the saccadic system, particularly increase in saccadic distractibility, and in smooth pursuit. Patients with TD show more saccadic distractibility than patients with schizophrenia who do not have dyskinesia, as evidenced by an increased error rate in the antisaccade task (150). This finding suggests a decrease in the tonic inhibition of the nigrotectal efferent that is mediated by GABA. Interestingly, the GABA agonist muscimol partly reverses the antisaccade deficit observed in patients with TD (54).

TARDIVE DYSKINESIA IN PSYCHOTIC AFFECTIVE DISORDERS

The use of antipsychotic medications is indicated in the treatment of PAD such as unipolar psychotic depression and bipolar depressed or manic states with psychotic features. Data from the mood disorders program at the McLean Hospital near Boston, Massachusetts, USA suggest that patients with unipolar or bipolar depression, whether psychotic or nonpsychotic, develop dyskinesia at a much higher rate than that seen in schizophrenia (151,152). This increased risk has been attributed to the administration of drug combinations (including lithium and fluoxetine), intermittent antipsychotic exposure, high doses of antipsychotics during manic or psychotic depressive states, and discontinuation of antipsychotic medications during depression (153–157). It has been reported that TD worsens during depression and diminishes or disappears during mania (158–160), and at least one report describes exacerbation of TD with mania (161, 162). Tardive dystonia has also been reported to diminish during mania and relapse during depressive episodes (163). However, the possibility that withdrawal dyskinesia occurs during the depressive episode of bipolar affective disorder following withdrawal of antipsychotics, and that TD is masked by reintroduction of neuroleptics during mania, cannot be excluded in all cases.

NEUROIMAGING IN TARDIVE DYSKINESIA

Since mid-1970s, more than a dozen studies have examined the morphologic changes in patients with schizophrenia who develop TD. The primary region of interest is obviously the basal ganglia.

Overall, these studies have provided rather inconsistent results. For instance, several studies have found reduced volumes of the caudate nucleus in patients with schizophrenia and TD (164–166), whereas one study found increased volume of the caudate nucleus in patients with TD (167), and most studies showed no considerable differences in the size of the caudate between patients with and without dyskinesia (168–172). Complicating the issue further, chronic antipsychotic treatment is thought to be associated with changes in sizes of basal ganglia (173,174). Therefore, determining whether any substantial morphologic difference in TD (or lack of such a difference) is an effect of antipsychotic medications *per se* becomes a critical issue.

Because spontaneous dyskinesia that is clinically indistinguishable from medication-induced dyskinesia can be observed in patients with schizophrenia who have never been medicated, the issue of potential confounding of antipsychotic medication can possibly be circumvented by examining these patients. An interesting study conducted in South India by McCreadie (175) recruited a large sample of patients with chronic schizophrenia and dyskinesias who had never been medicated (n = 31); the sample was then matched with 31 patients who did not have dyskinesia and who also had never been medicated. The author, assessing 12 measures including caudate and lentiform nucleus, hemisphere and ventricular volumes, and ventricle–hemisphere ratio, found no significant differences between the two treatment-naïve groups in any measures (175). Barring a number of measurement limitations in the study, it seems that the theory that morphologic changes in the basal ganglia is an index of dyskinesia is not supported, at least in antipsychotic-naïve patients.

Although the morphologic studies of basal ganglia involvement in patients with TD are inconclusive, functional imaging may offer new ways of studying the involvement of the basal ganglia *in vivo* in patients with antipsychotic-induced dyskinesia. However, direct evidence about receptor or hemodynamic functions in patients with TD is currently minimal. One of the first studies of the dopamine supersensitivity hypothesis evaluated dopamine D_2 receptor binding in five patients with TD and in three patients without TD using positron emission tomography (PET) (43). The researchers found no differences in striatal D_2 receptor binding between patients with and patients without dyskinesia, casting doubt on the dopamine D_2 hypothesis of TD. Similarly, another PET study using ^{76}Br-bromospiperone as the ligand also did not detect significant differences in D_2 receptor density in the striatum between patients with TD and controls (176).

However, in another study, Silvestri et al. (177) also measured dopamine D_2 receptor binding after long-term antipsychotic treatment in nine subjects (without TD) using [^{11}C] raclopride in PET (177). These researchers found, for the first time, that dopamine D_2 receptor binding was increased in the striatum in five of the nine subjects studied. Interestingly, the subject who showed the greatest amount of D_2 receptor binding went on to develop severe and persistent dyskinesia symptoms when treated with quetiapine. Although this case offers an *in vivo* link between dyskinesia and dopamine receptor supersensitivity caused by prolonged dopamine receptor blockade, the following issues remain to be determined: why only some patients showed upregulation of D_2 receptors after long-term antipsychotic exposure; whether all patients with upregulated D_2 receptors are at higher risk of developing dyskinesia; and why the upregulation is evident in one study but not in the others. In the study by Silvestri et al., (177) the extent of D_2 upregulation was similar in all patients, whether they had previously been treated with first-generation or new-generation antipsychotic medication. This finding is also not consistent with the clinical observation of reduced risk of TD in patients treated with new-generation antipsychotic medications.

As discussed earlier, prolonged dopamine receptor blockade by antipsychotic medications is also hypothesized to cause neurotoxicity (and possibly TD) by increasing dopamine turnover, thus increasing amounts of free radicals. *In vivo* neuroimaging may offer evidence of damage to dopaminergic neurons. In a preliminary study, Lavalaye et al. (178) hypothesized that a marker for the integrity of the dopaminergic neurons and changes in the density of the dopamine transporter in patients with TD may provide supportive evidence for their neurotoxicity theory (178). They used single photon emission computed tomography (SPECT) with ^{123}I-labeled N-(3-fluoropropyl)-2β-carbomethoxy-3β-(4-iodophenyl) nortropane (^{123}FP-CIT) ioflupane to investigate the integrity of striatal dopamine terminals. Comparing seven schizophrenic patients with TD and eight healthy controls, they found no differences in striatal dopamine transporter density between the two groups.

At this stage, the use of *in vivo* neuroimaging techniques to investigate the etiology of TD is relatively limited. However, further development in neuroimaging should help clarify the pharmacodynamic effects of antipsychotic medications and the etiology of TD.

SUMMARY

Even though new cases of TD are on the decline in North America and other western countries, TD remains a public health concern for patients with chronic schizophrenia, PAD, and for nonpsychiatric patients treated with dopamine receptor antagonists. The new generation of atypical antipsychotic medications is believed to pose less risk for TD. However, identifying the cognitive and disease-related correlates of TD should equip clinicians with the necessary tools to reduce the prevalence of this iatrogenic movement disorder. No effective treatments for TD are available. This lack of effective therapy is problematic, especially in the few patients in whom the disorder causes functional impairment and other complications, and in whom it may be irreversible.

ACKNOWLEDGMENTS

This work is supported in part by the NIMH Grants MH45074, MH49826, MH68580, and the Baltimore VA MIRECC. The authors thank Dawn Detamore for her administrative assistance on the chapter.

REFERENCES

1. Kane JM, Woerner M, Weinhold P, et al. Incidence of tardive dyskinesia: five-year data from a prospective study. *Psychopharmacol Bull* 1984;20:39–40.
2. Morgenstern H, Glazer WM. Identifying risk factors for tardive dyskinesia among long-term outpatients maintained with neuroleptic medications. Results of the Yale Tardive Dyskinesia Study. *Arch Gen Psychiatry* 1993;50:723–733.
3. Yassa R, Jeste DV. Gender differences in tardive dyskinesia: a critical review of the literature. *Schizophr Bull* 1992;18:701–715.
4. Gerlach J. Tardive dyskinesia. *Dan Med Bull* 1979;26: 209–245.
5. Kane JM, Smith JM. Tardive dyskinesia: prevalence and risk factors, 1959 to 1979. *Arch Gen Psychiatry* 1982;39:473–481.
6. Thaker GK, Hare TA, Tamminga CA. GABA system: clinical research and treatment of tardive dyskinesia. *Mod Probl Pharmacopsychiatry* 1983;21:155–167.
7. Tamminga CA, Thaker GK, Nguyen JA. GABA mimetic treatments for tardive dyskinesia: efficacy and mechanism. *Psychopharmacol Bull* 1989;25:43–46.
8. Arango C, Adami H, Sherr JD, et al. Relationship of awareness of dyskinesia in schizophrenia to insight into mental illness. *Am J Psychiatry* 1999;156: 1097–1099.
9. American Psychiatric Association. Tardive dyskinesia: a task force report of the American Psychiatric Association. Washington, DC, 1992.
10. Barnes TR, Liddle PF. Evidence for the validity of negative symptoms. *Mod Probl Pharmacopsychiatry* 1990; 24:43–72.
11. Swartz JR, Burgoyne K, Smith M, et al. Tardive dyskinesia and ethnicity: review of the literature. *Ann Clin Psychiatry* 1997;9:53–59.
12. Wonodi I, Hong LE, Avila MT, et al. Rating scales for drug-induced movement disorders. *Drug-induced movement disorder*, 2nd ed. (Editors Factor, Lang Weiner) 2004, Futura Publishing Company.
13. Bergen JA, Eyland EA, Campbell JA, et al. The course of tardive dyskinesia in patients on long-term neuroleptics. *Br J Psychiatry* 1989;154:523–528.
14. Delay J, Deniker P, Harl J. Utilization therpeutique psychiatrique d'une phenothiazine d'action centrale elective. *Ann Med Psychol* 1952;110:112–117.
15. Schonecker M. Ein eigentumliches syndrom im oralen bereich bei megaphen application. *Nervenartz* 1957; 28:35.
16. Kruse W. Treatment of drug-induced extrapyramidal symptoms. (A comparative study of three antiparkinson agents). *Dis Nerv Syst* 1960;21:79–81.
17. Casey DE, Rabins P. Tardive dyskinesia as a life-threatening illness. *Am J Psychiatry* 1978;135:486–488.
18. Keegan DL, Rajput AH. Drug-induced dystonia tarda: treatment with L-dopa. *Dis Nerv Syst* 1973;34:167–169.
19. Tarsy D. History and definition of tardive dyskinesia. *Clin Neuropharmacol* 1983;6:91–99.
20. Tarsy D, Granacher R, Bralower M. Tardive dyskinesia in young adults. *Am J Psychiatry* 1977;134:1032–1034.
21. Hunter R, Earl CJ, Thronicroft C. An apparently irreversible syndrome of abnormal movements following phenothiazine medication. *Proc R Soc Med* 1964;57: 758–762.
22. Gardos G, Cole JO, Haskell D, et al. The natural history of tardive dyskinesia. *J Clin Psychopharmacol* 1988;8:31S–37S.
23. Egan MF, Apud J, Wyatt RJ. Treatment of tardive dyskinesia. *Schizophr Bull* 1997;23:583–609.
24. Jeste DV, Wyatt RJ. Changing epidemiology of tardive dyskinesia: an overview. *Am J Psychiatry* 1981;138: 297–309.

25. Kane JM, Woerner M, Lieberman J. Tardive dyskinesia: prevalence, incidence, and risk factors. *J Clin Psychopharmacol* 1988;8:52S–56S.
26. Sherr JD, Myers C, Avila MT, et al. The effects of nicotine on specific eye tracking measures in schizophrenia. *Biol Psychiatry* 2002;52:721–728.
27. Simpson GM. Pharmacological treatments of schizophrenia. *Psychopharmacol Bull* 1986;22:33.
28. Smith JM, Baldessarini RJ. Changes in prevalence, severity, and recovery in tardive dyskinesia with age. *Arch Gen Psychiatry* 1980;37:1368–1373.
29. van Harten PN, Hoek HW, Matroos GE, et al. Intermittent neuroleptic treatment and risk for tardive dyskinesia: Curacao Extrapyramidal Syndromes Study III. *Am J Psychiatry* 1998;155:565–567.
30. Wonodi I, Adami H, Sherr J, et al. Naltrexone treatment of tardive dyskinesia in patients with schizophrenia. *J Clin Psychopharmacol* 2004;24:441–445.
31. Caligiuri MP, Jeste DV. Association of diabetes with dyskinesia in older psychotic patients. *Psychopharmacology (Berl)* 2004;176(3-4):281–286.
32. Edwards H. The significance of brain damage in persistent oral dyskinesia. *Br J Psychiatry* 1970;116:271–275.
33. Olivera AA, Kiefer MW, Manley NK. Tardive dyskinesia in psychiatric patients with substance use disorders. *Am J Drug Alcohol Abuse* 1990;16:57–66.
34. Schultz SK, Miller DD, Arndt S, et al. Withdrawal-emergent dyskinesia in patients with schizophrenia during antipsychotic discontinuation. *Biol Psychiatry* 1995;38:713–719.
35. Waddington JL, Youssef HA. The expression of schizophrenia, affective disorder and vulnerability to tardive dyskinesia in an extensive pedigree. *Br J Psychiatry* 1988;153:376–381.
36. Waddington JL, Youssef HA, Molloy AG, et al. Association of intellectual impairment, negative symptoms, and aging with tardive dyskinesia: clinical and animal studies. *J Clin Psychiatry* 1985;46:29–33.
37. Woerner MG, Saltz BL, Kane JM, et al. Diabetes and development of tardive dyskinesia. *Am J Psychiatry* 1993;150:966–968.
38. Stahl SM. *Essential psychopharmacology*, 2nd ed. New York: Cambridge University Press, 2000.
39. Halliday J, Farrington S, Macdonald S, et al. Nithsdale schizophrenia surveys 23: movement disorders. 20-year review. *Br J Psychiatry* 2002;181:422–427.
40. Luby E. Reserpine-like-drugs-clinical efficacy, in *Psychopharmacology: a review of progress*. 1957–1967. Washington, DC: Government Printing Office, 1968.
41. May P. *Treatment of schizophrenia: a comparative study of five treatment Methods*. New York: Science House, 1968.
42. Klawans HL, Rubovits R. Effect of cholinergic and anticholinergic agents on tardive dyskinesia. *J Neurol Neurosurg Psychiatry* 1974;27:941–947.
43. Andersson U, Eckernas SA, Hartvig P, et al. Striatal binding of 11C-NMSP studied with positron emission tomography in patients with persistent tardive dyskinesia: no evidence for altered dopamine D2 receptor binding. *J Neural Transm Gen Sect* 1990;79:215–226.
44. Pind K, Faurbye A. Concentration of homovanillic acid and 5-hydroxyindoleacetic acid in the cerebrospinal fluid after treatment with probenecid in patients with drug-induced tardive dyskinesia. *Acta Psychiatr Scand* 1970;46:323–326.
45. Crow TJ. Abnormal involuntary movements in schizophrenia: Are they related to the disease process of its treatment? Are they associated with changes indopamine receptors? *J Clin Psychopharmacol* 1982;2:336–340.
46. Mao CC, Marco E, Revuelta A, et al. The turnover rate of gamma-aminobutyric acid in the nuclei of telencephalon: implications in the pharmacology of antipsychotics and of a minor tranquilizer. *Biol Psychiatry* 1977;12:359–371.
47. Scheel-Kruger J. Dopamine-GABA interactions: evidence that GABA transmits, modulates and mediates dopaminergic functions in the basal ganglia and the limbic system. *Acta Neurol Scand Suppl* 1986;107:1–54.
48. Thaker GK, Tamminga CA, Alphs LD, et al. Brain gamma-aminobutyric acid abnormality in tardive dyskinesia. Reduction in cerebrospinal fluid GABA levels and therapeutic response to GABA agonist treatment. *Arch Gen Psychiatry* 1987;44:522–529.
49. Bolam JP, Hanley JJ, Booth PA, et al. Synaptic organisation of the basal ganglia. *J Anat* 2000;196(Pt 4):527–542.
50. Hikosaka O, Wurtz RH. Effects on eye movements of a GABA agonist and antagonist injected into monkey superior colliculus. *Brain Res* 1983;272:368–372.
51. Albin RL, Aldridge JW, Young AB, et al. Feline subthalamic nucleus neurons contain glutamate-like but not GABA-like or glycine-like immunoreactivity. *Brain Res* 1989;491:185–188.
52. Albin RL, Young AB, Penney JB. The functional anatomy of disorders of the basal ganglia. *Trends Neurosci* 1995;18:63–64.
53. DeLong MR. Primate models of movement disorders of basal ganglia origin [Review]. *Trends Neurosci* 1990;13:281–285.
54. Cassady SL, Thaker GK, Moran M, et al. GABA agonist-induced changes in motor, oculomotor, and attention measures correlate in schizophrenics with tardive dyskinesia. *Biol Psychiatry* 1992;32:302–311.
55. Thaker GK, Nguyen JA, Tamminga CA. Increased saccadic distractibility in tardive dyskinesia: functional evidence for subcortical GABA dysfunction. *Biol Psychiatry* 1989;25:49–59.
56. Cassady SL, Thaker GK, Tamminga CA. Pharmacologic relationship of antisaccade and dyskinesia in schizophrenic patients. *Psychopharmacol Bull* 1993;29:235–240.
57. Bourgoin S, Cesselin F, Artaud F, et al. In vivo modulations by GABA-related drugs of met-enkephalin release in basal ganglia of the cat brain. *Brain Res* 1982;248:321–330.
58. Maneuf YP, Mitchell IJ, Crossman AR, et al. On the role of enkephalin cotransmission in the GABAergic striatal efferents to the globus pallidus. *Exp Neurol* 1994;125:65–71.
59. Iakimovskii AF, Bobrova IV. Neuromotor dyskinesia occurring during repeated injections of enkephalins into the rat striatum. *Patol Fiziol Eksp Ter* 1991;(6):20–22.
60. McCormick SE, Stoessl AJ. Blockade of nigral and pallidal opioid receptors suppresses vacuous chewing movements in a rodent model of tardive dyskinesia. *Neuroscience* 2002;112:851–859.
61. Egan MF, Hurd Y, Hyde TM, et al. Alterations in mRNA levels of D_2 receptors and neuropeptides in striatonigral and striatopallidal neurons of rats with neuroleptic-induced dyskinesias. *Synapse* 1994;18:178–189.

62. Andreassen OA, Finsen B, Ostergaard K, et al. The relationship between oral dyskinesias produced by long-term haloperidol treatment, the density of striatal preproenkephalin messenger RNA and enkephalin peptide, and the number of striatal neurons expressing preproenkephalin messenger RNA in rats. *Neuroscience* 1999;88:27–35.

63. Andreassen OA, Waage J, Finsen B, et al. Memantine attenuates the increase in striatal preproenkephalin mRNA expression and development of haloperidol-induced persistent oral dyskinesias in rats. *Brain Res* 2003;994:188–192.

64. Blum I, Nisipeanu PF, Roberts E. Naloxone in tardive dyskinesia. *Psychopharmacology (Berl)* 1987;93:538.

65. Rascol O, Fabre N, Blin O, et al. Naltrexone, an opiate antagonist, fails to modify motor symptoms in patients with Parkinson's disease. *Mov Disord* 1994;9:437–440.

66. Cadet JL, Lohr JB. Possible involvement of free radicals in neuroleptic-induced movement disorders. Evidence from treatment of tardive dyskinesia with vitamin E. *Ann NY Acad Sci* 1989;570:176–185.

67. Lohr JB. Oxygen radicals and neuropsychiatric illness. Some speculations. *Arch Gen Psychiatry* 1991;48:1097–1106.

68. Tsai G, Goff DC, Chang RW, et al. Markers of glutamatergic neurotransmission and oxidative stress associated with tardive dyskinesia. *Am J Psychiatry* 1998;155:1207–1213.

69. Zhang ZJ, Zhang XB, Hou G, et al. Interaction between polymorphisms of the dopamine D3 receptor and manganese superoxide dismutase genes in susceptibility to tardive dyskinesia. *Psychiatr Genet* 2003;13:187–192.

70. Lohr JB, Browning JA. Free radical involvement in neuropsychiatric illnesses. *Psychopharmacol Bull* 1995;31:159–165.

71. Mahadik SP, Mukherjee S. Free radical pathology and antioxidant defense in schizophrenia: a review. *Schizophr Res* 1996;19:1–17.

72. Coyle JT, Puttfarcken P. Oxidative stress, glutamate, and neurodegenerative disorders [Review]. *Science* 1993;262:689–695.

73. Perry TL, Kish SJ, Hansen S. Gamma-vinyl GABA: effects of chronic administration on the metabolism of GABA and other amino compounds in rat brain. *J Neurochem* 1979;32:1641–1645.

74. Adler LA, Rotrosen J, Edson R et al., Veterans Affairs Cooperative Study #394 Study Group. Vitamin E treatment for tardive dyskinesia. *Arch Gen Psychiatry* 1999;56:836–841.

75. Barak Y, Swartz M, Shamir E, et al. Vitamin E (alpha-tocopherol) in the treatment of tardive dyskinesia: a statistical meta-analysis. *Ann Clin Psychiatry* 1998;10:101–105.

76. Egan MF, Hyde TM, Albers GW, et al. Treatment of tardive dyskinesia with vitamin E. *Am J Psychiatry* 1992;149:773–777.

77. Lohr JB, Cadet JL, Lohr MA, et al. Alpha-tocopherol in tardive dyskinesia. *Lancet* 1987;1:913–914.

78. Vatassery GT, Fahn S, Kuskowski MA, Parkinson Study Group. Alpha tocopherol in CSF of subjects taking high-dose vitamin E in the DATATOP study. *Neurology* 1998;50:1900–1902.

79. Zhang XY, Zhou DF, Cao LY, et al. The effect of vitamin E treatment on tardive dyskinesia and blood superoxide dismutase: a double-blind placebo-controlled trial. *J Clin Psychopharmacol* 2004;24:83–86.

80. Richardson MA, Reilly MA, Read LL, et al. Phenylalanine kinetics are associated with tardive dyskinesia in men but not in women. *Psychopharmacology (Berl)* 1999;143:347–357.

81. Alexander GE, DeLong MR, Strick PL. Parallel organization of functionally segregated circuits linking basal ganglia and cortex. *Annu Rev Neurosci* 1986;9:357–381.

82. Brown LL, Schneider JS, Lidsky TI. Sensory and cognitive functions of the basal ganglia. *Curr Opin Neurobiol* 1997;7:157–163.

83. Mega MS, Cummings JL. Frontal-subcortical circuits and neuropsychiatric disorders. *J Neuropsychiatry Clin Neurosci* 1994;6:358–370.

84. Alexander GE, Crutcher MD. Functional architecture of basal ganglia circuits: neural substrates of parallel processing [Review]. *Trends Neurosci* 1990;13:266–271.

85. Javoy-Agid F, Agid Y. Is the mesocortical dopaminergic system involved in Parkinson disease? *Neurology* 1980;30:1326–1330.

86. Lee TH, Smith TW. Serum digoxin concentration and diagnosis of digitalis toxicity. Current concepts. *Clin Pharmacokinet* 1983;8:279–285.

87. Lieberman A, Ransohoff J. Treatment of primary brain tumors. *Med Clin North Am* 1979;63:835–848.

88. Waddington JL, Brown K, O'Neill J, et al. Cognitive impairment, clinical course and treatment history in outpatients with bipolar affective disorder: relationship to tardive dyskinesia. *Psychol Med* 1989;19:897–902.

89. Waddington JL, O'Callaghan E, Buckley P, et al. Tardive dyskinesia in schizophrenia. Relationship to minor physical anomalies, frontal lobe dysfunction and cerebral structure on magnetic resonance imaging. *Br J Psychiatry* 1995;167:41–44.

90. Farran-Ridge C. Some symptoms referable to the basal ganglia occurring in dementia praecox and epidemic encephalitis. *J Med Sci* 1926;72:513–523.

91. Kraepelin E. *Dementia praecox and paraphrenia*. Huntington, NY: Krieger, 1919.

92. Waddington JL, Crow TJ. Abnormal involuntary movements and psychosis in the preneuroleptic era and in unmedication patients: implications for the concept of tardive dyskinesia. In: Wolf ME, Mosnaim AD, eds. *Tardive dyskinesia:biological mechanisms and clinical aspects*. Washington, DC: American Psychiatric Press, 1988:51–66.

93. Davis EJ, Borde M, Sharma LN. Tardive dyskinesia and type II schizophrenia. *Br J Psychiatry* 1992;160:253–256.

94. Fenton WS, Wyatt RJ, McGlashan TH. Risk factors for spontaneous dyskinesia in schizophrenia. *Arch Gen Psychiatry* 1994;51:643–650.

95. Owens DG, Johnstone EC, Frith CD. Spontaneous involuntary disorders of movement: their prevalence, severity, and distribution in chronic schizophrenics with and without treatment with neuroleptics. *Arch Gen Psychiatry* 1982;39:452–461.

96. Cassady SL, Adami HM, Moran MJ, et al. Spontaneous dyskinesia in schizophrenia spectrum personality. *Am J Psychiatry* 1998;155:70–75.

97. Myslobodsky MS. Anosognosia in tardive dyskinesia: "tardive dysmentia" or "tardive dementia"? *Schizophr Bull* 1986;12:1–6.

98. Myslobodsky MS. Central determinants of attention and mood disorder in tardive dyskinesia ("tardive dysmentia"). *Brain Cogn* 1993;23:88–101.
99. Perenyi A, Norman T, Burrows GD. Relationship of symptomatology of schizophrenia and tardive dyskinesia. *Eur Neuropsychopharmacol* 1992;2:51–55.
100. Richardson MA, Pass R, Bregman Z, et al. Tardive dyskinesia and depressive symptoms in schizophrenics. *Psychopharmacol Bull* 1985;21:130–135.
101. Albus M, Naber D, Muller-Spahn F, et al. Tardive dyskinesia: relation to computer-tomographic, endocrine, and psychopathological variables. *Biol Psychiatry* 1985;20:1082–1089.
102. Macpherson R, Collis R. Tardive dyskinesia. Patients' lack of awareness of movement disorder. *Br J Psychiatry* 1992;160:110–112.
103. Cuesta MJ, Peralta V. Lack of insight in schizophrenia. *Schizophr Bull* 1994;20:359–366.
104. Carpenter WT Jr, Heinrichs DW, Wagman AM. Deficit and nondeficit forms of schizophrenia: the concept. *Am J Psychiatry* 1988;145:578–583.
105. Gerlach J, Casey DE. Tardive dyskinesia. *Acta Psychiatr Scand* 1988;77:369–378.
106. Stone RK, May JE, Alvarez WF, et al. Prevalence of dyskinesia and related movement disorders in a developmentally disabled population. *J Ment Defic Res* 1989;33(Pt 1):41–53.
107. Wszola BA, Newell KM, Sprague RL. Risk factors for tardive dyskinesia in a large population of youths and adults. *Exp Clin Psychopharmacol* 2001;9:285–296.
108. Green MF. What are the functional consequences of neurocognitive deficits in schizophrenia? *Am J Psychiatry* 1996;153:321–330.
109. Green MF, Marder SR, Fenton W, et al. Overcoming obstacles in treating cognitive deficits in schizophrenia. *Biol Psychiatry* 2003;53:158S.
110. Gold JM, Randolph C, Carpenter CJ, et al. Forms of memory failure in schizophrenia. *J Abnorm Psychol* 1992;101:487–494.
111. Goldberg TE, Weinberger DR. Probing prefrontal function in schizophrenia with neuropsychological paradigms. *Schizophr Bull* 1988;14:179–183.
112. Goldberg TE, Weinberger DR, Berman KF, et al. Further evidence for dementia of the prefrontal type in schizophrenia? A controlled study of teaching the Wisconsin card sorting test. *Arch Gen Psychiatry* 1987;44:1008–1014.
113. Carlsson A. The current status of the dopamine hypothesis of schizophrenia. *Neuropsychopharmacology* 1988;1:179–186.
114. Meltzer HY. Effect of neuroleptics on the schizophrenic syndrome. *Psychopharmacol Ser* 1987;3:255–265.
115. Weinberger DR. Implications of normal brain development for the pathogenesis of schizophrenia. *Arch Gen Psychiatry* 1987;44:660–669.
116. Gold JM, Goldberg TE, Kleinman JE, et al. The effects of symptomatic state and pharmacological treatment on the neuropsychological test performance of patients with schizophrenia and affective disorders. In: Mohr E, Brouwers P, eds. *Handbook of clinical trials: the neurobehavioral approach*. Swets and Zeitlinger, 1991:185–216.
117. Waddington JL, Youssef HA. An unusual cluster of tardive dyskinesia in schizophrenia: association with cognitive dysfunction and negative symptoms. *Am J Psychiatry* 1986;143:1162–1165.
118. Waddington JL, Youssef HA, Dolphin C, et al. Cognitive dysfunction, negative symptoms, and tardive dyskinesia in schizophrenia. Their association in relation to topography of involuntary movements and criterion of their abnormality. *Arch Gen Psychiatry* 1987;44:907–912.
119. Hinton J, Withers E. The usefulness of the clinical tests of the sensorium. *Br J Psychiatry* 1971;119:9–18.
120. Famuyiwa OO, Eccleston D, Donaldson AA, et al. Tardive dyskinesia and dementia. *Br J Psychiatry* 1979;135:500–504.
121. Wolf ME, Ryan JJ, Mosnaim AD. Cognitive functions in tardive dyskinesia. *Psychol Med* 1983;13:671–674.
122. Collerton D, Fairbairn A, Britton P. Cognitive performance of medicated schizophrenics with tardive dyskinesia. *Psychol Med* 1985;15:311–315.
123. Hoffman WF, Labs SM, Casey DE. Neuroleptic-induced parkinsonism in older schizophrenics. *Biol Psychiatry* 1987;22:427–439.
124. Struve FA, Willner AE. Cognitive dysfunction and tardive dyskinesia. *Br J Psychiatry* 1983;143:597–600.
125. Collinson SC, Pantelis C, Barnes TR. Abnormal involuntary movements in schizophrenia and their association with cognitive impairment in schizophrenia. In: Pantev C, Nelson HE, Barnes TR, eds. *A neuropsychological perspective*. London: John Wiley & Sons, 1996:237–258.
126. Krabbendam L, Derix MM, Honig A, et al. Cognitive performance in relation to MRI temporal lobe volume in schizophrenic patients and healthy control subjects. *J Neuropsychiatry Clin Neurosci* 2000;12:251–256.
127. Myslobodsky MS, Tomer R, Holden T, et al. Cognitive impairments in patients with tardive dyskinesia. *J Nerv Ment Dis* 1985 Mar;173(3):156–160.
128. Granholm E, Bartzokis G, Asarnow RF, et al. Preliminary associations between motor procedural learning, basal ganglia T2 relaxation times, and tardive dyskinesia in schizophrenia. *Psychiatry Res* 1993;50:33–44.
129. Pantelis C, Barnes TR, Nelson HE. Is the concept of frontal-subcortical dementia relevant to schizophrenia? *Br J Psychiatry* 1992;160:442–460.
130. Pantelis C, Brewer W. Neuropsychological and olfactory dysfunction in schizophrenia: relationship of frontal syndromes to syndromes of schizophrenia. *Schizophr Res* 1995;17:35–45.
131. Pantelis C, Stuart GW, Nelson HE, et al. Spatial working memory deficits in schizophrenia: relationship with tardive dyskinesia and negative symptoms. *Am J Psychiatry* 2001;158:1276–1285.
132. Waddington JL, Youssef HA. Cognitive dysfunction in chronic schizophrenia followed prospectively over 10 years and its longitudinal relationship to the emergence of tardive dyskinesia. *Psychol Med* 1996;26:681–688.
133. Liddle PF, Barnes TR, Speller J, et al. Negative symptoms as a risk factor for tardive dyskinesia in schizophrenia. *Br J Psychiatry* 1993;163:776–780.
134. Barnes TRE & Liddle PF (1985). Tardive dyskinesia: Implications for schizophrenia? In schizophrenia: New Pharmacological and Clinical Developments (eds. Schiff AA, Roth M & Freeman H) London: Royal Society of Medicine.
135. Brown KW, White T. The association among negative symptoms, movement disorders, and frontal lobe psychological deficits in schizophrenic patients. *Biol Psychiatry* 1991;30:1182–1190.
136. Kidger T, Barnes TR, Trauer T, et al. Sub-syndromes of tardive dyskinesia. *Psychol Med* 1980;10:513–520.
137. Barnes TR, Kidger T, Gore SM. Tardive dyskinesia: a 3-year follow-up study. *Psychol Med* 1983;13:71–81.
138. Sachdev P, Hume F, Toohey P, et al. Negative symptoms, cognitive dysfunction, tardive akathisia and tardive dyskinesia. *Acta Psychiatr Scand* 1996;93:451–459.

139. Csernansky JG, Yesavage JA, Maloney W, et al. The treatment response scale: a retrospective method of assessing response to neuroleptics. *Am J Psychiatry* 1983; 140:1210–1213.
140. Gureje O. The significance of subtyping tardive dyskinesia: a study of prevalence and associated factors. *Psychol Med* 1989;19:121–128.
141. Karson CN, Jeste DV, Bigelow LB. Tardive dyskinesia and psychopathology in chronic schizophrenia: a cross-sectional study. *Compr Psychiatry* 1985;26: 388–391.
142. King RA, Riddle MA, Chappell PB, et al. Emergence of self-destructive phenomena in children and adolescents during fluoxetine treatment. *J Am Acad Child Adolesc Psychiatry* 1991;30:179–186.
143. Sandyk R, Kay SR. The relationship of tardive dyskinesia to positive schizophrenia. *Int J Neurosci* 1991;56: 107–139.
144. Liddle PF, Friston KJ, Frith CD, et al. Patterns of cerebral blood flow in schizophrenia. *Br J Psychiatry* 1992; 160:179–186.
145. Brown KW, White T. The influence of topography on the cognitive and psychopathological effects of tardive dyskinesia. *Am J Psychiatry* 1992;149:1385–1389.
146. White T, Brown KW, Woods JP. Tardive dyskinesia and positive symptoms of schizophrenia. *Acta Psychiatr Scand* 1991;83:377–379.
147. Cui DM, Yan YJ, Lynch JC. The pursuit subregion of the frontal eye field projects to the caudate nucleus in monkeys. *J Neurophysiol* 2003;89(5):2678–2684.
148. Hikosaka O, Wurtz RH. The basal ganglia. *Rev Oculomot Res* 1989;3:257–281.
149. Pokorny J, Basso MA. Participation of basal ganglia nucleus neurons in smooth pursuit eye movements. *Soc Neural Control Mov* 2003;8:E-02.
150. Thaker GK, Kirkpatrick B, Buchanan RW, et al. Oculomotor abnormalities and their clinical correlates in schizophrenia. *Psychopharmacol Bull* 1989;25:491–497.
151. Gardos G, Casey D. *Tardive dyskinesia and affective disorders*. Washington, DC: American Psychiatric Press, 1984.
152. Schatzberg AF, Cole JO, Battista C. *Manual of clinical psychopharmacology*, 4th ed. Washington, DC, London, UK: American Psychiatric Press, 2003.
153. Dubovsky SL, Thomas M. Tardive dyskinesia associated with fluoxetine. *Psychiatr Serv* 1996;47:991–993.
154. Hunt N, Silverstone T. Tardive dyskinesia in bipolar affective disorder: a catchment area study. *Int Clin Psychopharmacol* 1991;6:45–50.
155. Lazarus A. Tardive dyskinesia-like syndrome associated with lithium and carbamazepine. *J Clin Psychopharmacol* 1994;14:146–147.
156. Rosenbaum AH, Niven RG, Hanson NP, et al. Tardive dyskinesia: relationship with a primary affective disorder. *Dis Nerv Syst* 1977;38:423–427.
157. Sternbach H, Jordan S. Lithium-associated tardive dyskinesia. *J Clin Psychopharmacol* 1990;10:143–144.
158. Cutler NR, Post RM, Rey AC, et al. Depression-dependent dyskinesias in two cases of manic-depressive illness. *N Engl J Med* 1981;304:1088–1089.
159. Scappa S, Teverbaugh P, Ananth J. Episodic tardive dyskinesia and parkinsonism in bipolar disorder patients. *Can J Psychiatry* 1993 Dec;38(10):633–634
160. Weiner WJ, Werner TR. Mania induced remission of tardive dyskinesia in manic-depressive illness. *Ann Neurol.* 1982 Aug;12(2):229–230.
161. Esel E, Turan MT, Oguz A, et al. Tardive dyskinesia exacerbating with mania in a bipolar patient. *Eur Psychiatry* 2001;16:257–258.
162. Yazici O, Kantemir E, Tastaban Y, et al. Spontaneous improvement of tardive dystonia during mania. *Br J Psychiatry* 1991;158:847–850.
163. Sachdev P. Drug-induced movement disorders in institutionalised adults with mental retardation: clinical characteristics and risk factors. *Aust N Z J Psychiatry* 1992;26:242–248.
164. Bartels M, Themelis J. Computerized tomography in tardive dyskinesia. Evidence of structural abnormalities in the basal ganglia system. *Arch Psychiatr Nervenkr* 1983;233:371–379.
165. Dalgalarrondo P, Gattaz WF. Basal ganglia abnormalities in tardive dyskinesia. Possible relationship with duration of neuroleptic treatment. *Eur Arch Psychiatry Clin Neurosci* 1994;244:272–277.
166. Hoffman RE, Buchsbaum MS, Escobar MD, et al. EEG coherence of prefrontal areas in normal and schizophrenic males during perceptual activation. *J Neuropsychiatry Clin Neurosci* 1991;3:169–175.
167. Brown KW, White T, Wardlaw JM, et al. Caudate nucleus morphology in tardive dyskinesia. *Br J Psychiatry* 1996;169:631–636.
168. Elkashef AM, Buchanan RW, Gellad F, et al. Basal ganglia pathology in schizophrenia and tardive dyskinesia: an MRI quantitative study. *Am J Psychiatry* 1994; 151:752–755.
169. Gelenberg AJ. Computerized tomography in patients with tardive dyskinesia. *Am J Psychiatry* 1976;133:578–579.
170. Harvey I, Ron MA, Murray R, et al. MRI in schizophrenia: basal ganglia and white matter T1 times. *Psychol Med* 1991;21:587–598.
171. Jeste DV, Wagner RL, Weinberger DR, et al. Evaluation of CT scans in tardive dyskinesia. *Am J Psychiatry* 1980; 137:247–248.
172. Swayze VW, Yates WR, Andreasen NC, et al. CT abnormalities in tardive dyskinesia. *Psychiatry Res* 1988;26: 51–58.
173. Chakos MH, Lieberman JA, Bilder RM, et al. Increase in caudate nuclei volumes of first-episode schizophrenic patients taking antipsychotic drugs. *Am J Psychiatry* 1994;151:1430–1436.
174. Keshavan MS, Bagwell WW, Haas GL, et al. Changes in caudate volume with neuroleptic treatment. *Lancet* 1994;344:1434.
175. McCreadie RG, Thara R, Padmavati R, et al. Structural brain difference between nerve-treated patients with schizophrenia, with and without dyskinesia, and normal control subjects. A magnetic resonance imaging study. *Arch Gen Psychiatry* 2002 Apr;59(4):332–336.
176. Blin J, Baron JC, Cambon H, et al. Striatal dopamine D2 receptors in tardive dyskinesia: PET study. *J Neurol Neurosurg Psychiatry* 1989;52:1248–1252.
177. Silvestri S, Seeman MV, Negrete JC, et al. Increased dopamine D2 receptor binding after long-term treatment with antipsychotics in humans: a clinical PET study. *Psychopharmacology (Berl)* 2000;152:174–180.
178. Lavalaye J, Sarlet A, Booij J, et al. Dopamine transporter density in patients with tardive dyskinesia: a single photon emission computed tomography study. *Psychopharmacology (Berl)* 2001;155:107–109.

25

Treatment Issues in Psychogenic-Neuropsychiatric Movement Disorders

Daniel T. Williams,[1] Blair Ford,[2] and Stanley Fahn[2]

[1]*Department of Psychiatry, Columbia University, New York, New York;*
[2]*Department of Neurology, Columbia University, New York, New York*

Physicians have long been fascinated and puzzled by physical symptoms that cannot be understood in rational physiologic or anatomic terms. Since the time of Charcot and Freud, clinicians have attempted to distinguish psychiatrically based symptoms from those produced by demonstrable brain lesions (1). Indeed, one of Freud's neurologic papers, commissioned by Charcot, was a comparison of organic and "hysterical" paralysis (2). Accumulated clinical experience has enabled clinicians to identify neurologic symptoms of nonneurologic origin. In recent decades, advances in diagnostic technology, chiefly neuroimaging and neurophysiologic techniques, have allowed clinicians to exclude the possibility that such syndromes are the result of discrete lesions within the nervous system.

The terminology used to describe symptoms of nonneurologic origin has evolved since the time of Freud and Charcot, when individuals with such symptoms were considered to be suffering from "hysteria" (2a). Recently, some advocate supplanting the descriptors "psychogenic" or "nonneurologic" with the term "neuropsychiatric," in part to provide a neutral and nondisparaging designation that reflects the complexity of a syndrome comprising both neurologic and psychiatric elements (3).

This chapter describes the diagnosis and treatment of psychogenic-neuropsychiatric movement disorders (PNMDs). These disorders produce abnormal movements that cannot be considered to result directly from organic disease and that derive primarily from psychological and psychiatric causes. As commonly employed by movement disorder specialists, the term tends to exclude movements caused by certain types of psychiatric illness, such as the psychomotor retardation or bradykinesia that may accompany depression, the bizarre movements and postures of schizophrenia, or the stereotyped movements of autism. Although some of these syndromes can reasonably be characterized as "neuropsychiatric," the term "psychogenic-neuropsychiatric movement disorders" is meant to convey additional specificity regarding the origin of these disorders. For reasons described later, clinicians might prefer to use the simpler term "neuropsychiatric" or the nonspecific term "stress-induced" when communicating with patients and their families.

PNMDs are difficult to diagnose with certainty because, at the initial assessment, there is generally no objective means of diagnostic confirmation; the best a clinician can do using initial diagnostic testing is to exclude contributing organic disease. PNMDs are challenging to treat because patients are often highly invested in the idea of a physical or an organic lesion and are therefore unwilling to consider or accept the notion that their dramatic and disabling symptoms are the result of a psychiatric disturbance. Therefore, the two central challenges to the clinician are (a) establishing with as much confidence as possible that the origin of the movements is psychogenic; and (b) arranging for appropriate psychiatric evaluation and treatment. Although psychogenic illness has long fascinated neurologists and psychiatrists alike, the pathogenesis remains obscure, and therapy for these disorders remains primarily empiric.

Determining whether abnormal movements are produced by psychiatric disease, an organic disorder, or both is not a trivial diagnostic task and represents an essential step in successful treatment. Physicians should not underestimate the magnitude of disability and suffering that patients with these syndromes endure. Failure to diagnose a psychogenic-neuropsychiatric movement disorder invariably delays treatment and may perpetuate a patient's cycle of disability (3a). In addition, some patients with unrecognized psychogenic symptoms have been subjected to inappropriate or dangerous testing and treatment, including unwarranted neurosurgery.

EPIDEMIOLOGY

Psychogenic neurologic symptoms have been estimated to account for between 1% and 9% of all neurologic diagnoses (4,5). Perhaps 10% to 15% of patients with a psychogenic movement disorder have an underlying organic movement disorder as well. This overlap between abnormal movements of psychogenic origin and abnormal movements of organic origin is also observed in patients with psychogenic nonepileptic seizures (6,7). Such overlap syndromes fully justify the term "neuropsychiatric" and can be especially difficult to delineate and treat.

NEUROLOGIC CONSIDERATIONS

The diagnosis of PNMDs is best viewed as a two-stage process. The first task is to rule out or limit the role of definable neurologic illness. The next task is to identify or confirm the presence of a psychiatric disorder. Because most patients with PNMDs will see a neurologist before they see a psychiatrist, and because neurologists are trained to identify the limits of neuropathology, the initial stage of diagnosis properly resides with the neurologist.

The diagnostic process in movement disorders involves categorization by phenomenology: abnormal movements are scrutinized by observation and by using clinical maneuvers in order to assign them to a class of abnormal movement. All of the major categories of abnormal movement, whether parkinsonism, tremor, myoclonus, dystonia, gait disorder, or other hyperkinetic disorders, are governed by clinical rules: characteristic anatomic, physiologic, and movement pattern constraints that reveal diagnostic associations to the experienced clinician. Nonneurologic neuropsychiatric movement disorders do not conform to the expected patterns of abnormal movement that result from neurologic lesions.

In one large series of 131 patients with psychogenic movement disorders, the abnormal movements could be initially categorized into dystonia, tremor, gait disturbances, paroxysmal dyskinesias, and myoclonus (8). Seventy-nine percent of patients had multiple types of abnormal movements, whereas only 21% had a single definable type. Moreover, and in contrast to most organic movement disorders, in 55% of the patients the movements were either intermittent or paroxysmal; only 45% of the patients had continuous movements. The onset was abrupt in 60% and usually followed a specific inciting event. In 43% of patients, the movements spread beyond the initial site of involvement.

PNMDs are usually identified on the basis of (a) symptoms and signs that are incompatible with disease of organic origin, (b) symptoms and signs that are inconsistent from moment to moment and fluctuate throughout the evaluation, (c) a discrepancy between the patient's disability and objective signs of motor deficit, and (d) the presence of other psychiatric abnormalities (30). Additional clinical clues include paroxysmal movements that begin suddenly, often in relation to a trivial injury or in the context of emotional stress.

Dramatic, paroxysmal symptoms with intervening normal periods constitute a typical pattern of PNMDs. However, some movement disorders of organic etiology, such as the paroxysmal dyskinesias or periodic ataxias, have an unusual appearance and a paroxysmal course. Thus, the presence of paroxysmal events and remissions does not *by itself* establish the diagnosis of a psychogenic disorder. Even the experienced clinician should not assume that a movement disorder is nonneurologic just because it has an unfamiliar presentation.

The literature on PNMDs includes many descriptions, series, and reviews of movement phenomenology and electrophysiology (8–20).

TABLE 25-1. *General clinical clues that suggest a nonneurological neuropsychiatric disorder*

1. Abrupt onset
2. Inconsistent movements that vary in severity, distribution, and pattern
3. Incongruous movements and postures that do not correspond to recognized disease patterns or physiology
4. Additional unexpected and unexplained ancillary movements, especially rhythmical shaking, bizarre gait, deliberate slowness, verbal gibberish, facial grimacing, and excessive startle
5. Spontaneous remissions
6. Movements decrease or disappear with distraction
7. Response to placebo, suggestion, or psychotherapy
8. Paroxysmal course, with sudden dramatic symptoms and intervening periods of normalcy

The most common type of psychogenic-neuropsychiatric movement, whether isolated or in the presence of other types of movements, is a shaking movement that resembles tremor (10,18). Another common accompaniment to nonneurologic movements is a peculiar, atypical gait that may reveal lurching, staggering, posturing, excessive slowness, or genuflection (9,21). General clues that a psychogenic movement disorder may be present are summarized in Tables 25-1 and 25-2.

The neurologist's role in establishing the first stage of diagnosis of PNMD is crucial. No mental health professional should commence treatment of such patients without fully understanding the level of confidence with which a neurologic diagnosis has been either ruled out or delimited. If the initial consulting neurologist is unclear about the diagnosis, consultation with a second neurologist who specializes in movement disorders is frequently helpful. It is common for clinicians without extensive experience in the field of movement disorders to attribute a previously unrecognized abnormal movement pattern as PNMD, even though it may actually be organic in etiology. Misdiagnosis in either direction can harm the patient.

TABLE 25-2. *Additional clues that might accompany a nonneurological neuropsychiatric movement disorder*

1. False weakness
2. False sensory complaints
3. Multiple somatizations or undiagnosed conditions
4. Self-inflicted injuries
5. Obvious psychiatric disturbances
6. Employed in the health profession or in health insurance claims
7. Presence of secondary gain, including continuing care by a "devoted" spouse
8. Litigation or compensation pending
9. Demonstrations of overwhelming exhaustion or fatigue

PSYCHIATRIC REFERRAL

The task of a consulting psychiatrist is to clarify the psychopathology present and determine its relevance to the presenting PNMD symptoms. If psychiatric consultation supports the premise of a psychiatrically-based neurologic syndrome, the psychiatrist is favorably situated to take the lead in treatment, with collaborative support from the neurologist. Because patients with PNMD often strongly resist the idea that psychogenic factors are contributing to their physical symptoms (22), collaboration between the referring neurologist and the consulting psychiatrist is crucial.

If the patient experiences the psychiatric referral as a rejection or dismissal and feels that his or her symptoms are presumed to be "purely psychological" and hence unworthy of serious medical attention, the likelihood of successful psychiatric referral is markedly impaired. However, if the neurologist can sympathetically convey to the patient the concept of "stress-related" symptoms, an effective referral to psychiatry may be easier.

Since the most recent review of this topic at our institution (8), the basic approach to engaging patients in the treatment process has diversified. Initially, hospitalizing patients with suspected PNMDs and providing a multidisciplinary treatment plan, including the movement disorder neurologist, the consulting psychiatrist, and often a physical therapist, was found to be highly effective in bringing about symptom remission in many individuals. Our group considered this approach to be the clinical intervention of choice to establish firm confidence regarding the diagnosis, both neurologically and psychiatrically, while enhancing the chances of overcoming the patient's resistance to psychiatric intervention. The patient's acceptance of psychiatric involvement in both diagnosis and treatment was facilitated by having the consulting psychiatrist present from the time of admission.

In recent years, admitting patients with suspected PNMDs to the hospital has become difficult because access to inpatient psychiatric care has become increasingly restricted. On the other hand, while responding to managed care pressures, we have been pleasantly surprised by some positive responses to our current format for outpatient psychiatric consultation and treatment. In this format, an outpatient psychiatric consultation is scheduled when the evaluating neurologist sees a patient with suspected PNMD, before a fully detailed diagnostic impression and treatment recommendation is communicated. The neurologist tells the patient that this psychiatric consultation is needed to evaluate the possible role of stress factors in the development of the symptoms. Then the neurologist and psychiatrist make a collaborative clinical judgment as to whether the patient's physical and psychiatric condition is good enough to sustain an outpatient treatment trial or whether admission to the hospital is required. No therapeutic approach to treating PNMDs has been rigorously evaluated in prospective treatment trials and, therefore, our recommendations remain empiric, the result of an evolving clinical experience.

PSYCHIATRIC DIAGNOSIS

The psychiatric diagnosis for every patient with a PNMD requires exploration of both individual psychodynamics and relevant environmental contingencies. After the initial psychiatric evaluation is completed, a full multiaxial delineation of relevant psychopathology, in accordance with the nomenclature of the latest edition of the *Diagnostic and Statistical Manual* (DSM) of the American Psychiatric Association (23), substantially facilitates the differential diagnosis and associated treatment recommendations.

A movement disorder is proved to be non-neurologic when it completely resolves by psychotherapy, physical therapy, or other supportive, suggestive measures. At times, the remission is sudden and dramatic, though commonly it proceeds gradually. Spontaneous remissions in movement disorders that have an organic basis, such as dystonia, essential tremors, myoclonic disorders, or parkinsonism, are rare. For patients with frequent, prolonged paroxysms of abnormal movements, repeated trials with placebo can be informative. If such trials consistently produce remissions, then one can be convinced that the diagnosis is a documented psychogenic disorder. However, controlled trials with the patient's informed consent are recommended when using placebos, to prevent the patient from losing trust in the treatment team.

The primary psychopathology underlying PNMDs can be subdivided into three categories: *somatoform disorders, factitious disorders,* and *malingering.*

Somatoform Disorders

A somatoform disorder is one in which physical symptoms that cannot be explained by a diagnosable medical condition appear, after careful clinical assessment, to be linked to psychological factors, yet the symptom production is not under voluntary control, that is, not consciously produced (23). The two main types of somatoform disorders that produce psychogenic neurologic problems are conversion disorder and somatization disorder, the latter also known historically as *hysteria* or *Briquet's syndrome*. Other somatoform subtypes are hypochondriasis, pain disorder, body dysmorphic disorder, and undifferentiated somatoform disorder.

In *conversion disorder*, one or more symptoms are present that affect voluntary motor or sensory function and suggest a neurologic or other medical condition. Psychological factors may be judged to play a primary etiologic role in a variety of ways. This role may be suggested by a temporal relationship between the onset or worsening of the symptoms and the presence of an environmental stimulus that activates a psychological conflict or need. Alternatively, the symptom may be noted to free the patient from a noxious activity or encounter. The symptom cannot, after appropriate investigation, be fully explained by a general medical condition, by the direct effects of a substance, or as a culturally sanctioned behavior or experience.

A *somatization disorder* involves recurrent and multiple complaints of several years' duration, for which medical care has been sought, but which are apparently not caused by any physical disorder. The dynamics are presumably the same as those of conversion disorder, and the symptoms may emerge from chronic, recurrent, and untreated conversion disorder (24). Four pain symptoms, two gastrointestinal symptoms, one sexual symptom, and one pseudoneurologic symptom must be present. Other requirements are onset at 30 years of age or younger and symptoms so severe that the patient has taken medications, consulted a physician, or altered his or her lifestyle because of symptoms. An *undifferentiated somatoform disorder* happens when one or more physical symptoms persist for at least 6 months and share somatoform characteristics described above, but the symptom pattern does not meet full criteria for a somatization disorder.

Factitious Disorder

A factitious disorder is one in which the physical symptoms are intentionally produced, and hence under voluntary control, because of a deep psychological need, such as a craving to be cared for by assuming the role of a patient. External incentives for the symptomatic behavior, such as economic gain or avoiding responsibility, are absent. This group of disorders includes Münchausen's syndrome and is generally associated with severe dependent, masochistic, or antisocial personality disorders. Consequently, treatment prognosis is generally less favorable than in cases of somatoform disorder. Features of somatoform and factitious disorder may coexist within the same patient.

Malingering

Malingering consists of physical symptoms voluntarily produced in pursuit of a recognizably pragmatic goal, such as gaining financial compensation, avoiding school or work, evading criminal prosecution, or acquiring drugs. Associated characteristics often include a medical–legal context (e.g., pending litigation), a notable lack of cooperation during diagnostic evaluation and treatment, and the presence of an antisocial personality disorder. Malingering is not considered to be a mental disorder, though it may incorporate extensive coexisting psychopathology.

When faced with a patient who has a psychogenic movement disorder, the distinction among somatoform, factitious, and malingering disorders is often initially uncertain. A patient's volitional intent is often impossible to determine, especially early in the course of assessment, though clarification will often emerge in the course of ongoing evaluation and treatment, depending on the patient's degree of candor and responsiveness. Avoiding a prematurely confrontational stance is important, because a broad spectrum of capacity exists among patients to grasp the hypothesis of unconsciously-based symptom formation. If the clinician erroneously concludes that the patient is being purposefully noncompliant and shifts inappropriately to the adversarial stance that may become inevitable in the case of malingering, the possibility for a therapeutic alliance may be irretrievably lost. Table 25-3 summarizes relevant differential diagnostic subtypes (25).

Comorbid Psychiatric Conditions

A full diagnostic assessment in accordance with the most recent available edition of the DSM will enhance the prospects of effective treatment intervention in patients with PNMD (23). In addition to a primary Axis I diagnosis, most patients with psychogenic movement disorders have a coexisting Axis I diagnosis such as affective disorder, anxiety disorder, or adjustment disorder (8). The lifetime incidence of major depression in somatization disorder is reportedly 80% to 90% (26). Axis II diagnoses, such as developmental disorder and personality disorder, are also common (8). One must, of course, be cognizant of possible coexisting medical illness (Axis III). Specific stressors; sources of personal, familial, or marital conflict; possible symptom modeling; secondary gain (including financial compensation); and other environmental influences must also be identified (Axis IV). A history of physical, sexual, or emotional abuse is often present in patients with conversion disorder (27). A global assessment of psychosocial functioning helps define the extent of functional impairment (Axis V).

An assessment of the relevant psychodynamic and symbolic factors that contribute to the

TABLE 25-3. *PNMDs: Psychiatric differential diagnosis*

	Conscious intentionality	Primary gain	Secondary gain	Coexisting psychopathology	Prognosis
Somatoform disorders	Absent	Repress unacceptable wishes, feelings, or conflicts	Any pragmatic benefits, if present, are secondary	Highly variable: May include affective, anxiety, dissociative, psychotic, developmental, or personality disorders	Highly variable: depending on chronicity, coexisting psychopathology, patient resilience, support network, and treatment
Factitious disorders	Present	Assume the sick role	Generally no major pragmatic benefits; if present, they are secondary	Often includes dependent, histrionic, borderline, or antisocial personality features	Often poor, especially if chronic
Malingering	Present	Pragmatic benefit: financial, legal, drugs	Circumvent authority	Often includes antisocial personality disorder	Symptoms are relinquished only when the goal is either obtained or seen as clearly unobtainable
Psychological factors affecting a medical condition	Variable	None	Any pragmatic benefits, if present, are secondary	Highly variable	Highly variable, depending on the medical condition, chronicity, patient resilience, support network, and treatment
Undiagnosed medical condition	Absent	None	Any pragmatic benefits, if present, are secondary	Highly variable	Depends on the medical condition and the stage at which it is diagnosed and treated

[From Williams, D. (in press) Somatoform disorders. In: Merritt's Neurology, 11th Ed., with permission.]

physical symptoms aids the diagnosis. In conversion disorder, the movement disorder symptoms often arise in relation to a specific stressor. The patient is often unable to appreciate or articulate the relationship between the inciting event and the psychological symptoms, however obvious this relationship may seem to the physician. Conversion symptoms can occur in predisposed individuals who are unable to cope with the everyday demands of life, as well as in healthy subjects who are subjected to unusually stressful situations, such as medical illness (26).

In a series of 24 patients with psychogenic movement disorders who underwent detailed psychiatric evaluation, the profile of a typical patient consisted of a young person (mean age, 36 years; age range, 11 to 60 years), most often female (79%), of average or above average intelligence, with a mean duration of symptoms of 5 years (range, less than 1 month to 23 years), and unable to work and on disability (70% of patients) (8). Dysthymia, as a secondary psychiatric diagnosis, was present in 67% of patients. The remaining diagnoses included a variety of different psychiatric conditions such as major depression, adjustment disorder, organic mood or organic delusional disorders, obsessive–compulsive disorder, panic attacks, bipolar disorder, and others.

A prospective follow-up study assessed psychiatric diagnoses of a series of 42 patients with "hyperkinetic" PNMD (i.e., tremor, dystonia, and myoclonus) an average of 3.2 years after they were first assessed at a tertiary clinic for patients with movement disorders (22). An Axis I diagnosis of mental illness was made in 95% of subjects. Thirty-eight percent of subjects with PNMD had developed additional unexplained medical symptoms at follow-up. Point and lifetime prevalence rates for other Axis I diagnoses were major depression, 12% and 43%; anxiety disorders, 38% and 62%; and comorbid major depression and anxiety disorders, 12% and 27%. Personality disorders were present in 45% of patients. None of the subjects viewed their PNMD as primarily psychiatric in origin.

PATHOPHYSIOLOGY

Little is known about the pathophysiology of PNMDs. Why these disorders occur in certain individuals and why they manifest in specific abnormal movements, is unknown. Freud and Breuer coined the term *conversion* to describe how certain individuals unconsciously repress feelings of extreme helplessness, distress, anger, or conflict by substituting physical symptoms. According to psychodynamic theory, the development of a physical symptom binds unconscious feelings of conflict, leading to a reduction of anxiety and psychological distress, termed *primary gain*. According to Freud and Breuer, the specific physical symptom often embodies the unconscious conflict in symbolic terms (28,29).

Another hypothesis for symptom formation in conversion disorder comes from behavioral learning theory. In this model, conversion symptoms are viewed as sick role behaviors, learned in childhood and unconsciously brought forth as a means of coping with unbearable psychological stress. Sociocultural views of somatoform disorders postulate that unconsciously produced physical symptoms serve to communicate emotionally charged feelings or ideas that would otherwise be unacceptable in the cultural context. Patients may obtain *secondary gain* by using physical symptoms to manipulate their environments so as to obtain recognizable benefits, such as solicitude and attention from a caretaker, or as a means to avoid unpleasant situations or responsibility.

Implicit in the idea of conversion symptoms is the concept of dissociation: a functional separation of aspects of identity, memory, experience, insight, self-perception, and bodily function from the mainstream of conscious awareness (30). The capacity for dissociation may be a precondition for the development of a somatoform disorder. Biologically based studies are beginning to probe the neurologic substrate of conversion and dissociation (30a). Hypnosis, an inducible state of dissociation, can be studied using imaging techniques. Positron emission tomography (PET) activation studies reveal metabolic changes in the anterior cingulate gyrus during hypnosis, a brain region that may play a role in the perceptual and cognitive processing involved in dissociation.

TREATMENT

In the absence of controlled clinical trials specifically for patients with psychogenic-neuropsychiatric movement disorders, empiric treatment has generally focused on those features of psychopathology that can be identified in these patients (31). Therefore, a comprehensive psychiatric assessment is a crucial prerequisite to effective treatment. Those considerations that would ordinarily pertain to treating each category of relevant psychopathology would naturally pertain as well when dealing with a PNMD. This section addresses associated considerations of particular relevance to treating PNMDs.

Traditional treatment strategies for conversion disorders include considerations of predisposition, precipitating factors, and perpetuating factors (29). Predisposition includes personality factors and past experiences that predispose the patient to somatization; intellectual, emotional, or social constraints that limit the patient's ability to communicate; and underlying psychiatric or neurologic disorders. Precipitating stressors may involve activation of psychological conflicts (e.g., regarding sexual, aggressive, or dependency issues) or traumatic events (e.g., those threatening the patient's physical integrity or self-esteem). Perpetuating factors include both the extent to which the symptom resolves the conflict that gave rise to the symptom (primary gain) and associated pragmatic benefits of the symptom (secondary gain).

The goal of effective treatment is not merely to provide symptom relief in the short term, which can often be achieved by suggestion or placebos, but also to consider the factors that produced the symptoms and to assess possible ways to remove them. Implicitly, this treatment involves evaluating the possibility of an underlying psychiatric or neurologic disorder, or both, of which the patient may be unaware (32). This possibility would include situations of past or present physical, emotional, or sexual abuse that may be either consciously suppressed or unconsciously repressed by the patient (33). Often, a combination of psychotherapy to deal with psychological conflicts and practical advice about removing environmental stressors or abusers is required for sustained symptom alleviation. Similarly, treatment must address secondary gains achieved by the symptom, which may contribute to the patient's resistance to relinquishing it.

One may conceptualize a conversion symptom as a "dissociative reaction" whereby the patient is overwhelmed with adversity beyond capacity for conscious processing or expression, leading to a more primitive communication of a "body language expression of distress" (24,34,35). Traditionally, psychodynamic theory focuses on forbidden sexual or aggressive impulses that arouse fears of punitive societal consequences as the predominant source of unconscious repression and conversion into physical symptom formation.

Contemporary perspectives expand the prospective areas of relevant conflict to include a broad array of emotional needs, including dependency, competitive strivings, and self-esteem. The presenting conversion symptom, by removing the patient from responsibility for negotiating an irresolvable conflict, serves a partially protective function, albeit in a regressive and often maladaptive way. If the conversion symptom abates spontaneously after a short-term precipitating stress is resolved, no formal treatment may be needed, and supportive reassurance or suggestion may suffice. Symptom persistence or exacerbation, however, clearly mandates therapeutic intervention to avoid potential chronicity that makes subsequent treatment intervention difficult.

Psychotherapeutic interventions must be mindful of the patient's self-esteem and help generate a more effective adaptive strategy for dealing with preexisting conflicts by a process of emotional and cognitive "restructuring," which enables the patient to cope more effectively, without need for the maladaptive symptom. Such treatment should ideally take into account as many relevant etiologic variables as possible and address them with a systems theory perspective that includes biologic, psychological, and social influences. This intervention is more palatable to the patient if it is presented supportively, with the therapist taking a collaborative stance in helping the patient to improve "stress management" strategies (31).

Hypnosis provides the advantage of giving the patient a direct experience of dissociation under the protective rubric of the therapy setting (30,36). The current tendency to assess hypnotizability with standard scales enables the patient initially to experience a structured "mind-body" dissociative experience of a benign nature in a therapeutic setting. This experience becomes a paradigm through which the patient can be brought to understand that this capacity for dissociation is both a vulnerability to symptom formation and also, when restructured under the guidance of the therapist, a potential conduit for symptom relinquishment. Thus, the therapist can first use the trance experience as an opportunity for transmitting a sophisticated understanding of the dynamics of symptom formation (37). Once this understanding has been achieved in a supportive therapeutic relationship, hypnosis can be used as a vehicle for positive suggestions to improve coping strategies and thereby achieve symptom attenuation (38).

One recent randomized controlled trial attempted to evaluate the additional effect of hypnosis in a comprehensive treatment program for inpatients with persistent conversion disorder of the motor type. Moene et al. (39) treated 45 inpatients between 18 and 65 years of age with these symptoms, using symptom-oriented and insight-oriented techniques. A randomly selected subsample was also treated with hypnosis to ascertain whether this approach would yield additional therapeutic benefits. The comprehensive treatment program, either with or without hypnosis, resulted in significant improvement on all clinical outcome measures for the patient group as a whole. The addition of hypnosis had no extra effect on treatment outcome, and hypnotizability did not predict patient outcome. Further systematic studies of this type with larger patient groups would clearly be of interest.

Behavior therapy has substantial advantages in addressing those contingencies of reinforcement that appear to have contributed to symptom formation and perpetuation. These advantages extend to both primary and secondary gain related to the symptom. Speed (40) has advocated that this approach be used, rather than insight-oriented psychotherapy of the type outlined above. Our preference has been to use both behavior therapy and psychodynamic approaches, in a complementary manner. In this regard, we have found it important to adapt to the intellectual capacities and belief system of the patient when determining what conceptual formulation to use in attempting to instill understanding of how mind-body interactions can evolve on an unconscious basis. Some patients need an intellectual framework to understand the puzzling psychodynamics of unconsciously based mind-body interaction. Others find such an approach irritating, implausible, or insulting. They prefer a structured approach built on a purely "somatic stress" model, with supportive reassurance regarding the "biological" components of their treatment, as a more palatable route to recovery. Our experience favors integrating a behaviorally oriented intervention with an explanatory formulation that is acceptable to the patient.

Physical therapy can be extremely valuable in situations of symptomatic weakness, fixed postures, or gait abnormalities. This approach is effective because it responds directly and supportively to the patient's physical symptom, while allowing psychotherapy to be more readily tolerated at the same time. The physical therapist provides encouragement, reassurance, hands-on intervention, and reinforcement for improvement. For patients who have difficulty grasping or accepting psychodynamic formulations, physical therapy can provide a face-saving mechanism of recovery, provided that other relevant treatment considerations of primary and secondary gain have been diplomatically and effectively dealt with. Physical therapy may also be essential in treating or preventing disuse atrophy or contractures that may develop with more persistent conversion symptoms, as may occur in somatization disorders or undifferentiated somatoform disorders (41).

Pharmacotherapy can serve two valuable functions in treating patients with psychogenic-neuropsychiatric movement disorders. Clearly, pharmacotherapy is indicated for coexisting and often contributory psychiatric conditions, such as depression, anxiety, or psychosis. In addition, the coexistence of identifiable life stressors can often legitimately enable the neurologist and psychiatrist to delineate to patients how stress-induced neurophysiologic alterations in the central nervous system can contribute to physical symptoms through perturbations of neurotransmitter balance in the brain. The clinician can then explain that neuropsychiatric medications have often been able to correct such perturbations and contribute to recovery. In this way, not only may pharmacologic treatment relieve an underlying psychiatric factor contributing to the conversion disorder, but it also can provide a conceptual bridge to help the patient accept a biologic rationale for recovery, even if the patient may not be receptive to postulated psychodynamic formulations.

A variety of other treatment interventions may each play a valuable role in selected patients with conversion-based neuropsychiatric movement disorders. These interventions include family therapy (to deal with contributory conflicts, abuse, dependency, or enabling issues); intravenous amobarbital infusions (particularly to evaluate the possible presence of contractures in cases of fixed, dystonic posturing; or for the differential diagnosis of catatonia); electroconvulsive therapy (for coexisting, treatment-resistant depression or mania); speech therapy (for aphonia, dysarthria, or other neuropsychiatric speech problems); or direct environmental intervention (to deal with contributory stressors or the influence of secondary gain).

Difficult challenges of treating patients with *somatization disorder* and *undifferentiated somatoform disorder* include the chronicity of the course and the proliferation of symptoms. These features frequently generate greater treatment resistance than a relatively short-term conversion disorder. Because relevant psychodynamics in these disorders appear to include intensive help-seeking behavior directed to physicians, one recommendation for general management of these patients is to schedule regular visits with a designated primary physician who can judiciously and supportively monitor presenting symptoms, provide appropriate reassurance, and avoid either ordering unnecessary tests or harshly rebuffing the patient's exaggerated concerns. Continuity with a consistent primary care physician or neurologist, preferably supplemented by regular psychological or psychiatric care, or both, increases the opportunity to provide the supportive measures that diminish anxiety-driven searching for additional medical evaluations (41).

The literature about specific treatment for these disorders is sparse. One randomized controlled trial studied primary care patients with medically unexplained symptoms, a group that presumably included some patients with chronic, polysymptomatic somatoform disorders, though the psychiatric diagnoses in this study are not specifically delineated (42). A greater proportion of patients treated with cognitive-behavioral therapy experienced a decrease in the intensity and number of symptoms, an improvement in functioning, and a decrease in illness behavior. The treatment was delivered in the primary care setting, involving 12 sessions over 8 weeks. Kashner et al. (43) conducted a randomized controlled trial that involved short-term cognitive-behavioral group therapy (8 sessions) for patients with somatization disorder. This treatment reportedly yielded better physical and mental health status than that achieved by the group who did not receive the group therapy. A stance of therapeutic positivism regarding the feasibility of clinical improvement is advisable, even though the extent of improvement varies greatly in this group of disorders.

Even more challenging is the group of *factitious disorders*, in which the patient is aware of his or her purposeful fabrication of physical signs and symptoms but is by definition not fully aware of the underlying pathologic motivation to engage in this self-defeating behavior pattern. In these patients, unlike malingering patients, external pragmatic incentives, if present, play only a secondary role in symptom genesis.

Perhaps the first task in treating patients with factitious disorder is dealing with their physicians' anger when they realize that they have been purposely deceived by a patient who has often consumed much time and other expensive medical resources with a self-inflicted illness (44). To combat the temptation to launch into an unhelpful "unmasking" confrontation, recall that the patient is at least in part a victim of life traumas and deprivations, and of intrinsic, severe psychopathology that led to the presenting, "sick," attention-seeking behavior as a misguided "cry for help." Therefore, humiliating and dismissing the patient will only reinforce the patient's existing assumption that honest exploration of psychological components of his or her illness is likely to be traumatic and disappointing. This kind of confrontation will be counterproductive and will cause the patient's duplicitous and self-defeating illness behavior to persist.

An understandable pessimism is associated with the most severe form of factitious disorder, Munchausen's syndrome, in which the patient relentlessly pursues a lifestyle of unceasing patienthood. However, Reich and Gottfried (45) and Kapfhammer (46) have reported that up to 90% of factitious disorder patients do not have the Munchausen's syndrome variant. This finding suggests the potential merits of supportively presenting a potentially efficacious treatment plan with judicious regard for the patient's self-esteem, so that the prospects of effective therapeutic engagement are enhanced.

When the diagnosis is clarified during a medical hospitalization, the merits of a nonconfrontational, supportive joint debriefing by the neurologist and psychiatrist can be helpful. If the patient is insufficiently insightful, capable, or motivated to respond to an individually oriented clarification of the diagnosis and related treatment recommendations, including (with the patient's consent) relevant family members may be helpful in addressing relevant dependency issues and other behavioral contingencies that require more leverage for effective implementation than the patient alone can provide. In all such discussions, efforts should be made to emphasize those factors that contributed to the patient's illness that were outside of the patient's awareness, control, or both, in the interest of preserving the patient's self-esteem and, ideally, cultivating a nascent therapeutic alliance. As with somatoform disorders, effectively treating coexisting depression, anxiety, psychosis, or other coexisting psychopathology substantially increases one's prospects of effectively alleviating the presenting PNMD symptoms. Also as with somatoform disorders, a variety of reorienting techniques, geared to replace regressive somatization with more appropriate coping strategies, are available. However, for some treatment-resistant patients who present a serious danger to themselves, initial transfer to a closed psychiatric unit may be essential to protect them.

With regard to *malingering*, addressing management, rather than treatment, is most appropriate, insofar as malingering is not considered to be a psychiatric disorder (44). We have already addressed the need to approach the diagnosis of malingering only after thoroughly exploring and excluding other treatable causes of presenting PNMD symptoms. Dealing with the malingering patient still presents considerable challenges. First, recall that angry confrontation of the patient is unlikely to help anyone and may be harmful to the physician, the patient, or both in a variety of ways. If the patient presents at the outset with a clear pending litigation issue, formally request, in writing, all prior medical information of relevance and obtain written permission to speak with the patient's attorney and to prepare a written report, before actually doing so. Making a tactful but forthright statement to the patient about one's findings is advisable, but it may be judicious to do so in the presence of a supportive independent observer, in case of an unanticipated angry reaction by the patient. Having access to the patient's attorney can have the added potential benefit of providing another route of influence to the patient, because malingering patients are unlikely to relinquish their symptoms until their pragmatic goal is either achieved or recognized as not realistically attainable. The patient's attorney potentially can be helpful in educating the patient about the chances of success.

PROGNOSIS

The prognosis for any particular patient with a psychogenic-neuropsychiatric movement disorder is influenced by a variety of factors, including the nature, chronicity, and severity of the underlying psychopathology and external stressors; the intrinsic strengths and resilience of the patient; and the effectiveness of the patient's support system, including the appropriateness and effectiveness of treatment. Neither published reports nor our clinical experience contain any indication that the physically presenting form of the movement disorder has influence on the prognosis.

Follow-up studies of patients with *untreated* somatoform disorder suggest that the general outcome in these patients is poor and that spontaneous resolution of symptoms is uncommon. One recent study of 73 patients with "unexplained medical symptoms" who were admitted to the hospital, with a presumed substantial representation of neuropsychiatric somatoform symptoms, found that the index symptom was unimproved or worse in more than half the patients after 6-years of follow-up (47). A comparable outcome was reported in a 4-year follow-up study of 70 patients with conversion disorder or somatization disorder (48). Indeed, the pattern of recurrent, undiagnosed, or untreated conversion disorder in childhood and adolescence has been postulated, on the basis of follow-up studies, to lead developmentally to the more chronic and treatment-resistant features of somatization disorder (24).

Relatively speaking, a better prognosis is associated with conversion disorder in patients who have been hospitalized if they are younger than 40, with a short duration of symptoms, have had a recent change in marital status, and experience expeditious symptom remission by the end of hospital admission (49). Several studies suggest that the presence of an underlying treatable psychiatric disorder, such as depressive disorder or anxiety disorder, connotes a more favorable prognosis (47,49). By contrast, the presence of a personality disorder, pending litigation, and current or prospective secondary gain in the form of financial compensation is associated with a poorer prognosis (50). Furthermore, simply receiving medical treatment does not by itself predict better outcome. A 10-year follow-up study of 73 patients with conversion disorder found that patients with the most primary physician contact had the least likelihood of symptom remission (50). Finally, Feinstein's (22) follow-up study of 42 patients who were reassessed an average of 3.2 years after initial diagnosis with PNMD, with no indication of intervening psychiatric treatment, found that abnormal movements and associated psychopathology persisted in 90% of subjects. Thus, the data currently available suggests that benign neglect of these patients, rather than providing referral for psychiatric treatment, is probably unwise.

A relatively sanguine prognosis is suggested for patients with neuropsychiatric somatoform disorder, when treated with the type of integrated and relatively intensive treatment strategy advocated in this chapter. In the series of 24 patients reported by our group (8), all patients who responded to treatment had conversion disorder or somatization disorder. None of those with factitious disorder or malingering improved. This was not a controlled, prospective study, however, and the diagnoses of some patients changed to a more pathologic variant during the course of evaluation and treatment, as signs of uncooperativeness, purposeful dissimulation, and personality disorder emerged. For patients with somatoform disorder, favorable outcome was not correlated with such variables as age at onset, gender, intelligence level, or specific movement disorder phenomenology. In this retrospective review, the integrated treatment strategy outlined in this chapter resulted in sustained improvement (longer than 1 year) in 54% of patients. Complete symptom resolution was achieved in 25%, considerable improvement in 21%, and moderate improvement in 8% by the end of active treatment. Patients considered not significantly improved included 22% with modest improvement and 12% with no improvement. Some relapse after initial improvement was observed over time in about 20% of patients, as determined when contacted at follow-up. Of those who were functioning actively before the onset of their neuropsychiatric symptoms, 25% were reemployed full-time at the conclusion of treatment, 10% were employed part-time, and 15% were normally functional as homemakers or students. Although a long duration of symptoms has been associated with less favorable prognoses in other series of such patients (14,49), we have encountered several patients with chronic illness who, with effective diagnostic clarification and active treatment, were able to achieve complete and sustained symptom resolution. We note this outcome in an effort to dispel a self-fulfilling therapeutic nihilism in approaching such patients.

SUMMARY

Patients with PNMDs pose a fascinating challenge to clinicians at the neurology-psychiatry interface. We have outlined a diagnostic and therapeutic approach to these complex disorders. Patients with PNMDs typically manifest abnormal movements and postures that do not fit expected patterns of movement disorder phenomenology. The first goal of neurologic consultation is to make an accurate diagnosis, with a view to either ruling out or defining the extent of any organic substrate. The next task is an effective referral to a psychiatrist capable of diagnosing relevant psychopathology and collaborating in a treatment plan. A supportive explanation of the diagnosis, one that is sensitive to the patient's intellectual capacity, conception of the illness, and self-esteem, appears to be a crucial determinant that influences the patient's capacity to be engaged effectively in treatment. The treatment for each patient with PNMD is individualized and may include psychotherapy, hypnosis, pharmacotherapy, physical therapy, and other approaches. To date, no treatment approach has been shown to be superior, and very few long-term outcome data are available. Although many factors influence response to treatment, those of particular importance are the effectiveness of communication among the neurologist, the psychiatrist, and the patient; the nature, severity, and chronicity of relevant psychopathology and environmental stressors; and the quality of external support and intrinsic resources available to the patient.

ACKNOWLEDGMENTS

The authors are indebted to Drs. Steven Frucht, Paul Greene, Pietro Mazzoni, and Amir Raz for their clinical collaboration and insights that contributed to this chapter.

REFERENCES

1. Okun MS, Koehler PJ. Babinski's clinical differentiation of organic paralysis from hysterical paralysis. *Arch Neurol* 2004;61:778–783.
2. Freud S. Quelques considerations pour une etude comparative des paralysies motrices organiques et hysteriques. *Arch Neurol (Paris)* 1893;26:29–43.
2a. Freud S. Studies on Hysteria. 1893.
3. Williams D, Fahn S, Ford B, et al. Natural history of neuropsychiatric movement disorders. In: Hallett M, Fahn S, Jankovic J et al., eds. *Psychogenic movement disorders: psychobiology and therapy of a functional disorder, Advances in neurology*. Philadelphia, PA: Lippincott Williams & Wilkins, 2005.
3a. Crimlisk HL, Bhatia KP, Cope H, et al. Patterns of referral in patients with unexplained medical symptoms. *J Psychosom Res* 2000;49:217–219.
4. Marsden CD. Hysteria—a neurologist's view. *Psychol Med* 1986;16:277–288.
5. Lempert T, Dietrich M, Huppert D, et al. Psychogenic disorders in neurology: frequency and clinical spectrum. *Acta Neurol Scand* 1990;82:335–340.
6. Krumholz A, Niedermeyer E. Psychogenic seizures: a clinical study with follow-up data. *Neurology* 1983;33:498–502.
7. Lesser RP, Lueders H, Dinner DS. Evidence for epilepsy is rare in patients with psychogenic seizures. *Neurology* 1983;33:502–504.
8. Williams DT, Ford B, Fahn S. Phenomenology and psychopathology related to psychogenic movement disorders. *Adv Neurol* 1995;65:231–257.
9. Keane JR. Hysterical gait disorders: 60 cases. *Neurology* 1989;39:586–589.
10. Koller W, Lang A, Vetere-Overfield B, et al. Psychogenic tremors. *Neurology* 1989;39:1094–1099.
11. Ranawaya R, Riley D, Lang A. Psychogenic dyskinesias in patients with organic movement disorders. *Mov Disord* 1990;5:127–133.
12. Dooley JM, Stokes A, Gordon KE. Pseudo-tics in Tourette syndrome. *J Child Neurol* 1994;9(2):50–51.
13. Monday K, Jankovic J. Psychogenic myoclonus. *Neurology* 1993;43:349–352.
14. Factor SA, Podskalny GD, Molho ES. Psychogenic movement disorders: frequency, clinical profile, and characteristics. *J Neurol Neurosurg Psychiatry* 1995;59:406–412.
15. Lang AE. Psychogenic dystonia: a review of 18 cases. *Can J Neurol Sci* 1995;22:136–143.
16. Lang AE, Koller WG, Fahn S. Psychogenic parkinsonism. *Arch Neurol* 1995a;52:802–810.
17. Deuschl G, Koster B, Lucking Ch, et al. Diagnostic and pathophysiological aspects of psychogenic tremors. *Mov Disord* 1998;13:294–302.
18. Kim YJ, Pakiam ASI, Lang AE. Historical and clinical features of psychogenic tremor: a review of 70 cases. *Can J Neurol Sci* 1999;26:190–195.
19. Miyasaki JM, Sa DS, Galvez-Jiminez M, et al. Psychogenic movement disorders. *Can J Neurol Sci* 2003;30(Suppl. 1):S94–S100.
20. Thomas M, Jankovic J. Psychogenic movement disorders: diagnosis and management. *CNS Drugs* 2004;18:437–452.
21. Vecht CJ, Meerwaldt JD, Lees AJ, et al. Unusual movement disorder, Case 1, 1991. Unusual tremor, myoclonus and a limping gait. *Mov Disord* 1991;6:371–375.
22. Feinstein A, Stergiopoulos V, Fine J, et al. Psychiatric outcome in patients with a psychogenic movement disorder: a prospective study. *Neuropsychiatry Neuropsychol Behav Neurol* 2001;14:169–176.
23. American Psychiatric Association. *Diagnostic and statistical manual of mental disorders*, 4th ed., Text Revision. Washington, DC: American Psychiatric Association, 2000.
24. Williams DT. Somatoform disorders, factitious disorders and malingering. In: Noshpitz J, ed. *Handbook of child and adolescent psychiatry*, Vol. 2. New York: John Wiley and Sons, 1997:563–578.
25. Williams DT. Somatoform disorders. In: Rowland LP, ed. *Merritt's neurology*, 11th ed. Philadelphia, PA: Lippincott Williams & Wilkins, 2005:1140–1145.
26. Kellner R. *Psychosomatic syndromes and somatic symptoms*. Washington, DC: American Psychiatric Press, 1991.
27. Lazare A. Conversion symptoms. *N Engl J Med* 1981;305(13):745–748.
28. Freud S. The etiology of hysteria (1896), in *Collected papers, Vol. 1*. Translated and edited by Strachey J. London: Hogaith Press, 1946:183–219.
29. Ford CV. Conversion disorder and somatoform disorder not otherwise specified. In: Gabbard GO. ed. *Treatment of psychiatric disorders*, 3rd ed., Vol. 2. Washington, DC: American Psychiatric Association, 2001:1755–1776.
30. Spiegel H, Spiegel D. *Trance and treatment: clinical uses of hypnosis*, 2nd ed. Washington, DC: American Psychiatric Publishing, 2004.
30a. Vuilleumier P, Chicerio C, Assal F, et al. Functional neuroanatomical correlates of hysterical sensorimotor loss. *Brain* 2001;124:1077–1090.
31. Ford B, Williams DT, Fahn S. Treatment of psychogenic movement disorders. In: Kurlan R, ed. *Treatment of movement disorders*. Philadelphia, PA: JB Lippincott Co, 1994:475–485.
32. Bowman ES. Pseudoseizures. *Psychiatr Cin North Am* 1998;21:649–657.
33. Roelofs K, Keijsers GP, Hoogduin KA, et al. Child abuse in patients with conversion disorder. *Am J Psychiatry* 2002a;159:1908–1913.
34. Spitzer C, Spelsberg B, Grabe HJ, et al. Dissociative experiences and psychopathology in conversion disorders. *J Psychosom Res* 1999;46:291–294.
35. Hallett M. Voluntary and involuntary movements in humans. In: Hallett M, Fahn S, Jankovic J et al., eds. *Psychogenic movement disorders: psychobiology and therapy of a functional disorder, Advances in neurology*. Philadelphia, PA: Lippincott Williams & Wilkins, 2005.

36. Raz A, Shapiro T. Hypnosis and neuroscience: a cross talk between clinical and cognitive research. *Arch Gen Psychiatry* 2002;59(1):85–90.
37. Roelofs K, Hoogduin KA, Keijsers GP, et al. Hypnotic susceptibility in patients with conversion disorder. *J Abnorm Psychol* 2002;111:390–395.
38. Williams DT. Hypnosis. In: Weiner J, Duncan M, eds. *Textbook of child & adolescent psychiatry*, 3rd ed. Washington, DC: American Psychiatric Press, 2004: 1043–1054.
39. Moene FC, Spinhoven P, Hoodguin KA, et al. A randomized clinical trial on the additional effect of hypnosis in a comprehensive treatment program for inpatients with conversion disorder of the motor type. *Psychother Psychosom* 2002;71:66–76.
40. Speed J. Behavioral management of conversion disorder: retrospective study. *Arch Phys Med Rehabil* 1996; 77:147–154.
41. Smith GR. Somatization disorder and undifferentiated somatoform disorder. In: Gabbard GO, ed. *Treatment of psychiatric disorders*, 3rd ed., Vol. 2. Washington, DC: American Psychiatric Association, 2001:1735–1753.
42. Speckens AE, van Hembert AM, Spinhoven P, et al. Cognitive behavioral therapy for medically unexplained physical symptoms: a randomized controlled trial. *Br Med J* 1995;311:1328–1332.
43. Kashner TM, Rost K, Cohen B, et al. Enhancing the health of somatization disorder patients: effectiveness of short-term group therapy. *Psychosomatics* 1995;36: 462–470.
44. Eisendrath SJ. Factitious disorders and malingering. In: Gabbard GO, ed. *Treatment of psychiatric disorders*, 3rd ed., Vol. 2. Washington, DC: American Psychiatric Association, 2001:1825–1842.
45. Reich P, Gottfried LA. Factitious disorders in a teaching hospital. *Ann Intern Med* 1983;99:240–247.
46. Kapfhammer HP, Rothenheausler HB, Dietrich E, et al. Artifactual disorders—between deception and self-mutilation: experiences in consultation psychiatry at a university clinic. *Nevenarzt* 1998;69:401–409.
47. Crimlisk HL, Bhatia K, Cope H, et al. 6 year follow-up study of patients with medically unexplained symptoms. *Br Med J* 1998;316:582–586.
48. Kent DA, Tomasson K, Corvell W. Course and outcome of conversion and somatization disorders: a four-year follow-up. *Psychosomatics* 1995;36:138–144.
49. Couprie W, Wijdicks EFM, Rooijmans HGM, et al. Outcome in conversion disorder: a follow up study. *J Neurol Neurosurg Psychiatry* 1995;58:750–752.
50. Mace CJ, Trimble MR. Ten year prognosis of conversion disorder. *Br J Psychiatry* 1996;169:282–288.

Subject Index

A

Activities of daily living, and depression in Parkinson's disease (PD), 29, 32, 78, 91
Acute disseminated encephalomyelitis, 329
Acute rheumatic fever, in autoimmune-mediated movement disorders, 323
Adolescents, with dystonia, 291, 292, 293, 294, 298
Affective disorders
    and basal ganglia dysfunction, 18
    in Huntington's disease (HD), 202
    tardive dyskinesia, 336–349, 343
Age factors in Parkinson's disease (PD)
    cognitive decline, 84–85, 97, 144
    dementia, 84, 156–157
    depression, 84
Aggression
    in Huntington's disease (HD), 201, 268, 269, 271
Agranulocytosis, clozapine therapy, 121
Akathisia, 50, 200
Akinesia, psychic, 8
    in Huntington's disease (HD), 201
Alcoholism
    essential tremor (ET), 288–289
    in Huntington's disease (HD), 204
    and Parkinson's disease (PD), 60, 125
Alien limb phenomenon, 176
Alzheimer's disease (AD)
    and dementia in Parkinson's disease (PD), 157
    language, 100
    and late Parkinson's disease (PD), 78
    Lewy bodies, 148
    in Parkinson's disease (PD), 98
    secondary parkinsonism, 160
    subcortical dementia, 104, 151, 168, 210
    visuospatial skills, 199
Amantadine
    and depression in Parkinson's disease (PD), 44, 49
    psychosis induced by, 120
Amygdala, and nucleus accumbens, 1, 2
Amyloid precursor protein (APP), in Lewy bodies, 153
Amyotrophic lateral sclerosis (ALS), 177–179
Anhedonia, in Parkinson's disease (PD), 8, 26, 29, 136
Anti-basal ganglia antibodies, in autoimmune-mediated movement disorders, 325
Anticholinergic therapy
    in Parkinson's disease (PD)
        cognitive decline, 85
        depression, 44, 48, 85
    psychosis induction, 115, 120
Anxiety
    in autoimmune-mediated movement disorders, 324
    drug-induced, in Parkinson's disease (PD), 119–120
    in Huntington's disease (HD), 203
    in Pediatric autoimmune neuropsychiatric disorders associated with streptococcal infections (PANDAS), 327
    in Sydenham's chorea, 324
    in tardive dyskinesia, 341
    in Tourette's syndrome (TS), 242
    in Wilson's disease, 267
Anxiety disorders, in Parkinson's disease (PD)
    and antiparkinsonian medications, 44–45
    Beck Anxiety Inventory (BAI), 51
    brain localization, 48
    criteria, 42
    and dementia, 46
    and depression, 45–46
    central nervous system (CNS), 51
    cholecystokinin (CCK), 47
    chronic obstructive pulmonary disease (COPD), 43
    deep brain stimulation (DBS), 51
    depressive symptoms, 49
    dopamine, 47
    DSM-IV criteria, 42
    essential tremor (ET), 50
    etiology, 46–48
    features of, 43–44
        generalized anxiety disorder (GAD), 43
        obsessive–compulsive disorder (OCD), 44
        panic disorder, 43
        range of disorders, 43
        social phobia, 43
    gamma-aminobutyric acid (GABA), 47
    generalized anxiety disorder (GAD), 42
    hydroxytryptamine (5-HT2), 47
    left-sided hemiparkinsonism (LHP), 48
    levodopa therapy, 44, 45
    monoamine oxidase (MAO), 49
    monoamine oxidase inhibitors (MAOI), 48
    and motor fluctuations, 45
    National Alliance for Research in Schizophrenia and Depression (NARSD), 52
    neuropsychiatric inventory (NPI), 50
    norepinephrine, 47
    obsessive–compulsive disorder (OCD), 43
    obsessive–compulsive personality disorder (OCP), 44
    obsessive–compulsive symptoms (OCS), 44
    Parkinson study group (PSG), 51
    prevalence of, 42
    rapid eye movement behavior disorder (RBD), 50
    right-sided hemiparkinsonism (RHP), 48
    selective serotonin reuptake inhibitors (SSRI), 48
    serotonin, 47

Anxiety disorders, in Parkinson's disease (PD) (contd.)
  single photon emission computed tomography
      (SPECT), 47
  traditional tricyclic antidepressants (TCA), 48
  treatment of, 48–51
    antiparkinsonian agents, 48
    benzodiazepines, 49
    buspirone, 49
    cholinesterase inhibitors, 50
    medication interactions, 50
    pharmacotherapy, 48
    serotonin norepinephrine reuptake inhibitors
        (SNRIs), 50
    selective serotonin reuptake inhibitors
        (SSRIs), 49
    surgery, 51
  Unified Parkinson's Disease Rating Scale
      (UPDRS), 46
Apathy
  in Huntington's disease (HD), 201–202
  in Parkinson's disease (PD), 56–57, 142
Apathy evaluation scale (AES), in Parkinson's disease
    (PD), 57
Aphasia
  in cortical-basal ganglionic degeneration, 176–177
  in early Parkinson's disease (PD), 86
  in Huntington's disease (HD), 210
Apraxia
  in cortical-basal ganglionic degeneration, 175–176
  in early Parkinson's disease (PD), 86
Aripiprazole, for Parkinson's disease (PD), 122
Arithmetic test, frontal lobe dysfunction, 20
Arthritis, comparison with Parkinson's disease (PD), 43
Ataxia
  hereditary, 275–281
  in olivopontocerebellar atrophy, 170
Atrophy
  in Huntington's disease (HD), 198
Attention
  in Huntington's disease (HD), 215
  in Sydenham's chorea, 324
Attention and memory functioning, in Parkinson's
    disease (PD), dementia, 100
Attention-deficit/hyperactivity disorder (ADHD), 242
  comorbidity with other behavior disorders, 242
  pharmacological treatment
    guanfacine, 256
  and Tourette's syndrome (TS), 242, 243, 244
Autoactivation deficit and basal ganglia dysfunction, 18
Autoaggressive immune-mediated disorders. (AAIMD).
    See Movement disorders
Autoimmune-mediated movement disorders, 320–335
  definition, 320
Autoimmunity, 320–323
Automated Psychological Test (APT), in Wilson's
    disease, 271
Autonomic nervous system dysfunction, in striatonigral
    degeneration, 172

Autosomal dominant ataxias, 275–280
  behavioral abnormalities, 275
  cerebellar degeneration
      and multisystem atrophy, 280
  cognition/psychiatric symptoms, cerebellar
      degeneration, 280
  dentatorubral–pallidosylvian atrophy, 279–280
  episodic, 280
  Friedreich's ataxia, 275
  Machado–Joseph's disease (MJD), 277
  spinocerebellar ataxia (SCAs), 275–279

B

Basal ganglia
  abnormalities, in Huntington's disease (HD), 221
  amnesic syndrome, 20
  anatomical framework, 2
  in autoimmune-mediated movement disorders, 320, 323
  behavioral domains, 1–10
  calcification, 166
  cholinergic stimulation in, 338
  cognitive domain models, 5
  cognitive system, 6
  corticobasal ganglionic degeneration
      and behavior, 1–10
  disturbances, 320
  dorsolateral prefrontal circuit, 2, 6
  in essential tremor, 286
  focal lesions
    behavioral disturbances, 17–19
      autoactivation deficit, 18
      blunted affect, 18
      frequency of, 18
      inertia, 17–18
      mental emptiness, 18
      stereotyped activities and compulsions, 19
    cognitive disturbances, 19–21
      instrumental activities, 19
      intellectual efficiency, 19
      learning, procedural, 20
      memory, explicit, 20
  focal lesions, 17–25
  functional imaging, 6–7
  functional magnetic resonance imaging (fMRI), 21
  in Huntington's disease (HD), 198, 199
  and magnetic resonance imaging (MRI), 19
  in obsessive–compulsive disorder (OCD), 254
  in paraneoplastic disorders, 331
  in Sydenham's chorea, 325
  in Tourette's syndrome (TS), 253
  lateral, medial orbitofrontal, and cingulate circuits, 21
  neuropsychiatric disorders, 17, 21
  memory domains, 5
  motor models, 4
  motor system, 6
  neurophysiology of, 4
  nonmotor sphere, 21
  obsessive–compulsive disorder (OCD), 6

SUBJECT INDEX

Basal ganglia (*contd.*)
  Parkinson's disease (PD), as paradigm, 7–9
  psychiatric models, 5
  Tourette's syndrome (TS), 6
Beck Depression Inventory (BDI)
  in dystonia, 295
  in Parkinson's disease (PD), 29, 91, 140, 174
Beck Rating Scales, in olivopontocerebellar atrophy, 171
Behavior therapy, for obsessive–compulsive disorder, (OCD), 257
Behavior, and basal ganglia lesions. *See* Basal ganglia
Behavioral abnormalities
  personality changes
    in Huntington's disease (HD), 201
Behavioral and psychiatric symptoms
  aggression, in Huntington's disease (HD), 201
  in Huntington's disease (HD), 197–205
  irritability, in Huntington's disease (HD), 199
  suicide rates in Huntington's disease (HD), 202
Behavioral changes
  in frontotemporal dementia, 187–195
  in parkinson-plus syndromes, 166–182
Behçet's syndrome, 331
Benton's Facial Recognition Task, 87
Beta-N-methylaminoalanine, 177
Bipolar disorders
  tardive dyskinesia, 341
Blepharospasm, in psychogenic movement disorders, 291
Blessed Information Memory Concentration (BIMC), 152
Blood flow, cerebral
  in Parkinson's disease (PD), 5
Blunted affect, and basal ganglia dysfunction, 18
Boston Naming Test
  in early Parkinson's disease (PD), 86
Botulinum injections, for torticollis, 301
Botulinum toxin, for dystonia, 313
Bradykinesia
  in autoimmune movement disorders, 330
  in early Parkinson's disease (PD), 90
  in psychogenic movement disorders, 350
Bradyphrenia, in Parkinson's disease (PD), 167
Brain imaging
  in Huntington's disease (HD), 198–199
Brain stem Lewy bodies, 148
Brain
  in autoimmune-mediated movement disorders, 323
  in Wilson's disease, 262, 263
Brief Test of Attention, in Huntington's disease (HD), 215
Briquet's syndrome, 353
Bromocriptine therapy
  in early Parkinson's disease (PD), 44, 85, 115, 126
Brown–Peterson Distractor Task, 88, 173
Buspirone, 256

C

CAG repeat in DNA, in Huntington's disease (HD), 197, 198, 209, 226
Carbidopa, and depression in Parkinson's disease (PD), 44, 71, 114, 121
Catatonia, 358
  in encephalitis lethargica, 330
Caudate nucleus
  in Huntington's disease (HD), 198, 215, 217
  lesions of, 19, 20
Central nervous system (CNS) lesions, psychotic symptoms, 180
Centre médian-parafascicular (CM/Pf), in basal ganglia, 3
Cerebellum, olivopontocerebellar atrophy, 172
Cerebrospinal fluid (CSF), in Parkinson's disease (PD), 29
Ceruloplasmin, in Wilson's disease, 262, 264, 265
Child Behavior Checklist (CBCL) in tics, 244
Children, with dystonia, 315
Chlorpromazine
  in tardive dyskinesia, 337
Choline acetyltransferase
  in diffuse Lewy body disease, 149
  in late Parkinson's disease (PD), 103
  in progressive supranuclear palsy, 169
Cholinesterase inhibitors, in Parkinson's disease (PD), 106
Chorea, 197
  absence of, in Huntington's disease (HD), 197
  in children, 324
  in systemic autoimmune disorders, 331
Chorea gravidarum, 331
Chorea insaniens, 325
Choreic temperament, in autoimmune-mediated movement disorders, 324
Chromosome 4, and Huntington's disease (HD), 197
Chronic neurodegenerative disease, as Parkinson's disease (PD), 65–81
Churg–Strauss syndrome, 331
Cigarette smoking, and Parkinson's disease (PD), 98
Circuits, basal ganglia, 3–5
Citalopram
  for obsessive–compulsive behavior (OCB), 255
Classification. *See also* DSM-IIIR criteria
  psychogenic movement disorders, 291
    clinically established, 308, 309
    documented, 308
    possible, 308
    probable, 308
Clomipramine, for obsessive–compulsive behavior (OCB), 200, 254, 255
Clonazepam
  for obsessive–compulsive disorder (OCD), 256
Clonidine
  for obsessive–compulsive disorder, 256
Clozapine, for Parkinson's disease (PD), 120–123
Cognitive function
  and basal ganglia. *See* Basal ganglia, focal lesions
  in cortical-basal ganglionic degeneration, 177
  impairment *vs.* dementia, 155–156
  in Parkinson's disease (PD), 29, 35, 46, 95, 105. *See also* Parkinson's disease (PD)
  in progressive supranuclear palsy, 167–170
  in tardive dyskinesia, 341–342
  in Wilson's disease, 268

Cognitive symptoms
  in Huntington's disease (HD), 199
Complete blood count (CBC), in clozapine therapy, 121
Comprehension
  in early Parkinson's disease (PD), 86
  in Huntington's disease (HD), 218
Comprehensive Psychopathological Rating Scale (CPRS)
  for obsessional–compulsive inventory 252
  in Wilson's disease, 271
Compulsions
  obsessive–compulsive disorder (OCD), and basal
    ganglia dysfunction, 19
Conduct disorder, in Huntington's disease (HD), 204
Contamination fears
  in autoimmune-mediated movement disorders, 327
  in obsessive–compulsive disorder (OCD), 251
  in pediatric autoimmune neuropsychiatric disorders
    associated with streptococcal infections
    (PANDAS), 327
Contrast sensitivity, in early Parkinson's disease (PD), 90
Conversion disorder, 353
Copper. *See* Wilson's disease
Core Assessment Program for Surgical Intervention
  Therapies in Parkinson's Disease
  (CAPSIT-PD), 140
Corneal copper, in Wilson's disease, 262
Cortical-basal ganglionic degeneration, 175–177, 195
  alien limb phenomenon, 176
  aphasia, 176
  apraxia, 175–176
  cognitive disturbances and dementia, 177
  cognitive dysfunction, 195
  features of, 195
  neglect, 177
  visuospatial and constructional deficits, 177
Corticostriatal–putaminal–thalamic–cortical (CSPTC),
    in Parkinson's disease (PD), 29
Counseling, risk groups for Huntington's disease (HD), 233
Creutzfeldt–Jakob disease (CJD), 180–181

D

Decision making, in Huntington's disease (HD), 215
Deep brain stimulation (DBS)
  in basal ganglia, 1
  for obsessive–compulsive disorder (OCD), 257
  in Parkinson's disease (PD), 130
  surgery, in Parkinson's disease (PD), 31
Delirium, drug-induced, 115–117, 123
Delusions
  drug-induced, 115–117
  in diffuse Lewy body disease, 152
  in Huntington's disease (HD), 203
  in tardive dyskinesia, 337, 342
Dementia
  cortical, in Huntington's disease (HD), 210
  vs. cognitive impairment, 155
  in cortical-basal ganglionic degeneration, 177
  definition of, 210
  in diffuse Lewy body disease, 150–151
  frontal system, 167
  frontotemporal, 214
  in Huntington's disease (HD). *See* Huntington's disease
    (HD)
  and Lewy bodies, 150
  in olivopontocerebellar atrophy, 170
  in Parkinson's disease (PD). *See* Parkinson's disease (PD)
  and parkinsonism-dementia/amyotrophic lateral
    sclerosis (ALS), 178
  subcortical, 17, 167, 168, 169, 172, 173, 178
    in Huntington's disease (HD), 210
Dementia Rating Scale, Huntington's disease (HD), 213
Dementia with Lewy bodies (DLB), 56, 116
Dementia
  anxiety, 46
  in Parkinson's disease (PD), 95–106
Dementia–disinhibition–parkinsonism–amyotrophy
    syndrome, 187
Depression
  in chorea gravidarum, 331
  in dystonia, 293, 294
  in early Parkinson's disease (PD), 91
  in essential tremor, 286–287
  in Huntington's disease (HD), 199, 212
  in olivopontocerebellar atrophy, 171
  in Parkinson's disease (PD), 6, 26–37
    biochemical and organic viewpoint
      unifying hypothesis, 34
    biological markers, 30–32
      neuroimaging, 31
      neuropathology, 30
      surgery, 31
    diagnosis, 29–30
    etiology, 32–35
      biological, 33
      reactive, 34
    psychosocial aspects
      disease-related factors
        age of onset, 84
        stage of illness, 66
        symptom severity, 27, 28, 46, 73, 84
    treatment, 35–37
  in tardive dyskinesia, 341
  in Tourette's syndrome (TS), 245
  in Wilson's disease, 267, 268
Diabetes, comparison with Parkinson's disease (PD), 71
Diagnostic Interview Schedule for Children (DISC),
    in tics, 244
Diagonal band of Broca (DBB), in Parkinson's
    disease (PD), 103
Diffuse cortical Lewy bodies, 148–160
  in neurodegenerative disorders, 148–160
Diffuse Lewy body disease. *See* Lewy bodies
Disability, and depression in Parkinson's disease (PD),
    28, 35, 174
DNA
  amplification, in Huntington's disease (HD), 198

SUBJECT INDEX

Dopamine
  in basal ganglia circuitry, 1
  in dystonia, 305
  in Parkinson's disease (PD), 1, 28, 30
  in progressive supranuclear palsy, 169
  in tardive dyskinesia, 338
Dopamine agonists (DA), in Parkinson's disease (PD), 124
Dopamine dysregulation syndrome, in Parkinson's disease (PD), 61
Dopamine supersensitivity, in tardive dyskinesia, 337–338
Dorsal raphe nuclei (DRN), in Parkinson's disease (PD), 104
Dorsolateral prefrontal circuit, 2, 6
Down's syndrome, and Parkinson's disease (PD), 157
Dreaming abnormalities, drug-induced, 117
Drug-induced psychosis (DIP), in Parkinson's disease (PD), 121
Drugs, in Parkinson's disease (PD), 35
DSM-IIIR criteria
  dementia
    vs. cognitive impairment, 155
    in obsessive–compulsive disorder (OCD), 324
    in Parkinson's disease (PD), 27, 42, 46, 84, 91, 95, 156, 173
  dystonia, 296
  psychiatric morbidity, 295
  tic disorders, 241
DSM-IV criteria
  dementia in Huntington's disease (HD), 210, 212
  obsessive–compulsive disorder (OCD), 252
DSM-IV-TR criteria, in Parkinson's disease (PD), 155
Dynorphin
  in basal ganglia circuitry, 2
  in Tourette's syndrome (TS), 2
Dysarthria
  in Huntington's disease (HD), 202, 218
  in Wilson's disease, 263
Dysexecutive syndrome
  basal ganglia, 17
Dysphonia, 20
Dysprosodia, 20
Dystonia
  in autoimmune-mediated movement disorders, 330
  definition, 291
  drug-induced, 291
  paraneoplastic, 332
    psychiatric disturbance in, 306–312
  psychiatric manifestations, 291
  psychiatric morbidity in, 305–306
  psychogenic, 306–312
    diagnosis of, 306–312
  in psychogenic movement disorders, 351.
    See also Psychogenic disorders
  psychosocial dysfunction in, 305–306
  psychosocial functioning, 298
  stigma in, 301–302
  types of, 291
  in Wilson's disease, 264
Dystonia Society in United Kingdom, 306

E

Electroconvulsive therapy
  in Parkinson's disease (PD), 37
  in late Parkinson's disease (PD), 170
  for psychosis in Parkinson's disease (PD), 120
Electroencephalogram (EEG)
  in diffuse Lewy body disease, 152
  psychogenic dystonia, 308
Electromyography (EMG)
  psychogenic movement disorders, 308
Encephalitis lethargica, 330
Encephalitis, and parkinsonism, 179–180
Enkephalin
  in basal ganglia circuitry, 2
  in tardive dyskinesia, 337
Environmental factors, and basal ganglia lesions, 5, 19
Epilepsy, psychogenic seizures, 309, 351
Escitalopram
  for obsessive–compulsive behavior (OCB), 255
Essential Tremor (ET), 284–289
  abnormality in, 286
  alcoholism, 288–289
  anxiety, 287
  ataxia, 284
  Beck Depression Inventory (BDI), 286
  behavioral symptoms, 284–289
  characteristics, 284
  cognition, 284–286
  cognitive impairment, 285
  dementia, 284
  depression, 286–287
  duration of, 285
  and ethanol, 288
  Geriatric Depression Scale (GDI), 286
  Hamilton Anxiety Rating Scale (HARS), 287
  kinetic tremor, 284
  Liebowitz Social Anxiety Scale, 287
  loss of body mass index, 284
  memory, 285
  Mini-Mental State Examination (MMSE), 285
  olfactory dysfunction, 284
  phobia, 287
  personality changes, 287–288
  Stroop test, 285
  substance abuse, 288–289
  Tridimensional Personality Questionnaire (TPQ), 287
  Wisconsin Card Sorting Test, 285
Estrogen receptor 1 (ESR 1), in Parkinson's disease (PD), 98
Event-related potentials (ERP), in progressive supranuclear palsy (PSP), 167
Excessive daytime sleepiness (EDS), in Parkinson's disease (PD), 59
Executive function
  and basal ganglia dysfunction, 20, 21
  in Huntington's disease (HD), 213–215
  in Parkinson's disease (PD), 89–90, 99
Extrapyramidal motor system, in basal ganglia, 7

Extrapyramidal side effects in tardive dyskinesia, 337
Extrapyramidal signs (EPS), in Parkinson's disease (PD), 97
Extrapyramidal symptoms (EPS)
　in diffuse Lewy body disease, 149
　in Parkinson's disease (PD), 120

F

Factitious disorder, 354
Family history
　and dementia in Parkinson's disease (PD), 157
　of Huntington's disease (HD), 237
　and poststreptococcal neuropsychiatric disorder, 329
Family members,
　of obsessive–compulsive disorders (OCD) and Tourette's syndrome (TS), 253
Fatigue
　in Parkinson's disease (PD), 57–58
Fidgeting, in Pediatric autoimmune neuropsychiatric disorders associated with streptococcal infections (PANDAS), 327
Finger tapping test, in Huntington's disease (HD), 220
Fluoxetine
　for obsessive–compulsive behavior (OCB), 200, 252, 254, 256
　in Parkinson's disease (PD), 170
Flutamide
　for obsessive–compulsive disorder (OCD), 256
Fluvoxamine
　for obsessive–compulsive behavior (OCB), 255, 256, 257
　in Parkinson's disease (PD), 36, 49
Forebrain Lewy bodies, 148
Free radicals and tardive dyskinesia, 339
Frontal lobe dysfunction
　and basal ganglia dysfunction, 7
　dementia, 167
　in olivopontocerebellar atrophy, 171
　in Parkinson's disease (PD), 57, 89, 98
　in striatonigral degeneration, 173
Frontotemporal dementia with parkinsonism, 187–195, 188–192
　behavioral changes in, 187–195
　behavioral features, 188–189
　cognitive features, 189–190
　vs. Huntington's disease (HD), 214
　motor symptoms, 190
　neuroanatomy, 190–192
Frontotemporal lobar degeneration, 187–195
　and Alzheimer's disease (AD), 187
　amyotrophic lateral sclerosis (ALS), 187
　behavioral disturbance, 187
　and chromosome 17, 187
　corticobasal degeneration, 187
　and dementia, 187
　diagnostic criteria, 187
　extrapyramidal signs, 187
　frontotemporal
　　behavioral changes, 189

　frontotemporal dementia, 188–192
　　antisocial behaviors, 188
　　characteristics of, 187
　　compulsive behaviors, 189
　　criteria for, 188
　　Mini-Mental State Examination (MMSE), 190
　　motor neuron disease, 191
　　motor neuron signs, 187
　　neurobehavioral syndromes, 187
　　neuropathology, 188
　　Pick-Complex, 188
　　progressive nonfluent aphasia, 192–193
　　　Broca's aphasia, 193
　　　characteristics, 187
　　progressive supranuclear palsy, 187
　　　features of, 195
　　semantic dementia, 193–194
　　　characteristics, 187, 193
　　spectrum disorders, comparison, 195
Functional Disability Questionnaire (FDQ), for dystonia, 299
Functional magnetic resonance imaging (fMRI)
　in basal ganglia, 6
　in obsessive–compulsive disorder (OCD), 254
　in Parkinson's disease (PD), 91

G

Gait disorder
　and dementia, 156
　in psychogenic movement disorders, 351
Gamma-aminobutyric acid (GABA)
　dysfunction, in tardive dyskinesia, 338
　in basal ganglia circuitry, 6
Gene mutation
　in Huntington's disease (HD), 209
　Wilson's disease, 262
Generalized anxiety disorder (GAD), in Parkinson's disease (PD), 142
Genetic discrimination in Huntington's disease (HD), 236
Genetics
　in Huntington's disease (HD), 197–198
　of Tourette's syndrome (TS), 253
　obsessive–compulsive disorders (OCD), 253
Geriatric Depression Inventory (GDI), in Parkinson's disease (PD), 140
Gerstmann–Strassler–Scheinker disease (GSS), 181–182
Gilles de la Tourette's syndrome. See Tourette's syndrome (TS)
Glial cytoplasmic inclusions (GCI), 159
Globus pallidus interna (GPi), in Parkinson's disease (PD), 31, 130
Globus pallidus lesions, and motor disorders, 2, 17
Glucose metabolism
　in Huntington's disease (HD), 221
　in Parkinson's disease (PD), 6

H

Hallervorden–Spatz disease
　dementia with extrapyramidal signs, 160
　subcortical dementia, 160

Hallucinations
  in diffuse Lewy body disease, 151, 152
  drug-induced, 115–117
  in Huntington's disease (HD), 203
  in tardive dyskinesia, 337, 342
Hamilton Rating Scale for Depression (HDRS), 91, 140
  in olivopontocerebellar atrophy, 171
  in Parkinson's disease (PD), 27, 29
Head trauma, and Parkinson's disease (PD), 157
Hemiballism, 331
Henoch–Schönlein syndrome, 331
Hepatitis, and Wilson's disease, 263
Hepatolenticular degeneration. *See* Wilson's disease
Hereditary ataxia, 275–281
  autosomal dominant ataxias, 275–280
  behavior of, 275–281
  genetic testing, 280–281
Hoehn and Yahr rating scale
  in Parkinson's disease (PD), 84
  in Parkinson's disease (PD), dementia, 101
Homovanillic acid, in Parkinson's disease (PD), 30
Hooper Visual Organization Task, 87, 171
Huntington, 197
Huntington Study Group (HSG), 219
Huntington's disease (HD), 197–205
  absence of chorea, 197
  affective disorders, 202
  anxiety disorders, 203
  apathy, 201–202
  atrophy in, 198
  basal ganglia domains, 7, 17, 19, 21
  behavioral abnormalities, 201
  behavioral and psychiatric symptoms
    depression and suicide, 202
    mania and hypomania, 202
    neuropsychiatric alterations, 201
    obsessive–compulsive disorder (OCD), 203
    personality changes, 201
    prosody, 218
    psychosis, 203
    sexual behavior, 203
  behavioral symptoms, 197–205
    aggression, 201
    irritability, 199
  brain imaging, 198–199
  characteristics, 197
  chorea in, 197
  cognitive disorders, 212
  cognitive symptoms, 199
    memory deficits, 199
  dementia and cognitive changes, 209–225
    executive function, 213–215
    language, 217–218
      motor aspects, 217–218
      prosody, 218
    memory, 215–216
    visuoperceptual function, 218
  depression. *See* Depression
  diagnosis of, 211
  genetic discrimination, 236
  genetics, 197–198
  inheritance, 197
  negative family history, 237
  neuroimaging, 220–222
  neurologic abnormalities in, 197
  neuropathologic change, 198
  obsessive–compulsive behavior (OCB), 253
  obsessive and compulsive symptoms in, 198
  odor recognition, 217
  predictive testing
    adverse events, 230
      predictors of, 230–231
      timing of, 231
    participation rate, 236
  predictive testing, psychological effects, 226–239
    as model for late onset illnesses, 237–238
    decreased risk result, 228
    early symptoms and signs, 233
    increased risk result, 228–229
    prenatal testing, 235–236
  procedural learning, 21
  psychiatric changes, 198
  psychiatric symptoms
    depression, 199
    effect on family members, 199
  psychiatric symptoms, 199
  research, 219
    cognitive changes, 219
    Predict-HD, 219–220
  sleep changes, 203
  stereotyped activities, 19
  subcortical dementia, 167, 168, 210
  treatment, 205
Hypomania, in Huntington's disease (HD), 202
Hypotension, orthostatic, in Parkinson's disease (PD), 35, 121, 153
Hysteria, 353

I

Illness, physical
  stages of, 66
Inertia, and basal ganglia dysfunction, 17–18
Influenza A virus
  and parkinsonism-dementia/amyotrophic lateral sclerosis (ALS), 177
  and postencephalitic parkinsonism, 179
Information processing
  in Huntington's disease (HD), 216
  in Parkinson's disease (PD), 5
Insomnia, in Parkinson's disease (PD), 36, 58, 72
Intellectual disability
  and basal ganglia dysfunction, 19
  in progressive supranuclear palsy, 167, 168
Irritability
  in Huntington's disease (HD), 199

J

Judgment of Line Orientation, 87

K

Karolinska Scales of Personality (KSP), in Wilson's disease, 271
Kayser–Fleischer rings, 264
Kindling phenomenon, 117

L

Language skills
  in early Parkinson's disease (PD), 86, 100
  in Huntington's disease (HD), 217–218
L-dopa–induced dyskinesia, 338
Learning
  in Huntington's disease (HD), 215–216
Learning disorders
  and basal ganglia dysfunction, 20
Left-sided hemiparkinsonism (LHP), in Parkinson's disease (PD), 91
Levodopa therapy, for Parkinson's disease (PD), 105, 124
  cognitive decline, 58, 59, 60
  and depression, 44, 71, 114, 121
  psychosis induction, 97, 115, 117
Lewy bodies
  cortical disease, 148–160
    clinical presentation, 151–155
    dementia in Parkinson's disease (PD), 155–158
    identification and composition, 148
  diffuse Lewy body disease, 150–151
    alpha-synuclein pathology, 159–160
    as cause of dementia, 155
    clinical characteristics, 151–152
    dementia, 151–155
    improving diagnostic accuracy, 152
    incidental bodies, 159
    management of patients, 158–160
    pathology, 150, 153–155
  in late Parkinson's disease (PD), 78
  Lewy body variant (LBV), 149
  pure diffuse Lewy body disease (pDLBD), 150
Leyton Obsessional Inventory (LOI), 251, 252
Limb movements
  and basal ganglia, 1
  in corticobasal ganglionic degeneration, 175
  in tardive dyskinesia, 336
Lisuride, psychosis induction, 115
Liver in Wilson's disease, 262, 263, 272
Locus ceruleus (LC), in Parkinson's disease (PD), 30, 31, 103, 148
Logical Memory Passages, 88

M

Machado–Joseph's disease (MJD), 174–175
Magnetic resonance imaging (MRI)
  in acute disseminated encephalomyelitis, 330
  in Huntington's disease (HD), 198, 222
  in neuropsychiatric lupus, 331
  in obsessive–compulsive disorder (OCD), 254
  in Parkinson's disease (PD), 101, 126
  in Sydenham's chorea, 325

Malingering, 354, 360
Mania
  in Huntington's disease (HD), 202
  in Parkinson's disease (PD), 59–60
  in Tourette's syndrome (TS), 250
Masked personality
  in Lewy bodies, 151
  in Parkinson's disease (PD), 27
Mattis Dementia Rating Scale, in Parkinson's disease (PD), 98
Maudsley Obsessional–Compulsive Inventory (MOCI), 252
Meige's syndrome, 291
Memory
  in Alzheimer's disease (AD), 154, 167
  in diffuse Lewy body disease, 151–155
  domains of, 5
  in early Parkinson's disease (PD), 88–90
  explicit, and basal ganglia dysfunction, 20
  in Huntington's disease (HD), 215–216, 215–216
  impairment, in Huntington's disease (HD), 212
  in late Parkinson's disease (PD), 78, 88
  in Parkinson's disease (PD), 88
  in progressive supranuclear palsy, 167, 169
Memory impairment, in Huntington's disease (HD), 212
Memory retention
  Huntington's disease (HD) vs. Alzheimer's (AD), 199
Mental emptiness, and basal ganglia dysfunction, 18
Mesencephalic locomotor region (MLR), in Parkinson's disease (PD), 5
Midbrain inflammation, in postencephalitic parkinsonism, 180
Mild cognitive impairment, in Huntington's disease (HD), 212
Mini-Mental State Examination (MMSE)
  in cortical-basal ganglionic degeneration, 176
  in Huntington's disease (HD), 213
  in late Parkinson's disease (PD), 95, 118
  in olivopontocerebellar atrophy, 171
  in Parkinson's disease (PD), 57
  in tardive dyskinesia, 341
Minnesota Multiphasic Personality Inventory (MMPI)
  dystonia, 293
  in Huntington's disease (HD), 204
Monoamine oxidase A (MOA-A), in Parkinson's disease (PD), 36
Monoamine oxidase B (MOA-B) inhibitors, in late Parkinson's disease, 36, 49
Montgomery–Asberg Depression Rating Scale (MADRS), in Parkinson's disease (PD), 27, 140
Mood Adjective Checklist (MACL), for dystonia, 301
Mood changes, in Parkinson's disease (PD), 9
Motor abnormalities
  in Huntington's disease (HD), 199
Motor symptoms
  and psychiatric states, 45
  in early Parkinson's disease (PD), 59
Movement disorders
  in Huntington's disease (HD), 197–205

Movement Disorders Society (MDS), in Parkinson's disease (PD), 121
Movement disorders, autoimmune-mediated, 320–335
 central nervous system in, 322
 in children, 326–328
 chorea gravidarum, 331
 lymphocytes in, 320
 postinfectious (poststreptococcal) disorders, 323
 principles of autoimmunity, 320–323
 psychiatric considerations
  comorbidity, 327
 streptococcal infection in, 321, 329
  children, 326–328
 tolerance, 320
Movement disorders, psychogenic, 306–312, 350–363
 diagnosis of, 306–312
  psychiatric, 353
  psychogenic, 292
 gait disturbance, 351
 myoclonus, 351
 parkinsonism, 305
 phenomenology, 351, 361
 psychiatric considerations, 351–352
  comorbidity, 311, 313, 354–356
  diagnosis and treatment, 310–312, 356
  etiology and pathogenesis, 294, 305, 356
  prognosis, 360–361
 psychiatric disturbance in, 306–312
 psychopathology, 353
 treatment, 350–363
Multiple sclerosis
 comparison with Parkinson's disease (PD), 42, 45, 58
Multiple system atrophy (MSA), 160
 alpha-synuclein, 159–160
 olivopontocerebellar atrophy, 173–174
 in Parkinson's disease (PD), 59
 Shy–Drager syndrome, 172–174
 striatonigral degeneration, 172–174
Münchausen's syndrome, 310, 354, 359
Myoclonus
 psychogenic, 351

N

N-acetylaspartate (NAA), in Parkinson's disease (PD), 102
Nazer index, in Wilson's disease, 266
Neglect, in cortical-basal ganglionic degeneration, 177
Neocortex, Lewy bodies, 148
Neurofibrillary tangles
 in Alzheimer's disease (AD), 149
 in Lewy bodies, 150
Neuroimaging
 in Huntington's disease (HD), 220–222
 in tardive dyskinesia, 343–345
Neuroleptic therapy
 and tardive dyskinesia. See Tardive dyskinesia, in schizophrenia
 in Parkinson's disease (PD), 120, 122. See also Clozapine

Neuroleptics, in tardive dyskinesia, 337
Neurologic abnormalities
 in Huntington's disease (HD), 197
Neuropeptide Y
 in basal ganglia circuitry, 2
Neuropsychiatric features
 of Parkinson's disease (PD), 106
Neuropsychiatric Inventory (NPI), in Parkinson's disease (PD), 56, 57
Neuropsychiatric lupus, 331
 chorea, 331
 comorbidity, 331
Neurosurgery, for obsessive–compulsive disorder (OCD), 257
Neurotransmitters
 in Tourette's syndrome (TS), 254
Neutrophil count, clozapine therapy, 121
New Adult Reading Test (NART), in early Parkinson's disease (PD), 86
National Institute of Mental Health (NIMH)-Global Obsessive–Compulsive Scale, 252
Nonamyloid component (NAC)
 Lewy bodies, 148
Norepinephrine Dopamine Reuptake Blockers (NDRIs), in Parkinson's disease (PD), 36
Norepinephrine
 in Parkinson's disease (PD), 31, 92
 in tardive dyskinesia, 337
Nucleus accumbens, and amygdala, 1, 2
Nucleus basalis of Meynert, and dementia in Parkinson's disease (PD), 103, 158

O

Obsessive and compulsive symptoms
 in Huntington's disease (HD), 198
Obsessive–compulsive behaviors (OCB), 249
Obsessive–compulsive disorder (OCD)
 basal ganglia pathology, 5, 6
 in Tourette's syndrome (TS), 249–258
  clinical features, 250–253
   assessment, 252–253
   epidemiology, 250–251
   phenomenology, 251–252
  genetics, 253
  neurobiology, 254
  treatment, 255–257
   behavior therapy, 257
   neurosurgery, 257
   pharmacotherapy, 255–257
 stereotyped activities, 19
 striatal dysfunction, 6–7
Oculomotor control, 4
 in progressive supranuclear palsy, 170
Oculomotor dysfunction, in tardive dyskinesia, 343
Odor recognition, in Huntington's disease (HD), 217
Olanzapine, for Parkinson's disease (PD), 122
Olfaction, in early Parkinson's disease (PD), 90
Olivopontocerebellar atrophy, 170–172
 dementia with extrapyramidal signs, 160, 170

Ondansetron, for psychosis in Parkinson's disease (PD), 118, 120
Oppositional defiant disorder, 245
Organic movement disorders, 351
  and psychogenic disorders, 351
Osteoarthritis, comparison with Parkinson's disease (PD), 42, 57
Oxidative stress and tardive dyskinesia, 339

P

Pediatric autoimmune neuropsychiatric disorders associated with streptococcal infections (PANDAS)
  diagnosis, 327
  etiology, 328
  Sydenham's chorea, comparison, 328
Panic attacks
  drug-induced, in Parkinson's disease (PD), 119
Paralysis agitans, 148
Paraneoplastic chorea, 332
Paraneoplastic disorders, 331–332
Paraneoplastic dystonia, 332
Parkinson's disease (PD), 7–9
  anxiety, 42–52
  basal ganglia domains, 1, 7–9
  in chronic neurodegenerative disease, 65–81
  dementia
    Alzheimer pathology, 104
    clinical and neuropsychological features, 99–101
    diagnosis, 105
    epidemiology, 95–99
    executive function, 99
    incidence of, 96
    language and praxis, 100
    Lewy body pathology, 104
    neuroimaging, 101
    neuropathology of, 102–105
    pathologic correlates, 157
    prevalence and incidence, 156
    prevalence of, 95
    prophylaxis of, 106
    psychiatric symptoms, 101
    restricted subcortical pathology, 102
    risk factors, 96, 156–157
    treatment considerations, 105–106
    visuospatial functioning, 100
    vs. cognitive impairment, 155–156
  depression. *See* Depression
  dopamine loss, 1, 28
  drug-induced psychiatric states, 114–126
    and motor fluctuations, 45
    anxiety, 119–120
    clinical features, 115–117
    cognition and dementia, 117–118
    epidemiology, 114–115
    other risk factors, 118
    psychotic symptoms, 114–123
    reward-based behaviors, 123–126
    risk factors and pathophysiology, 117
    sleep disorders, 118
    treatment, 119–120

    clozapine and other neuroleptics, 120–123
    side effects of, 123
  DSM-IV, 26
  early stage of, 66–71
    dependency fears and conflicts, 68
    effect on relationships, 69
  early cognitive changes and nondementing behavior, 84–92
    clinical correlates
      age factors, 84–85
      medication effects, 85
      motor symptomatology and side of onset, 85
      motor symptoms, 85
    clinical correlates, 84–88
    cognitive processing time, 90
    depression, 91
    executive functions, 89–90
    language, 86
    memory impairment, 88–90
    neurochemical correlates, 91
    sensory changes, 90
    visuospatial skills, 86–88
  5-Hydroxy-indoleacetic acid (5-HIAA), 29, 30, 101
  5-hydroxytryptamine (5-HT3), 118
  late cognitive changes and dementia, 95–106
    pathophysiology
      locus ceruleus, 31, 148
      nucleus basalis of Meynert, 103, 158
    types of changes
      visuospatial changes, 88
  late stage of, 75–78
    dementia, 78
    drooling, 76
    facial masking, 76
    hallucinations and paranoia, 77
  middle stage of, 71–75
    daytime somnolence, 72
    effect on relationships, 73
    insomnia, 72
  as model for degenerative disease of basal ganglia, 7–9
  motivation/sexual conduct/sleep disorders, 56–61
  neurosurgical treatment, 8
  obsessive–compulsive behavior (OCB), 253
  procedural learning, 21
  psychiatric symptoms
    subthalamic stimulation
      causes, 130
  psychiatric symptoms following subthalamic stimulation, 130–144
  psychogenic movements, 305
  subthalamic stimulation
    depression, 134–137
    mania, 137–138
    postoperative management, 141–144
      anxiety, 142
      apathy, 142
      cognitive symptoms, 144

Parkinson's disease (PD) (contd.)
    depression, 141
        emotional reactivity, 143
        levodopa, nonmotor effects, 142
        mania/hallucinations, 141
        obsessive–compulsive symptoms (OCS), 144
        social outcome, 143
        suicidal ideation, 143
    preoperative assessment, 139–141
        absolute contraindications, 139
        depression, 140
    symptoms of mood elevation, 137–138
    visual hallucinations, 138–139
Parkinson-dementia complex of Guam, 160
Parkinson-plus syndromes, 166–182
    cortical-basal ganglionic degeneration
        alien limb phenomenon, 176
        apraxia, 175–176
        neglect, 177
        visuospatial and constructional deficits, 177
    Machado–Joseph's disease (MJD), 174–175
    multiple system atrophy, 170–174
        olivopontocerebellar atrophy, 170–172
        Shy–Drager syndrome, 172–174
        striatonigral degeneration, 172–174
    parkinsonism-dementia/amyotrophic lateral sclerosis (ALS), 177–179
    postencephalitic parkinsonism, 179–180
    prion-related diseases, 180–182
        Creutzfeldt–Jakob disease (CJD), 180
        Gerstmann–Straussler–Scheinker disease (GSS), 181–182
    progressive supranuclear palsy, 167–170
Paroxetine (Paxil), 255
Paroxysmal dyskinesia, 351
Participation rate in predictive testing, for Huntington's disease (HD), 236
Pathologic gambling and abuse
    in Parkinson's disease (PD), 60–61
Pediatric autoimmune neuropsychiatric disorders associated with streptococcal infections (PANDAS), 326–328
Pedunculopontine nucleus, in late Parkinson's disease (PD), 136
Penicillamine, for Wilson's disease, 262, 265, 266
Pergolide, 115, 126, 141
Personality changes
    in Huntington's disease (HD), 201
    in Parkinson-plus syndromes, 167
    and postencephalitic parkinsonism, 179
    in Wilson's disease, 267, 269
Personality, in Parkinson's disease (PD), 60
Phenylalanine and tardive dyskinesia, 339
Phobia, in essential tremor, 287
Physostigmine, 169
Picture Arrangement Task, in cortical-basal ganglionic degeneration, 176
Positron emission tomography (PET)
    in Huntington's disease (HD), 198, 221
    in Parkinson's disease (PD), 30, 31, 60, 101, 102
    in striatonigral degeneration, 173
    in Sydenham's chorea, 325
    motor learning, 6, 21
    in obsessive–compulsive disorder (OCD), 254
    parkinsonism-dementia/amyotrophic lateral sclerosis (ALS), 178
    in Parkinson's disease, 136
    progressive supranuclear palsy, 169
    psychogenic parkinsonism, 356
    tardive dyskinesia, 344
Postencephalitic parkinsonism
    extrapyramidal syndrome, 179
Postural instability and gait disorder (PIGD), 156
Posture, in psychogenic movement disorders, 358
Praxis, in early Parkinson's disease (PD), 86
Predict-HD, 219–220
Predictive testing for Huntington's disease (HD)
    as model for late onset illnesses, 237–238
    decreased risk result, 228
    increased risk result, 228–229
    participation rate, 236
    persons with disease, 233–235
    prenatal testing, 235–236
    psychological effects, 226–239
Prenatal testing, for Huntington's disease (HD), 235–236
Present State Examination (PSE), 91
Primary antiphospholipid syndrome, 331
Prion-related diseases, 180–182
Processing time, cognitive, in early Parkinson's disease (PD), 90
Progressive nonfluent aphasia, 192–193
    behavioral changes, 193
Prosody, in Huntington's disease (HD), 218
Prozac. *See* Fluoxetine
Psychiatric symptoms
    depression, in Huntington's disease (HD), 199
Psychiatric symptoms relationship, in Huntington's disease (HD), 204
Psychogenic disorders
    dystonia
        in children, 315
        definition, 291
        management, 312
        psychological consequences, 315
    movement disorders. *See* Movement disorders, psychogenic
Psychosis
    in Chorea gravidarum, 331
    drug-induced, in Parkinson's disease (PD). *See* Parkinson's disease (PD)
    in postencephalitic parkinsonism, 181
    in Wilson's disease, 267
Psychosocial aspects of depression. *See* Depression, in Parkinson's disease (PD)
Psychotherapy, for psychogenic movement disorders, 308, 311
Purdue Pegboard Test, in Wilson's disease, 268

Q

Quality of life (QOL), in Parkinson's disease (PD), 95
Quetiapine, for Parkinson's disease (PD), 121

R

Raphe nuclei, in late Parkinson's disease (PD), 92
Rapid eye movement (REM)
  in Parkinson's disease (PD), 58, 73, 118
Rapid eye movement behavior disorder (RBD),
    in Parkinson's disease (PD), 58
Rating scales, in Parkinson's disease (PD), 29
Recall performance, basal ganglia lesions, 20
Relative risk (RR), in Parkinson's disease (PD), 96
Reporter's Test, in early Parkinson's disease (PD), 86
Retirement age, and depression in Parkinson's disease (PD), 73
Rey Osterreith Complex Figure, 87
Rheumatic carditis, 325
Rheumatic fever, in autoimmune-mediated movement disorders, 323, 324, 325
Right hemiparkinsonism (RHP), in Parkinson's disease (PD), 91
Risk factors
  dementia in Parkinson's disease (PD), 156–157
  for diffuse Lewy body disease, 153
  for Parkinson's disease (PD), 28–29
Risperidone, for psychosis in Parkinson's disease (PD), 122
Rituals, obsessional, 255, 258

S

Schizophrenia
  basal ganglia pathology, 5
  clozapine therapy, 120, 121
  striatal dysfunction, 5
  and tardive dyskinesia. *See* Tardive dyskinesia in schizophrenia
Seizures
  and clozapine therapy, 121
  psychogenic, 309, 351
Selective Reminding Test, 98
Selective serotonin reuptake inhibitors (SSRI),
    in Parkinson's disease (PD), 31, 68
Selegiline, in Parkinson's disease (PD), 44
Semantic dementia, 193–194
Senile plaques (SP), in Lewy bodies, 149
Sensory phenomena
  in early Parkinson's disease (PD), 90
Seroton in Norepinephrine Reuptake Inhibitors (SNRIs),
    in Parkinson's disease (PD), 36
Serotonin
  in Parkinson's disease (PD), 30, 119
  reuptake inhibitors, for obsessive–compulsive behavior (OCB), 254, 255
Serotonin 2 Antagonist/Reuptake Inhibitors (SARIs),
    in Parkinson's disease (PD), 36
Serotonin, in tardive dyskinesia, 337
Sertraline (Zoloft), 255
Set shifting, 198
Sexual behavior
  in Huntington's disease (HD), 203
  in Wilson's disease, 267
Sexual disturbances
  in Parkinson's disease (PD), 58
Shy–Drager syndrome, 172–174
Single photon emission computed tomography
  in Parkinson's disease (PD), 101
  in progressive supranuclear palsy, 169
  in Sydenham's chorea, 325
Sjögren's syndrome, 331
Sleep changes
  in Huntington's disease (HD), 203
Sleep disturbances
  drug-induced, 117
  in Machado–Joseph's disease (MJD), 174
  in Parkinson's disease (PD), 27, 35, 43, 58
  and parkinsonism-dementia/ALS, 178
  and postencephalitic parkinsonism, 179
  in Wilson's disease, 271
Smell, sense of, in early Parkinson's disease (PD), 90
Social support network, risk groups for Huntington's disease (HD), 233
Somatization disorder, 353
Somatoform disorders, 353–354
Somatostatin
  in basal ganglia circuitry, 2
Somnolence, and postencephalitic parkinsonism, 179
Spasmodic dysphonia, 302
Spatial–perceptual skill, in Huntington's disease (HD), 217
Specific Serotonin Reuptake Inhibitors (SSRIs),
    in Parkinson's disease (PD), 36
Speech
  in tardive dyskinesia, 342
  motor aspects of, 217–218
Spielberger Trait Anxiety Scale
  in dystonia, 295
Spinocerebellar ataxia (SCAs), 275–279
  in olivopontocerebellar atrophy, 171
  subcortical dementia, 172
Split-brain syndrome, 176
Startle reflex, 307, 352
Stereotyped activity
  and basal ganglia dysfunction, 19
Stress
  risk groups for Huntington's disease (HD), 228
Striatonigral degeneration, 172–174
Striatopallidal complex, 18, 20, 22
Striatum
  and neuropsychiatric disorders, 17, 21
  and substantia nigra, 2
Stroop Color Word Test, in Huntington's disease (HD), 213
Structured Clinical Interview for DSM-III-R (SCID)
  in dystonia, 295
Subcortical dementia, 17, 167, 168, 169, 172, 173, 178
  in Huntington's disease (HD), 210
Substance abuse, in Wilson's disease, 268
Substance P, in basal ganglia circuitry, 2

Substantia nigra
    and dementia in Parkinson's disease (PD), 150
    in Parkinson's disease (PD), 136
    and striatum, 2
    dementia with extrapyramidal signs, 150
Subthalamic nucleus (STN)
    in basal ganglia, 1
    in Parkinson's disease (PD), 31, 130
Suicidal ideation
    in Huntington's disease (HD), 202
    in Parkinson's disease (PD), 26, 27, 67, 139, 141, 143
Suicides
    after predictive testing, 230
    in Huntington's disease (HD), 202
Supranuclear palsy, progressive
    and basal ganglia dysfunction, 17, 19, 20, 21
    cognitive and behavioral changes, 167–170
    subcortical dementia, 167
Sydenham's chorea, 323–326
    and ADHD symptoms, 324
    chorea insaniens, 325
Sydenham's chorea, 253
Systemic autoimmune disorders, 330–331
    neuropsychiatric lupus, 331
    primary antiphospholipid syndrome, 331
    systemic lupus erythematosus, 331
Systemic lupus erythematosus, 331
    autoantibodies in, 331
    parkinsonian signs, 331

T

Tardive dyskinesia
    basal ganglia pathology, 340
    dopamine supersensitivity, 338
    GABA dysfunction, 338
    neuroleptics in, 337
    oculomotor dysfunction, 343
    oxidative stress, 339
    pathophysiology of, 337–339
    in schizophrenia, 341
        cognitive dysfunction, 341–342
        psychiatric diagnosis, 337
        psychopathology, 341
            negative symptomatology, 342–343
            positive psychotic symptomatology, 342–343
        synthesis and speculation
            pathophysiologic basis, 336, 342
            vulnerability, 341
Tardive dysmentia, 341
Tegmento pedunculo pontinus (TPC), in basal ganglia, 3
Tetrathiomolybdate, for Wilson's disease, 266
Thalamus, in behavioral activation, 19
Thought disorder, in tardive dyskinesia, 343
Thyroid disease
    and Parkinson's disease (PD), 157
Tic disorders, 240–248
    definition, 241

Tics. *See also* Tourette's syndrome (TS)
    behavioral problems, 242
    decline, 240
    prevalence, 241
    psychiatric problems, 243
    in Sydenham's chorea, 324
Time perception, in Huntington's disease (HD), 218
Tonically Active Neurons (TAN), in basal ganglia, 2
Toronto Western Spasmodic Torticollis Rating Scale (TWSTRS), in dystonia, 303
Torticollis, 302
    in dystonia, 292, 312, 313, 314, 315
    spasmodic, 291
Tourette's syndrome (TS)
    basal ganglia pathology, 6, 19
    behavior disorders, 240–248
        attention-deficit/hyperactivity disorder, 242, 243, 244
        comorbidity of, 242
        oppositional defiant disorder, 245
    behavioral spectrum disorder, 240
    depression. *See* Depression
    epidemiology, 240
    genetic factors, 240
    obsessive–compulsive disorder (OCD), 249–258
        behavior therapy, 257
        clinical features, 250–253
        genetic studies, 253
        neurobiological features, 253–255
        neurosurgery, 257
        treatment, 255–257
            pharmacotherapy, 255–257
    pediatric neuropsychiatric disorder, 256
    stereotyped activities, 19
Tower of London, 168, 173
    in early Parkinson's disease (PD), 89
    in Huntington's disease (HD), 213
Tower of London test, 213
Transcranial magnetic stimulation (TMS)
    for obsessive–compulsive disorder (OCD), 257
    in Parkinson's disease (PD), 37
Tremors
    in early Parkinson's disease (PD), 67
    in psychogenic movement disorders, 351, 352
    in Wilson's disease, 263
Tricyclic antidepressants (TCAs)
    for obsessive–compulsive behavior (OCB), 255
    in Parkinson's disease (PD), 31, 35
Trientine, for Wilson's disease, 266
Trinucleotide repeats, in Huntington's disease (HD), 197, 226
Tryptophan, in Parkinson's disease (PD), 31
Twin studies, obsessive–compulsive disorders (OCD) and Tourette's syndrome (TS), 253

U

Unified Huntington's disease Rating Scale (UHDRS)
    in Huntington's disease (HD), 209
    in Parkinson's disease (PD), 46, 97, 115

Unipolar illness, tardive dyskinesia, 341
University of Pennsylvania Smell Identification Test (UPSIT), 90
  in Huntington's disease (HD), 217

V

Ventral tegmental area (VTA)
  in Parkinson's disease (PD), 137
  dopamine neurons, 30
Video monitoring, psychogenic movement disorders, 312
Vigilance
  in Huntington's disease (HD), 215
Visual hallucinations (VH), in Parkinson's disease (PD), 139
Visuospatial skills
  in cortical-basal ganglionic degeneration, 177
  in early Parkinson's disease (PD), 86–88
  in Huntington's disease (HD), 211, 217
von Economo's encephalitis, 253
Voon, 130

W

Wechsler Adult Intelligence Scale (WAIS)
  diffuse Lewy body disease, 152
  in early Parkinson's disease (PD), 86
  in Huntington's disease (HD), 215
  in olivopontocerebellar atrophy, 171
  in progressive supranuclear palsy, 169
Wechsler Intelligence Scale for Children-Revised (WISC-R), 152
Wechsler Memory Scale (WMS)
  in progressive supranuclear palsy, 169
Weschler Adult Intelligence Scale-Revised (WAIS-R),
  in Parkinson's disease (PD), 98
White blood cells, clozapine therapy, 121
Wilson's disease
  anticopper therapy, 270–271
  delayed recognition, 264–265
  dementia with extrapyramidal signs, 160
  diagnosis, 265
  etiology and pathogenesis, 262
  prognosis, 267
  psychiatric and behavioral abnormalities, 261–274
    as initial manifestations of disease, 267–272
    cognitive impairment, 268, 269, 270
    personality changes, 267
    psychosis, 267
    treatment, 265–266
  screening, 264–265
  subcortical dementia, 160
  tremor, 264
Wisconsin Card Sorting Test (WCST)
  in early Parkinson's disease (PD), 89
  frontal lobe dysfunction, 22
  in Huntington's disease (HD), 213
  in Parkinson's disease (PD), 20, 89
  in progressive supranuclear palsy, 167
Word fluency, in early Parkinson's disease (PD), 86
Work capacity
  in Wilson's disease, 268

Y

Yale-Brown Obsessive–Compulsive Scale (Y-BOCS), 252

Z

Zinc therapy, for Wilson's disease, 262, 265
Ziprasidone, for Parkinson's disease (PD), 122
Zung Scale of Depression, 172